Practical Issues in Geriatrics

Series Editor

Stefania Maggi, Aging Branch, CNR-Neuroscience Institute
Padua, Italy

This practically oriented series presents state of the art knowledge on the principal diseases encountered in older persons and addresses all aspects of management, including current multidisciplinary diagnostic and therapeutic approaches. It is intended as an educational tool that will enhance the everyday clinical practice of both young geriatricians and residents and also assist other specialists who deal with aged patients. Each volume is designed to provide comprehensive information on the topic that it covers, and whenever appropriate the text is complemented by additional material of high educational and practical value, including informative video-clips, standardized diagnostic flow charts and descriptive clinical cases. Practical Issues in Geriatrics will be of value to the scientific and professional community worldwide, improving understanding of the many clinical and social issues in Geriatrics and assisting in the delivery of optimal clinical care.

Antonio Cherubini • Arduino A. Mangoni
Denis O'Mahony • Mirko Petrovic
Editors

Optimizing Pharmacotherapy in Older Patients

An Interdisciplinary Approach

Springer

Editors
Antonio Cherubini
Geriatric
Geriatric Admissions and Aging Research
Center, IRCCS INRCA
Ancona, Italy

Arduino A. Mangoni
Discipline of Clinical Pharmacology
College of Medicine and Public Health,
Flinders University
Bedford Park, SA, Australia

Denis O'Mahony
Department of Medicine, and Department
of Geriatric Medicine
Cork University Hospital
Cork, Ireland

Mirko Petrovic
Section of Geriatrics, Department of
Internal Medicine and Paediatrics
Ghent University
Gent, Belgium

ISSN 2509-6060 ISSN 2509-6079 (electronic)
Practical Issues in Geriatrics
ISBN 978-3-031-28060-3 ISBN 978-3-031-28061-0 (eBook)
https://doi.org/10.1007/978-3-031-28061-0

This Springer imprint is published by the registered company Springer Nature Switzerland AG
The registered company address is: Gewerbestrasse 11, 6330 Cham, Switzerland

Foreword

Aging seems to be a longer lasting pandemic than COVID. Older people enjoy living happily despite a rapidly increasing disease burden, and this has to do with the robust and expanding achievements of hygiene and medicine. This may or may not include the most important option for treatment in almost all therapeutic areas, which is the prescription of drugs. Medication can positively contribute to disease prevention and mitigation, but due to inevitable side effects it could also be limiting the enjoyment of life or even end it.

This topic of medication in older people thus is of paramount importance for this steadily growing population part of our industrial societies. The new book on *Optimizing pharmacotherapy in older patients* is one of the very few attempts to condense our knowledge on this issue and comprehensively detail the dimensions, implications, and technical accommodations for coping with this challenging aspect of medicine. In its 29 chapters, the book deals with the epidemiology of "polypharmacy" (a widely used, but incorrect term which should rather be multimedication), the detrimental impact of some pharmacodynamic and pharmacokinetic features of the aging body on therapeutic outcomes and on instruments, practices, and tools to optimize medication use in older people. Catchwords like "deprescribing" or "potentially inappropriate medications" (PIM) are defined and discussed in the current scientific context. Drug–drug, drug–nutrient, and drug–disease interactions are being exemplified, issues of adherence and the roles of potential networking partners such as pharmacists addressed in chapters by outstanding researchers in the area.

The content of this first section on general issues is applied to geriatric syndromes such as frailty or falls, and to special aspects of medications for frequent diseases in older people (e.g., hypertension or heart failure) in the second main part of the book.

It thus does not only provide the theoretical background but also practical, disease-oriented solutions to medication-related problems in older people.

In its comprehensive approach, this book provides all relevant information for enabling a better and more appropriate medication process in the geriatric population. The book, thus, addresses physicians both in ambulatory and clinical care, pharmacists, nursing staff, and all care providers involved in the complex process of individualized medication in older people. Only few similar books have been published on this important issue to date, but none is comparably actual and comprehensive.

We are convinced that this new book is instructive, helpful, and protective in this context by not only showing the risks, but also the opportunities by the correct application of drugs in older people. It clearly conveys that drugs may harm, but also successfully treat older people if chosen correctly. The current FORTA-list contains 41% of positively labelled drugs. Thus, the right drug for the right patient is still a very good option for older people to live longer and/or better.

In the name of all those patients benefitting from the book, we sincerely thank the editors and authors for the creation of this important work.

Co-leader EuGMS Special Interest Group on Pharmacology Rob van Marum
Amsterdam, The Netherlands

Department of General Practice and Elderly Care Medicine
Amsterdam Public Health Research Institute
Amsterdam UMC, VUmc
Amsterdam, The Netherlands

Departments of Clinical Pharmacology and Geriatrics
Jeroen Bosch Hospital
's-Hertogenbosch, The Netherlands

Co-leader EuGMS Special Interest Group on Pharmacology Martin Wehling
Mannheim, Germany

Institut für Experimentelle und Klinische Pharmakologie
und Toxikologie Klinische Pharmakologie Mannheim
Medizinische Fakultät Mannheim der Universität
Heidelberg, Germany
December 2022

Contents

Part I

General Issues

1 The Impact of Ageing on Pharmacokinetics

Arduino A. Mangoni and Elzbieta A. Jarmuzewska

1.1 Introduction

The age-associated accumulation and coexistence of disease states and the increasingly proactive approach towards disease management by healthcare professionals have led to an increased medication use in the older patient population [1, 2]. However, a concomitant increasing exposure to drugs that are potentially inappropriate has also been extensively reported, with the consequent risk of toxicity and its clinical sequelae, for example, falls, cognitive impairment, hospitalisation and death [3–8]. The predisposition of older people to the unintended effects of drug exposure is largely due to specific alterations in body composition, organ function and homeostatic capacity, both at the cellular and the system level, that may influence the pharmacokinetics of several drugs [9]. Such alterations, in turn, lead to excessive drug accumulation and an increased risk of drug–drug and drug–disease interactions, particularly in the context of inappropriate prescribing and polypharmacy [9]. A better understanding of the main pharmacokinetic changes associated with advancing age might play an important role in minimising the burden of inappropriate polypharmacy. This burden is particularly high in frail patients, an ever-growing subgroup characterised by reduced functional capacity and marked vulnerability to adverse health outcomes [10].

A. A. Mangoni (✉)
Discipline of Clinical Pharmacology, College of Medicine and Public Health, Flinders University and Flinders Medical Centre, Adelaide, SA, Australia

Department of Clinical Pharmacology, Flinders Medical Centre, Southern Adelaide Local Health Network, Adelaide, Australia
e-mail: arduino.mangoni@flinders.edu.au

E. A. Jarmuzewska
Department of Internal Medicine, Polyclinic IRCCS, Ospedale Maggiore, University of Milan, Milan, Italy
e-mail: elzbieta.jarmuzewska@unimi.it

A. Cherubini et al. (eds.), *Optimizing Pharmacotherapy in Older Patients*, Practical Issues in Geriatrics, https://doi.org/10.1007/978-3-031-28061-0_1

This chapter describes the main physiological and pathophysiological changes in organ function and homoeostatic capacity occurring with human ageing and the current knowledge on the effects of advancing age on the four pillars of pharmacokinetics, that is, absorption, distribution, metabolism and elimination. A critical appraisal of the available evidence and the potential use of pharmacokinetic data in the routine care of older patients are also discussed. In particular, the development of robust, yet relatively simple, pharmacokinetic-based prescribing tools that assist with therapeutic decisions are likely to augment therapeutic efficacy and minimise toxicity in this highly heterogeneous patient group.

1.2 Age-Associated Changes in Organs and Systems

A critical determinant of the pharmacokinetic changes observed with advancing age is the occurrence of structural and/or functional alterations in the body overall, that is, body composition as well as specific organs and systems, that is, cardiovascular system, kidney and gastrointestinal system (Table 1.1).

1.2.1 Body Composition

Under physiological circumstances, the fat mass, body mass index (BMI) and percentage of body fat progressively increase from age 20 and tend to level off at approximately 80 years in men. By contrast, the fat-free mass increases slightly from age 20 to 47 and then declines with advancing age [11]. Similar observations have been reported in other studies, although women have been shown to have higher percentage body mass values than men across different age groups [12]. Furthermore, the actual age-related increase in fat mass and decrease in lean mass appear to be somewhat attenuated in women [13]. The possible implications of gender-associated differences in body composition trajectories across age groups, both in terms of pharmacokinetics and clinical effects, require further studies.

1.2.2 Cardiovascular System

Left ventricular ejection fraction and cardiac output at rest are both preserved in healthy older adults. However, the increase in left ventricular ejection fraction that is normally observed during exercise is blunted in old age, mainly due to a reduction

Table 1.1 Main age-associated structural and functional changes in organs and systems

• Relative increase in body fat and reduction in lean mass
• Blunted cardiac output and heart rate response during exercise
• Reduction in kidney volume and glomerular filtration rate
• Reduction in liver volume and hepatic blood flow

in ejection fraction reserve [14]. Similarly, although the resting heart rate is not significantly different compared to younger cohorts, a significant reduction in the maximal, exercise-induced heart rate is observed with advancing age [14]. The latter is primarily responsible for the age-associated reduction in maximal cardiac output, in the presence of a preserved stroke volume [14]. Therefore, physiological ageing is not associated with significant changes in cardiac function under resting conditions. Rather, it is characterised by a diminished overall cardiac reserve and cardiac output during stress, which might adversely affect the perfusion to critical organs, for example, the liver and the kidney, involved in drug metabolism and elimination. The prevalence of heart failure, particularly the subtype with left ventricular dysfunction and reduced ejection fraction, increases significantly with advancing age [15]. In these patients, the reduced peripheral organ perfusion and increased venous pressure, with or without concomitant kidney and/or liver disease, might exert significant effects on pharmacokinetics [16, 17].

1.2.3 Kidney

A progressive volume loss of the kidneys, primarily affecting the cortex, is typically observed after the age of 50 [18]. There is also a concomitant reduction in glomerular filtration rate (GFR), approximately 1 mL/min per year, after the age of 40 [19]. These processes can be accelerated by conditions such as hypertension and diabetes, the main causes of chronic kidney disease (CKD) worldwide [20]. Additionally, age-associated alterations in tubular structure and function can impair the capacity to reabsorb sodium and secrete hydrogen and potassium, increasing the risk of fluid, electrolyte and acid–base abnormalities in older adults [21].

1.2.4 Gastrointestinal System

There is no convincing evidence that advancing age per se is associated with significant changes in gastric emptying, intestinal transit or absorptive capacity of the small intestine and the colon, despite a reduced gastric secretion of hydrochloride acid and the presence of morphological changes in enterocytes [22–24]. By contrast, a significant age-related reduction, between 20 and 50%, in liver mass and hepatic blood flow has been reported [25].

1.3 Age-Associated Changes in Pharmacokinetics

1.3.1 Absorption

The absorption process for drugs administered orally predominantly occurs in the small intestine through passive diffusion or active transport [26]. With advancing age, drug absorption via passive diffusion across the gastrointestinal epithelium seems to be relatively preserved [27], whilst a reduction in the active transport of iron, calcium and vitamin B_{12} has been reported [28]. Similarly, the function and the expression of p-glycoprotein, the main intestinal efflux transporter, seems to be preserved in older age [29]. Whilst more research is required to investigate the effects of ageing, with or without concomitant disease states, on intestinal absorption, the reported age-related reduction in gastric acid production might affect the dissolution of drugs in the stomach [30]. This effect is likely augmented by the common, albeit often inappropriate, use of proton pump inhibitors in the older population [5, 31]. The consequent increase in gastric pH may facilitate the absorption of weakly acidic drugs, a result of increased dissolution, and reduce the absorption of weakly basic drugs, due to decreased dissolution. By contrast, gastric emptying does not seem to be significantly altered in older adults, in absence of comorbidities such as diabetes and Parkinson's disease [27]. For drugs that are administered via non-oral routes, there is virtually no information available regarding possible age-related alterations in absorption. Therefore, research is warranted to investigate the effects of advancing age, if any, on the extent and the rate of non-oral drug absorption.

1.3.2 Distribution

In line with the previously described age-related changes in body composition, that is, relative reduction in total body water and lean muscle mass and concomitant increase in body fat, the volume of distribution of highly lipophilic drugs, for example, benzodiazepines, significantly increases in older adults [32]. As a result, there is a prolongation in the elimination half-life, in absence of significant changes in clearance (see formula below), with the risk of drug accumulation and toxicity [33]:

$$t½ = \frac{0.693 \times V_{\mathrm{d}}}{\mathrm{CL}},$$

where $t½$ is the half-life, V_{d} is the volume of distribution and CL is the clearance.

For example, in a study in healthy subjects divided in two age groups (young adults, $n = 7$, age 28 ± 4 years; older adults, $n = 8$, age 69 ± 6 years), the half-life of diazepam in older adults was nearly three times that of younger participants (86 ± 36 vs. 31 ± 12 h, $p < 0.005$) [34]. By contrast, the volume of distribution of highly hydrophilic medications, for example, digoxin, tends to decrease in the older patient population. In a pharmacokinetic study, the volume of distribution of digoxin in older and younger participants was 4.1 ± 0.9 L/kg and 5.3 ± 0.6 L/kg, respectively [35].

A progressive reduction in the serum concentrations of the drug-binding protein albumin has been reported with advancing age [36, 37]. Such changes may theoretically affect the active, unbound, portion of highly protein-bound drugs, for example, warfarin and phenytoin. However, the rapid equilibrium occurring through drug elimination significantly limits this phenomenon's biological and clinical significance, therefore, minimising fluctuations in the concentrations of the unbound fraction [38].

1.3.3 Metabolism

The process of drug metabolism occurs primarily in the liver and involves the biotransformation of active drugs into more soluble inactive or active metabolites that subsequently undergo renal elimination [39]. These reactions include Phase I functionalisation (i.e. oxidation, reduction and hydrolysis, mediated by the cytochrome P450 enzyme superfamily) and Phase II conjugation (i.e. acetylation, glucuronidation and sulphation, mediated by transferases) [40]. Phase I and II reactions have also been described in the intestine, lung and kidney. However, the biological and clinical significance of these extra-hepatic reactions are not fully established [41].

1.3.3.1 Hepatic Blood Flow

The previously described age-related decrease in liver mass and hepatic blood flow can potentially reduce the metabolism, particularly first-pass, of drugs with high (>0.7) extraction ratio, defined as the ratio between hepatic clearance and hepatic blood flow. The reduction in metabolism is likely to be clinically significant (>50%) with amitriptyline and fentanyl [42]. Consequently, both the loading and the maintenance dose of such drugs should be decreased in older age [43]. By contrast, drugs with relatively low extraction ratio are not significantly affected by alterations in hepatic blood flow; however, they can be affected by modifications in the intrinsic metabolising capacity of the liver (see below).

1.3.3.2 Phase I–II Metabolism

Studies have shown a 30–50% reduction in the clearance of several drugs undergoing Phase I metabolism; however, it is unclear whether this is due to a reduction in the expression and/or activity of specific cytochrome P450 isoforms, hepatic blood flow or a combination of both [44–47]. This issue notwithstanding, caution is recommended when prescribing high- and low-extraction drugs undergoing significant Phase I metabolism in older patients. Examples of such drugs include clozapine (metabolised by CYP1A2), citalopram (metabolised by CYP2C19) and carbamazepine (metabolised by CYP3A4).

In contrast to Phase I metabolism, there is no clear evidence that advancing age affects Phase II metabolism in healthy individuals [48–51]. However, a reduction in Phase II metabolism of paracetamol, metoclopramide and aspirin has been reported in frail older patients when compared to fit age-matched and younger healthy controls [52–54]. The effect of frailty on Phase II metabolism might have additional adverse clinical consequences that are independent of reduced drug elimination. For example, the reduced Phase II conjugation of paracetamol results in the synthesis of *N*-acetyl-*p*-benzoquinone imine, a highly toxic metabolite. The impaired detoxification of *N*-acetyl-*p*-benzoquinone imine in frail subjects, secondary to the reduced production of the antioxidant glutathione, might significantly increase the risk of paracetamol-induced hepatotoxicity [55, 56].

1.3.4 Drug Elimination

The kidneys are the main site of elimination of soluble drugs and their metabolites. Renal clearance is considered to be the net result of glomerular filtration, tubular excretion and tubular reabsorption [57]. The previously reported decline in GFR with advancing age inevitably leads to impaired drug elimination and consequent accumulation. This is particularly relevant for drugs that have a narrow therapeutic index, for example, digoxin, lithium and gentamicin [58]. The dose of such drugs should be reduced proportionally to the reduction in renal clearance and regularly monitored [59].

The direct calculation of the GFR by measuring the renal clearance of inulin has been replaced by formulae that estimate either the creatinine clearance or the GFR (eGFR), the Cockcroft–Gault formula, the Modification of Diet in Renal Disease formula and the CKD Epidemiology Collaboration formula [60–62]. However, the available evidence regarding dose adjustment according to renal function is still largely based on the Cockcroft–Gault formula.

There is increasing evidence that an impairment in renal function can also influence absorption, distribution and non-renal elimination. The accumulation of uremic toxins in CKD can inhibit the expression and/or activity of CYP3A4, CYP1A2, CYP2B6, CYP2C9 and CYP2D6 [63, 64]. Examples of drugs with reduced extra-renal clearance include carvedilol (CYP3A4, CYP2C9 and CYP2D6), ciprofloxacin (CYP1A), cyclophosphamide (CYP2B6, CYP2C9 and CYP3A4), duloxetine (CYP1A and CYP2D6), erythromycin (CYP3A4), solifenacin (CYP3A4) and tadalafil (CYP3A4) [64]. In some cases, for example, intravenous midazolam (CYP3A4), the increase in exposure, expressed as area under the concentration curve, can be as high as sixfold in patients with renal failure when compared with healthy controls [65].

1.4 General Considerations

The available evidence regarding the impact of ageing on pharmacokinetics, albeit useful, needs to be interpreted with some caution (Table 1.2). Studies addressing this issue have generally been conducted in relatively healthy older participants. However, the age-related pharmacokinetic changes observed in clinical practice are likely to be the result of complex organ–organ and/or drug–disease interactions in patients with extensive medication exposure and comorbidity. This requires the conduct of studies in cohorts that are better representative of patients that are routinely managed in clinical practice. Furthermore, most pharmacokinetic studies have investigated relatively old drugs that are rarely prescribed in current medical practice [9, 16, 33, 66]. Therefore, additional research is warranted to investigate the potential pharmacokinetic alterations of newer drugs, particularly cardiovascular, anti-cancer and immunomodulating agents. Finally, there is emerging evidence that frailty can affect Phase II metabolism, as previously discussed, and drug elimination, although other studies have reported negative results [53, 67–69]. The potential influence of frailty on drug metabolism and elimination further justifies the need

Table 1.2 Key changes in drug metabolism and elimination in older adults

• Reduction in phase I metabolism, with consequent reduction in first-pass metabolism and clearance
• Reduction in phase II metabolism, with consequent reduction in clearance, in frail subjects
• Reduction in the clearance of renally excreted drugs
• Reduction in non-renal drug elimination, through impaired phase I metabolism, in patients with renal disease

Table 1.3 Areas requiring further pharmacokinetic studies in older age

• Impact of frailty
• Role of pharmacogenomics and ethnicity
• Study of subjects >80 years
• Impact of renal disease on extra-renal metabolism
• Assessment of drugs prescribed in current practice

for pre- and/or post-marketing studies that also include frail older participants (Table 1.3) [70, 69].

1.5 Pharmacokinetic Data for Personalised Prescribing

The incorporation of pharmacokinetic parameters, particularly those pertaining to drug metabolism and elimination, into electronic tools can potentially assist with the practice of personalised prescribing in a highly complex and heterogeneous patient population. The difficulties in routinely assessing hepatic blood flow and the impact of advancing age on Phase I and Phase II metabolism currently prevent the use of these parameters for optimal selection of drugs and dose regimens in individual patients. By contrast, an increasing contribution of the eGFR, an easily measurable and robust marker of renal drug elimination, in personalised prescribing decisions is anticipated. eGFR-based decisions are likely to assist not only with the selection of specific treatments but also with dose adjustments over time. The increasing evidence of a significant association between CKD and impairment in Phase I metabolism suggests that eGFR-based prescribing decisions might not only be limited to the use of renally cleared drugs but also include those undergoing significant Phase I metabolism. However, any new prescribing tool that incorporates pharmacokinetic parameters will require robust evidence of superiority versus standard of care or existing tools, in terms of practicality, accessibility, risk of adverse drug reactions and clinical and patient-centred outcomes [71], in adequately designed intervention trials.

1.6 Conclusions

The available evidence suggests that human ageing is characterised by several pharmacokinetic changes, particularly an increased volume of distribution for highly lipophilic drugs, a reduction in Phase I metabolism, a reduction in Phase II metabolism in the presence of frailty and a reduction in the clearance of renally excreted drugs. Another potentially relevant age-related effect is the impaired Phase I metabolism in older patient with chronic kidney disease. Whilst the routine use of this information may, in principle, improve the quality and safety of drug prescribing, more research is warranted to investigate the specific impact of frailty, pharmacogenomics and drug–drug, drug–disease and organ–organ interactions. The results of these studies will further assist with the development of personalised prescribing tools that are likely to improve the quality of life and clinical outcomes in this ever-expanding patient population.

References

1. Qato DM, Wilder J, Schumm LP, Gillet V, Alexander GC. Changes in prescription and over-the-counter medication and dietary supplement use among older adults in the United States, 2005 vs 2011. JAMA Intern Med. 2016;176(4):473–82. https://doi.org/10.1001/jamainternmed.2015.8581.
2. Gao L, Maidment I, Matthews FE, Robinson L, Brayne C, Medical Research Council Cognitive Function and Ageing Study, et al. Medication usage change in older people (65+) in England over 20 years: findings from CFAS I and CFAS II. Age Ageing. 2018;47(2):220–5. https://doi.org/10.1093/ageing/afx158.
3. Bostock CV, Soiza RL, Mangoni AA. Association between prescribing of antimuscarinic drugs and antimuscarinic adverse effects in older people. Expert Rev Clin Pharmacol. 2010;3(4):441–52. https://doi.org/10.1586/ecp.10.34.
4. Ruxton K, Woodman RJ, Mangoni AA. Drugs with anticholinergic effects and cognitive impairment, falls and all-cause mortality in older adults: a systematic review and meta-analysis. Br J Clin Pharmacol. 2015;80(2):209–20. https://doi.org/10.1111/bcp.12617.
5. Hamzat H, Sun H, Ford JC, Macleod J, Soiza RL, Mangoni AA. Inappropriate prescribing of proton pump inhibitors in older patients: effects of an educational strategy. Drugs Aging. 2012;29(8):681–90. https://doi.org/10.2165/11632700-000000000-00000.
6. Maes ML, Fixen DR, Linnebur SA. Adverse effects of proton-pump inhibitor use in older adults: a review of the evidence. Ther Adv Drug Saf. 2017;8(9):273–97. https://doi.org/10.1177/2042098617715381.
7. Abrahami D, McDonald EG, Schnitzer M, Azoulay L. Trends in prescribing patterns of proton pump inhibitors surrounding new guidelines. Ann Epidemiol. 2021;55:24–6. https://doi.org/10.1016/j.annepidem.2020.12.002.
8. Sumukadas D, McMurdo ME, Mangoni AA, Guthrie B. Temporal trends in anticholinergic medication prescription in older people: repeated cross-sectional analysis of population prescribing data. Age Ageing. 2014;43(4):515–21. https://doi.org/10.1093/ageing/aft199.
9. Reeve E, Wiese MD, Mangoni AA. Alterations in drug disposition in older adults. Expert Opin Drug Metab Toxicol. 2015;11(4):491–508. https://doi.org/10.1517/17425255.2015.1004310.
10. Fried LP, Tangen CM, Walston J, Newman AB, Hirsch C, Gottdiener J, et al. Frailty in older adults: evidence for a phenotype. J Gerontol A Biol Sci Med Sci. 2001;56(3):M146–56. https://doi.org/10.1093/gerona/56.3.m146.
11. Jackson AS, Janssen I, Sui X, Church TS, Blair SN. Longitudinal changes in body composition associated with healthy ageing: men, aged 20–96 years. Br J Nutr. 2012;107(7):1085–91. https://doi.org/10.1017/S0007114511003886.
12. He X, Li Z, Tang X, Zhang L, Wang L, He Y, et al. Age- and sex-related differences in body composition in healthy subjects aged 18–82 years. Medicine (Baltimore). 2018;97(25):e11152. https://doi.org/10.1097/MD.0000000000011152.

13. Bazzocchi A, Diano D, Ponti F, Andreone A, Sassi C, Albisinni U, et al. Health and ageing: a cross-sectional study of body composition. Clin Nutr. 2013;32(4):569–78. https://doi.org/10.1016/j.clnu.2012.10.004.
14. Lakatta EG, Levy D. Arterial and cardiac aging: major shareholders in cardiovascular disease enterprises: part II: the aging heart in health: links to heart disease. Circulation. 2003;107(2):346–54. https://doi.org/10.1161/01.cir.0000048893.62841.f7.
15. Savarese G, Lund LH. Global public health burden of heart failure. Card Fail Rev. 2017;3(1):7–11. https://doi.org/10.15420/cfr.2016:25:2.
16. Mangoni AA, Jarmuzewska EA. The influence of heart failure on the pharmacokinetics of cardiovascular and non-cardiovascular drugs: a critical appraisal of the evidence. Br J Clin Pharmacol. 2019;85(1):20–36. https://doi.org/10.1111/bcp.13760.
17. Ergatoudes C, Schaufelberger M, Andersson B, Pivodic A, Dahlstrom U, Fu M. Non-cardiac comorbidities and mortality in patients with heart failure with reduced vs. preserved ejection fraction: a study using the Swedish heart failure registry. Clin Res Cardiol. 2019;108(9):1025–33. https://doi.org/10.1007/s00392-019-01430-0.
18. Dunnill MS, Halley W. Some observations on the quantitative anatomy of the kidney. J Pathol. 1973;110(2):113–21. https://doi.org/10.1002/path.1711100202.
19. Brenner BM, Meyer TW, Hostetter TH. Dietary protein intake and the progressive nature of kidney disease: the role of hemodynamically mediated glomerular injury in the pathogenesis of progressive glomerular sclerosis in aging, renal ablation, and intrinsic renal disease. N Engl J Med. 1982;307(11):652–9. https://doi.org/10.1056/NEJM198209093071104.
20. Sasaki T, Tsuboi N, Okabayashi Y, Haruhara K, Kanzaki G, Koike K, et al. Synergistic impact of diabetes and hypertension on the progression and distribution of glomerular histopathological lesions. Am J Hypertens. 2019;32(9):900–8. https://doi.org/10.1093/ajh/hpz059.
21. Denic A, Glassock RJ, Rule AD. Structural and functional changes with the aging kidney. Adv Chronic Kidney Dis. 2016;23(1):19–28. https://doi.org/10.1053/j.ackd.2015.08.004.
22. Madsen JL, Graff J. Effects of ageing on gastrointestinal motor function. Age Ageing. 2004;33(2):154–9. https://doi.org/10.1093/ageing/afh040.
23. Dumic I, Nordin T, Jecmenica M, Stojkovic Lalosevic M, Milosavljevic T, Milovanovic T. Gastrointestinal tract disorders in older age. Can J Gastroenterol Hepatol. 2019;2019:6757524. https://doi.org/10.1155/2019/6757524.
24. Warren PM, Pepperman MA, Montgomery RD. Age changes in small-intestinal mucosa. Lancet. 1978;2(8094):849–50. https://doi.org/10.1016/s0140-6736(78)92639-9.
25. Wynne HA, Cope LH, Mutch E, Rawlins MD, Woodhouse KW, James OF. The effect of age upon liver volume and apparent liver blood flow in healthy man. Hepatology. 1989;9(2):297–301. https://doi.org/10.1002/hep.1840090222.
26. Vertzoni M, Augustijns P, Grimm M, Koziolek M, Lemmens G, Parrott N, et al. Impact of regional differences along the gastrointestinal tract of healthy adults on oral drug absorption: an UNGAP review. Eur J Pharm Sci. 2019;134:153–75. https://doi.org/10.1016/j.ejps.2019.04.013.
27. Maher D, Ailabouni N, Mangoni AA, Wiese MD, Reeve E. Alterations in drug disposition in older adults: a focus on geriatric syndromes. Expert Opin Drug Metab Toxicol. 2021;17(1):41–52. https://doi.org/10.1080/17425255.2021.1839413.
28. Russell RM. Changes in gastrointestinal function attributed to aging. Am J Clin Nutr. 1992;55(6 Suppl):1203S–7S. https://doi.org/10.1093/ajcn/55.6.1203S.
29. Mangoni AA. The impact of advancing age on P-glycoprotein expression and activity: current knowledge and future directions. Expert Opin Drug Metab Toxicol. 2007;3(3):315–20. https://doi.org/10.1517/17425255.3.3.315.
30. Soenen S, Rayner CK, Jones KL, Horowitz M. The ageing gastrointestinal tract. Curr Opin Clin Nutr Metab Care. 2016;19(1):12–8. https://doi.org/10.1097/MCO.0000000000000238.
31. Jarchow-Macdonald AA, Mangoni AA. Prescribing patterns of proton pump inhibitors in older hospitalized patients in a Scottish health board. Geriatr Gerontol Int. 2013;13(4):1002–9. https://doi.org/10.1111/ggi.12047.

32. Herman RJ, Wilkinson GR. Disposition of diazepam in young and elderly subjects after acute and chronic dosing. Br J Clin Pharmacol. 1996;42(2):147–55. https://doi.org/10.1046/j.1365-2125.1996.03642.x.
33. Mangoni AA, Jackson SH. Age-related changes in pharmacokinetics and pharmacodynamics: basic principles and practical applications. Br J Clin Pharmacol. 2004;57(1):6–14. https://doi.org/10.1046/j.1365-2125.2003.02007.x.
34. Greenblatt DJ, Harmatz JS, Zhang Q, Chen Y, Shader RI. Slow accumulation and elimination of diazepam and its active metabolite with extended treatment in the elderly. J Clin Pharmacol. 2021;61(2):193–203. https://doi.org/10.1002/jcph.1726.
35. Cusack B, Kelly J, O'Malley K, Noel J, Lavan J, Horgan J. Digoxin in the elderly: pharmacokinetic consequences of old age. Clin Pharmacol Ther. 1979;25(6):772–6. https://doi.org/10.1002/cpt1979256772.
36. Weaving G, Batstone GF, Jones RG. Age and sex variation in serum albumin concentration: an observational study. Ann Clin Biochem. 2016;53(Pt 1):106–11. https://doi.org/10.1177/0004563215593561.
37. Gom I, Fukushima H, Shiraki M, Miwa Y, Ando T, Takai K, et al. Relationship between serum albumin level and aging in community-dwelling self-supported elderly population. J Nutr Sci Vitaminol (Tokyo). 2007;53(1):37–42. https://doi.org/10.3177/jnsv.53.37.
38. Grandison MK, Boudinot FD. Age-related changes in protein binding of drugs: implications for therapy. Clin Pharmacokinet. 2000;38(3):271–90. https://doi.org/10.2165/00003088-200038030-00005.
39. Kinirons MT, O'Mahony MS. Drug metabolism and ageing. Br J Clin Pharmacol. 2004;57(5):540–4. https://doi.org/10.1111/j.1365-2125.2004.02096.x.
40. Klotz U. Pharmacokinetics and drug metabolism in the elderly. Drug Metab Rev. 2009;41(2):67–76. https://doi.org/10.1080/03602530902722679.
41. Gundert-Remy U, Bernauer U, Blomeke B, Doring B, Fabian E, Goebel C, et al. Extrahepatic metabolism at the body's internal–external interfaces. Drug Metab Rev. 2014;46(3):291–324. https://doi.org/10.3109/03602532.2014.900565.
42. Butler JM, Begg EJ. Free drug metabolic clearance in elderly people. Clin Pharmacokinet. 2008;47(5):297–321. https://doi.org/10.2165/00003088-200847050-00002.
43. Pirmohamed M. Prescribing in liver disease. Medicine. 2019;47(11):718–22. https://doi.org/10.1016/j.mpmed.2019.08.012.
44. Schmucker DL. Liver function and phase I drug metabolism in the elderly: a paradox. Drugs Aging. 2001;18(11):837–51. https://doi.org/10.2165/00002512-200118110-00005.
45. Le Couteur DG, McLean AJ. The aging liver. Drug clearance and an oxygen diffusion barrier hypothesis. Clin Pharmacokinet. 1998;34(5):359–73. https://doi.org/10.2165/00003088-199834050-00003.
46. Battino D, Croci D, Mamoli D, Messina S, Perucca E. Influence of aging on serum phenytoin concentrations: a pharmacokinetic analysis based on therapeutic drug monitoring data. Epilepsy Res. 2004;59(2–3):155–65. https://doi.org/10.1016/j.eplepsyres.2004.04.006.
47. Bebia Z, Buch SC, Wilson JW, Frye RF, Romkes M, Cecchetti A, et al. Bioequivalence revisited: influence of age and sex on CYP enzymes. Clin Pharmacol Ther. 2004;76(6):618–27. https://doi.org/10.1016/j.clpt.2004.08.021.
48. Herd B, Wynne H, Wright P, James O, Woodhouse K. The effect of age on glucuronidation and sulphation of paracetamol by human liver fractions. Br J Clin Pharmacol. 1991;32(6):768–70.
49. Court MH. Interindividual variability in hepatic drug glucuronidation: studies into the role of age, sex, enzyme inducers, and genetic polymorphism using the human liver bank as a model system. Drug Metab Rev. 2010;42(1):209–24. https://doi.org/10.3109/03602530903209288.
50. Thompson CM, Johns DO, Sonawane B, Barton HA, Hattis D, Tardif R, et al. Database for physiologically based pharmacokinetic (PBPK) modeling: physiological data for healthy and health-impaired elderly. J Toxicol Environ Health B Crit Rev. 2009;12(1):1–24. https://doi.org/10.1080/10937400802545060.

51. Ginsberg G, Hattis D, Russ A, Sonawane B. Pharmacokinetic and pharmacodynamic factors that can affect sensitivity to neurotoxic sequelae in elderly individuals. Environ Health Perspect. 2005;113(9):1243–9. https://doi.org/10.1289/ehp.7568.
52. Wynne HA, Cope LH, Herd B, Rawlins MD, James OF, Woodhouse KW. The association of age and frailty with paracetamol conjugation in man. Age Ageing. 1990;19(6):419–24. https://doi.org/10.1093/ageing/19.6.419.
53. Wynne HA, Yelland C, Cope LH, Boddy A, Woodhouse KW, Bateman DN. The association of age and frailty with the pharmacokinetics and pharmacodynamics of metoclopramide. Age Ageing. 1993;22(5):354–9. https://doi.org/10.1093/ageing/22.5.354.
54. Williams FM, Wynne H, Woodhouse KW, Rawlins MD. Plasma aspirin esterase: the influence of old age and frailty. Age Ageing. 1989;18(1):39–42. https://doi.org/10.1093/ageing/18.1.39.
55. Serviddio G, Romano AD, Greco A, Rollo T, Bellanti F, Altomare E, et al. Frailty syndrome is associated with altered circulating redox balance and increased markers of oxidative stress. Int J Immunopathol Pharmacol. 2009;22(3):819–27. https://doi.org/10.1177/039463200902200328.
56. Ging P, Mikulich O, O'Reilly KM. Unexpected paracetamol (acetaminophen) hepatotoxicity at standard dosage in two older patients: time to rethink 1 g four times daily? Age Ageing. 2016;45(4):566–7. https://doi.org/10.1093/ageing/afw067.
57. Miners JO, Yang X, Knights KM, Zhang L. The role of the kidney in drug elimination: transport, metabolism, and the impact of kidney disease on drug clearance. Clin Pharmacol Ther. 2017;102(3):436–49. https://doi.org/10.1002/cpt.757.
58. Olyaei AJ, Steffl JL. A quantitative approach to drug dosing in chronic kidney disease. Blood Purif. 2011;31(1–3):138–45. https://doi.org/10.1159/000321857.
59. Doogue MP, Polasek TM. Drug dosing in renal disease. Clin Biochem Rev. 2011;32(2):69–73.
60. Willems JM, Vlasveld T, den Elzen WP, Westendorp RG, Rabelink TJ, de Craen AJ, et al. Performance of Cockcroft–Gault, MDRD, and CKD-EPI in estimating prevalence of renal function and predicting survival in the oldest old. BMC Geriatr. 2013;13:113. https://doi.org/10.1186/1471-2318-13-113.
61. Raman M, Middleton RJ, Kalra PA, Green D. Estimating renal function in old people: an in-depth review. Int Urol Nephrol. 2017;49(11):1979–88. https://doi.org/10.1007/s11255-017-1682-z.
62. Elinder CG, Barany P, Heimburger O. The use of estimated glomerular filtration rate for dose adjustment of medications in the elderly. Drugs Aging. 2014;31(7):493–9. https://doi.org/10.1007/s40266-014-0187-z.
63. Tieu A, House AA, Urquhart BL. Drug disposition issues in CKD: implications for drug discovery and regulatory approval. Adv Chronic Kidney Dis. 2016;23(2):63–6. https://doi.org/10.1053/j.ackd.2016.01.013.
64. Ladda MA, Goralski KB. The effects of CKD on cytochrome P450-mediated drug metabolism. Adv Chronic Kidney Dis. 2016;23(2):67–75. https://doi.org/10.1053/j.ackd.2015.10.002.
65. Thomson BK, Nolin TD, Velenosi TJ, Feere DA, Knauer MJ, Asher LJ, et al. Effect of CKD and dialysis modality on exposure to drugs cleared by nonrenal mechanisms. Am J Kidney Dis. 2015;65(4):574–82. https://doi.org/10.1053/j.ajkd.2014.09.015.
66. Mangoni AA. Cardiovascular drug therapy in elderly patients: specific age-related pharmacokinetic, pharmacodynamic and therapeutic considerations. Drugs Aging. 2005;22(11):913–41. https://doi.org/10.2165/00002512-200522110-00003.
67. Johnston C, Hilmer SN, McLachlan AJ, Matthews ST, Carroll PR, Kirkpatrick CM. The impact of frailty on pharmacokinetics in older people: using gentamicin population pharmacokinetic modeling to investigate changes in renal drug clearance by glomerular filtration. Eur J Clin Pharmacol. 2014;70(5):549–55. https://doi.org/10.1007/s00228-014-1652-7.
68. Opdam FL, Modak AS, Mooijaart SP, Louwerens M, de Waal MW, Gelderblom H, et al. CYP2D6 metabolism in frail elderly compared to non-frail elderly: a pilot feasibility study. Drugs Aging. 2015;32(12):1019–27. https://doi.org/10.1007/s40266-015-0319-0.

69. Hilmer SN, Kirkpatrick CMJ. New horizons in the impact of frailty on pharmacokinetics: latest developments. Age Ageing. 2021;50(4):1054–63. https://doi.org/10.1093/ageing/afab003.
70. Mangoni AA, Jansen PA, Jackson SH. Under-representation of older adults in pharmacokinetic and pharmacodynamic studies: a solvable problem? Expert Rev Clin Pharmacol. 2013;6(1):35–9. https://doi.org/10.1586/ecp.12.75.
71. Mangoni AA, Pilotto A. New drugs and patient-centred end-points in old age: setting the wheels in motion. Expert Rev Clin Pharmacol. 2016;9(1):81–9. https://doi.org/10.1586/17512433.2016.1100074.

2 Polypharmacy: Definition, Epidemiology, Consequences and Solutions

Donal Fitzpatrick and Paul F. Gallagher

Sample Case Scenario

Ms. PP is an 82-year-old woman with the following past medical history and regular medications:

Past medical history	Current medications
• Epilepsy	1. Valproate (slow release) 400 mg od
• Ischaemic heart disease	2. Amlodipine 5 mg od
• Hypertension	3. Amitriptyline 10 mg od
• Mild cognitive impairment	4. Clopidogrel 75 mg od
• Cervical spondylosis	5. Omeprazole 20 mg od

She attends her general practitioner (GP) for a routine visit and is noted to be hypertensive. Amlodipine is prescribed. A few weeks later, she returns to her GP with bilateral lower limb swelling. The GP prescribes furosemide. She then develops urinary frequency and is prescribed fesoterodine. She becomes delirious and is admitted to the hospital. She becomes agitated and is prescribed haloperidol. She develops constipation, urinary retention and a urinary tract infection. She has several non-convulsive vacant episodes which are diagnosed as partial seizures. Her medications are reviewed, and potentially inappropriate medications are deprescribed. Her delirium slowly resolves, and after a short period of rehabilitation, she is discharged home.

Questions

1. What drug–disease interaction is illustrated in this case?
2. What drug–drug interactions (DDIs) are illustrated in this case?
3. Can you identify the prescribing cascade in this case?

D. Fitzpatrick
Department of Geriatric Medicine, Cork University Hospital, Cork, Ireland

P. F. Gallagher (✉)
Department of Geriatric Medicine, Bon Secours Hospital, Cork, Ireland

A. Cherubini et al. (eds.), *Optimizing Pharmacotherapy in Older Patients*, Practical Issues in Geriatrics, https://doi.org/10.1007/978-3-031-28061-0_2

2.1 Introduction

The increasing age profile and consequent rising prevalence of multimorbidity means that older people are taking more medications than ever before [1, 2]. The concurrent use of multiple medications is referred to as polypharmacy, multimorbidity being the principal cause. Complex combinations of drugs are often hazardous in older adults. Pharmacodynamic and pharmacokinetic changes in older adults increases the risk of adverse drug interactions and adverse drug events [3–5].

In many cases, polypharmacy is justified. For example, after a myocardial infarction, a patient may require multiple medications for acute treatment and for secondary prevention [6]. It is therefore important to differentiate between appropriate and inappropriate polypharmacy (Box 2.1).

Box 2.1 Definitions

Appropriate polypharmacy

Appropriate polypharmacy is present, when (a) all medicines are prescribed for the purpose of achieving specific therapeutic objectives; (b) therapeutic objectives are actually being achieved or there is a high probability that they will be achieved in the future; (c) medication therapy has been optimised to minimise the risk of adverse drug reactions (ADRs) and adverse drug events (ADEs); and (d) the patient is motivated and able to take all medicines as intended [7].

Inappropriate polypharmacy

Inappropriate polypharmacy is defined as the prescribing of multiple medicines inappropriately, or where the intended benefit of the medication is not realised. It pertains to the prescription of drugs that:

- have no indication or an incorrect indication
- have a high risk of ADRs and ADEs
- are unnecessarily expensive
- are used for inappropriate duration (for too short or too long a time period)

2.2 Epidemiology of Polypharmacy

The prevalence of polypharmacy in older adults has uniformly increased across Europe and in the United States over the last two decades [8–16]. This is intrinsically associated with rising prevalence of multimorbidity. Two-thirds of the European older adult population have two or more chronic diseases [17]. A cross-sectional analysis of the Survey of Health, Ageing and Retirement in Europe (SHARE) database found 20% of people aged 70–74 years were prescribed 10 or more medicines [11], often referred to as 'hyperpolypharmacy'.

Despite multimorbidity being the rule rather than the exception in older people, clinical guidelines often follow a single disease approach with each comorbidity generating prescription of additional medications without consideration of other health conditions or medications. Certain chronic conditions are particularly associated with polypharmacy including chronic obstructive pulmonary disease, atrial fibrillation, hypertension, ischaemic heart disease, obesity and depression [9].

Inappropriate polypharmacy is associated with significant morbidity through drug–drug interactions, drug–disease interactions, adverse clinical events and non-adherence. Up to 11% of all unplanned hospital admissions are attributable to medicine-related harm [18].

2.3 Age-Related Changes in Pharmacokinetics and Pharmacodynamics

Ageing is associated with physiological changes which affect drug pharmacokinetics (what the body does to the drug i.e. absorption, distribution, metabolism and excretion) and pharmacodynamics (the effect of the drug on the body) [19]. There is significant variability in the ageing process amongst individuals. This variability is accentuated by the presence of chronic disease and the use of other medications. Biochemical processes and organ function can often vary substantially between individuals of the same age. This heterogeneity extends to drug pharmacokinetics and pharmacodynamics, meaning that the clinical effects and adverse event profile of medications are less predictable in older adults [5].

2.3.1 Pharmacokinetics

2.3.1.1 Absorption and Bioavailability

Normal ageing has minimal impact on drug absorption, which takes place predominantly in the small bowel. Prokinetic drugs such as domperidone and erythromycin increase gastric emptying, potentially increasing the rate at which a drug is absorbed after ingestion. Anticholinergic drugs can decrease saliva production, reducing the rate but not necessarily the extent of drug absorption through the buccal mucosa, for example, glyceryl trinitrate and midazolam.

The bioavailability of most drugs is not affected by normal ageing. However, drugs such as morphine, buprenorphine, midazolam, propranolol, nitrates, verapamil and tricyclic antidepressants undergo substantial first-pass hepatic metabolism. Age-related reductions in liver volume and blood flow result in reduced first-pass hepatic extraction leading to higher systemic bioavailability. For example, the greater bioavailability of nitrates and verapamil in older patients can lead to significant first-dose hypotension. Initial doses of these drugs should therefore be reduced in older patients ("start low and go slow").

2.3.2 Distribution

Ageing is associated with an increased volume of distribution (*Vd*) of lipid soluble drugs. Older people generally have reduced lean muscle mass and therefore a relative increase in total body fat. This larger *V*d results in longer elimination half-lives and a tendency to accumulation of lipid soluble drugs such as morphine, benzodiazepines, antipsychotics and amitriptyline. This increases the risk of toxicity and adverse events such as falls and oversedation from these drugs. Smaller doses and a slower up-titration should therefore be used in older people.

Conversely, the lower lean body mass in older patients means that for water-soluble drugs, the *V*d is smaller than in younger adults leading to higher plasma concentrations, and therefore, lower doses are necessary. For example, *V*d of digoxin falls with age, and the loading dose should be reduced in older adults [4]. Other examples of this reduced *V*d phenomenon include lithium, theophylline and gentamicin.

Most drugs are inactive when they are bound to circulating plasma proteins (e.g. albumin and α-1 glycoprotein). Serum albumin concentration decreases slightly in older age [20]. More significant reductions in albumin are found in chronic disease states, which can lead to higher concentrations of unbound (active) drug. This can result in clinically significant effects for drugs, which are heavily protein bound, for example, benzodiazepines, antipsychotics, non-steroidal anti-inflammatory drugs (NSAIDs), warfarin and phenytoin. These drugs have a higher *V*d in patients with hypoalbuminaemia leading to longer half-lives and higher potential for toxicity [19].

2.3.2.1 Metabolism

Liver enzyme activity is preserved in ageing. However, many drug interactions of patients affected by polypharmacy are mediated through inhibition and induction of hepatic cytochrome p450 metabolising enzymes. Cytochrome p450 enzyme inhibition can cause a significant reduction in drug metabolism leading to toxic accumulation. For example, haloperidol inhibits cytochrome p450 2D6, which is responsible for the metabolism of amitriptyline. Therefore, haloperidol can exacerbate the potential for anticholinergic side effects of amitriptyline by increasing its active drug concentration. Similarly, clarithromycin can inhibit the metabolism of statins leading to statin toxicity, including myositis and hepatitis.

Conversely, drugs such as carbamazepine and phenytoin can induce cytochrome p450 enzymes, which can accelerate the metabolism and clearance of other drugs. Clinically relevant examples of cytochrome p450 enzyme inhibitors include antimicrobials, antiarrhythmics and some anticoagulants (see Table 2.1) [19].

Table 2.1 Cytochrome p450 inducers and inhibitors

Enzyme	Inducers	Inhibitors
CYP1A2	Phenytoin, rifampin	Ciprofloxacin, fluvoxamine
CYP2C9	Carbamazepine, rifampin	Fluconazole
CYP2D6		Bupropion, fluoxetine, paroxetine
CYP3A	Carbamazepine, phenytoin, rifampicin, St John's wort	Macrolides (e.g. erythromycin, clarithromycin), azole antifungals (e.g. voriconazole, itraconazole, ketoconazole, fluconazole), protease inhibitors (e.g. indinavir, ritonavir, saquinavir), cimetidine, grapefruit juice

2.3.2.2 Elimination

The kidneys are primarily responsible for the removal of drugs and their metabolites from the body. Ageing is associated with reduced renal size, perfusion and urine concentrating capability, and even in healthy ageing, glomerular filtration rate (GFR) begins to decline progressively from the age of 30 years onwards [21]. Chronic diseases such as hypertension and diabetes mellitus and the use of nephrotoxic medications such as NSAIDs accelerate this decline in GFR.

Serum creatinine concentration should not be used as the sole measure to estimate renal function in older adults, because production of creatinine is related to muscle mass which, as discussed earlier, is significantly reduced in older adults. Approximately 50% of older patients have a normal serum creatinine level but a reduced creatinine clearance estimate. The Cockcroft–Gault formula [22], based on serum creatinine, age, weight and sex, has been the most common method of estimating GFR. This formula underestimates GFR in older adults and newer formulas such as the CKD Epidemiology Collaboration (CKD-EPI, based on serum creatinine, age and sex) [23], are likely more accurate in older individuals. However, many dosing recommendations are based on the Cockcroft–Gault formula.

Older adults frequently develop acute kidney injury (AKI) in the context of acute illness and premorbid chronic kidney disease (CKD). Precipitating factors include hypotension, dehydration, sepsis, cardiorenal syndrome and cardiac failure. Drugs often mediate or exacerbate AKI in older adults especially NSAIDs, diuretics, ACE inhibitors and angiotensin receptor blockers. These drugs often need to be stopped temporarily in patients with an AKI or those at high risk of an AKI. Other drugs may need to be reduced or stopped because of the risk of toxic accumulation during an AKI or in the context of CKD, for example, lithium and metformin.

2.3.3 Pharmacodynamics

Pharmacodynamics is the study of the physiologic effect of drugs on the body. Drugs mediate their effects by binding to receptors and target molecules within the body. Ageing is associated with changes in receptor expression, activity and affinity resulting in altered (usually increased) pharmacodynamic effects of commonly prescribed drugs (Table 2.2). In practice, this means that older patients are more sensitive to medications (obtain clinical effects and experience adverse effects) at doses that produce a therapeutic effect and are normally used in younger patients, for example, the anticoagulant response to warfarin is proportionately more potent in older patients resulting in a greater risk of bleeding than in younger patients receiving the same dose.

Similarly, older patients are often more susceptible to the effects of drugs acting on the central nervous system than younger patients. Reduced integrity of the blood brain barrier and reduced cholinergic neurotransmission make older adults more sensitive to the effects of anticholinergic drugs, benzodiazepines, opioids, antidepressants and antipsychotics.

Table 2.2 Medications with altered pharmacodynamics in older patients

Drug	Age-related pharmacodynamic change	Clinical consequences	Recommendation for use
Antipsychotics Typical: Haloperidol, chlorpromazine Atypical: Quetiapine, risperidone, olanzapine	Increased sensitivity to antipsychotics, reduced dopamine reserve, loss of integrity of blood brain barrier	*Typical* • Impaired mobility and balance, gait disorders: extrapyramidal effects: Parkinsonism (tremor, rigidity, bradykinesia) dystonia, akathisia—more commonly with typical than atypical drugs *Atypical* • Orthostatic hypotension • Sedation and cognitive impairment • Weight gain • Incontinence • Anticholinergic	Limit use if possible and review need for ongoing prescription regularly Use smallest possible dose and titrate up slowly Avoid co-prescription of anticholinergic medications and sedative medications
Benzodiazepines	Greater sensitivity of older patients to the effects of benzodiazepines	• Sedation and cognitive impairment • Mobility and balance impairment with increased falls risk • Drug dependence • Impaired consciousness and respiratory depression in toxicity	Avoid use if possible. Use for shortest duration possible
Calcium channel blockers	Reduced baroreceptor response to low blood pressure Greater sinoatrial suppressive effect (verapamil, diltiazem)	• Greater hypotensive effect—especially first dose • Bradycardia	'Start low, go slow' with dose Apply caution if using concurrently with other antihypertensives or heart rate-lowering medications
Diuretics	Reduced diuretic response due to reduced tubular secretion of drug and reduced GFR	• Reduced efficacy at conventional doses. Increased risk of hypokalaemia, hypomagnesaemia	May need higher doses. Need to use cautiously as more susceptible to hypotensive effects and dehydration. Use cautiously with other antihypertensives, ACE inhibitors, NSAID's

(continued)

Table 2.2 (continued)

Drug	Age-related pharmacodynamic change	Clinical consequences	Recommendation for use
Opioids	Greater sensitivity to opioids, more prone to accumulation and toxicity	• Sedation, cognitive impairment, hallucinations • Nausea, vomiting, constipation • Mobility and balance impairment with increased falls risk • Respiratory depression in toxicity • Drug dependence • Orthostatic hypotension especially with tramadol	Use lower doses and titrate up cautiously according to effect and tolerability

Antihypertensive medications can be more challenging to use in older adults. Altered autonomic regulation including reduced baroreceptor sensitivity to changes in posture, combined with loss of elasticity in large arteries, means that older patients are more likely to experience orthostatic hypotension, which is associated with falls, injuries and reduced mobility. Alpha-1 adrenergic receptor antagonists, such as doxazosin, are especially likely to induce orthostatic hypotension as they counteract the reflex vasoconstriction that occurs normally when a person stands up. Other drugs with anticholinergic properties such as tricyclic antidepressants and first-generation antihistamines may also exacerbate orthostatic hypotension.

In general, in older patients, it is wise to commence a new drug at a low dose and titrate the dose upward with caution, that is, 'start low and go slow'.

2.3.4 Consequences of Polypharmacy

Clearly, some instances of polypharmacy are appropriate and justified. However inappropriate polypharmacy leads to a range of potentially harmful consequences. Each additional drug prescribed adds to the potential adverse effects he/she may experience. The interplay of multiple drugs and comorbidities in an older person with altered pharmacokinetics and pharmacodynamics often leads to drug–drug interactions and drug–disease interactions with increased risk of adverse outcomes.

2.3.4.1 Drug–Drug Interactions

The potential for drug–drug interactions rises almost exponentially with the number of prescribed medications [24]. The drugs most frequently involved with DDIs are diuretics, antihypertensive drugs, anticoagulants, cardiac glycoside drugs and antithrombotic agents. Clinically significant drug–drug interactions are found in 80–90% of older patients hospitalised in geriatric units [25].

Drug–drug interactions can be pharmacokinetic where one drug affects the absorption, distribution, metabolism or excretion of another drug or pharmacodynamic, where a drug directly influences the effect of another drug on its receptor or target molecule. Many of the common and significant drug–drug interactions are pharmacokinetic, mediated through the cytochrome p450 system. Table 2.3 illustrates frequently encountered important drug–drug interactions.

Table 2.3 Examples of common and important drug–drug interactions

Drug interaction	Mechanism	Clinical significance
Lithium plus NSAIDs	NSAIDs reduce prostaglandin synthesis leading to vasoconstriction of the afferent arteriole of the glomerulus reducing GFR	NSAIDs increase the potential for lithium toxicity
Nitrates plus phosphodiesterase type-5 inhibitors (e.g. sildenafil, tadalafil)	Increased cyclic guanosine monophosphate (GMP) in smooth muscle. Combined effect leads to excessive vasodilation	Concurrent use is contraindicated, risk of severe hypotension
Potassium sparing diuretics plus ACE inhibitor	Both drugs increase serum potassium levels	Combined effect leads to dangerous hyperkalaemia
Tamoxifen plus Paroxetine	Tamoxifen is a prodrug metabolised to its active form by CYP2D6. Paroxetine inhibits CYP2D6	Paroxetine reduces the level of active tamoxifen reducing its clinical effect
Olanzapine plus tricyclic antidepressants	Using multiple drugs with anticholinergic properties increases the risk of anticholinergic toxicity	May cause confusion, urinary retention, dry mouth, and constipation. Many medications have anticholinergic side properties. The cumulative clinical effect of taking more than one of these medications is referred to as anticholinergic burden
Haloperidol plus macrolide antibiotic e.g. clarithromycin	Both drugs prolong the QT interval	Use of multiple QT prolonging drugs increases the risk of arrhythmias and sudden cardiac death
Phenytoin plus carbamazepine	Both drugs are inducers of cytochrome p450	Both drugs reduce the plasma concentrations of each other and if used in combination, increased risk of seizures such that more therapeutic monitoring is needed
Allopurinol plus azathioprine	Allopurinol is a xanthine oxidase inhibitor which breaks down 6-mercaptopurine, the active metabolite of azathioprine	Toxic levels of 6-mercaptopurine lead to bone marrow suppression. These two drugs should not be used together
Valproate plus carbapenems	Carbapenems inhibit acylpeptide hydrolase, an enzyme that converts inactive valproate-glucuronide to active valproate	Carbapenems substantially reduce the therapeutic efficacy of valproate and co-administration of these two drugs should be avoided if possible

Table 2.4 Clinically significant drug–disease interactions in older patients

Drug	Disease or condition	Drug–disease interaction
Benzodiazepines Antipsychotics Antihypertensives Anticholinergics	Falls	Increased risk of falls, gait instability
Benzodiazepines Anticholinergics Antipsychotics Corticosteroids Opioids	Cognitive impairment/dementia	Increased confusion, delirium
Diuretics Anticholinergics Peripheral vasodilators Nitrates Levodopa	Orthostatic hypotension	Syncope, falls, hip fracture
Corticosteroids Antiepileptics such as carbamazepine, valproate and Phenytoin Proton pump inhibitors Aromatase inhibitors SSRI's	Osteopenia/osteoporosis	Fragility facture
NSAIDs Dihydropyridine calcium channel blockers	Heart failure	Cause sodium retention (NSAIDs), and increased incidence of heart failure
Anticholinergics Alpha agonists	Benign prostate Hyperplasia	Urinary retention
NSAIDS	Renal failure	Particularly in combination with other drugs harmful to the kidney
Metoclopramide Prochlorperazine Antipsychotics	Parkinsonism	Extrapyramidal side effects

2.3.4.2 Drug–Disease Interactions

Drug–disease interactions are present when a drug prescribed for one disease exacerbates a concomitant disease. Drug–disease interactions in older adults have been associated with increased risk of functional decline, health services use and adverse drug events [25, 26]. Potentially inappropriate medications should be minimised, and safer alternatives should be prescribed instead if possible. Drug–disease interactions are more common in frailer older adults who have reduced physiologic reserve. The major geriatric syndromes of dementia, delirium, incontinence and falls can frequently be caused or exacerbated by medications (Table 2.4).

2.3.4.3 Prescribing Cascades

A prescribing cascade occurs when a medication generates an adverse drug reaction, and instead of the culpable medication being stopped, a new medication is added to manage the symptoms of the adverse drug reaction. In this way, the patient continues to be exposed to further potential adverse drug reactions, which may in turn be managed by further medications. (See Fig. 3 in the case answers at the end of the chapter for an example of a prescribing cascade). Prescribing cascades are discussed and illustrated in detail in Chap. 5.

2.3.4.4 Falls, Immobility and Fractures

Falls and subsequent fractures have been linked to polypharmacy in numerous studies [27–29]. Amongst the most common culprits are antihypertensives, which are often used in combination. Whilst having therapeutic and mortality benefits for many, older patients are more likely to experience orthostatic hypotension and falls. Other drugs such as psychotropics, anticholinergics, benzodiazepines and opioids can cause sedation and cognitive impairment, increasing falls risk.

As people age, bone mineral density reduces. Osteoporosis is highly prevalent in older people and is associated with a much higher incidence of fractures after relatively low impact trauma [30]. Several medications, including corticosteroids, anti-epileptic drugs, selective serotonin receptor inhibitors and proton pump inhibitors can accelerate osteoporosis.

2.3.4.5 Cognitive Impairment

Polypharmacy is often associated with impaired cognitive function and dementia [31, 32]. Drugs with anticholinergic properties are associated with cognitive impairment in older patients [33]. Drugs with anticholinergic properties are used to treat a wide variety of common chronic diseases including depression, psychosis, overactive bladder, Parkinson's disease and COPD. It is common for older patients to be prescribed more than one anticholinergic drug. Various anticholinergic burden scales have been developed to quantify the cumulative effect of multiple anticholinergic medications [34]. Benzodiazepines and antipsychotics also cause cognitive impairment and should be avoided if possible [35]. These drugs, especially benzodiazepines, often need to be reduced very gradually to avoid withdrawal reactions.

2.3.4.6 Frailty, Physical Function, and Disability

Polypharmacy is associated with impaired physical function in older patients with reductions in gait speed and grip strength [3]. Older patients with polypharmacy are more likely to be frail and to have functional impairments. It is inherently difficult to prove a causal relationship between polypharmacy and these variables as patients who are frail and have functional and physical impairments are more likely to have higher levels of multimorbidity and be taking multiple medications.

2.3.4.7 Medication Errors

The greater the number of medications a patient takes the higher the potential for medication errors [36]. Transitions of care, such as admission to and discharge from hospital are particularly hazardous for patients with polypharmacy such that meticulous medication reconciliation is vital at points of care transition.

2.3.4.8 Economic Cost of Polypharmacy

Adverse drug events (ADEs) and unnecessary prescriptions resulting from inappropriate polypharmacy represents an enormous public health cost. It is estimated that

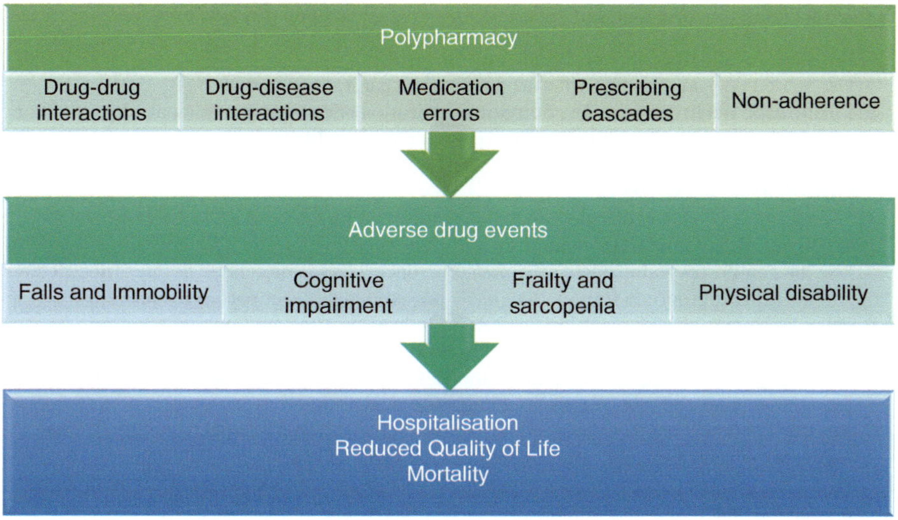

Fig. 2.1 Consequences of polypharmacy in older people

18 billion US dollars, 0.3% of the global total health expenditure, could be saved by avoidance of inappropriate prescribing [37]. Avoiding ADEs would not only improve safety outcomes for patients but would also reduce costs in terms of fewer hospital admissions, readmissions and shorter length of stay. National campaigns promoting appropriate prescribing and reducing inappropriate polypharmacy have demonstrated significant cost savings and economic benefits in Sweden [38] and Scotland [39] (Fig. 2.1).

2.3.5 Optimising Medications in Patients with Polypharmacy

Addressing polypharmacy has the potential to reduce an older person's risk of ADEs, improve treatment of their underlying comorbidities, reduce medication burden and substantially reduce costs for both the patient and the healthcare system in general. These are summarised in Table 2.5.

2.3.5.1 Use of Nonpharmacological Options

When making treatment decisions, doctors frequently underuse nonpharmacological options. For example, cognitive behavioural therapy reduces the need for antidepressants and anxiolytics in many cases. Implementing good sleep hygiene practices is more effective that sedative medications. Diet and exercise can reduce the need for diabetes medications [40].

2.3.5.2 Medication Reconciliation

The first step in optimising a patient's medications is drawing up an accurate list of the medications a patient is actually taking—a process known as medication

Table 2.5 Summary of recommendations for prescribing in older adults

1. Prioritise nonpharmacological treatment when possible
2. Use shared decision-making with the patient (and carer if appropriate)
3. Ensure each medication has an appropriate indication, clear therapeutic goal, clear duration of treatment and consideration is given to the patient's individual goals of care and life expectancy. Prescribing tools such as STOPP/START criteria are useful when evaluating prescribing appropriateness
4. 'START low, go slow', that is, initiate medications at the lowest dose and titrate up slowly according to response and tolerability
5. Use the simplest possible dosing regimen (e.g. once a day is preferable to three times a day) and the most appropriate formulation; use a pre-prepared blister pack if available
6. Provide the patient with clear instructions on indication, time and route of administration and potential adverse effects of each medication
7. Maintain an up-to-date list of all medications being taken by the patient, including over-the-counter and complementary/alternative medicines
8. Review a patient's medications regularly in the context of coexisting disease states, drug interactions, functional and cognitive status, and goals of care
9. Be aware that newly presenting symptoms may be due to an existing medication, drug–drug interaction or drug–disease interaction (avoid prescribing cascades)
10. When stopping a medication, check that it can be stopped immediately or whether it needs to be reduced gradually, for example, long-term steroids, benzodiazepines

reconciliation. This is all the more likely in older patients who may be on many different medications and are not able to reliably discuss their medication regimens. Transitions in care represent an opportunity for medication errors with potentially serious adverse outcomes to occur [41, 42]. Careful medication reconciliation is vital to reduce these errors. Medication reconciliation is dealt with in more detail in Chap. 8.

2.3.5.3 Adherence

Non-adherence with prescribed medication is a major public health issue and is closely associated with polypharmacy [17]. It is estimated that between 50 and 80% of patients with chronic conditions are non-adherent with their medications. Non-adherence has been estimated to contribute to 48% of asthma deaths, an 80% increased risk of death in diabetes and a 3.8-fold increased mortality following myocardial infarction [43]. It is estimated that non-adherence to medicines costs the European Union 125 billion euros per year [17].

Adherence may be intentional or nonintentional. Barriers to non-adherence should be addressed. For example, a patient with cognitive impairment may simply forget to take their medications or make mistakes in their administration. Medication blister packs or reminder alarms are simple ways to overcome some to these barriers (Fig. 2.2).

2.3.5.4 Medication Review

Medication review is an integral component of comprehensive geriatric assessment in which a holistic multidisciplinary systematic approach should be used. It is important to ascertain the patient's goals and expectations regarding their

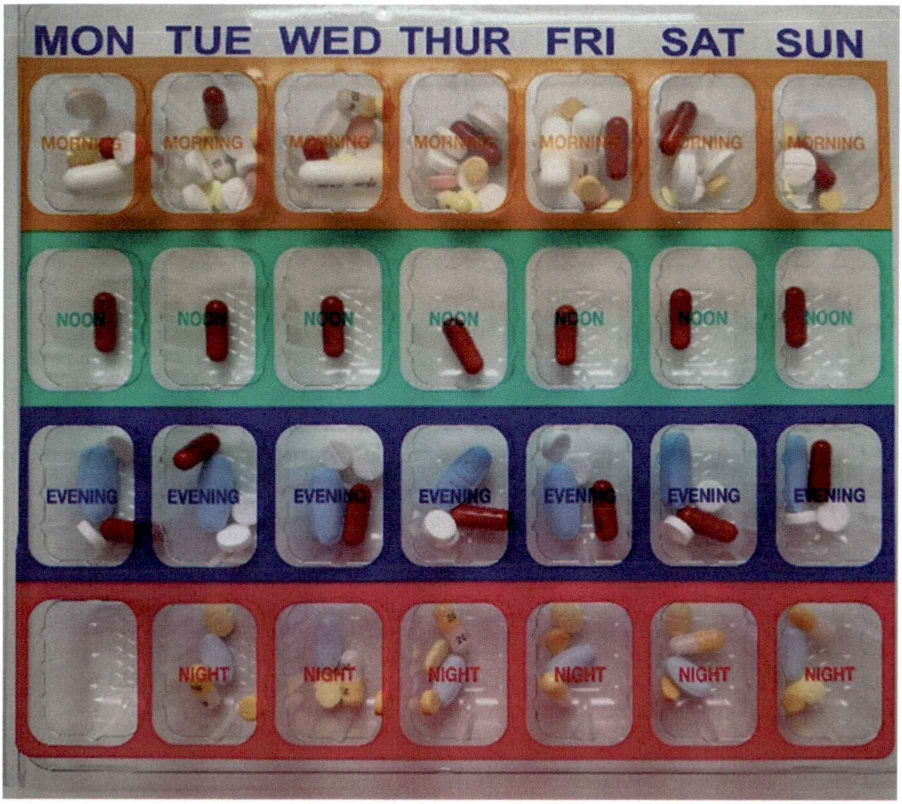

Fig. 2.2 Example of blister packed medications

medications and to individualise treatment accordingly. Shared decision-making is likely to improve adherence. It is important to educate patients about the medications they are taking, the purpose of each medication and associated common potential adverse side-effects. The indication, efficacy, safety and the cost of each drug should be assessed during each review. The medications should then be assessed for potential drug–drug interactions and drug–disease interactions.

2.3.5.5 Medication Review Tools

Recognition of the impact of polypharmacy on older individuals and on public health at large has led to the development of multiple medication review tools.

Beers criteria, originally drafted in 1991 and more recently modified in 2019, comprises a list of medications that are considered potentially inappropriate and a list of medications to avoid in certain conditions. STOPP/START criteria, initially published in 2008 [44] and revised in 2015 [45], appraise an older patient's medications in the context of their clinical conditions. The tool is organised by physiological system. STOPP criteria describe specific contexts where medications would be potentially inappropriate to prescribe for an older person, so-called potentially inappropriate medications or PIMs. START criteria identify potential prescribing omissions (PPOs), that is, where evidence-based medications likely to provide benefit to older patients for specific indications should be initiated rather than withheld for irrational or ageist reasons. This tool has been demonstrated to improve medication appropriateness and reduce adverse drug reactions [46]. Inappropriate prescribing is described in greater detail in Chap. 4.

2.3.6 Polypharmacy in the Frailest Adults

Frailty and polypharmacy are clearly linked in a bidirectional way, that is, frailty reflects multimorbidity, which generates polypharmacy, whilst polypharmacy engenders PIMs and ADRs/ADEs which often exacerbate frailty. The severely frail older person cohort is especially vulnerable to the adverse effects of polypharmacy [47]. The goals of medication in this group are often directed toward symptomatic benefit rather than prolonging life and long-term disease prevention. Despite this, the SHELTER study reported rates of polypharmacy (defined as 5–9 long-term drugs daily) and excessive polypharmacy (≥10 drugs) in nursing home residents to be 48.7% and 24.3%, respectively [44].

In patients with frailty and limited life expectancy, medication review should focus on reducing medication burden and optimising symptom management, rather than long-term preventative strategies. The STOPPFrail criteria provide a list of medications that should be discontinued or withdrawn in certain settings for older people who meet all the following criteria: 'end stage irreversible pathology, poor 1-year survival prognosis, severe functional impairment or severe cognitive impairment or both, [in whom] symptom control is the priority rather than prevention of disease progression' [48, 49].

Whilst medication review tools are helpful in this group, it is important to recognise that this is a heterogeneous group and prescribing decisions should be individualised, and the patient (and carer when appropriate) should be involved as much as possible.

Sample Case Answers

Question 1: What drug–disease interaction is illustrated in this case?

Answer: Ciprofloxacin lowers the seizure threshold, and an alternative antibiotic should be used for patients in epilepsy. Fluoroquinolones would usually not be first line for uncomplicated cystitis due to significant adverse effects including clostridium difficile infection, tendinopathy, neuropathy and QT prolongation. Haloperidol also lowers the seizure threshold.

Question 2: What drug–drug interactions are illustrated in this case?

Answer: Omeprazole and clopidogrel: see Table 2.4. There is also no clear indication for a proton pump inhibitor. Amitriptyline, festerodine and haloperidol have anticholinergic properties. Combining anticholinergics increases the likelihood of anticholinergic side effects such as delirium, constipation, urinary retention, and dry mouth. She is also taking multiple QT prolonging agents which when combined increase the risk of dangerous arrhythmias: ciprofloxacin, haloperidol and amitriptyline.

Question 3: Can you identify the prescribing cascade in this case?

Amlodipine causes lower limb swelling, which is inappropriately managed with diuretics. The diuretic causes urinary frequency, which is mismanaged with an anti-cholinergic medication which causes delirium, constipation and urinary retention and leads the patient to be admitted to hospital with exposure to multiple other drugs and drug interactions.

Author Declaration The above chapter is, in its entirety, the work of the listed authors. It does not contain any third party material or any material under copyright.

References

1. Corselli-Nordblad L, Strandell H. Ageing Europe—Looking at the lives of older people in the EU 2020 edition. Luxembourg: Eurostat; 2020. https://doi.org/10.2785/628105.
2. United Nations Department of Economic and Social Affairs Population Division. The world population ageing 2020 highlights: living arrangements of older persons. New York: United Nations; 2020.
3. Wastesson JW, Morin L, Tan ECK, Johnell K. An update on the clinical consequences of polypharmacy in older adults: a narrative review. Expert Opin Drug Saf. 2018;17:1185–96. https://doi.org/10.1080/14740338.2018.1546841.
4. Reeve E, Wiese MD, Mangoni AA. Alterations in drug disposition in older adults. Expert Opin Drug Metab Toxicol. 2015;11:491–508.
5. Maher D, Ailabouni N, Mangoni AA, Wiese MD, Reeve E. Alterations in drug disposition in older adults: a focus on geriatric syndromes. Expert Opin Drug Metab Toxicol. 2020;17:41–52. https://doi.org/10.1080/17425255.2021.1839413.
6. Ibanez B, James S, Agewall S, et al. 2017 ESC guidelines for the management of acute myocardial infarction in patients presenting with ST-segment elevation. The task force for the management of acute myocardial infarction in patients presenting with ST-segment elevation of the European Society of Cardiology (ESC). Eur Heart J. 2018;39:119–77.
7. Scottish Government Polypharmacy Model of Care Group. Polypharmacy guidance, realistic prescribing. 3rd ed. Edinburgh: NHS; 2018.
8. Kantor ED, Rehm CD, Haas JS, Chan AT, Giovannucci EL. Trends in prescription drug use among adults in the United States from 1999 to 2012. JAMA. 2015;314:1818–30.
9. Khezrian M, McNeil CJ, Murray AD, Myint PK. An overview of prevalence, determinants and health outcomes of polypharmacy. Ther Adv Drug Saf. 2020;11:2042098620933741. https://doi.org/10.1177/2042098620933741.
10. Moriarty F, Hardy C, Bennett K, Smith SM, Fahey T. Trends and interaction of polypharmacy and potentially inappropriate prescribing in primary care over 15 years in Ireland: a repeated cross-sectional study. BMJ Open. 2015;5:e008656.
11. Midão L, Giardini A, Menditto E, et al. Polypharmacy prevalence among older adults based on the survey of health, ageing and retirement in Europe. Arch Gerontol Geriatr. 2018;78:213–20.
12. Wastesson JW, Fastbom J, Johnell K. Expanding the proportion of life with polypharmacy in Sweden: 2006–2013. J Am Med Dir Assoc. 2016;17:957–8.
13. Hernández-Rodríguez MÁ, Sempere-Verdú E, Vicens-Caldentey C, et al. Evolution of polypharmacy in a Spanish population (2005–2015): a database study. Pharmacoepidemiol Drug Saf. 2020;29:433–43.

14. Lukačišinová A, Fialová D, Peel NM, et al. The prevalence and prescribing patterns of benzodiazepines and Z-drugs in older nursing home residents in different European countries and Israel: retrospective results from the EU SHELTER study. BMC Geriatr. 2021;211(21):1–16.
15. Toepfer S, Bolbrinker J, König M, Steinhagen-Thiessen E, Kreutz R, Demuth I. Potentially inappropriate medication in older participants of the Berlin Aging Study II (BASE-II)—sex differences and associations with morbidity and medication use. PLoS One. 2019;14:e0226511.
16. Franchi C, Tettamanti M, Pasina L, Djignefa CD, Fortino I, Bortolotti A, Merlino L, Nobili A. Changes in drug prescribing to Italian community-dwelling elderly people: the EPIFARM-elderly project 2000–2010. Eur J Clin Pharmacol. 2014;70:437–43.
17. Mair A, Fernandez-Llimos F, Alonso A, Harrison C, Hurding S, Kempen T, Kinnear M, Michael N, McIntosh J, Wilson M. Polypharmacy management by 2030: a patient safety challenge. 2nd ed. Coimbra: Simpathy; 2017.
18. Kongkaew C, Hann M, Mandal J, Williams SD, Metcalfe D, Noyce PR, Ashcroft DM. Risk factors for hospital admissions associated with adverse drug events. Pharmacotherapy. 2013;33:827–37.
19. Mangoni AA, Jackson SHD. Age-related changes in pharmacokinetics and pharmacodynamics: basic principles and practical applications. Br J Clin Pharmacol. 2004;57:6.
20. Weaving G, Batstone GF, Jones RG. Age and sex variation in serum albumin concentration: an observational study. Ann Clin Biochem. 2015;53:106–11. https://doi.org/10.1177/0004563215593561.
21. Glassock RJ, Winearls C. Ageing and the glomerular filtration rate: truths and consequences. Trans Am Clin Climatol Assoc. 2009;120:419.
22. Cockcroft DW, Gault MH. Prediction of creatinine clearance from serum creatinine. Nephron. 1976;16:31–41.
23. Levey AS, Stevens LA, Schmid CH, et al. A new equation to estimate glomerular filtration rate. Ann Intern Med. 2009;150:604–12.
24. Johnell K, Klarin I. The relationship between number of drugs and potential drug–drug interactions in the elderly: a study of over 600,000 elderly patients from the Swedish Prescribed Drug Register. Drug Saf. 2007;30:911–8.
25. de Oliveira LM, Diel JD, Nunes A, Dal Pizzol TD. Prevalence of drug interactions in hospitalised elderly patients: a systematic review. Eur J Hosp Pharm. 2021;28:4–9.
26. Danijea G, Kristina J. Clinical implications from drug–drug and drug–disease interactions in older people. Clin Exp Pharmacol Physiol. 2013;40:320–5.
27. Fried TR, O'Leary J, Towle V, Goldstein MK, Trentalange M, Martin DK. Health outcomes associated with polypharmacy in community-dwelling older adults: a systematic review. J Am Geriatr Soc. 2014;62:2261–72.
28. Laflamme L, Monárrez-Espino J, Johnell K, Elling B, Möller J. Type, number or both? A population-based matched case-control study on the risk of fall injuries among older people and number of medications beyond fall-inducing drugs. PLoS One. 2015;10(3):e0123390. https://doi.org/10.1371/JOURNAL.PONE.0123390.
29. Ambrose AF, Paul G, Hausdorff JM. Risk factors for falls among older adults: a review of the literature. Maturitas. 2013;75:51–61.
30. Compston J, Cooper A, Cooper C, et al. UK clinical guideline for the prevention and treatment of osteoporosis. Arch Osteoporos. 2017;12:43.
31. Niikawa H, Okamura T, Ito K, Ura C, Miyamae F, Sakuma N, Ijuin M, Inagaki H, Sugiyama M, Awata S. Association between polypharmacy and cognitive impairment in an elderly Japanese population residing in an urban community. Geriatr Gerontol Int. 2017;17:1286–93.
32. Rawle MJ, Cooper R, Kuh D, Richards M. Associations between polypharmacy and cognitive and physical capability: a British birth cohort study. J Am Geriatr Soc. 2018;66:916–23.
33. Fox C, Richardson K, Maidment ID, Savva GM, Matthews FE, Smithard D, Coulton S, Katona C, Boustani MA, Brayne C. Anticholinergic medication use and cognitive impairment in the older population: the Medical Research Council Cognitive Function and Ageing Study. J Am Geriatr Soc. 2011;59:1477–83.

34. Welsh TJ, van der Wardt V, Ojo G, Gordon AL, Gladman JRF. Anticholinergic drug burden tools/scales and adverse outcomes in different clinical settings: a systematic review of reviews. Drugs Aging. 2018;356(35):523–38.
35. Drake MJ, Nixon PM, Crew JP. Drug-induced bladder and urinary disorders. Drug Saf. 1998;19:45–55.
36. Calderón-Larrañaga A, Poblador-Plou B, González-Rubio F, Gimeno-Feliu LA, Abad-Díez JM, Prados-Torres A. Multimorbidity, polypharmacy, referrals, and adverse drug events: are we doing things well? Br J Gen Pract. 2012;62:e821–6.
37. Aitken M, Gorokhovich L. Advancing the responsible use of medicines: applying levers for change. SSRN Electron J. 2012;2012:2222541. https://doi.org/10.2139/SSRN.2222541.
38. Kempen TGH, Bertilsson M, Hadziosmanovic N, Lindner K-J, Melhus H, Nielsen EI, Sulku J, Gillespie U. Effects of hospital-based comprehensive medication reviews including postdischarge follow-up on older patients' use of health care: a cluster randomized clinical trial. JAMA Netw Open. 2021;4(4):e216303. https://doi.org/10.1001/JAMANETWORKOPEN.2021.6303.
39. Mair A, Wilson M, Dreischulte T. The polypharmacy programme in Scotland: realistic prescribing. Prescriber. 2019;30:10–6.
40. Rochon PA, Petrovic M, Cherubini A, Onder G, O'Mahony D, Sternberg SA, Stall NM, Gurwitz JH. Polypharmacy, inappropriate prescribing, and deprescribing in older people: through a sex and gender lens. Lancet Health Longev. 2021;2:e290–300.
41. Wheeler AJ, Scahill S, Hopcroft D, Stapleton H. Reducing medication errors at transitions of care is everyone's business. Aust Prescr. 2018;41:73.
42. Gleason KM, McDaniel MR, Feinglass J, Baker DW, Lindquist L, Liss D, Noskin GA. Results of the medications at transitions and clinical handoffs (MATCH) study: an analysis of medication reconciliation errors and risk factors at hospital admission. J Gen Intern Med. 2010;25:441–7.
43. Rachel E. Non-adherence to medicines: not solved but solvable. J Health Serv Res Policy. 2009;14:58–61.
44. Paul G, Cristin R, Stephen B, Julia K, Denis O. STOPP (screening tool of older person's prescriptions) and START (screening tool to alert doctors to right treatment). Consensus validation. Int J Clin Pharmacol Ther. 2008;46:72–83.
45. O'Mahony D, O'Sullivan D, Byrne S, O'Connor MN, Ryan C, Gallagher P. STOPP/START criteria for potentially inappropriate prescribing in older people: version 2. Age Ageing. 2015;44:213–8.
46. O'Connor MN, O'Sullivan D, Gallagher PF, Eustace J, Byrne S, O'Mahony D. Prevention of hospital-acquired adverse drug reactions in older people using screening tool of older persons' prescriptions and screening tool to alert to right treatment criteria: a cluster randomized controlled trial. J Am Geriatr Soc. 2016;64:1558–66.
47. Lavan AH, Gallagher P. Predicting risk of adverse drug reactions in older adults. Ther Adv Drug Saf. 2016;7:11.
48. Lavan AH, Gallagher P, Parsons C, O'Mahony D. STOPPFrail (screening tool of older persons prescriptions in frail adults with limited life expectancy): consensus validation. Age Ageing. 2017;46:600–7.
49. Curtin D, Gallagher P, O'Mahony D. Deprescribing in older people approaching end-of-life: development and validation of STOPPFrail version 2. Age Ageing. 2021;50:465–71.

3 Drug–Drug and Drug–Nutrients Interactions: From Theory to Clinical Relevance

Eline M. de Koning, Jeannine Huisbrink, and Wilma Knol

3.1 Introduction

The ageing of the population is accompanied by the development of a growing number of chronic diseases. This multimorbidity increases the prevalence of polypharmacy, which is often defined as using five or more medications daily [1]. An expanding number of prescribed drugs is one of the most important risk factors for drug–drug interactions (DDIs) [2, 3]. A drug–drug interaction is defined as an interaction between two or more drugs on a pharmacokinetic and/or a pharmacodynamic level, with the risk of increasing the toxicity or reducing the intended effect of one or more of the involved drugs [4, 5]. Not only multimorbidity and polypharmacy increase the susceptibility to DDI's, but also age-related changes in pharmacokinetics and pharmacodynamics are involved.

DDIs are associated with an elevated risk of adverse drug reactions, worsening of functional status, mortality and are responsible for approximately 5% of hospital admissions in older patients [6–11].

E. M. de Koning
Department of Hospital Pharmacy, Medisch Spectrum Twente, Enschede, The Netherlands
e-mail: Eline.deKoning@mst.nl

J. Huisbrink
Department of Hospital Pharmacy, Franciscus Gasthuis en Vlietland, Schiedam/Rotterdam, The Netherlands
e-mail: j.palsgraaf-huisbrink@Franciscus.nl

W. Knol (✉)
Department of Geriatric Medicine and Expertise Centre Pharmacotherapy in Old Persons, University Medical Center Utrecht, Utrecht University, Utrecht, The Netherlands
e-mail: w.knol@umcutrecht.nl

A. Cherubini et al. (eds.), *Optimizing Pharmacotherapy in Older Patients*, Practical Issues in Geriatrics, https://doi.org/10.1007/978-3-031-28061-0_3

Not only interactions between drugs are prevalent. Drugs can also interfere with certain foods or enteral feeding (drug–nutrition interactions or DNIs), herbs or fluids like alcohol. Drug–nutrition interactions are defined as modifications of pharmacokinetics or pharmacodynamics of a drug because of nutrients or a modification in nutritional status because of the addition of a drug [12].

This chapter will focus on drug–drug interactions and drug–nutrition interactions.

3.2 Theory

Drugs may interact on a pharmaceutical, pharmacokinetic or pharmacodynamic basis. Pharmaceutical interactions emerge when two drugs are mixed in IV fluids or syringes and chemically react, which may affect the safety, efficacy and stability of the drug. This could also occur with the combination of a drug and a nutrient, for example, in an enteral feeding tube. For instance sucralfate, when given simultaneously with enteral nutrition, binds to proteins within the enteral feed, leading to a change in consistency and possibly tube blockage.

Enteral feeding could be applied in cases of malnourishment or when swallowing is no longer possible or recommended. If given continuously or over large parts of the day, problems may arise when medication needs to be administered. This chapter will address pharmacokinetic (PK) and pharmacodynamic (PD) interactions.

3.2.1 Pharmacokinetic Interactions

Pharmacokinetic interactions are defined as interactions where a drug or nutrient affects the absorption, distribution, metabolism or excretion of another drug. These interactions can lead to changes in serum drug concentrations, which might alter clinical response. We will discuss the most important elements of pharmacokinetics.

3.2.1.1 Absorption

Absorption defines the uptake of a substance into the systemic circulation. Several factors influence the degree of absorption, such as physiochemical properties (e.g. drug solubility, lipophilicity of the drug), drug formulation, route of administration and patient factors (e.g. gastrointestinal pH). Additionally, the presence of food could affect drug absorption, for example, by decreasing gastric emptying, changing the pH of the stomach and decreasing gut motility [13–15].

An active substance can become unsuitable for absorption due to chemical reaction with another active substance within the gastrointestinal tract. This happens for example when iron is given simultaneously with quinolones, such as ciprofloxacin. The latter drugs form an insoluble complex, which reduces the bioavailability of ciprofloxacin. This interaction could be avoided by prolonging the interval of administration. Furthermore, calcium ions in milk or other dairy products could form insoluble complexes with ciprofloxacin and also with bisphosphonates, which should, therefore, be taken on an empty stomach. Ciprofloxacin absorption is also significantly decreased when combined with enteral feed [16]. Another example is the combination of phenytoin with enteral formulations. Phenytoin is known to bind certain components of the enteral formulations, particularly proteins and calcium salts, reducing drug absorption. Given that it is not always possible to have intermittent feeding, the doctor could consult a pharmacist to provide advice about an alternative drug or feeding regimen.

Another type of interaction could emerge when one drug or nutrient causes a change in pH of the stomach. Some drugs, such as itraconazole, require an acidic environment in order for the drug to be converted to a soluble salt form. Drugs that increase the pH of the stomach, such as proton pump inhibitors, diminish the absorption of those drugs. It is, therefore, recommended to administer drugs such as itraconazole with an acidic substance to decrease the pH. Drugs that have an enteric coating could dissolve too early when acidity is changed. This coating normally protects the drug from early degradation or protects the stomach from damaging effects of the drug itself.

The rate of absorption could also be influenced by agents that alter the rate of gastric emptying. The intestinal motility could be altered by anticholinergic drugs, opioids or metoclopramide, thus leading to delayed absorption. This might enhance the emergence of DDIs and DNIs.

3.2.1.2 Distribution

The absorbed drug will be distributed after entering the general circulation. Drugs can bind to several proteins in the bloodstream or diffuse to tissues located outside the bloodstream. Many drugs are highly bound to plasma proteins, such as albumin or alpha-1-acid glycoprotein. An interaction may emerge if one agent displaces another agent from its plasma binding site. By displacement, more unbound drug becomes available. Such protein binding interactions hardly ever lead to clinically significant changes in efficacy, since there will be further distribution or elimination of the drug. In theory, the interaction could become relevant if one agent has a small volume of distribution, a narrow therapeutic index and high plasma protein binding properties.

3.2.1.3 Metabolism

The cytochrome P450 (CYP) enzyme family plays a very important role in catalysing the biotransformation of certain drugs and other xenobiotic agents. Approximately half of the 200 most commonly used drugs undergo CYP-mediated metabolism [17]. CYP3A4/5, CYP2D6, CYP2C9, CYP2B6 and CYP2C19 are mostly involved in this metabolism [18].

Drug metabolism occurs mainly within the liver and kidney, but could also take place inside the lungs or gastro-intestinal tract, where CYP3A4 is present in the gut wall.

Hepatic metabolism incorporates two types of biochemical reactions to create more water-soluble compounds, phase I and phase II reactions. Phase I reactions include minor molecular modifications, where hydrophilic groups are added to the drug molecule. Phase II reactions cover conjugation reactions.

Many pharmacokinetic-based interactions emerge through the altered function of drug-metabolising enzymes (e.g. phase I CYP enzymes) and transporters [e.g. P-glycoprotein (P-gp)].

The risk of a clinical relevant interaction increases if the substrate (= the agent whose metabolism is affected) has only one metabolism pathway, and the corresponding enzyme is strongly inhibited or induced by another substance.

For example, grapefruit juice is well known for inhibiting intestinal CYP3A4, thereby reducing the metabolism of CYP3A4 substrates, such as simvastatin. CYP1A2 is involved in the metabolism of clozapine. Smoking has an inducing effect on CYP1A2. When a patient is using drugs that are metabolised by CYP1A2, quitting smoking could have a considerable inducing effect on their metabolism.

Inhibition of CYP enzymes occurs rapidly and is generally reversible. After discontinuation, the inhibitory effect is mainly dependent on the (elimination) half-life of the inhibitor. By inducing CYP enzymes, more additional enzymes will be formed. Hence, the inducing effect sets in more gradually (over days to weeks). Following withdrawal of the enzyme-inducing agent, the disappearance of the inducing effect depends on the (elimination) half-life of the inducer and on the degradation of enzymes additionally produced by the induction. The inducing effect will, therefore, diminish gradually (usually in a few weeks).

3.2.1.4 Elimination

Elimination is a process of clearance of the drug, mostly by the kidney or via bile. There are also other routes of elimination, such as pulmonary or dermal elimination.

Drug-induced changes in hepatic blood flow could affect certain drugs that have high hepatic extraction ratios, such as propranolol. Drugs that increase hepatic blood flow, such as glucagon and verapamil, accelerate elimination of drugs like propranolol. This, however, has an unknown clinical relevance.

Renal elimination of drugs may be diminished by agents that decrease glomerular filtration rate, such as aminoglycoside antibiotics or angiotensin-converting enzyme (ACE)-inhibitors. Drug-induced renal impairment may be aggravated by concomitantly prescribing drugs that enhance renal impairment. A combination of non-steroidal anti-inflammatory drugs (NSAIDs) and ACE-inhibitors could lead to renal failure.

A third mechanism that could lead to interactions is competition for tubular active transport. One substance could disrupt renal excretion of another agent, possibly leading to accumulation and toxicity. For example, the body recognizes lithium as sodium and is, therefore, processed in similar ways. Drugs that induce reabsorption of sodium could also provoke reabsorption of lithium, resulting in toxicity.

3.2.2 Pharmacodynamic Interactions

Pharmacodynamic interactions include interactions of drugs acting on the same receptors, site of action or physiological systems. These interactions could result in additive, synergistic or antagonistic effects. Interactions at the receptor site arise when one agent has a higher affinity for the receptor than the other agent, leading to competition. This could occur at opioid receptors when combining a partial opioid agonist and a full opioid agonist or at beta-adrenoceptors with non-selective beta-antagonists such as propranolol together with beta-agonists such as salbutamol. Furthermore, a diet or enteral feed rich of vitamin K antagonizes the therapeutic effect of vitamin K antagonists, such as warfarin.

Moreover, some drugs can change the pharmacodynamic effects of another drug by altering receptor sensitivity. Drugs can also influence PD by acting on another receptor resulting in synergistic or antagonistic effects within that cell or at another downstream site. For example, opioids enhance the sedative response to benzodiazepines.

Additionally, drugs that act on the same physiological system may enhance their mutual effect. The combination of an angiotensin receptor blocker with an ACE-inhibitor potentiates a stronger lowering of blood pressure, but can also lead to a reduction in kidney function. Both drugs act on the renin–angiotensin–aldosterone system (RAAS), but through a different mechanism. Furthermore, prescribing two different drugs effecting the central nervous system causes more sedation.

Changes in fluid and electrolyte balance may alter the effects of drug action on the kidney, myocardium and on neuromuscular transmission. For example, if a patient is using digoxin and becomes hypokalaemic, which could be induced by diuretics, the action of digoxin is altered. Digoxin inhibits the exchange of sodium and potassium by acting on the sodium–potassium pump (Na-K-ATP-ase). This increases the concentration of intracellular sodium ions and decreases the concentration of intracellular potassium ions. Potassium and digoxin compete for binding on the Na-K-ATP-ase pump. Hypokalaemia, therefore, results in increased binding of digoxin, increasing its therapeutic effect and possibly enhancing toxicity.

3.3 Age-Related Changes in Pharmacokinetics

There are minor changes regarding absorption in the older patient. The absorption is slightly slowed, but total drug absorption does not change. There is a higher availability for drugs with very large first pass effect. The gastric pH is higher, which could lead to a variable absorption of tablets requiring low pH. However, most of these changes do not lead to clinically relevant alterations in drug levels.

Older patients hold more fat, less muscle tissue and less body water. Hydrophilic drugs with a high volume of distribution (e.g. digoxin) have a smaller volume of distribution due to less fluid and muscle tissue. Thus, a lower loading dose of digoxin should be given to avoid toxicity. On the contrary, lipophilic drugs have a larger volume of distribution. Therefore, accumulation of lipophilic drugs (e.g. diazepam) could occur, and such drugs may cause prolongation of action and adverse effects.

Phase I metabolism is reduced in older people (approximately 30%), especially regarding CYP1A2 and CYP3A4. Phase II metabolism remains intact. Clinical consequences regarding altered phase I metabolism remain unknown.

The age-related changes concerning elimination are of highest relevance. Kidney function decreases with age but is also affected by comorbidities such as hypertension or diabetes. In case of renal insufficiency, dose adjustments are frequently necessary for drugs that are cleared renally.

3.4 Clinically Relevant PK Interactions

PK interactions that could become clinically relevant are mostly due to CYP-related metabolism. For example, the use of ciprofloxacin (CYP1A2 inhibitor) in older patients treated with clozapine (CYP1A2 substrate) leads to a decreased metabolism of clozapine. Moreover, phase I metabolism by CYP1A2 is shown to be reduced by aging. Additionally, CYP1A2 activity is known to be reduced during infection. These combined effects may further enhance the therapeutic effects or even toxicity of clozapine.

Another example is the combination of simvastatin or atorvastatin and CYP3A4 inhibitors. Increased statin exposure due to the inhibition of CYP3A4-mediated metabolism by, for example, verapamil and grapefruit juice could lead to severe myopathy and rhabdomyolysis, which, in turn, may lead to acute renal failure. On the contrary, prescribing simvastatin with CYP3A4 inducers such as carbamazepine (70–80% reduction of plasma concentration) or St John's wort (60% reduction) could lead to higher cholesterol concentrations [19, 20].

A third example is the combination of lithium with an ACE-inhibitor or diuretic. Diuretics or ACE-inhibitors enhance sodium loss. Because of this, there will be a compensatory distal reabsorption of sodium and lithium, leading to lithium toxicity.

3.5 Age-Related Changes in Pharmacodynamics

Older patients have an increased vulnerability because of a decline in physiological reserve [less functional homoeostatic mechanisms (e.g. reduced sense of thirst with a risk of dehydration)] and a decline across multiple organ systems (reduced ability to excrete free water). Furthermore, older patients are known to have a lower receptor responsiveness (e.g. beta-adrenoceptor), which could lead to an altered sensitivity to drugs [21–25].

Older people are more sensitive to adverse effects of psychotherapeutic drugs. A decline of central receptors (e.g. dopamine D2) with age and a greater affinity, for example, for antipsychotics may account for this increased risk.

3.6 Clinically Relevant PD Interactions

The most clinically relevant changes in pharmacodynamics are increased susceptibility to certain drugs, for example, central acting drugs. Research has shown that most clinically relevant interactions are of pharmacodynamic origin [26–29]. These interactions concern drugs that are often used by older patients to treat age-related conditions, as cardiovascular or neurological conditions. For example, prescribing a combination of psychotropic medication may enhance sedation, apathy or falls. Multiple agents that act on haemostasis, such as oral anticoagulants in combination with antiplatelet drugs potentially increase the risk of bleeding. The risk of (mainly gastrointestinal) bleeding also increases with concomitant use of NSAIDs with a serotonin-selective reuptake inhibitor (SSRI) or serotonin–noradrenalin reuptake inhibitor (SNRI), by additive effects on platelet inhibition.

Combining two drugs with potassium sparing effects (e.g. triamterene, spironolactone, ACE-inhibitors, cotrimoxazole) may enhance additive potassium retention leading to hyperkalaemia.

Combining drugs that reduce potassium (e.g. beta 2-agonists, thiazides, loop diuretics, corticosteroids) could, however, also be potentially dangerous, especially if a patient is also on digoxin.

Furthermore, if an older patient is using a diuretic agent or inhibitor of the RAAS system and is prescribed an NSAID, the patient is at risk of renal failure. NSAIDs negatively influence the compensatory mechanism that is activated to maintain adequate renal blood flow, when renal perfusion seems to decrease.

A clinically relevant pharmacodynamic DNI could occur if a patient is prescribed paroxetine whilst using St John's wort. When St John's wort is used in conjunction with paroxetine, an additive serotonergic effect may occur, which could lead to serotonin syndrome.

Table 3.1 provides an overview of DDIs and DNIs that are commonly clinically relevant in older adults.

Table 3.1 Most common drug–drug and drug–nutrient interactions in older people

Drug class	Drug/nutrient	Drug/nutrient	Impact/mechanism	Type of IA
Cardiovascular	ACE-inhibitors	Potassium supplements/ aldosterone antagonists/ potassium sparing diuretics	Elevated serum potassium	PD
	ACE-inhibitor	ARB	Risk of renal failure by additive or synergistic effects on renal blood flow and blood pressure	PD
	Digoxin	Amiodarone	Digoxin toxicity due to p-gp inhibition; both drugs suppress the SA node, resulting in bradycardia	PK + PD
	Digoxin	Verapamil	PK: Verapamil inhibits both renal tubular secretion and non-renal excretion of digoxin. Diltiazem decreases the clearance and/or volume of distribution of digoxin PD: The slowing effects of verapamil or diltiazem and digoxin on atrioventricular conduction may be additive	PK + PD
	Verapamil/diltiazem	CYP3A4 substrates (e.g. carbamazepine, simvastatin, midazolam)	Inhibition metabolism of substrates, therefore higher concentrations	PK
	Dabigatran/edoxaban	P-gp inhibitor	Higher risk of bleeding	PK
	Rivaroxaban/apixaban	P-gp inhibitor or CYP3A4 inhibitor	Higher risk of bleeding	PK
	Oral anticoagulant	Antiplatelet drug	Higher risk of bleeding	PD
	Antiplatelet drugs	Ginkgo biloba	Increased risk of bleeding. Mechanism remains unknown	PD
	Beta-blocker	Verapamil/diltiazem	Increased effect on AV nodal conduction, heart rate or cardiac contractility, resulting in bradycardia, AV block and hypotension	PD
	Beta-blocker	Beta2-agonist	Beta-blockers may diminish the bronchodilatory effect of beta2-agonists. Of particular concern with non-selective beta-blockers or higher doses of the beta1 selective beta-blockers	PD

	Diuretics	RAAS-inhibitors	Volume depletion induced by diuretic therapy, combined with the peripheral vasodilation and initial decrease in renal blood flow produced by the RAAS-inhibitor, leading to exaggerated hypotensive response and possible renal injury	PD
	Vitamin K antagonists	Vitamin K-rich foods/vitamin K supplements/vitamin K-rich enteral nutrition formulations	Vitamin K antagonists interfere with the ability of the body to effectively use vitamin K in the production of certain clotting factors (II, VII, IX, X). This interference can be overcome by administering adequate quantities of exogenous vitamin K	PD
	Warfarin	Enteral nutrition formulations	Warfarin could bind to proteins in enteral nutrition formulations, reducing bioavailability	PK
	Simvastatin/atorvastatin/nifedipine	Grapefruit juice	Inhibition of CYP3A4-mediated metabolism, resulting in an increased bioavailability and AUC	PK
Central nervous system	Lithium	Thiazide diuretic	Thiazide diuretics enhance proximal tubular reabsorption of lithium, leading to elevated lithium serum concentrations	PK
	Lithium	ACE-inhibitor/ARB	Lowered levels of angiotensin II lead to lower circulating levels of aldosterone. Subsequently, sodium and water excretion increase possibly causing greater renal retention of the lithium ion	PK
	Lithium	NSAID	NSAIDs inhibit the synthesis of prostaglandins (PGE2) in the kidneys. As a result, the blood flow to the kidneys is inhibited, and thus, lithium excretion is reduced. This will cause the lithium concentration to rise	PK
	Levodopa	High-protein diet	High-protein diets have the potential to impair levodopa absorption; levodopa competes with certain amino acids for transport across the gut wall or across the BBB	PK
	Levodopa	Iron	Reduced absorption due to complexation	PK
	Levodopa	Metoclopramide	Diminished effect levodopa due to D2 blockage	PD

(continued)

Table 3.1 (continued)

Drug class	Drug/nutrient	Drug/nutrient	Impact/mechanism	Type of IA
	MAO-inhibitors	SSRI/opioid	Serotonin syndrome or opioid toxicity by enhancing the serotonergic effect of MAO inhibitors	PD
	MAO-inhibitors	Tyramine-rich foods	Severe hypertensive episodes by inhibiting tyramine metabolism, leading to increased biosynthesis of catecholamines	PK
	Phenytoin	Enteral nutrition formulations	Phenytoin binds proteins and calcium salts in enteral nutrition formulations, leading to reduced absorption	PK
	Paroxetine/fluoxetine	Metoprolol	Increase in metoprolol concentrations due to CYP2D6 inhibition, possibly resulting in bradycardia	PK
	Fluoxetine	Tricyclic antidepressant	Risk of serotonin syndrome by additive serotonergic effects or tricyclic antidepressant toxicity due to fluoxetine-mediated inhibition of CYP2D6 and/or CYP2C19, enzymes responsible for the metabolism of tricyclic antidepressants	PK + PD
	Paroxetine/fluoxetine	St John's wort	St John's wort may enhance the serotonergic effect of paroxetine or fluoxetine, which could result in serotonin syndrome	PD
	Concomitant use of ≥3 centrally acting drugs (e.g. opioids, antipsychotics, benzodiazepines, antidepressants or antiepileptics)		Increased risk of falling, possibly leading to fractures and impaired cognition	PD
	Clozapine	CYP1A2 inducers/inhibitors (e.g. carbamazepine/ciprofloxacin)	Influences on clozapine concentrations due to induction or inhibition of CYP1A2, leading to loss of effect or toxicity	PK
Anti-infective agents	Fluoroquinolones/doxycyclin	Calcium/dairy products/iron/cations in enteral nutrition	Reduced absorption due to complexation	PK
	Antifungal agents e.g. miconazole	Warfarin/acenocoumarol/fenprocoumon	Increased serum concentrations of vitamin K antagonists by inhibition of CYP2C9 enzymes	PK

	Itraconazole	Proton pump inhibitors	Decreased bioavailability because of increased gastric pH	PK
Endocrine	Metformin	Proton pump inhibitors	Malabsorption of vitamin B12, possibly leading to vitamin B12 deficiency Most probably, metformin may interfere with the active calcium dependent absorption of the vitamin B12-intrinsic factor complex	PK
	Levothyroxine	Calcium/dairy products/iron/ cations in enteral nutrition	Reduced absorption due to complexation	PK
Pain medication	Oxycodone	CYP3A4 inhibitors (e.g. voriconazole)	Increase in serum concentration of oxycodone. Serum concentrations of the active metabolite oxymorphone may also be increased	PK
	Opioid agonist	Mixed opioid agonist/ antagonist (e.g. buprenorphine)	Reduced effects of pure opioid agonists via competition/ antagonism at opioid receptor sites. This could precipitate withdrawal symptoms, necessitate unusually high doses, or lead to therapeutic failure	PD
	NSAID	SSRI/SNRI	Increased risk of gastrointestinal bleeding by additive inhibitory effects on platelet aggregation	PD
	NSAID	ACE-inhibitor/ARB	Significant decrease in renal function and risk of renal failure due to the ability of NSAIDs to reduce the synthesis of vasodilating renal prostaglandins. This would affect vascular tone and fluid homoeostasis	PD
Immunosuppressive agents	Methotrexate	Trimethoprim/cotrimoxazole	Methotrexate toxicity (e.g. bone marrow suppression). Both drugs contribute to folate deficiency (via suppression of dihydrofolate reductase)	PD
Respiratory	Theophylline	Ciprofloxacin (or other moderate to strong CYP1A2 inhibitors)	Theophyllin toxicity due to inhibition of CYP1A2-mediated metabolism of theophylline	PK

(continued)

Table 3.1 (continued)

Drug class	Drug/nutrient	Drug/nutrient	Impact/mechanism	Type of IA
Gastro-intestinal	Proton pump inhibitor	Vitamin B12	Malabsorption of vitamin B12 due to inhibition of intrinsic factor	PK
	Sucralfate	Enteral nutrition formulations	Sucralfate binds proteins within the enteral feed, leading to a change in consistency and possible feeding tube blockage	PC
Other	Bisphosphonate	Calcium/dairy products/iron/cations in enteral nutrition	Reduced absorption due to complexation	PK
	St John's wort	CYP3A4 substrate (e.g. verapamil)	Reduced efficacy due to induction of CYP3A4	PK

ACE angiotensin-converting enzyme, *ARB* angiotensin II receptor blocker, *AV* atrioventricular, *AUC* area under the curve, *BBB* blood–brain barrier, *CYP* cytochrome P450, *D2* dopamine 2 receptor, *IA* interaction, *MAO* monoamine oxidase, *NSAID* non-steroidal anti-inflammatory drug, *PC* pharmaceutical, *PD* pharmacodynamic, *P-gp* P-glycoprotein, *PK* pharmacokinetic, *RAAS* renin–angiotensin–aldosterone-system, *SA* sinoatrial, *SNRI* serotonin and noradrenalin reuptake inhibitor, *SSRI* selective serotonin reuptake inhibitor

References

1. Masnoon N, Shakib S, Kalisch-Ellett L, Caughey GE. What is polypharmacy? A systematic review of definitions. BMC Geriatr. 2017;17(1):230. https://doi.org/10.1186/s12877-017-0621-2.
2. Salazar JA, Poon I, Nair M. Clinical consequences of polypharmacy in elderly: expect the unexpected, think the unthinkable. Expert Opin Drug Saf. 2007;6(6):695–704.
3. Shetty V, Chowta MN, Chowta KN, Shenoy A, Kamath A, Kamath P. Evaluation of potential drug–drug interactions with medications prescribed to geriatric patients in a tertiary care hospital. J Aging Res. 2018;2018:5728957.
4. Bjerrum L, Andersen M, Petersen G, Kragstrup J. Exposure to potential drug interactions in primary health care. Scand J Prim Health Care. 2003;21:153–8.
5. Magro L, Moretti U, Leone R. Epidemiology and characteristics of adverse drug reactions caused by drug–drug interactions. Expert Opin Drug Saf. 2012;11:83–94.
6. Mallet L, Spinewine A, Huang A. The challenge of managing drug interactions in elderly people. Lancet. 2007;370:185–91.
7. Hines LE, Murphy JE. Potentially harmful drug–drug interactions in the elderly: a review. Am J Geriatr Pharmacother. 2011;9:364–77.
8. Gnjidic D, Johnell K. Clinical implications from drug–drug and drug–disease interactions in older people. Clin Exp Pharmacol Physiol. 2013;40:320–5.
9. Bykov K, Gagne JJ. Generating evidence of clinical outcomes of drug–drug interactions. Drug Saf. 2017;40:101–3.
10. Swart F, Bianchi G, Lenzi J, Iommi M, Maestri L, Raschi E, et al. Risk of hospitalization from drug–drug interactions in the elderly: real-world evidence in a large administrative database. Aging. 2020;12(19):711–39.
11. Dechanont S, Maphanta S, Butthum B, Kongkaew C. Hospital admissions/visits associated with drug–drug interactions: a systematic review and meta-analysis. Pharmacoepidemiol Drug Saf. 2014;23:489–97.
12. Genser D. Food and drug interaction: consequences for the nutrition/health status. Ann Nutr Metab. 2008;52:29–32.
13. Amadi CN, Mgbahurike AA. Selected food/herb–drug interactions: mechanisms and clinical relevance. Am J Ther. 2018;25(4):e423–33.
14. Akamine D, Filho MK, Peres CM. Drug–nutrient interactions in elderly people. Curr Opin Clin Nutr Metab Care. 2007;10(3):304–10.
15. Briguglio M, Hrelia S, Malaguti M, Serpe L, Canaparo R, Dell'Osso B, Galentino R, De Michele S, Dina CZ, Porta M, Banfi G. Food bioactive compounds and their interference in drug pharmacokinetic/pharmacodynamic profiles. Pharmaceutics. 2018;10(4):277.
16. White R, Bradnam V. Handbook of drug administration via enteral feeding tubes. London: Pharmaceutical Press; 2015.
17. Williams JA, Hyland R, Jones BC, Smith DA, Hurst S, Goosen TC, et al. Drug–drug interactions for UDP-glucuronosyltransferase substrates: a pharmacokinetic explanation for typically observed low exposure (AUCi/AUC) ratios. Drug Metab Dispos. 2004;32(11):1201–8.
18. Zanger UM, Schwab M. Cytochrome P450 enzymes in drug metabolism: regulation of gene expression, enzyme activities, and impact of genetic variation. Pharmacol Ther. 2013;138(1):103–41.
19. Ucar M, et al. Carbamazepine markedly reduces serum concentrations of simvastatin and simvastatin acid. Eur J Clin Pharmacol. 2004;59:879–82.
20. Eggertsen R, et al. Effects of treatment with a commercially available St John's Wort product (Movina) on cholesterol levels in patients with hypercholesterolemia treated with simvastatin. Scand J Prim Health Care. 2007;25:154–9.
21. Bowie MW, Slattum PW. Pharmacodynamics in older adults: a review. Am J Geriatr Pharmacother. 2007;5(3):263–303.

22. Vestal RE, Wood AJJ, Shand DG. Reduced β-adrenoceptor sensitivity in the elderly. Clin Pharmacol Ther. 1979;26(2):181–6.
23. Ferrara N, Komici K, Corbi G, Pagano G, Furgi G, Rengo C, Femminella GD, Leosco D, Bonaduce D. β-Adrenergic receptor responsiveness in aging heart and clinical implications. Front Physiol. 2014;9(4):396.
24. White M, Roden R, Minobe W, Khan MF, Larrabee P, Wollmering M, et al. Age-related changes in β-adrenergic neuroeffectors system in the human heart. Circulation. 1994;90:1225–38.
25. Scarpace PJ, Turner N, Mader SL. β-Adrenergic function in aging. Drugs Aging. 1991;1:116–29.
26. Zerah L, Henrard S, Wilting I, O'Mahony D, Rodondi N, Dalleur O, Dalton K, Knol W, Haschke M, Spinewine A. Prevalence of drug–drug interactions in older people before and after hospital admission: analysis from the OPERAM trial. BMC Geriatr. 2021;21(1):571.
27. Tulner LR, Frankfort SV, Gijsen GJ, van Campen JP, Koks CH, Beijnen JH. Drug–drug interactions in a geriatric outpatient cohort: prevalence and relevance. Drugs Aging. 2008;25(4):343–55.
28. Anrys P, Petit AE, Thevelin S, Sallevelt B, Drenth C, Soiza RL, Correa-Pérez A, Dalleur O, De Brauwer I, Petrovic M, Coleman JJ, Dalton K, O'Mahony D, Löwe A, Thürig S, Gudmundsson A, Cherubini A, Panos A, Mavridis D, Rodondi N, Spinewine A. An international consensus list of potentially clinically significant drug–drug interactions in older people. J Am Med Dir Assoc. 2021;22(10):2121–2133.e24.
29. Vonbach P, Dubied A, Krähenbühl S, Beer JH. Prevalence of drug–drug interactions at hospital entry and during hospital stay of patients in internal medicine. Eur J Intern Med. 2008;19(6):4123–0.

Inappropriate Prescription of Medicines

4

Denis O'Mahony

4.1 Introduction

Inappropriate prescribing (IP) of medication to patients of any age refers to any one or more of the following patterns:

1. Prescribing that increases the risk of adverse drug–drug interactions to an unacceptably high level.
2. Prescribing that increases the risk of adverse drug–disease interactions to an unacceptably high level.
3. Prescribing of medications at too high a dose.
4. Prescribing of medications for too long or too short a duration.
5. Prescribing of medications that are too expensive when cheaper alternatives exist.
6. Failure to prescribe appropriate medications for irrational or ageist reasons when they are clearly indicated.

Instances of IP that fall into categories (1)–(5) are generally referred to as 'potentially inappropriate medications' or PIMs; instances of category (6) are termed 'potential prescribing omissions' or PPOs.

PIMs and PPOs are important in older people because they are associated with significant adversity, that is, increased risk of adverse drug reactions (ADRs) and adverse drug events (ADEs), greater levels of unscheduled hospitalization, more healthcare utilization (mostly through primary care physician consultation), poorer quality of life and increased mortality. It is estimated that more than half of all instances of PIMs and PPOs are avoidable; this has highly significant economic, as

D. O'Mahony (✉)
Department of Medicine, University College Cork, Cork, Ireland

Department of Geriatric Medicine, Cork University Hospital, Cork, Ireland
e-mail: denis.omahony@ucc.ie

A. Cherubini et al. (eds.), *Optimizing Pharmacotherapy in Older Patients*, Practical Issues in Geriatrics, https://doi.org/10.1007/978-3-031-28061-0_4

well as individual patient, implications in the context of rapidly ageing populations in most countries globally.

There are a number of important risk factors for IP which every prescriber should be aware of, principally polypharmacy (i.e. where patients take ≥5 long-term daily medications), age-related changes in pharmacokinetics and pharmacodynamics, cognitive impairment, reduced functional capacity and higher levels of overall frailty. In addition, certain classes of drugs carry inherently higher risks of medication-related morbidity in older people, such as non-steroidal anti-inflammatory drugs, anticoagulants, insulin and other hypoglycaemic agents, antipsychotic drugs, benzodiazepines and loop diuretics.

In this chapter, we will examine the challenge of IP in general, important instances of PIMs and PPOs in particular and how IP can be systematically detected and addressed during routine medication review of older people. There will be specific focus on the multimorbid older person because multimorbidity is the rule rather than the exception amongst people aged over 70 years and because polypharmacy occurs as a result of multimorbidity. The central aim in detecting PIMs and PPOs is for the prescriber to consider the following issues carefully:

1. Which medications are essential for symptom control?
2. Which medications are essential for short-term and long-term prevention?
3. Which medications are safest in individual patients?
4. Which medications address the issues that matter most to the patient?
5. Which combination of medications is most acceptable and manageable for the patient?

4.2 Inappropriate Prescribing Criteria

There are several sets of criteria for defining IP in older people in the literature. These are broadly classified as 'implicit criteria' and 'explicit criteria'.

Implicit IP criteria are usually based on decision algorithms without specific reference to any one drug or drug class; well-cited examples include ACOVE criteria and the Medication Appropriateness Index (MAI) [1, 2]. In general, implicit IP criteria have remained in the research domain and have not been deployed in routine clinical practice to any significant extent.

Explicit IP criteria, in contrast, have had much greater application in the clinical arena. The first of the explicit IP criteria sets was published in 1991 by Mark Beers and colleagues [3]. This first iteration of Beers criteria provided for the first time a list of drugs and drug doses that should be avoided in older nursing home residents in all circumstances and certain drugs that should be avoided in certain disease groups. Since the first iteration of Beers criteria, there have been five subsequent updated versions; the most recent of which was published in 2019 [4]. Beers criteria, as the longest established explicit IP criteria, are the most widely cited in the literature. One limitation of Beers criteria is that they do not include instances of

PPOs. In contrast, STOPP/START criteria deal both with PIMs and PPOs arranged by physiological system, as one finds in drug formularies. STOPP/START criteria were first published in 2008 [5] revised in 2015 [6] and again in 2023 [in press].

There are over 30 other explicit PIM criteria sets in the literature, which describe a variety of approaches to PIM detection [7]. FORTA criteria, PRISCUS criteria, French Consensus criteria and NORGEP criteria have all gained significant attention in the literature. However, Beers criteria and STOPP/START criteria are the most cited in mainstream online bibliographies. They have also had the most traction in terms of clinical application in routine practice.

4.3 Clinical Relevance of PIMs and PPOs

There would be little point in looking for PIMs and PPOs if they were not clinically relevant or avoidable. However, the literature demonstrates clearly that PIMs and PPOs are both associated with significant adversity for older people and for the most part readily detectable and, therefore, preventable. In a prospective study of 600 unselected older patients presenting to hospital with acute illness, Hamilton et al. showed that ADEs occurred significantly more often in those who were prescribed STOPP criteria-defined PIMs; in contrast, patients taking Beers version 3 criteria-defined PIMs had no significant increase in ADEs [8]. Previous studies had shown a lack of association between Beers criteria and ADEs [9–11].

The increased risk of ADRs and ADEs arising from PIMs are associated with several related adverse outcomes for older people, including increased incidence of acute hospitalization, increased physician consultation, increased healthcare costs and diminished quality of life [12–14]. Risk factors for PIMs include polypharmacy, poor functional status and depression [15].

4.4 Clinical Trials of STOPP/START Criteria as an Intervention

Given the significantly increased risk of ADEs (approximately 85%) when STOPP-defined PIMs were prescribed to multimorbid older people [8], a series of single-centre intervention clinical trials were undertaken to test the clinical efficacy of STOPP/START criteria. These trials are summarized in Table 4.1. They demonstrated that STOPP/START criteria as an intervention had the following benefits compared to standard pharmaceutical care:

1. Reduced prevalence of PIMs and PPOs.
2. Reduced polypharmacy.
3. Improved medication appropriateness.
4. Reduced incident ADRs.
5. Reduced monthly medication costs.
6. Reduced incident falls.

Table 4.1 Single-centre clinical trials in which STOPP/START criteria were used as an intervention in multimorbid older people with polypharmacy

Trial authors, year of publication	Target patient population (number of patients randomized)	Impact of intervention compared to usual pharmaceutical care (control) group that was statistically significant
Gallagher et al. [16]	Acutely ill hospitalized multimorbid, aged (400)	Unnecessary polypharmacy, the use of drugs at incorrect doses and potential drug–drug and drug–disease interactions were less frequent in the intervention group at discharge (absolute risk reduction 35.7%); underutilization of clinically indicated medications was also reduced (absolute risk reduction 21.2%)
Dalleur et al. [17]	Hospitalized 'frail' (146)	Approximately twice as many PIMs removed at discharge in the intervention group compared to the control group
Frankenthal et al. [18]	Chronic care geriatric facility residents (359)	Fewer drugs, lower care costs and reduced incidence of falls
O'Connor et al. [19]	Acutely ill hospitalized multimorbid (732)	Reduced ADR incidence in hospital; reduced median monthly medication cost (physician-delivered intervention)
O'Sullivan et al. [20]	Acutely ill hospitalized multimorbid (737)	Reduced ADR incidence (pharmacist-delivered intervention)

These benefits were demonstrated from single-centre, unblinded clinical trials. However, two subsequent multi-centre, partially blinded clinical trials (SENATOR [21] and OPERAM [22]) have not shown significant benefit from STOPP/START application in multimorbid older patients exposed to polypharmacy. The primary endpoint in the SENATOR trial was incident ADRs within 14 days of randomization to STOPP/START criteria application (with drug–drug and drug–disease interaction screening) and feedback to attending clinicians or standard pharmaceutical care. A total of 1537 patients were randomized in a 1:1 ratio in SENATOR. Incident ADRs within 14 days of randomization occurred in 24.5% of intervention patients and in 24.8% of control patients; however, the overall uptake of STOPP/START recommendations by attending clinician prescribers was poor, that is, approximately 15%.

The OPERAM trial was designed to maximize the uptake of STOPP/START recommendations by attending clinicians of older multimorbid patients in hospital. The intervention with details of the prescribing changes was further supported following discharge through contact with patients' primary care physicians and community pharmacists as well as follow-up with the patients and their carers. In all, 2008 patients were cluster randomized in OPERAM in a 1:1 ratio. With these additional features in the OPERAM intervention, the adherence with one or more proposed medication changes was approximately 62%. The primary endpoint in OPERAM was drug-related admissions (DRAs) within 12 months of randomization to STOPP/START intervention or standard pharmaceutical care; DRAs occurred in 21.9% of intervention patients and in 22.4% of control patients, that is, despite greater adherence with STOPP/START prescribing recommendations, there was no significant reduction in DRAs.

4.5 Other Clinical Trials of PIM Criteria as an Intervention

Another set of PIM criteria called FORTA (Fit fOR The Aged) criteria devised and validated by Wehling and colleagues in Germany have also been assessed by clinical trial. FORTA criteria are divided into four categories: A (indispensable), B (beneficial), C (questionable) or D (avoid). In the VALFORTA clinical trial [23], 409 multimorbid patients (cared for in two specialist geriatric medicine units in Mannheim and Essen) were randomized to a control unit with standard pharmaceutical care or to an intervention unit where a FORTA team instructed attending physicians on FORTA assessment of each prescribed medication. The primary endpoint, that is, the FORTA score was the sum of medication errors, defined as over-, under-, or incorrect treatment with prescribed medication. Enrolled patients were randomized to intervention or control trial arms in a 1:1 ratio. They had a mean age of 81.5 years; 64% were female, and the mean hospital length of stay was 17.4 days. The trial results showed a greater reduction of medication errors in the intervention group versus the control group, with a mean (± SD) FORTA score difference between admission and discharge in the intervention group of 2.7 (± 2.25) versus 1.0 (± 1.8) in the control group, which was highly significant ($p < 0.0001$). In addition, ADRs (not a pre-specified endpoint) were significantly reduced in the intervention group compared to the control group; the absolute risk reduction for incident ADRs was 19.8%, equating to a number needed to treat of 5 which was once again statistically significant ($p < 0.05$). These results are certainly interesting and of potential clinical importance; however, the VALFORTA trial was a validation trial, treatment groups not blinded and, to date, results have not been replicated.

4.6 Clinical Trials Using Pharmacist-Driven Interventions to Optimize Medication in Multimorbid Older People

A number of other interventions have been designed to minimize IP in multimorbid older people that are not based on the application of IP criteria. Principally, these involve structured medication review and feedback to attending physician prescribers. There is evidence that medication review by an appropriately trained pharmacist with feedback to the attending physician can minimize medication errors and improve medication appropriateness [24]. However, evidence of clear clinical benefit to older multimorbid patients from pharmacist-driven structured medication review and feedback is lacking [25].

The OPTIMIST trial [26], carried out in four Danish hospitals, addressed these issues where 1467 patients (median age 72 years) were randomized to one of three trial arms: (1) standard pharmaceutical care (control), (2) limited pharmacist-driven medication optimization or (3) extended pharmacist-driven medication optimization. The trial endpoints were (i) readmission within 30 days, (ii) readmission within 180 days and (iii) number of emergency department (ED) visits within 180 days; the composite primary endpoint was hospital readmission or ED visit within 180 days. Readmissions at 30 days and at 180 days were significantly reduced in the extended intervention group, but not in the basic intervention group, compared to controls. For the primary composite endpoint, once again patients in the extended intervention group but not those in the basic intervention group experienced a significant benefit compared to control patients. The hazard ratio (95% CI) for experiencing the composite primary endpoint was 0.77 (0.64–0.93) representing a number needed to treat with the extended intervention of 12, that is, a clinically relevant intervention. The basic pharmacist intervention included structured detailed medication review with particular focus on aspirin, diuretics, anticoagulants and NSAIDs followed by a structured report placed in electronic medical record with medication adjustment recommendations and one-to-one contact with the attending physician. The extended intervention in the OPTIMIST trial included the basic intervention with the following elements added:

- Medication reconciliation on discharge.
- A 30-min interview with the patient ("motivational approach").
- A comprehensive summary of changes in medication during hospitalization.
- A report with details of all recommended medication changes implemented or not sent to the patient's primary care physician post-discharge.
- A follow-up telephone contact with (1) the patient's primary care physician, (2) the patient's principal carer and (3) the community pharmacist at 72 hours post-discharge.
- A follow-up motivational interview with the patient's primary care physician, caregiver and community pharmacist at 1 week and 6 months post-discharge.

The extended intervention that yielded significant benefit to the patients in OPTIMIST in terms of unscheduled hospital readmissions and ED attendances was complex, multifaceted and challenging to implement, with uncertain cost-effectiveness. Very likely, elements of the pharmacist intervention are clinically relevant. However, the transferability of the extended intervention in OPTIMIST to routine clinical practice for the purpose of minimizing IP in older people is, therefore, uncertain.

4.7 Clinical Manifestations of IP in Older People

Inappropriate prescribing in older people is commonplace but avoidable. It is clinically and economically important to minimize IP, as IP is intimately associated with medication-related morbidity which, in turn, is the primary reason for admission in approximately 10% of unselected older people who are hospitalized with acute illness. A recent systematic review and meta-analysis provides important clarity on IP-related ADRs in older people in the hospital setting [27]. The study showed that approximately one in six older people will experience a non-trivial ADR during hospitalization for acute illness.

The most commonly reported ADRs in older people and their presentations are listed in Table 4.2. As can be seen, many of these ADR presentations mimic

Table 4.2 Common adverse drug reaction (ADR) presentations in older people in order of frequency (after Jennings et al. [27])

ADR type	Frequency	Clinical or laboratory manifestation
Fluid and electrolyte derangement	17.3%	Hypokalaemia, hyperkalaemia, hyponatraemia, hypernatraemia, fluid volume overload, fluid volume depletion
Gastrointestinal motility disorders	14.8%	Constipation, diarrhoea
Renal function impairment	8.2%	Acute kidney injury, renal failure complications
Blood pressure derangement	5.5%	Hypotension, orthostatic symptoms
Delirium	4.1%	New onset confusion
Injuries	3.8%	Falls
Cardiac arrhythmias	3.7%	Bradycardia, atrioventricular block, tachycardia
Other cardiovascular disorders	3.4%	Various
Coagulopathy/bleeding	3.0%	Increased INR[a], increased APTT[b], increased prothrombin time
Other gastrointestinal disorders	2.8%	Various
Vascular haemorrhagic disorders	2.7%	Overt bleeding, haematoma
Gastrointestinal haemorrhage	2.6%	Overt bleeding, malaena
Neurological disorder (unspecified)	2.5%	Various
Glucose derangement	2.3%	Hypoglycaemia, hyperglycaemia
Skin disorder	2.2%	Rash, exanthems and other eruptions
Other gastrointestinal disorders	2.2%	Nausea/vomiting, dyspepsia, abdominal pain

[a]*INR* international normalized ratio
[b]*APTT* activated partial thromboplastin time

common symptom presentations in older people; consequently, prescribers must always consider the possibility of medication being the basis for symptoms such as constipation, diarrhoea, hypotension, acute confusion and so forth.

This analysis of ADR presentations in older people has formed the basis of an ADR 'Trigger List', which can be helpful in clinical practice based on the fact that approximately 90% of all ADRs result from 16 medication classes, that is, occurrence of any of the clinical manifestations of ADRs summarized in Table 4.2 should make prescribers consider the possibility of an underlying ADR.

4.8 Medication Review Aimed at Minimizing IP and Its Consequences: A Practical Approach

In the current literature, there are numerous described methods for identifying or minimizing IP. In a recent review by Rochon et al. [28], a practical method for performing medication review in a way that is designed to minimize IP and its

Table 4.3 DRUGS guide to minimizing IP and optimizing medication safety for older adults (after Rochon et al. [28])

***D*iscuss goals of care and what matters most to the patient**
Include patients and caregivers in deprescribing discussions to ensure decisions focus on goals of care
***R*eview medications**
• Encourage patients to bring all prescribed and over-the-counter medications to their appointment
• Review medications on an ongoing basis and when clinical conditions or goals of care change
• Discontinue potentially unnecessary drugs
• Consider drug side effects as a potential cause for a new symptom
• Consider non-pharmacological options
• Change for safer alternatives
• Lower the dose
• To identify possible prescribing cascades, determine when the medication was started and why
***U*se tools and frameworks**
• Identify drugs from the inappropriate prescribing tools, including Beers criteria or STOPP criteria
• Use the STOPPFrail list when the individual is extremely frail and approaching the end of life
• Consider whether the new or existing medical condition could be the result of a prescribing cascade[a] and ask:
– Is a new drug being prescribed to manage a side effect from another prescribed drug?
– Could the initial drug be replaced with a safer drug or could the dose be reduced?
– Does the patient need the first drug or could this drug be stopped?
– Pay attention to older people who are receiving so-called good drugs with narrow therapeutic windows that might no longer be needed or for whom dose reduction might be beneficial
***G*eriatric medicine approach**
Geriatricians carefully consider how multiple medical problems, frailty, cognitive impairment and limited life expectancy reduce medication benefit, increase adverse events or interfere with medication adherence
***S*TOP the medications**
Consider the algorithm created by Scott [29] or the Good Palliative–Geriatric Practice algorithm to guide deprescribing [30]

[a]'Prescribing cascades' refer to inappropriate prescription of drugs for symptoms arising from side-effects of medications that are misinterpreted as new conditions

consequences has been described. This approach is usefully summarized under the acronym DRUGS, that is, (1) *D*iscuss goals of care and what matters most to the patient, (2) *R*eview medications, (3) *U*se tools and frameworks, (4) *G*eriatric medicine approach and (5) *S*top the medications. More specific details of this approach are shown in Table 4.3.

Rochon et al. also stressed the importance of patient sex and gender considerations when reviewing and optimizing older people's medications. Some of these considerations include the following:

- Older women consume more non-prescription ("over-the-counter") medications than older men.
- Older women receive more psychotropic prescriptions than older men.

- Older men receive more preventive medication than older women.
- Older women tend to experience higher levels of chronic multimorbidity, greater degrees of frailty and more ADEs than older men.
- Older men are less likely to discuss deprescribing with their physicians than older women.
- Older men are more likely to have their chronic medical conditions managed more aggressively than older women, for example, ischaemic heart disease, urinary incontinence and osteoarthritis.

A constant awareness of sex-determined differences in pharmacokinetics and pharmacodynamics is necessary in the selection of well-balanced and safer polypharmacy for older multimorbid patients. These differences are discussed in Chap. 1.

4.9 Minimizing IP in Older People with Marked Frailty Approaching End-of-Life

With the rapid growth of the frail older person population aged over 80 years (predominantly female) in most countries, physicians encounter the challenge of medication optimization in those older people with a poor 1-year survival prognosis. These older patients usually have complex multimorbid illness, often have major impairment of physiological homoeostatic reserve in more than one physiological system and are usually exposed to high-level polypharmacy. In one study, the association between the extent of chronic multimorbid illness (measured by the Cumulative Index Rating Scale—Geriatric, CIRS-G) and number of daily prescription drugs was a linear one with a high correlation *R* value of 0.726 [31], i.e. cause-and-effect is manifest.

Deprescribing in these frailer older people is generally considered desirable in order to minimize risk of adverse drug–drug and drug–disease interactions as well as to lessen medication burden for the patients and their carers. Various approaches to deprescribing have been tried, from implicit criteria algorithms to explicit criteria for deprescribing of several medication classes, mostly prescribed initially for long-term disease prevention, in end-of-life situations. In small-scale clinical trials, both approaches been shown to be both feasible and effective in reducing polypharmacy and medication burden in multimorbid frailer older people [32–34]. The impact of deprescribing interventions on clinical outcomes, like incident ADEs, rehospitalization and quality of life, however, remains unclear. Approaches to structured deprescribing are discussed in greater detail in Chap. 10.

4.10 Inappropriate Medication Avoidance: Summary and Practical Points

PIMs and PPOs are highly prevalent in older people in all clinical settings. Because they have clear cut and often serious negative consequences for older people, PIMs and PPOs should be looked for using appropriate explicit criteria screening tools during routine medication review particularly in multimorbid older people with polypharmacy. Whilst large scale multi-centre trials do not show significant patient outcome benefit from application of STOPP/START criteria in hospitalized older people with multimorbidity and polypharmacy in terms of ADR incidence or rehospitalization, there are nevertheless good reasons to minimize PIMs and PPOs in these at-risk patients. Consideration of older frailer patients' life expectancy is critically important in decision-making relating to medication. Patients who are unlikely to survive beyond 12 months should have their long-term preventive medications reviewed carefully and possibly deprescribed, and their overall medication list rationalized with a focus on symptom management. Explicit STOPPFrail criteria can assist prescribers with choosing which medications to discontinue in frailer older people with very limited life expectancy.

In addition to the patients themselves and their principal carers, involvement of all relevant healthcare professionals involved in prescribing, dispensing and monitoring older people's medication is important for medication optimization and achieving therapeutic targets, that is, patients' primary care physicians, community pharmacists and community nurses.

It is likely that in the future as the information technology support for medication prescribing, dispensing and monitoring becomes more sophisticated, PIM and PPO detection software will become more user friendly and effective in terms of enhancing patient safety. However, this is also contingent on health service providers investing meaningfully in the software systems necessary to deploy and support PIM/PPO detection criteria. Systematic review evidence indicates that computerized prescribing systems can significantly reduce PIMs; however, evidence is lacking for PPO prevention because PPO prevalence is not currently defined as an outcome measure [35]. Future studies will need to address this deficiency in the literature, since the presence of two or more START criteria PPOs predicts hospitalization at least as effectively as the presence of PIMs [36].

References

1. Hanlon JT, Schmader KE. The medication appropriateness index at 20: where it started, where it has been, and where it may be going. Drugs Aging. 2013;30(11):893–900.
2. Bulloch MN, Olin JL. Instruments for evaluating medication use and prescribing in older adults. J Am Pharm Assoc (2003). 2014;54(5):530–7.
3. Beers MH, Ouslander JG, Rollingher I, Reuben DB, Brooks J, Beck JC. Explicit criteria for determining inappropriate medication use in nursing home residents. UCLA Division of Geriatric Medicine. Arch Intern Med. 1991;151(9):1825–32.
4. By the 2019 American Geriatrics Society Beers Criteria® Update Expert Panel. American Geriatrics Society 2019 updated AGS Beers Criteria® for potentially inappropriate medication use in older adults. J Am Geriatr Soc. 2019;67(4):674–94.
5. Gallagher P, Ryan C, Byrne S, Kennedy J, O'Mahony D. STOPP (screening tool of older Person's prescriptions) and START (screening tool to alert doctors to right treatment). Consensus validation. Int J Clin Pharmacol Ther. 2008;46(2):72–83.
6. O'Mahony D, O'Sullivan D, Byrne S, O'Connor MN, Ryan C, Gallagher P. STOPP/START criteria for potentially inappropriate prescribing in older people: version 2. Age Ageing. 2015;44(2):213–8.

7. Motter FR, Fritzen JS, Hilmer SN, Paniz ÉV, Paniz VMV. Potentially inappropriate medication in the elderly: a systematic review of validated explicit criteria. Eur J Clin Pharmacol. 2018;74(6):679–700.
8. Hamilton H, Gallagher P, Ryan C, Byrne S, O'Mahony D. Potentially inappropriate medications defined by STOPP criteria and the risk of adverse drug events in older hospitalized patients. Arch Intern Med. 2011;171(11):1013–9.
9. Onder G, Landi F, Liperoti R, Fialova D, Gambassi G, Bernabei R. Impact of inappropriate drug use among hospitalized older adults. Eur J Clin Pharmacol. 2005;61(5–6):453–9.
10. Laroche ML, Charmes JP, Nouaille Y, Picard N, Merle L. Is inappropriate medication use a major cause of adverse drug reactions in the elderly? Br J Clin Pharmacol. 2007;63(2):177–86.
11. Budnitz DS, Shehab N, Kegler SR, Richards CL. Medication use leading to emergency department visits for adverse drug events in older adults. Ann Intern Med. 2007;147(11):755–65.
12. Davies LE, Spiers G, Kingston A, Todd A, Adamson J, Hanratty B. Adverse outcomes of polypharmacy in older people: systematic review of reviews. J Am Med Dir Assoc. 2020;21(2):181–7.
13. Xing XX, Zhu C, Liang HY, Wang K, Chu YQ, Zhao LB, Jiang C, Wang YQ, Yan SY. Associations between potentially inappropriate medications and adverse health outcomes in the elderly: a systematic review and meta-analysis. Ann Pharmacother. 2019;53(10):1005–19.
14. Hyttinen V, Jyrkkä J, Valtonen H. A systematic review of the impact of potentially inappropriate medication on health care utilization and costs among older adults. Med Care. 2016;54(10):950–64.
15. Tommelein E, Mehuys E, Petrovic M, Somers A, Colin P, Boussery K. Potentially inappropriate prescribing in community-dwelling older people across Europe: a systematic literature review. Eur J Clin Pharmacol. 2015;71(12):1415–27.
16. Gallagher PF, O'Connor MN, O'Mahony D. Prevention of potentially inappropriate prescribing for elderly patients: a randomized controlled trial using STOPP/START criteria. Clin Pharmacol Ther. 2011;89(6):845–54.
17. Dalleur O, Boland B, Losseau C, Henrard S, Wouters D, Speybroeck N, Degryse JM, Spinewine A. Reduction of potentially inappropriate medications using the STOPP criteria in frail older inpatients: a randomised controlled study. Drugs Aging. 2014;31(4):291–8.
18. Frankenthal D, Lerman Y, Kalendaryev E, Lerman Y. Intervention with the screening tool of older persons potentially inappropriate prescriptions/screening tool to alert doctors to right treatment criteria in elderly residents of a chronic geriatric facility: a randomized clinical trial. J Am Geriatr Soc. 2014;62(9):1658–65.
19. O'Connor MN, O'Sullivan D, Gallagher PF, Eustace J, Byrne S, O'Mahony D. Prevention of hospital-acquired adverse drug reactions in older people using screening tool of older persons' prescriptions and screening tool to alert to right treatment criteria: a cluster randomized controlled trial. J Am Geriatr Soc. 2016;64(8):1558–66.
20. O'Sullivan D, O'Mahony D, O'Connor MN, Gallagher P, Gallagher J, Cullinan S, O'Sullivan R, Eustace J, Byrne S. Prevention of adverse drug reactions in hospitalised older patients using a software-supported structured pharmacist intervention: a cluster randomised controlled trial. Drugs Aging. 2016;33(1):63–73.
21. O'Mahony D, Gudmundsson A, Soiza RL, Petrovic M, Jose Cruz-Jentoft A, Cherubini A, Fordham R, Byrne S, Dahly D, Gallagher P, Lavan A, Curtin D, Dalton K, Cullinan S, Flanagan E, Shiely F, Samuelsson O, Sverrisdottir A, Subbarayan S, Vandaele L, Meireson E, Montero-Errasquin B, Rexach-Cano A, Correa Perez A, Lozano-Montoya I, Vélez-Díaz-Pallarés M, Cerenzia A, Corradi S, Soledad Cotorruelo Ferreiro M, Dimitri F, Marinelli P, Martelli G, Fong Soe Khioe R, Eustace J. Prevention of adverse drug reactions in hospitalized older patients with multi-morbidity and polypharmacy: the SENATOR* randomized controlled clinical trial. Age Ageing. 2020;49(4):605–14.
22. Blum MR, Sallevelt BTGM, Spinewine A, O'Mahony D, Moutzouri E, Feller M, Baumgartner C, Roumet M, Jungo KT, Schwab N, Bretagne L, Beglinger S, Aubert CE, Wilting I, Thevelin S, Murphy K, Huibers CJA, Drenth-van Maanen AC, Boland B, Crowley E, Eichenberger A, Meulendijk M, Jennings E, Adam L, Roos MJ, Gleeson L, Shen Z, Marien S, Meinders AJ,

Baretella O, Netzer S, de Montmollin M, Fournier A, Mouzon A, O'Mahony C, Aujesky D, Mavridis D, Byrne S, Jansen PAF, Schwenkglenks M, Spruit M, Dalleur O, Knol W, Trelle S, Rodondi N. Optimizing therapy to prevent avoidable hospital admissions in multimorbid older adults (OPERAM): cluster randomised controlled trial. BMJ. 2021;374:n1585.
23. Wehling M, Burkhardt H, Kuhn-Thiel A, Pazan F, Throm C, Weiss C, Frohnhofen H. VALFORTA: a randomised trial to validate the FORTA (fit fOR the aged) classification. Age Ageing. 2016;45(2):262–7.
24. Walsh KA, O'Riordan D, Kearney PM, Timmons S, Byrne S. Improving the appropriateness of prescribing in older patients: a systematic review and meta-analysis of pharmacists' interventions in secondary care. Age Ageing. 2016;45(2):201–9.
25. Holland R, Desborough J, Goodyer L, Hall S, Wright D, Loke YK. Does pharmacist-led medication review help to reduce hospital admissions and deaths in older people? A systematic review and meta-analysis. Br J Clin Pharmacol. 2008;65(3):303–16.
26. Ravn-Nielsen LV, Duckert ML, Lund ML, Henriksen JP, Nielsen ML, Eriksen CS, Buck TC, Pottegård A, Hansen MR, Hallas J. Effect of an in-hospital multifaceted clinical pharmacist intervention on the risk of readmission: a randomized clinical trial. JAMA Intern Med. 2018;178(3):375–82.
27. Jennings ELM, Murphy KD, Gallagher P, O'Mahony D. In-hospital adverse drug reactions in older adults; prevalence, presentation and associated drugs—a systematic review and meta-analysis. Age Ageing. 2020;49(6):948–58.
28. Rochon PA, Petrovic M, Cherubini A, Onder G, O'Mahony D, Sternberg SA, Stall NM, Gurwitz JH. Polypharmacy, inappropriate prescribing, and deprescribing in old age: through a sex and gender lens. Lancet Healthy Longev. 2021;2:e290–300.
29. Scott IA, Hilmer SN, Reeve E, et al. Reducing inappropriate polypharmacy: the process of deprescribing. JAMA Intern Med. 2015;175:827–34.
30. Garfinkel D, Zur-Gil S, Ben-Israel J. The war against polypharmacy: a new cost-effective geriatric-palliative approach for improving drug therapy in disabled elderly people. Isr Med Assoc J. 2007;9:430–4.
31. Gilmartin D, O'Mahony D. Polypharmacy and potentially inappropriate prescribing in hospitalised older Irish adults. Age Ageing. 2012;41(Suppl 2):278.
32. Thillainadesan J, Gnjidic D, Green S, Hilmer SN. Impact of deprescribing interventions in older hospitalised patients on prescribing and clinical outcomes: a systematic review of randomised trials. Drugs Aging. 2018;35(4):303–19.
33. Anderson K, Freeman C, Foster M, Scott I. GP-Led deprescribing in community-living older Australians: an exploratory controlled trial. J Am Geriatr Soc. 2020;68(2):403–10.
34. Curtin D, Jennings E, Daunt R, Curtin S, Randles M, Gallagher P, O'Mahony D. Deprescribing in older people approaching end of life: a randomized controlled trial using STOPPFrail criteria. J Am Geriatr Soc. 2020;68(4):762–9.
35. Dalton K, O'Brien G, O'Mahony D, Byrne S. Computerised interventions designed to reduce potentially inappropriate prescribing in hospitalised older adults: a systematic review and meta-analysis. Age Ageing. 2018;47(5):670–8.
36. Moriarty F, Bennett K, Cahir C, Kenny RA, Fahey T. Potentially inappropriate prescribing according to STOPP and START and adverse outcomes in community-dwelling older people: a prospective cohort study. Br J Clin Pharmacol. 2016;82(3):849–57.

Prescribing Cascades

5

Shelley A. Sternberg, Jerry H. Gurwitz,
and Paula A. Rochon

5.1 Introduction

Prescribing cascades are important contributors to drug-related harm in older adults. A prescribing cascade occurs when a healthcare provider misinterprets the side effect of a drug as a new medical condition and prescribes a second, potentially unnecessary drug therapy to address the side effect [1–3]. Many prescribing cascades have been described in the literature [4–6]. The ageing of the population with its associated multimorbidity and polypharmacy highlights the importance of considering prescribing cascades and their impact on the health of older people at an international level [7]. As a result, many countries have addressed the need to decrease the risk of drug-related harm in older adults specifically targeting prescribing cascades [8, 9].

S. A. Sternberg
Department of Geriatric Medicine, Maccabi Healthcare Services, Modiin, Israel

J. H. Gurwitz
Division of Geriatric Medicine and Meyers Primary Care Institute, University of Massachusetts Medical School, Worcester, MA, USA
e-mail: Jerry.Gurwitz@umassmed.edu

P. A. Rochon (✉)
Women's Age Lab, Women's College Hospital, Toronto, ON, Canada

Department of Medicine, University of Toronto, Toronto, ON, Canada

Institute of Health Policy, Management and Evaluation, Dalla Lana School of Public Health, University of Toronto, Toronto, ON, Canada
e-mail: Paula.Rochon@wchospital.ca

A. Cherubini et al. (eds.), *Optimizing Pharmacotherapy in Older Patients*,
Practical Issues in Geriatrics, https://doi.org/10.1007/978-3-031-28061-0_5

Providers can prevent prescribing cascades by asking a few simple questions at the time of prescribing [10]. In addition, the identification of prescribing cascades during medication review, especially in older women, can provide an opportunity to deprescribe and to optimize drug therapy [11]. These interventions to prevent and interrupt prescribing cascades can lead to improved quality of care and patient safety in older adults.

5.2 Definition of Prescribing Cascades

Prescribing cascades were described by Rochon and Gurwitz in the 1990s [1, 2]. One typical example of a prescribing cascade is a non-steroidal anti-inflammatory drug (NSAID) leading to hypertension and subsequently leading to the initiation of a new anti-hypertensive medication prescription [2]. This definition was expanded in 2017 [3] to include the prescribing of potentially unnecessary over-the-counter drug therapies and medical devices such as permanent pacemaker devices to counteract severe bradyarrhythmias unrecognized as being caused by cardiovascular drugs like beta-blockers, digoxin and verapamil. Prescribing cascades must, by definition, reflect inappropriate prescribing (Fig. 5.1).

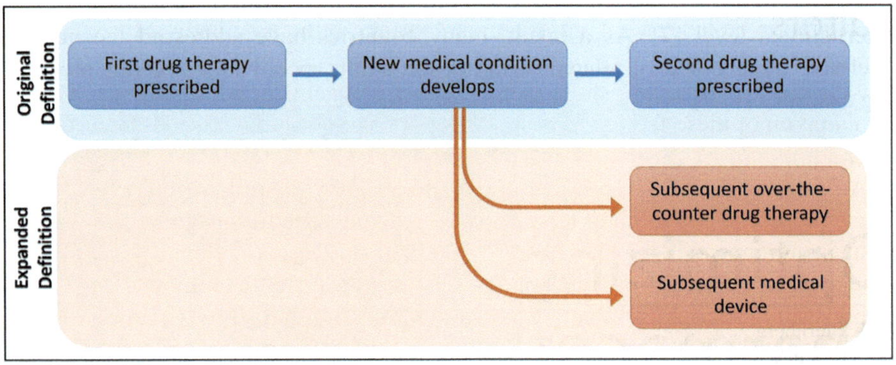

*Adapted from: **The prescribing cascade revisited,** Rochon, Paula A et al. (2017) The Lancet, Volume 389, Issue 10081, 1778 - 1780

Fig. 5.1 Expanded prescribing cascade definition

5.3 Why Prescribing Cascades are Important for Older Adults

Older adults are particularly at risk for prescribing cascades and drug-related harm due to the high prevalence of multimorbidity and associated polypharmacy. Most older adults have multiple medical conditions and drug therapies that are used to treat these conditions [11]. Polypharmacy is also extremely common in older adults, especially in the long-term care setting [12]. In the United States, the use of five or more medications by older adults over age 65 has increased from 13% in 1988 to 39% in 2010 [13]. The prevalence of polypharmacy in European older adults ranged from 26% in Switzerland to 40% in the Czech Republic, as reported by the Survey of Health, Ageing and Retirement in Europe (SHARE) based on 2015 data from 17 countries [14]. Among older adults living in long-term care in Europe and Israel, almost half used between five and nine daily drug therapies, and almost a quarter used ten or more drugs [15]. For older adults living in long-term care homes in Canada, where almost 70% of residents are women [16], almost 50% were prescribed medications from ten or more drug classes [12]. This high rate of hyperpolypharmacy (i.e. ten or more daily drugs) is related not only to multimorbidity but is also a consequence of multiple prescribers caring for older people without adequate communication between the prescribers. In addition, clinical guidelines tend to focus on single diseases without taking into consideration that two-thirds of adults over the age of 65 have multiple chronic conditions requiring the use of numerous medications [11]. Finally, current prescribing guidelines do not routinely take into consideration an older adult's goals of care or their remaining life expectancy [17]. Important factors such as a person's cognitive and frailty status are insufficiently considered when assessing the potential risks and benefits of a medication [18]. The combination of these factors increases the risk of prescribing cascades occurring in older adults.

Among older adults, prescribing cascades may disproportionately impact older women. Older women have the most chronic conditions and often use the greatest number of drug therapies [19]. In addition, sex (female biology) and gender (sociocultural construct), in combination, contribute to this increased risk of prescribing cascades. The pharmacokinetic and pharmacodynamic changes associated with the female sex and older age contribute to the increased prevalence of adverse drug events in women compared to men [20–23]. Furthermore, it was found that older European women were more likely than men to have multimorbidity and as a result were more likely to be prescribed multiple medications [24]. In summary, differences in pharmacokinetics and pharmacodynamics as well as patterns of multimorbidity put older women at higher risk for prescribing cascades.

Gender (sociocultural factors) impacts both the patients and the prescribers and contributes to the risk of prescribing cascades. On the patients' side, women are more likely than men to seek medical care and to follow recommendations from their providers [25]. Older women are less likely than older men to have pensions or drug benefit plans because they were less likely to have been part of the formal work force [26] and, therefore, may have less ability to pay for medications. On the prescribers' side, there is evidence that physicians may treat female patients differently from male patients [27]. For example, women are more likely to be prescribed psychotropic medications, whereas men are more likely to receive drug therapy for physical disorders, particularly cardiovascular conditions [28]. These sex and gender factors all contribute to placing older women at increased risk for prescribing cascades.

5.4 Original Investigations to Identify Prescribing Cascades

In 1997, three initial prescribing cascades were described [2]. The original examples were: NSAIDs leading to a prostaglandin-mediated rise in blood pressure with the subsequent prescription of antihypertensive therapy in older people; thiazide diuretics prescribed to treat hypertension leading to hyperuricemia and the subsequent prescription of colchicine for gout; and the initiation of antipsychotic drug therapy followed by the development of Parkinsonism, which was misinterpreted as Parkinson's disease and treated with levodopa/carbidopa. As awareness has increased, so have the number of prescribing cascades. In 2017 [3], there were 20 examples of prescribing cascades, and recently, more than 100 prescribing cascades have been identified as part of an international project [7]. Examples of prescribing cascades can be seen in Table 5.1.

One notable example of a prescribing cascade is a cholinesterase inhibitor (e.g. donepezil) prescribed to manage the symptoms of dementia leading to the development of urinary incontinence with the subsequent initiation of a urinary anticholinergic drug to treat the incontinence [6]. The concern about starting a urinary anticholinergic agent is that this therapy can lead to additional side effects, including dry mouth, constipation and confusion. Another example of a prescribing cascade is a calcium channel blocker (CCB) leading to ankle oedema and the subsequent prescribing of loop diuretics [4]. This cascade was described in a large population-based cohort study that included 41,000 adults over age 65 (59% women) who were newly prescribed a CCB. After adjustment, individuals who were newly dispensed a CCB had significantly increased relative rates of being dispensed a loop diuretic compared with individuals who were newly dispensed an angiotensin-converting enzyme inhibitor or angiotensin II receptor blocker. Given that calcium channel blockers are among the top ten prescribed medications, and that 2–25% of CCBs

Table 5.1 Examples of prescribing cascades commonly encountered in clinical practice

Initial drug therapy prescribed	Adverse event misinterpreted as a new medical condition	New drug therapy prescribed
Prescribing cascades: drug classes		
ACE inhibitor [33, 34]	Cough	Antibiotic
Anticholinergic [35]	Lowered oesophageal sphincter pressure (GERD)	Proton pump inhibitors
Antiepileptic [33]	Nausea	Metoclopramide
Antipsychotic[a] [33, 36–38]	Parkinsonism	Anti-Parkinsonian agents
Beta-blocker [36]	Depression	Antidepressant
Calcium[a] channel blocker [4, 39–41]	Edema	Diuretics
Cholinesterase[a] inhibitor [6, 33, 36]	Urinary incontinence	Urinary anticholinergics
NSAID [2, 33, 36]	Hypertension	Antihypertensive
Sodium[a] glucose cotransporter 2 inhibitors (SGLT-2) [29]	Genital mycotic infection	Antifungals
	Urinary tract infection	Antibiotics
Thiazide and thiazide-like diuretics [2, 33]	Gout	Anti-gout
Prescribing cascades: individual drug therapy		
Amitriptyline [36]	Decreased cognition	Donepezil
Amlodipine [36]	Oedema	Furosemide
Bupropion [36]	Insomnia	Mirtazapine
Ciprofloxacin [36]	Delirium	Risperidone
Gabapentin[a] [5, 36]	Oedema	Furosemide
Metoclopramide [2, 33, 36, 42]	Parkinsonism	Levodopa/carbidopa
	Diarrhoea	Loperamide
Omeprazole [36]	Low B12	B12 supplement

This table is an expansion of a table which appeared in our recent Commentary in The Lancet
ACE inhibitor angiotensin converting enzyme inhibitor, *NSAID* non-steroidal anti-inflammatory drug
[a]Prescribing cascades supported by large population-based studies

cause peripheral oedema, this prescribing cascade has the potential to cause important drug-related harm to older adults.

Another population-based study investigated the prescribing cascade of sodium glucose cotransporter 2 inhibitor (SGLT2) medications leading to genital fungal infection and the subsequent initiation of an anti-fungal medication to treat this SGLT2 side effect [29]. It compared 21,444 new users of SGLT2 inhibitors to 22,463 incident users of dipeptidyl-peptidase-4 (DPP4) inhibitors. After adjusting for propensity score, age, sex and recent urinary tract infection, there was a 2.47-fold increased risk of genital fungal infection (determined by the use of antimycotic medication) with incident use of SGLT2 inhibitors within 30 days compared to incident use of DPP4 inhibitors. This prescribing cascade should be an important consideration when using SGLT2 medications for older adults with diabetes and cardiovascular disease.

In the expanded version of the prescribing cascade definition, over-the-counter (OTC) drugs and medical devices were also included (Table 5.2). One case study

Table 5.2 Examples of the expanded definition of prescribing cascades involving over-the-counter therapies and medical devices

Over-the-counter therapy		
Initial drug therapy prescribed	Adverse event misinterpreted as a new medical condition	Subsequent over-the-counter drug therapy
Cholinesterase inhibitor [30]	Gastrointestinal symptoms	Bismuth subsalicylate
Cholinesterase inhibitor [43]	Rhinorrhoea	Diphenhydramine
Enalapril [36]	Cough	Dextromethorphan
Bupropion [44]	Insomnia	Sleep medication
Ramipril [44]	Cough	Cough syrup
Medical device		
Initial drug therapy prescribed	**Adverse event misinterpreted as a new medical condition**	**Medical device**
Cholinesterase inhibitors[a] [45]	Bradycardia	Pacemaker device

[a] *The article did not mention the term prescribing cascade in the text, but described the concept of a prescribing cascade*

[30] example involved an acetylcholinesterase that was prescribed for dementia and subsequently led to abdominal discomfort. The patient self-medicated with large quantities of bismuth salicylate causing him to suffer from salicylate toxicity and bismuth neurotoxicity, leading to a fall and hospitalization for subdural haemorrhage and bilateral frontal contusions. This case illustrates that prescribing cascades can occur with OTC drugs and with prescription medications. In addition, prescribing cascades can increase the risk of serious consequences such as morbidity and hospitalization.

5.5 The Application of Prescribing Cascades to Inform Better Clinical Care and Deprescribing Initiatives

Identifying and preventing prescribing cascades can inform better clinical care. Many tools and frameworks have been described to identify inappropriate prescribing [11] including the prescribing cascade framework. Providing a detailed medication history, particularly when a medication was started, would help clinicians determine the drug prescribing sequence and facilitate the early recognition of a prescribing cascade. One such tool includes four simple questions to help physicians identify and interrupt prescribing cascades [10]. These questions were developed to raise awareness of prescribing cascades each time a new drug is prescribed. Providers need to think of prescribing cascades and be adept at identifying when they occur, in order to prevent them (Box 5.1).

Box 5.1 Questions to help identify and prevent prescribing cascades

Questions to help identify and prevent prescribing cascades
1. Is the patient reporting a symptom that could represent a drug side effect?
2. Is a new drug being prescribed to address an adverse event from a previously prescribed drug therapy?
3. Could the initial drug be substituted for a safer alternative, or could the dose be reduced, potentially eliminating the need for the subsequent drug therapy?
4. Does the patient really need the initial drug therapy, so could it be stopped?

Physicians are often confronted with prescribing cascades in their clinical practice. For example, enalapril is prescribed for hypertension leading to a persistent dry cough and an antibiotic such as levofloxocin is prescribed for suspected underlying respiratory infection. Atenolol, a beta-blocker, is prescribed after a cardiac event, leading to depression, and escitalopram is prescribed to treat the depression. Table 5.1 presents examples of drug classes and specific examples of prescribing cascades reported by physicians in clinical practice, and Table 5.2 provides some examples of prescribing cascades involving OTC medications and medical devices, as described in the expanded definition (see Fig. 5.1). Prescribing cascades have also been incorporated into many deprescribing protocols [11]. Deprescribing is the process of tapering or stopping medications that may not be indicated, in accordance with the patients' preferences, to minimize polypharmacy and improve patient outcomes [31]. Most deprescribing protocols review all medications and indications for use, consider each drugs risk/benefit profile and then develop a prioritized plan for deprescribing. The medication review stage provides an opportunity to identify prescribing cascades and then determine their potential for deprescribing. Process mapping is another tool that can be used by clinicians to identify prescribing cascades in their patients [32]. A clinical process map is a tool designed to graphically illustrate a patient's presentation, symptoms, medications, possible side effects and interventions. This is generated quickly at the bedside by the clinician to help visualize the sequence of events leading to the development of the prescribing cascade and to understand its consequences.

5.6 Conclusions

Prescribing cascades are well documented in the literature and are an important cause of drug-related harm in older adults. Older women are at higher risk for drug-related harm than older men. Prescribing cascades can be prevented by implementing interventions at each stage of drug prescription and use. At the time of prescribing, the provider should be aware of potential prescribing cascades that may arise from the drug being initiated and carefully document the date that each new drug was started. At regular follow-up, providers should question whether a new complaint could be a medication side effect and whether a new prescription is really necessary. At medication review, validated tools and frameworks should be applied to identify inappropriate prescribing and to recognize opportunities for deprescribing. Preventing, detecting and reversing prescribing cascades provide an opportunity to improve quality of care for older adults and reduce drug-related harm.

References

1. Rochon PA, Gurwitz JH. Drug therapy. Lancet. 1995;346(8966):32–6.
2. Rochon PA, Gurwitz JH. Optimising drug treatment for elderly people: the prescribing cascade. BMJ. 1997;315(7115):1096–9.
3. Rochon PA, Gurwitz JH. The prescribing cascade revisited. Lancet. 2017;389(10081):1778–80.
4. Savage RD, Visentin JD, Bronskill SE, et al. Evaluation of a common prescribing cascade of calcium channel blockers and diuretics in older adults with hypertension. JAMA Intern Med. 2020;180(5):643–51.
5. Read SH, Giannakeas V, Pop P, et al. Evidence of a gabapentinoid and diuretic prescribing cascade among older adults with lower back pain. J Am Geriatr Soc. 2021;69(10):2842–50.
6. Gill SS, Mamdani M, Naglie G, et al. A prescribing cascade involving cholinesterase inhibitors and anticholinergic drugs. Arch Intern Med. 2005;165(7):808–13.
7. Sternberg SA, Petrovic M, Onder G, et al. Identifying key prescribing cascades in older people (iKascade): a transnational initiative on drug safety through a sex and gender lens—rationale and design. Eur Geriatr Med. 2021;12(3):475–83.
8. Choosing Wisely Australia. 5 Things clinicians and consumers should question. Developed by the Australasian Society of Clinical and Experimental Pharmacologists and Toxicologists. 2016. http://www.choosingwisely.org.au/recommendations/ascept. Accessed 9 July 2021.
9. Onder G, Bonassi S, Abbatecola AM, et al. High prevalence of poor quality drug prescribing in older individuals: a nationwide report from the Italian Medicines Agency (AIFA). J Gerontol A Biol Sci Med Sci. 2014;69(4):430–7.
10. Sternberg SA, Guy-Alfandary S, Rochon PA. Prescribing cascades in older adults. CMAJ. 2021;193(6):E215.
11. Rochon PA, Petrovic M, Cherubini A, et al. Polypharmacy, inappropriate prescribing, and deprescribing in old age:through a sex and gender lens. Lancet Healthy Longev. 2021;2(5):E290–300.
12. Canadian Institute for Health Information. Drug use among seniors in Canada, 2016. Ottawa: CIHI; 2018. https://secure.cihi.ca/free_products/drug-use-among-seniors-2016-en-web.pdf. Accessed 9 July 2021
13. Guthrie B, Makubate B, Hernandez-Santiago V, Dreischulte T. The rising tide of polypharmacy and drug–drug interactions: population database analysis 1995–2010. BMC Med. 2015;13:74.
14. Midao L, Giardini A, Menditto E, Kardas P, Costa E. Polypharmacy prevalence among older adults based on the survey of health, ageing and retirement in Europe. Arch Gerontol Geriatr. 2018;78:213–20.
15. Onder G, Liperoti R, Fialova D, et al. Polypharmacy in nursing home in Europe: results from the SHELTER study. J Gerontol A Biol Sci Med Sci. 2012;67(6):698–704.
16. Statistics Canada. 2016 Census of population, statistics Canada catalogue no. 98-400-X2016018. 2019. https://www12.statcan.gc.ca/census-recensement/2016/geo/geosearch-georecherche/ips/index.cfm?q=98-400-X2016018&l=en&g=2016A000011124. Accessed 9 Sept 2021.
17. Stall NM, Fischer HD, Fung K, et al. Sex-specific differences in end-of-life burdensome interventions and antibiotic therapy in nursing home residents with advanced dementia. JAMA Netw Open. 2019;2(8):e199557.
18. Holmes HM, Hayley DC, Alexander GC, Sachs GA. Reconsidering medication appropriateness for patients late in life. Arch Intern Med. 2006;166(6):605–9.

19. Gurwitz JH. The age/gender interface in geriatric pharmacotherapy. J Womens Health (Larchmt). 2005;14(1):68–72.
20. Watson S, Caster O, Rochon PA, den Ruijter H. Reported adverse drug reactions in women and men: aggregated evidence from globally collected individual case reports during half a century. EClinicalMedicine. 2019;17:100188.
21. Alturki A, Alaama T, Alomran Y, Al-Jedai A, Almudaiheem H, Watfa G. Potentially inappropriate medications in older patients based on beers criteria: a cross-sectional study of a family medicine practice in Saudi Arabia. BJGP Open. 2020;4(1):bjgpopen20X101009.
22. Rydberg DM, Mejyr S, Loikas D, Schenck-Gustafsson K, von Euler M, Malmström RE. Sex differences in spontaneous reports on adverse drug events for common antihypertensive drugs. Eur J Clin Pharmacol. 2018;74(9):1165–73.
23. Sørup FKH, Eriksson R, Westergaard D, Hallas J, Brunak S, Ejdrup AS. Sex differences in text-mined possible adverse drug events associated with drugs for psychosis. J Psychopharmacol (Oxford, England). 2020;34(5):532–9.
24. Bezerra de Souza DL, Oliveras-Fabregas A, Espelt A, et al. Multimorbidity and its associated factors among adults aged 50 and over: a cross-sectional study in 17 European countries. PLoS One. 2021;16(2):e0246623.
25. McCormick A, Charlton J. Morbidity statistics from general practice. In: Fourth national study 1991–1992. OPCS series MB5 no. 3. London: HMSO; 1995.
26. Cheff R, Hill M, Iveniuk J. Who benefits? Gaps in medication coverage for Ontario workers. Toronto: Wellesley Institute; 2019. https://www.wellesleyinstitute.com/wp-content/uploads/2019/12/Coverage-Gaps-for-Ontario-Workers_EMBARGO_27.11.19.pdf. Accessed 9 July 2021
27. Mauvais-Jarvis F, Bairey Merz N, Barnes PJ, et al. Sex and gender: modifiers of health, disease, and medicine. Lancet (London, England). 2020;396(10250):565–82.
28. Regitz-Zagrosek V. Sex and gender differences in pharmacology. Berlin: Springer; 2012.
29. Lega IC, Bronskill SE, Campitelli MA, et al. Sodium glucose cotransporter 2 inhibitors and risk of genital mycotic and urinary tract infection: a population-based study of older women and men with diabetes. Diabetes Obes Metab. 2019;21(11):2394–404.
30. Rosenberg J, Rochon PA, Gill SS. Unveiling a prescribing cascade in an older man. J Am Geriatr Soc. 2014;62(3):580–1.
31. Frank C, Weir E. Deprescribing for older patients. CMAJ. 2014;186(18):1369–76.
32. Piggott KL, Mehta N, Wong CL, Rochon PA. Using a clinical process map to identify prescribing cascades in your patient. BMJ. 2020;368:m261.
33. Kalisch LM, Caughey GE, Roughead EE, Gilbert AL. The prescribing cascade. Aust Prescr. 2011;34(6):162–6.
34. Liu PT, Argento VS, Skudlarska BA. Prescribing cascade in an 80-year-old Japanese immigrant. Geriatr Gerontol Int. 2009;9(4):402–4.
35. Rababa M, Al-Ghassani AA, Kovach CR, Dyer EM. Proton pump inhibitors and the prescribing cascade. J Gerontol Nurs. 2016;42(4):23–31.
36. Kwan D, Farrell B. Polypharmcy: optimizing medication use in elderly patients. CGS J CME. 2014;4(1):21–7.
37. Rochon PA, Stukel TA, Sykora K, et al. Atypical antipsychotics and Parkinsonism. Arch Intern Med. 2005;165(16):1882–8.
38. Singh S, Cocoros NM, Haynes K, et al. Antidopaminergic–antiparkinsonian medication prescribing cascade in persons with Alzheimer's disease. J Am Geriatr Soc. 2021;69(5):1328–33.
39. Singh S, Cocoros NM, Haynes K, et al. Identifying prescribing cascades in Alzheimer's disease and related dementias: the calcium channel blocker-diuretic prescribing cascade. Pharmacoepidemiol Drug Saf. 2021;30(8):1066–73.
40. Trenaman SC, Bowles SK, Kirkland S, Andrew MK. An examination of three prescribing cascades in a cohort of older adults with dementia. BMC Geriatr. 2021;21(1):297.
41. Vouri SM, van Tuyl JS, Olsen MA, Xian H, Schootman M. An evaluation of a potential calcium channel blocker-lower-extremity edema-loop diuretic prescribing cascade. J Am Pharm Assoc (2003). 2018;58(5):534–9 e4.

42. Ponte ML, Wachs L, Wachs A, Serra HA. Prescribing cascade. A proposed new way to evaluate it. Medicina (B Aires). 2017;77(1):13–6.
43. Vouri SM, Chung JM, Binder EF. Successful intervention to mitigate an acetylcholinesterase inhibitor-induced rhinorrhea prescribing cascade: a case report. J Clin Pharm Ther. 2017;42(3):370–1.
44. Gnon C, Currie J, Trimble J. Are you the victim of a prescribing cascades? Candian deprescribing network. 2020. https://www.deprescribingnetwork.ca/blog/prescribing-cascade. Accessed 28 Sept 2021.
45. Gill SS, Anderson GM, Fischer HD, et al. Syncope and its consequences in patients with dementia receiving cholinesterase inhibitors: a population-based cohort study. Arch Intern Med. 2009;169(9):867–73.

6 Adverse Drug Reactions in Older People: A Twenty-First Century View

Mary Randles and Denis O'Mahony

6.1 Introduction

The unprecedented number of adults living beyond 65 years is one of the great success stories of modern civilisation and modern medicine. Over the past century, the proportion of older adults in the United States of America has increased threefold, similar to like western Europe and most developed countries globally, leading to an increase in life expectancy that has not yet reached a plateau [1, 2]. The proportion of adults over 65 years in the United States was recently calculated at 20.3%, representing an increase of 2.9% over the 10 years to 2019. While these increases in longevity represent progress in relation to societal health in general, they also pose many challenges currently and in the future in terms of growing levels of comorbidity and frailty accompanied by higher prevalence of polypharmacy and adverse drug reactions in the population of any country observing societal ageing.

The success of medical management and pharmacotherapy in this population is not straightforward. It is generally accepted that medical interventions have facilitated older people to increase their longevity and maintain generally better health. However, greater exposure to polypharmacy has resulted in an ever-increasing potential for adverse drug reactions (ADRs), adverse drug events (ADEs) and adverse drug withdrawal events (ADWEs).

M. Randles · D. O'Mahony (✉)
Department of Medicine (Geriatrics), University College Cork, Cork, Ireland

Department of Geriatric Medicine, Cork University Hospital, Cork, Ireland
e-mail: mary.randles@ucc.ie; denis.omahony@ucc.ie

A. Cherubini et al. (eds.), *Optimizing Pharmacotherapy in Older Patients*, Practical Issues in Geriatrics, https://doi.org/10.1007/978-3-031-28061-0_6

6.2 Definition of Adverse Drug Reactions

An adverse drug reaction was originally defined by the World Health Organisation (WHO) over 50 years ago as: "A response to a drug that is noxious and unintended and occurs at doses normally used in man for the prophylaxis, diagnosis or therapy of disease, or for the modification of physiological function" [3]. This WHO definition was developed with the aim of monitoring ADRs, particularly in drug development trials and soon after approval of drugs for marketing for general use. Edwards and Aronson further defined an ADR as: "An appreciably harmful or unpleasant reaction, resulting from an intervention related to the use of a medicinal product, which predicts hazard from future administration and warrants prevention or specific treatment, or the alteration of the dosage regimen, or withdrawal of the product" [4]. They further point out that while an adverse drug effect and adverse drug reaction are often used interchangeably, an adverse drug effect is seen from the point of view of the drug, whereas the adverse drug reaction is seen from the point of view of the patient [4]. Edwards and Aronson's definition was further expanded in 2010 to include reactions occurring as a result of error, misuse or abuse and to suspected reactions to medicines that are unlicensed or used off label in addition to the authorised use of a medicinal product in normal doses [5].

When discussing ADRs, some experts emphasise the need to differentiate between ADRs and ADEs. The difference depends essentially on the adverse effect. While we can define an ADE as an adverse outcome that occurs while a patient is taking a drug, it is not necessarily directly attributable to the drug [4], such as the increased incidence of falls and fractures when older people are taking benzodiazepines.

6.3 Prevalence and Cost of ADRs in Older Adults

While historically there has been little interest in the specific effect of ADRs in older adults, over the past two decades, there has been increasing focus on the prevalence, incidence, clinical effect and cost of ADRs in older adults. In the general adult hospitalised population, ADRs account for approximately 6% of all admissions [6]. Furthermore, prospective analysis of inpatient episodes demonstrated that 14.7% (95% CI, 13.6–15.9%) of patients experienced at least one incident ADR [6, 7]. Given the increased complexity of comorbid diseases and polypharmacy in older people, it is unsurprising that a systematic review and meta-analysis [8] found the prevalence of ADRs in older adults in acute care settings was greater than in the general adult population. The overall mean prevalence of ADRs in the same review was 11.0% (95% CI: 5.1–16.8) with 11.5% occurring during hospitalisation. This meta-analysis demonstrated a wide variation of overall ADR prevalence across the included studies, that is, from 5.8% [8] to 46.3% [9]. The authors note that prospective studies and larger scale studies generally found higher ADR prevalence rates [10] in studies of ADRs in 'old old' adults (i.e. over 80 years), reporting an average in-hospital ADR incidence of 13%. Although the large variance in the prevalence of

ADRs observed in older hospitalised adults has been attributed to the difference in sample sizes and different admission settings within hospitals (general unselected medical acute admissions versus dedicated geriatric medicine unit admissions) [11], it remains very clear that ADRs are a common problem faced by all clinicians treating older adults.

Highly variable prevalence rates of ADRs have been reported in community-dwelling older adults also, varying from 6.5% in one prospective study [6] to 78% in a retrospective cohort of older adults where the ADRs were self-reported by patients and corroborated by clinician review [12]; the latter study also included drug events that may not have resulted in the index hospitalisation. Older adults in long-term care settings were found to have an ADR prevalence of 14% with other studies reporting an ADR incidence in long-term care older patients between 1.19 and 7.26 per 100 resident-months [12]. It is estimated that older adults are approximately seven times more likely to experience an ADR requiring hospital admission, and when hospitalised they are substantially more likely to experience ADRs during their hospital admission than younger patients [13, 14].

ADRs in older adults result in excess economic costs during hospital admissions, increased length of stay, additional cost of care and increased mortality. A French study evaluating the cost of ADRs with the aim of assessing the additional financial resource utilisation arising from ADRs found that the ADR incidence increased with age and that half of the ADRs led to additional investigations and increased median length of stay, that is, 11 days versus 7 days in those patients who did not experience ADRs. This increase in length of stay resulted in a mean cost of approximately €1800 per ADR [15], similar to the cost of €2128 per ADR-related hospitalisation calculated by Beijer and Blaey [16]. ADRs have a significant impact on hospital running costs accounting for 5% of overall hospital running costs in the USA, estimated at between $3.5 billion and $30 billion per annum [13–15, 17]. The fatality rate from ADRs has been reported as 0.15% in a larger scale, retrospective, population-based study and 0.44% in older adults in one meta-analysis [6, 18].

6.4 Why Do ADRs Occur More Commonly in Older People?

As discussed in previous chapters, old age results in diminished ability to maintain homoeostasis with a concomitant decrease in the functional capacity of multiple organ systems leading to changes in absorption, distribution, metabolism and excretion of some drugs [19]. Older age is associated with delayed gastric emptying, decreased splanchnic blood flow and reduced surface area for absorption, coupled with increased gastric pH. Older people often have a greater body fat to lean body mass ratio with an overall reduction in body total water and serum albumin concentration. This leads to a relative increase of the volume of distribution such that the half-life for lipophilic drugs such as benzodiazepines is prolonged; there is an increased concentration of water-soluble drugs like lithium and an increased proportion of free unbound highly protein-bound drugs like Ibuprofen and phenytoin [19].

Metabolism of drugs may be altered with ageing also due to reductions in hepatic volume, renal and hepatic perfusion, and protein binding. Older people who experience polypharmacy are more likely to take drugs that cause inhibition or activation of the CYP pathway [11, 20]. Normal physiological ageing and common disorders such as cardiovascular disease, diabetes, heart failure and hypertension can all lead to reduced renal clearance and excretion of drugs [20].

Multimorbidity, the co-occurrence of two or more coinciding medical conditions was shown to affect up to 95.1% of patients aged over 65 in the primary care setting in a systematic review of 39 studies [21]. Older people are at considerably higher risk of experiencing polypharmacy due to a much higher burden of multimorbidity than is encountered in younger people. Polypharmacy, as the principal risk factor for ADRs, may be engendered and exacerbated by older people attending multiple specialists for individual diseases or conditions, leading to more evidence-based drug therapies.

In one study [22], researchers found that taking five or more daily medications was associated with an odds ratio for ADEs of 1.88 (95% CI, 1.58–2.25) compared to patients taking zero to four daily medications). Over the last 20 years, there has been a notable increase in treatment guidelines for many common conditions, particularly in cardiovascular disease and diabetes where treatment guidelines recommend multiple drugs for secondary prevention and ongoing management of these conditions. Worryingly, studies demonstrate that polypharmacy has increased in the last decade, particularly after hospital admissions [23, 24]. Higher levels of polypharmacy increase the risk of both drug–disease interactions and drug–drug interactions [25].

Although older patients experience most of the burden of multimorbidity and polypharmacy and are the largest group of patients receiving evidence-based pharmacotherapies, paradoxically, they are often excluded from clinical drug trials because of their multimorbidity. An example of this discrepancy can be seen in cancer drug trials. While people over 65 years represent over 60% of new cancer cases in Europe and the US annually, they only account for 22% of patients recruited into cancer trials; this proportion drops to 8–13% in those aged over 70 years [26]. This degree of older patient exclusion from clinical trials is further illustrated in a review of 440 trials of drugs for type 2 diabetes [27]. Despite being the most common long-term metabolic condition experienced by older adults, only six trials were specifically designed to study older adults; 289 trials excluded individuals based on an arbitrary age cut-off and a further 76.8% of trials excluded people with comorbidities.

6.5 Types of ADRs

Historically, ADRs were classified as Type A and Type B reactions. In Rawlins and Thompson's classification, Type A reactions were typically associated with drug doses and were predictable from the pharmacological properties and physiological actions of the drug. Type B or "Bizarre" reactions were not seen as dose related, such as idiosyncratic hypersensitivity reactions [28]. Over time, these categorical ADR types were expanded to include further four categories; (Table 6.1) Type C

Table 6.1 Classifications of adverse drug reactions

Reaction type	Type of effect	Common	Characteristics	Example	Management
A	Augmented	Yes	**Dose related** • Related to the pharmacological action of the drug • Predictable • Low mortality	• Side effects: orthostatic hypotension with anti-hypertensives • Toxic effects: serotonin syndrome with SSRIs, digoxin toxicity	• Dose reduction • Withdrawal of drug if necessary • Review for drug–drug interactions
B	Bizarre	No	**Non-dose related** • Not related to pharmacological action of the drug • Unpredictable • High mortality	• Immunological reactions: anaphylaxis to penicillin • Idiosyncratic reactions: malignant hyperthermia with anaesthetics, acute porphyria	• Immediate withdrawal of drug and avoidance in the future
C	Chronic	No	**Dose-related and time-related** • Related to cumulative dose of the drug	• Hypothalamic–pituitary–adrenal axis suppression by corticosteroids	• Dose reduction • Withdrawal, if necessary, often over a prolonged period of time
D	Delayed	No	**Time related** • Often also dose related • Occurs some time after the use of the drug	• Traditive dyskinesia • Carcinogenesis • Teratogenesis	• Often non-treatable
E	End-of-use	No	**Withdrawal** • Occurs soon after withdrawal of drug	• Withdrawal syndrome after discontinuation of opiates or benzodiazepines • Myocardial ischemia after withdrawal of beta-blockers	• Reintroduction of drug • Slow withdrawal
F	Failure	Yes	**Unexpected failure of therapy** • Dose related • Drug interaction related	• Inadequate anticoagulation effect from warfarin with carbamazipine	• Increase in dosage • Review of effects of concomitant therapy

(Adapted from Edwards & Aronson, 2000)

[dose- and time-dependent (chronic) reactions], Type D (delayed reactions), Type E (withdrawal reactions) and Type F (failure of therapy) [4].

Aronson and Ferner proposed the DoTS (**Do**se-related/**T**ime-related/**S**usceptibility-related) system of classification to incorporate the temporal relationship and susceptibility of the individual to the reaction [29]. They argue that the Type A–F classification is defined only by the properties of the drug and its known pharmacology and dose-dependent effects. They proposed a classification system that takes account of the time course and severity of a reaction and the genetic, pathological and biological differences of the individual, which may make them more susceptible to an adverse reaction.

In the DoTS classification, dose relatedness divides ADRs into reactions that occur at supratherapeutic doses (toxic effects), ADRs that occur at standard therapeutic doses (collateral effects) and ADRs that occur at subtherapeutic doses in sensitive individuals, that is, hyper-susceptibility reactions. They distinguish two distinct patterns of time course for ADRs, i.e. one that is dependent on the time exposed to the drug and one that is time independent, occurring at any time during drug treatment. Time-dependent reactions range from rapid to delayed and can be seen in greater detail in Table 6.2.

This classification also acknowledges that different individuals will have different levels of susceptibility to particular ADRs based on their genetics, age, sex, disease profile and drug or food interactions, for example, older women are considered to be more susceptible to ADRs from hypnotics than younger adults. The three elements of dose, time and susceptibility can be combined to give greater information about an ADR and also guide future prescribing to prevent further ADRs.

Table 6.2 Types of time-dependent drug reactions based of Aronson and Ferner ADR classification [29]

Time-dependant reactions		
Type of reaction	Features	Example
Rapid reactions	Occur only when a drug is administered too quickly	Vancomycin → red man syndrome
First dose reactions	Occur after the first dose of a certain treatment. May or may not occur again	Ace inhibitor-hypotension Type I hypersensitivity reaction to penicillin
Early reactions	Occur early in treatment but abate as treatment progresses	Acetylcholinesterase inhibitors → gastrointestinal disturbance or nausea
Intermediate reactions	Occur after some delay, however if a reaction hasn't occurred after a certain time, the population risk falls	Type II–IV hypersensitivity reactions
Late reactions	Risk increases with repeated exposure Also includes withdrawal reactions	Dopamine receptor antagonists → tardive dyskinesias Corticosteroids → osteoporosis
Delayed reactions	Effects are observed at some time after exposure, even if the drug has been withdrawn	Carcinogens

6.6 Recognising ADRs in Older Adults

Recognising ADRs in older adults can present a particular challenge to clinicians. ADRs have been described as one of the great mimics in healthcare due to their propensity to present in a similar manner to other common age-related disorders, often with non-specific symptoms [30]. Acute kidney injury, electrolyte disturbance, falls, orthostatic hypotension, symptomatic bradycardia, gastrointestinal upset and bleeding are familiar presentations of acute illness to clinicians caring for older people. However, these presentations were also found to be the most common presentations of ADRs in a study of 513 older adults during their hospital stay for acute illness [31]. Medications that were associated with these common clinical problems included diuretics, benzodiazepines, opioids, antihypertensives, antiplatelet/anticoagulants, antidiabetic drugs and NSAIDs [31–33], that is, medications that are commonly utilised in the care of older adults. Recognising non-specific symptoms such as fatigue, cognitive decline, new onset of falls and constipation as potential ADRs is important to prevent potential prescribing cascades (see Chap. 5).

Reliably defining and classifying ADRs in practice can be challenging in due to heterogeneity of ADR risk assessment and causality tools [34]. Despite the high prevalence of ADRs in older adults, none of the most frequently used ADR assessment tools was developed specifically with older patients in mind. The WHO–UMC assessment matrix (Table 6.3) relies on expert judgement, knowledge of the medical conditions, understanding of comorbid illness and laboratory results. It considers drug–drug interactions, which is advantageous when assessing causality in comorbid older adults. Algorithm or probability-based methods such as the Naranjo ADR probability [35] algorithm are less reliant on expert judgement; however, they use some criteria such as response to placebo and drug rechallenge to confirm suspected ADRs, which could pose practical and ethical difficulties in the management of older adults in routine clinical practice.

Once the causality of an ADR has been established, a severity rating can be applied such as that proposed by Hartwig and Siegal (1992). This scale assigns severity of ADRs into seven categories depending on the clinical consequences to the patient (Table 6.4). The Hallas ADR avoidability criteria are also illustrated in Table 6.4.

While the tools discussed in this section may be of benefit in assessing ADRs at a population level, they may not be practical for routine clinical use. Nevertheless,

Table 6.3 Adverse drug reactions (ADR) causality matrix adapted from World Health Organisation–Upsala Monitoring Centre (WHO–UMC) ADR causality criteria [36]

Categories of ADR attribution	Time sequence consistent with ADR	Other drugs/ diseases ruled out as causative	Dechallenge response, that is, clinical improvement	Rechallenge response, that is, clinical relapse
Certain	Yes	Yes	Yes	Yes
Probable	Yes	Yes	Yes	No
Possible	Yes	No	No	No
Unlikely	No	No	No	No

Table 6.4 Hartwig adverse drug reactions (ADR) severity scale and Hallas ADR avoidability criteria

Hartwig ADR severity grade (Hartwig et al. 1992) [37]		Hallas ADR avoidability criteria (Hallas et al. 1990) [38]	
1	An ADR occurred but no change in treatment with suspected drug	Definitely avoidable	The drug event was due to a drug treatment procedure inconsistent with present-day knowledge of good medical practice or was clearly unrealistic, taking the known circumstances into account
2	The ADR required that treatment with the suspected drug be held, discontinued or otherwise changed (no antidote required and no increase in length of stay)	Possibly avoidable	The prescription was not erroneous, but the drug event could have been avoided by an effort exceeding the obligatory demands
3	The ADR required that treatment with the suspected drug be held, discontinued or otherwise changed or and an antidote or other treatment was required	Unavoidable	The drug event could not have been avoided by any reasonable means, or it was an unpredictable event in the course of a treatment fully in accordance with good medical practice
4	Any level 3 ADR which resulted in admission or increased length of stay by at least 1 day	Unclassifiable	The data for rating could not be obtained or the evidence was conflicting
5	Any level 4 ADR which required intensive medical care		
6	Any ADR causing permanent harm to the patient		
7a	The ADR indirectly linked to death in the patient		
7b	The ADR was directly linked to death in the patient		

clinicians caring for older patients need to maintain a heightened vigilance for detection of possible ADRs and to carefully examine all presentations to ensure that ADRs are not overlooked as a diagnosis.

6.7 Preventing ADRs in Older People

ADRs are a potentially preventable form of iatrogenic harm. In the past decade, interest in developing new clinical tools designed to reduce and prevent ADRs in older people has grown. Given the association between inappropriate prescribing (IP) and ADRs, explicit IP assessment tools such as STOPP/START criteria and Beers criteria, although developed to identify and reduce IP, may have potential to reduce ADRs. In one single-centre, single-blinded study, application of STOPP/START criteria (version 1) to the medication lists of acutely hospitalised older adults was associated with a 9.3% absolute risk reduction in hospital-acquired ADRs compared to standard pharmaceutical care [39]. In contrast, the larger scale, multi-centre OPERAM trial examining the impact of application of STOPP/START criteria (version 2) on drug-related admissions (DRAs) in older hospitalised patients compared with standard pharmaceutical care did not show any significant beneficial impact on DRAs in the 12 months post-intervention [40].

ADR risk assessment tools designed specifically for use in older people have appeared in the literature in recent years, such as the GerontoNet ADR risk score [41] the BADRI score [42] and the ADRROP score [43]. In each model, researchers have attempted to prioritise and quantify the main risk factors for ADRs in multimorbid older people leading to an ADR risk score that might be applicable in routine clinical practice. However, none of these ADR risk scores has through prospective validation assessment been sufficiently robust to recommend their routine use.

More recently, Jennings et al. (2019) have identified the need for an ADR risk prediction tool that looks beyond the individual patient factors and suggest a shift in focus to the drugs that carry higher risk for ADRs in older people [44]. In a recent systematic review and meta-analysis [44], the same group has identified those drug classes that are most associated with ADRs in older people in hospital [43]; these higher risk drug classes are listed in Table 6.5. Given the doubt about benefit from applying ADR risk tools, clinician awareness and vigilance remain fundamental to ADR detection and avoidance. By applying knowledge of the physiological changes associated with ageing and remaining vigilant to the risks of inappropriate prescribing and drug–drug and drug–disease interactions, clinicians can reduce the risk of ADRs. Increased awareness of common ADRs and a high index of suspicion when

Table 6.5 The ten most common drug classes causing adverse drug reactions (ADRs) in hospitalised older patients [43]

Drug class (in rank order of frequency)	Proportion of total reported ADRs	Most commonly reported pharmacological subgroup
Diuretics	19.83%	Loop (high ceiling) diuretics
Antibacterials (systemic use)	14.84%	Beta-lactams (penicillins, cephalosporins), macrolides, quinolones
Antithrombotics	12.24%	VKAs[a], heparin and heparinoids, antiplatelet agents
Analgesics	10.90%	Opioids
Drugs for obstructive airways disease	4.74%	Beta-2 adrenergic agonists, xanthines (e.g. theophylline)
Renin–angiotensin system antagonists	4.11%	ACE inhibitors, angiotensin-II receptor blockers
Psychotropics	3.86%	Benzodiazepines, antipsychotics
Corticosteroids (systemic use)	3.23%	Glucocorticoids
Cardiac drugs	2.98%	Cardiac glycosides, vasodilators, class I and III antiarrhythmics
Antidiabetic drugs	2.56%	Insulin and insulin analogues, oral antidiabetics

[a]Vitamin K antagonists, for example, warfarin

new symptoms develop in an older person, particularly after commencing or changing medications, could help reduce ADR risk.

Advanced (electronic) medication reconciliation at points of transition care can also reduce medication errors and ADEs by identifying prescribing errors or discrepancies or dose errors in patients' prescriptions [45]. Deprescribing of unnecessary or inappropriate medications with particular focus on attainable therapeutic goals coupled with incorporating the wishes of the patient could reduce the number of drugs prescribed, particularly those drugs with minimal benefit to the patient that are repeatedly prescribed.

Routine review of regular medications for appropriateness, drug–drug and drug–disease interactions is recommended, incorporating specific enquiry about over-the-counter (OTC) medication use and medication adherence.

6.8 Conclusion

As multimorbidity and polypharmacy become more prevalent in tandem with societal ageing, risk of ADRs in older people increases. Clinicians must seek to achieve a balance between potentially beneficial medications and risk of ADRs. Acknowledging that older people are a heterogeneous group with varying degrees of physiological and physical function, prescribers should be vigilant in order to minimise risk of iatrogenic harm. It is imperative that clinicians caring for older adults are aware of ADRs, the main risk factors for ADRs and the often-non-specific clinical presentations of ADRs in order to reduce ADR risk while maintaining beneficial medications. Careful assessment of the individual older patient, his/her goals and expectations from pharmacotherapy and careful review of medications at each healthcare encounter, with a focus on potentially inappropriate medications helps to minimise ADR risk in older adults.

References

1. Eurostat. Population structure and aging 2020. https://ec.europa.eu/eurostat/statistics-explained/index.php/Population_structure_and_ageing#Past_and_future_population_ageing_trends_in_the_EU-27.
2. Anderson LA, Goodman RA, Holtzman D, Posner SF, Northridge ME. Aging in the United States: opportunities and challenges for public health. Am J Public Health. 2012;102(3):393–5.
3. World Health Organization. International drug monitoring: the role of national centres, report of a WHO meeting [held in Geneva from 20 to 25 September 1971]. Geneva: World Health Organization; 1972.
4. Edwards IR, Aronson JK. Adverse drug reactions: definitions, diagnosis, and management. Lancet. 2000;356(9237):1255–9.
5. Parliament E, December Co. Directive 2010/84/EU of The European Parliament and of the Council of 15 December 2010, amending, as regards to pharmacovigilance, Directive 2001/83/EC on the Community Code relating to medicinal products for human use. 2010.

6. Pirmohamed M, James S, Meakin S, Green C, Scott AK, Walley TJ, et al. Adverse drug reactions as cause of admission to hospital: prospective analysis of 18,820 patients. BMJ. 2004;329(7456):15–9.
7. Davies EC, Green CF, Taylor S, Williamson PR, Mottram DR, Pirmohamed M. Adverse drug reactions in hospital in-patients: a prospective analysis of 3695 patient-episodes. PLoS One. 2009;4(2):e4439.
8. Franceschi M, Scarcelli C, Niro V, Seripa D, Pazienza AM, Pepe G, et al. Prevalence, clinical features and avoidability of adverse drug reactions as cause of admission to a geriatric unit. Drug Saf. 2008;31(6):545–56.
9. De Paepe P, Petrovic M, Outtier L, Van Maele G, Buylaert W. Drug interactions and adverse drug reactions in the older patients admitted to the emergency department. Acta Clin Belg. 2013;68(1):15–21.
10. Alhawassi TM, Krass I, Bajorek BV, Pont LG. A systematic review of the prevalence and risk factors for adverse drug reactions in the elderly in the acute care setting. Clin Interv Aging. 2014;9:2079–86.
11. Davies EA, O'Mahony MS. Adverse drug reactions in special populations—the elderly. Br J Clin Pharmacol. 2015;80(4):796–807.
12. Handler SM, Wright RM, Ruby CM, Hanlon JT. Epidemiology of medication-related adverse events in nursing homes. Am J Geriatr Pharmacother. 2006;4(3):264–72.
13. Tangiisuran B, Gozzoli M, Davies J, Rajkumar C. Adverse drug reactions in older people. Rev Clin Gerontol. 2010;20(3):246.
14. White TJ, Arakelian A, Rho JP. Counting the costs of drug-related adverse events. PharmacoEconomics. 1999;15(5):445–58.
15. Patel K, Kedia M, Bajpai D, Mehta S, Kshirsagar N, Gogtay N. Evaluation of the prevalence and economic burden of adverse drug reactions presenting to the medical emergency department of a tertiary referral centre: a prospective study. BMC Clin Pharmacol. 2007;7(1):1–5.
16. Beijer H, De Blaey C. Hospitalisations caused by adverse drug reactions (ADR): a meta-analysis of observational studies. Pharm World Sci. 2002;24(2):46–54.
17. Cronenwett LR, Bootman JL, Wolcott J, Aspden P. Preventing medication errors. Washington, DC: National Academies Press; 2007.
18. Patel TK, Patel PB. Mortality among patients due to adverse drug reactions that lead to hospitalization: a meta-analysis. Eur J Clin Pharmacol. 2018;74(6):819–32.
19. Corsonello A, Pedone C, Incalzi RA. Age-related pharmacokinetic and pharmacodynamic changes and related risk of adverse drug reactions. Curr Med Chem. 2010;17(6):571–84.
20. Corsonello A, Pedone C, Lattanzio F, Onder G, Incalzi RA. Association between glomerular filtration rate and adverse drug reactions in elderly hospitalized patients. Drugs Aging. 2011;28(5):379–90.
21. Violan C, Foguet-Boreu Q, Flores-Mateo G, Salisbury C, Blom J, Freitag M, et al. Prevalence, determinants and patterns of multimorbidity in primary care: a systematic review of observational studies. PLoS One. 2014;9(7):e102149.
22. Bourgeois FT, Shannon MW, Valim C, Mandl KD. Adverse drug events in the outpatient setting: an 11-year national analysis. Pharmacoepidemiol Drug Saf. 2010;19(9):901–10.
23. Corsonello A, Pedone C, Corica F, Incalzi RA. Polypharmacy in elderly patients at discharge from the acute care hospital. Ther Clin Risk Manag. 2007;3(1):197.
24. Guthrie B, Makubate B, Hernandez-Santiago V, Dreischulte T. The rising tide of polypharmacy and drug–drug interactions: population database analysis 1995–2010. BMC Med. 2015;13(1):74.
25. Johnell K, Klarin I. The relationship between number of drugs and potential drug–drug interactions in the elderly. Drug Saf. 2007;30(10):911–8.
26. Aapro MS, Köhne C-H, Cohen HJ, Extermann M. Never too old? Age should not be a barrier to enrollment in cancer clinical trials. Oncologist. 2005;10(3):198–204.
27. Cruz-Jentoft AJ, Carpena-Ruiz M, Montero-Errasquín B, Sánchez-Castellano C, Sánchez-García E. Exclusion of older adults from ongoing clinical trials about type 2 diabetes mellitus. J Am Geriatr Soc. 2013;61(5):734–8.

28. Rawlins M, Thompson J. Pathogenesis of adverse drug reactions. In: Davies D, editor. Textbook of adverse drug reactions. Oxford: Oxford University Press; 1977. p. 10.
29. Aronson JK, Ferner RE. Joining the DoTS: new approach to classifying adverse drug reactions. BMJ. 2003;327(7425):1222–5.
30. Coleman JJ, Pontefract SK. Adverse drug reactions. Clin Med (Lond). 2016;16(5):481–5.
31. O'Connor MN, Gallagher P, Byrne S, O'Mahony D. Adverse drug reactions in older patients during hospitalisation: are they predictable? Age Ageing. 2012;41(6):771–6.
32. Budnitz DS, Lovegrove MC, Shehab N, Richards CL. Emergency hospitalizations for adverse drug events in older Americans. N Engl J Med. 2011;365(21):2002–12.
33. Howard RL, Avery AJ, Slavenburg S, Royal S, Pipe G, Lucassen P, et al. Which drugs cause preventable admissions to hospital? A systematic review. Br J Clin Pharmacol. 2007;63(2):136–47.
34. Lavan AH, Gallagher P. Predicting risk of adverse drug reactions in older adults. Ther Adv Drug Saf. 2016;7(1):11–22.
35. Naranjo CA, Busto U, Sellers EM, Sandor P, Ruiz I, Roberts EA, et al. A method for estimating the probability of adverse drug reactions. Clin Pharmacol Ther. 1981;30(2):239–45.
36. WHO. The use of the WHO–UMC system for standardised case causality assessment: World Health Organisation. https://www.who.int/medicines/areas/quality_safety/safety_efficacy/WHOcausality_assessment.pdf.
37. Hartwig SC, Siegel J, Schneider PJ. Preventability and severity assessment in reporting adverse drug reactions. Am J Hosp Pharm. 1992;49(9):2229–32.
38. Hallas J, Harvald B, Gram L, Grodum E, Brøsen K, Haghfelt T, et al. Drug related hospital admissions: the role of definitions and intensity of data collection, and the possibility of prevention. J Intern Med. 1990;228(2):83–90.
39. O'Connor MN, O'Sullivan D, Gallagher PF, Eustace J, Byrne S, O'Mahony D. Prevention of hospital-acquired adverse drug reactions in older people using screening tool of older persons' prescriptions and screening tool to alert to right treatment criteria: a cluster randomized controlled trial. J Am Geriatr Soc. 2016;64(8):1558–66.
40. Blum MR, Sallevelt BT, Spinewine A, O'Mahony D, Moutzouri E, Feller M, et al. Optimizing therapy to prevent avoidable hospital admissions in multimorbid older adults (OPERAM): cluster randomised controlled trial. BMJ. 2021;374:n1585.
41. Onder G, Petrovic M, Tangiisuran B, Meinardi MC, Markito-Notenboom WP, Somers A, et al. Development and validation of a score to assess risk of adverse drug reactions among in-hospital patients 65 years or older: the GerontoNet ADR risk score. Arch Intern Med. 2010;170(13):1142–8.
42. Tangiisuran B, Scutt G, Stevenson J, Wright J, Onder G, Petrovic M, et al. Development and validation of a risk model for predicting adverse drug reactions in older people during hospital stay: Brighton adverse drug reactions risk (BADRI) model. PLoS One. 2014;9(10):e111254.
43. O'Mahony D, O'Connor MN, Eustace J, Byrne S, Petrovic M, Gallagher P. The adverse drug reaction risk in older persons (ADRROP) prediction scale: derivation and prospective validation of an ADR risk assessment tool in older multi-morbid patients. Eur Geriatr Med. 2018;9(2):191–9.
44. Jennings E, Gallagher P, O'Mahony D. Detection and prevention of adverse drug reactions in multi-morbid older patients. Age Ageing. 2018;48(1):10–3.
45. Killin L, Hezam A, Anderson KK, Welk B. Advanced medication reconciliation: a systematic review of the impact on medication errors and adverse drug events associated with transitions of care. Jt Comm J Qual Patient Saf. 2021;47(7):438–51.

Adherence: How to Measure and Improve It

7

Alessandra Marengoni and Laura J. Sahm

7.1 State of the Art

Older adults are typically affected by multimorbidity, the co-occurrence of multiple diseases, which makes their care complex, and the use of medications, a challenging task [1]. More than 90% of older adults receive drug prescriptions according to guidelines for specific diseases; it has been shown that around 50% of older adults chronically receive polypharmacy (≥5 drugs) and about 10% excessive polypharmacy (≥10 drugs) [2]. The mean number of prescribed medications progressively rises from the age group with less than 65 years to the 80–84-year age group [3] and is higher among patients affected by dementia [4].

Polypharmacy is one of the main determinants of poor adherence to treatment in older patients. The World Health Organization defines adherence as the extent to which a person's behavior—taking medication, following a diet and/or executing lifestyle changes—corresponds with agreed recommendations from a healthcare provider [5]. When limiting to medication adherence, the latter is usually defined as the proportion of days covered of more than 80%. Adherence can be split into three phases: initiation (taking the first dose of prescribed drug), implementation (taking the prescribed dosing regimen from the initiation on) and persistence (time between initiation and the last dose); each of them presents specific issues and challenges. Non-adherence may be intentional (when the patient decides not to take treatment or to take it in a way that differs from the one suggested by the care provider) or unintentional (when the patient is willing to take his/her treatment but cannot due to

A. Marengoni (✉)
Department of Clinical and Experimental Sciences, University of Brescia, Brescia, Italy
e-mail: alessandra.marengoni@unibs.it

L. J. Sahm
School of Pharmacy, University College Cork, Cork, Ireland

Department of Pharmacy, Mercy University Hospital, Cork, Ireland
e-mail: L.Sahm@ucc.ie

A. Cherubini et al. (eds.), *Optimizing Pharmacotherapy in Older Patients*, Practical Issues in Geriatrics, https://doi.org/10.1007/978-3-031-28061-0_7

Table 7.1 Determinants of non-adherence

	Patient-related	Therapy-related	Condition-related	Health-system related	Social and economical
Forgetfulness	x		x		
Lack of information	x			x	
Length of treatment		x	x		
Number of drugs		x	x		
Previous adverse drug reactions	x	x	x		
Therapeutic failures		x	x		
Poor education	x			x	x
Reimbursement system		x		x	x
Cultural beliefs	x				x

limitations in mental or physical capacity or resources). In older persons, unintentional adherence is very often due to cognitive and psychological problems, visual and motor impairments and inadequate caregivers or social support [6].

Overall, a number of studies have found that, in developed countries, adherence among older patients suffering chronic diseases averages only 50% [7], and it is even less in developing countries.

According to the World Health Organization (WHO), determinants of non-adherence can be aggregated into five dimensions: patient-related, therapy-related, condition-related, health system-related, and socio-economic [8] (Table 7.1). Several initiatives have been taken worldwide in order to better understand factors of non-adherence and possible interventions to improve it, especially in older persons. For instance, the European Innovation Partnership on Active and Healthy Ageing Action Group A1 focused on "Adherence to prescriptions" bringing together partners representing multi-stakeholder commitments from national, regional and local authorities, academic and non-academic research centres, industries and enterprises across the European Union. As a general aim, the Action Group A1 has to contribute to the improvement of adherence to medical plans and medication at European level [9]. Still, at present, poor adherence is the main factor underlying the failure of patients and healthcare systems to achieve treatment outcomes.

7.2 How to Assess Adherence

Measuring medication adherence is important to clinicians and researchers, and there is no "one size fits all" approach. The methods used should be tailored to the question being asked and in the specific population and should consider the severity of the consequences of non-adherence. There are many ways to measure medication adherence, and they usually fall into direct or indirect methods. The World Health Organization (WHO) delineates these into subjective and objective measures [8]. We know from listening to our patients that whilst they may not have taken the medication, they would also not like to admit this as it may cause some embarrassment or perhaps a fear of disappointing the prescriber. In addition, we know that the more medications a patient needs, due to multimorbidity and/or older adult with polypharmacy, the more likely that medication adherence will be suboptimal [10].

7.2.1 Let Us Look First at the Direct Methods

There can be the direct measurement of the amount of drug in the patient at a particular point in time, for example, by taking a blood sample. This is commonly used when dealing with narrow therapeutic index drugs, for example, digoxin or theophylline, and there is a need to establish the therapeutic drug concentration, to avoid sub- or supra- therapeutic doses. This can also be used to measure adherence but is not done routinely in practice due to its cumbersome and costly nature, in addition to the fact that parameters such as the absorption, distribution, metabolism and elimination of the drug (or indeed its metabolites) may have individual variation. Also, bearing in mind that the patient may have taken this drug with food or other drugs, there may well be drug–drug or drug–food or indeed drug–herbal interactions. These interactions may result in the faster/slower elimination of the drug and, therefore, muddy the water.

At best these drug levels provide a snapshot of what is happening in the body at the time and do not offer a view as to the long-term medication adherence. This is analogous to the doctor who relies on a fasting blood glucose to indicate the adherence of a patient to their antidiabetic agents rather than seeking to review the glycosylated haemoglobin. This method may be appropriate for the measurement of adherence to single drug therapy but does little to offer explanations as to why the patient may not be adhering to therapy or any indication of whether this non-adherence is a single event or indicative of someone who is persistently non-adherent. The simplistic nature of this result, that is, plasma level of drug detected, also fails to consider the myriad factors that go into the patient's intentional or unintentional non-adherence to the prescribed regimen.

I remember a specific instance when I was monitoring warfarin (vitamin K antagonist) for a patient, and this is commonly done with the aid of an automated decision-making tool to aid dose adjustment. The patient had a target Internationalized Normalized Ratio (INR) of 2.5 with a range of 2–3. On this occasion, the patient said that he was wondering whether he could consume alcohol. I answered with my usual "warfarin loves everything but change" and that a moderate amount of alcohol (less than two units per day) should be fine. The following week, the patient presented with an INR of 4.5. I asked whether there had been any variations in diet/coprescribed medications/taking too many tablets and of course alcohol consumption. The patient told me that he had stuck with the guidance and that he had saved up his two units of alcohol per day and had consumed 14 units of alcohol the night before; this was a big lesson for me and one that helps to illustrate the importance of clear communication with our patients. Needless to say, I modified this message going forward!

Another method of directly measuring adherence is Directly Observed Therapy (DOT). As the name implies, the healthcare worker (HCW) (doctor, nurse, pharmacist) observes the patient ingesting (or simulating ingestion) the medicine. This is seen when patients have to follow complex regimens, for example, those with tuberculosis, and according to the Centre for Disease Control this is an effective strategy to ensure adherence [11]. Again, here the question remains as to whether this is a measure of adherence or whether it may promote adherence at a certain time. This is true of drug rounds in hospitals where patients may be asked to take their medication as soon as they receive it from the HCW, and the HCW documents this as having successfully administered the medication, but there have been instances whereby patients have simulated this medication-taking behaviour but not swallowed the medication.

7.2.2 Indirect Measures

These tend to be more widely used research and include the use of electronic health records (EHR) electronic monitoring devices, pill count and self-reported measures.

From an adherence point of view, we talk about primary and secondary non-adherence. Primary non-adherence would be the patient who visits their physician and receives a prescription for medication but does not take this to be dispensed. In other words, the non-adherence is clear from the first point in the sequence. Secondary non-adherence is whereby this patient does go to the pharmacy and gets the medication order filled, but having brought the medications home, the medication is not taken at all or not taken as directed.

If we look at the data available from pharmacy claims databases, we can estimate what is often termed the Medication Possession Ration (MPR). The MPR has been defined as the proportion (or percentage) of days' supply obtained during a specified time or over a period of refill intervals [4]. Another method, the Proportion of Days Covered (PDC) is the number of days when the medication was available divided by the number of days in the study period. A cut-off point is commonly advised (e.g. at least 80% adherent), and this allows the group to be divided into adherent and non-adherent [12]. For both the MPR and the PDC, it is important to be clear on how the calculation is performed as this can vary between studies. These measures of adherence may be useful for seeing trends in a particular population, but as we know just because a patient has collected the medicine, it does not mean that it will be taken. The MPR and PDC determine the maximum adherence possible; in other words, if a patient has only collected 30 days of medication in the last 60 days, they are unable to be more than 50% adherent. Conversely, if pharmacists were to interrogate their own data, they would be able to find individual patients who may benefit from a medicine use review (MUR).

A MUR is a planned face-to-face consultation between a pharmacist and a patient to discuss their medicines, both prescribed and non-prescribed. The review is medication adherence-centred and aims to help increase patients' knowledge and understanding of their medicines, including how and why they should be taken. It also provides an opportunity to highlight any medication adherence questions, side effects or other medicine-related problems from the patient's perspective and propose solutions where appropriate [13]. It should be noted, however, that whilst it is relatively common, in some jurisdictions, for pharmacists to perform MUR, other healthcare professionals, for example, nurses, also have a crucial role to play. A recent systematic review by Mardani and colleagues in 2020 highlights the role that nurses play in the medication management process at transitions of care, including, but not limited to, medication reconciliation and monitoring of adverse effects. This review included ten studies conducted between 2014 and 2020, seven studies from the USA, one from Canada, one from Oman and one from Australia. They discuss the role of communication within the multidisciplinary team in the optimization of medication and, thus, better outcomes for patients [14].

There are also electronic monitoring (EM) devices, such as Medication Event Monitoring System (MEMS). The most often used EM device consists of a medication vial cap that has the same appearance as regular medication bottle caps but electronically records the date and time of bottle opening [15]. This has proven useful for those with mental health disorders with one study finding that the greater mean EM adherence was significantly related to lower mean symptom severity in their study population of patients with schizophrenia or schizoaffective disorder [16].

Newer developments in this space include the Ingestible event marker also termed digital health feedback systems. One of the first to be marketed and approved by the Food and Drug Administration (FDA) in 2012 was the Proteus ingestible sensor [17]. These sensors are formulated within the medication and give real-time, data-driven healthcare. The sensor communicates this information regarding ingestion time and other variables (e.g. heart rate) to a patch on the skin which is then communicated to an external electronic device such as mobile phone. Whilst the advantage of having this information accessible to the prescriber is clear, what is not so clear is whether this technology would suit all patient groups.

Pill count is a straightforward process that literally requires the counting of tablets from one appointment to the next. If a patient was due to take one tablet in the morning and one in the evening for 30 days, then the patient receives 60 tablets. If the researcher/clinician wants to check, after 10 days, for example, then they know that there should be 40 tablets remaining and compare this to actual number thereby calculating an adherence ratio. Whilst this is a simple method and one that can be used for different formulations, for example, a pill count can also be used with inhalers to assess the remaining actuations left, nonetheless it also is associated with certain assumptions. There is an assumption that if the tablet is missing that it has been ingested and that this occurred at the correct time.

7.2.3 Subjective Measures

These measures include written questionnaires, semi-structured interviews or perhaps online assessments, and there are over 40 available. I refer the reader to the review article by Nguyen et al. in which the authors have summarized the main measures as well as their advantages and disadvantages for different cohorts [18]. Many of these questionnaires require the patient to self-complete introducing more variability and challenges. If we consider those who are (1) non-native speakers, (2) have low health literacy and/or specifically in the older adult, practicalities such as being able to read the font size and/or ability to accurately recall when and how many medications were taken in the last day(s), we can see that likelihood of having any meaningful data is quite low. Certainly, these measures may be useful in clinical practice by providing an opportunity to discuss any obstacles to medication adherence; however, they would likely lead to inaccuracies and probable overestimation of medication adherence due to the challenges mentioned above and social desirability reporting bias. In addition, not all these questionnaires are free from restrictions regarding their use even for research purposes, so readers should consult the copyright and licensing rules prior to any inclusion in a protocol.

In summary, it is likely that a multi-modal approach encompassing objective and subjective measures will likely yield the most accurate estimate of adherence.

7.3 How to Improve Adherence

The benefits of proper adherence to treatment are several, including preventing diseases, improvement of health, better quality of life and a more cost-effective use of healthcare resources [19]. To date, no single intervention strategy has proven effectiveness in enhancing adherence across all patients, clinical conditions and settings. Unfortunately, a number of knowledge gaps still exist and limit previous clinical trials aiming to improve adherence as well as adherence in the real world population; for instance, poor understanding of the interplay between adherence, multimorbidity and polypharmacy, fragmentation of care and poor communication among care players, the lack of definition of a specific target population, absence of validated information on new technologies and lack of standardized information systems [6].

In a Cochrane review including randomized clinical trials of interventions to improve adherence, measuring both medication adherence and clinical outcome, with at least 80% follow-up of each group studied and at least 6 months' follow-up for studies with positive findings at earlier time points, only few randomized clinical studies showed a low risk of bias and among them only five improved both adherence and clinical outcome [20]. A narrative review focused on the most frequent interventions employed to improve medication adherence and the outcomes achieved, with a special eye on factors associated with ageing and with cognitive impairment or dementia [21]. The authors underlined that older persons have been systematically excluded from randomized clinical trials especially if affected by multimorbidity and prescribed with polypharmacy. As a consequence, the onset of unknown adverse drug reactions during the marketing of the drugs limit adherence in this group of patients. Regarding cognition and drug consumption, a systematic evidence-based review showed the importance of relational aspects in improving adherence in patients with dementia, which may benefit more from human communication as reminder than technology [22]. Indeed, in the same review, only three studies met inclusion criteria of interventional, two evaluated reminder systems and showed no benefit, whereas one study improved adherence through telephone and televideo reminders at each dosing interval. Another reason of poor adherence in older persons living in countries without welfare is the limitation to medications access, the so-called cost-related non-adherence. The Medicare Current Beneficiary Survey showed that in 2016, 34.5% of enrollees under 65 years with disability and 14.4% of those 65 years and older did not take their medications as prescribed due to high costs [23]. Three indicators of worse health (general health status, functional limits and count of conditions) were all independently associated with higher risk of cost-related non-adherence. Strategies that effectively improve adherence could produce financial benefits by attenuating the effect of risk factors and preventing disease progression in a wide number of patients and different settings [24].

A few years ago, a group of professionals with expertise in geriatrics, pharmacology, epidemiology and public health reached a consensus on the possible best interventions to improve adherence in older individuals. Seven strategies were identified and classified based on their target (patient, therapy and public health/society) (Table 7.2): (1) Comprehensive Geriatric Assessment (CGA)—CGA should be administered to all older adults participating in a program aimed at improving medication adherence because it identifies their needs and priorities; (2) patient and caregiver education—educational programs should account for health literacy level and include lifestyle recommendations in order to improve patient empowerment; (3) optimization of treatment—optimized treatment should be reached through clinical decision, use of criteria for appropriate prescription and computerized prescription support systems; (4) use of adherence aids—electronic support devices for patients, particularly alerting non-adherence systems, web-based software tools and wearable units need to be implemented; (5) physicians and other healthcare professionals should be trained by educational professionals through a cascade model and regular meetings focused on improving both medication knowledge and communication skills; (6) adherence assessment—adherence assessment should be mostly objective (e.g. drug refill, clinical assays) and continuous; (7) facilitating access to medicine by service integration by medication delivery and general practitioner pharmacist bidirectional consultation [6]. The authors suggested that the reasons of non-adherence are so multifactorial that interventions to improve it should be patient-centred, involving multiple stakeholders, with the different players providing different services, but integrated with one another. Further, in the near future, information and communication technology (ICT) systems may become particularly relevant for improving adherence, through the use of Tele-Medicine and Internet-linked clinical support models, wireless sensor networks and so forth. ICT technologies may provide self-management utilities for patients and caregivers; education modules for patients, caregivers, and health professionals; and information integration for patient care by physicians and nurses.

At present, another important issue that may limit adherence improvement at population level is the wide variability in methodology used to evaluate adherence

Table 7.2 Interventions to improve adherence [6]

	Definition	Target population	Health professional involved	How	Time
Intervention 1	Comprehensive geriatric Assessment (including adherence behaviour)	All older adults	GP + healthcare assistant	InterRai + tools to assess adherence (i.e. MARS)	Program entry and then every year or if change in health status occurs
Intervention 2	Patient (and caregiver if needed) education to improve patient empowerment	Patients and caregivers or all older and willing to receive the intervention	GP + healthcare assistant, pharmacist, healthcare system, patients associations	Health beliefs model, training, multilevel interventions	Continuously
Intervention 3	Optimization of treatment (reduction of polypharmacy)	All older adults	GP + healthcare assistant	Software (i.e. CDSS) + clinical judgement	Program entry and then every year or if change in health status occurs
Intervention 4	Use of adherence aids	Older adults with cognitive impairment; disability; social isolation; polypharmacy; unintended non-adherence	Pharmacist, ICT company, pharma company	Pillboxes, reminders, blistering by the pharmacy	Continuously
Intervention 5	Physician and other healthcare professional education	Physician and other healthcare professional	Educational professional and professional associations	Cascade model; circle meetings (both focused on improved medication knowledge and communication skill)	Continuously
Intervention 6	Adherence assessment	All older adults	GP + healthcare assistant; pharmacist	Objective (drug refill; drug count; clinical assays) and subjective (i.e. MARS/communication) evaluation	Continuously
Intervention 7	Facilitating access to medicine by service integration	All older adults	GP and pharmacists	ICT, medication delivery, GP-pharmacist bidirectional consultation	Continuously

and poor reporting of findings from research on this topic. An international panel of experts elaborated guidelines to improve the quality of drug adherence research reporting, the ESPACOM Medication Adherence Reporting Guidelines (EMERGE) [25], where ESPACOM is the European Society for Patient Adherence (www.espacom.eu). EMERGE provides guidance on reporting observational and interventional studies on medication adherence useful for different stakeholders, such as investigators, authors, journal editors and health policy decision makers.

Finally, a relevant question to be answered is whether higher adherence to medical prescription would produce better outcomes in older subjects, not only in term of length of life, symptoms control and healthcare utilization [26], but also as beneficial on functional outcomes, such as falls and cognitive decline. In a study of community-dwelling older people presenting a prescription for antihypertensive medication to 106 community pharmacies in Ireland, with no evidence of cognitive impairment, taking antihypertensive medication for ≥1 year ($n = 938$), each 5-day gap in antihypertensive refill adherence increased the risk of self-reported injurious falls by 18% [27].

7.4 Conclusions

Despite being a major cause of morbidity, medication non-adherence in older persons is not well described in the literature, and thus, it is difficult to draw final conclusions on potential barriers and improvements. Future research should focus on standardizing medication adherence measurements and better scientific reporting as well as on clinical trials based on multifactorial interventions.

References

1. Marengoni A, Onder G. Guidelines, polypharmacy, and drug–drug interactions in patients with multimorbidity. BMJ. 2015;350:h1059.
2. Onder G, Bonassi S, Abbatecola AM, Folino-Gallo P, Lapi F, Marchionni N, Geriatrics Working Group of the Italian Medicines Agency, et al. High prevalence of poor-quality drug prescribing in older individuals: a nationwide report from the Italian Medicines Agency (AIFA). J Gerontol A Biol Sci Med Sci. 2014;69(4):430–7.
3. Onder G, Marengoni A, Russo P, Degli Esposti L, Fini M, Monaco A, Geriatrics Working Group of the Italian Medicines Agency (Agenzia Italiana del Farmaco, AIFA), Medicines Utilization Monitoring Center Health Database Network, et al. Advanced age and medication prescription: more years, less medications? A nationwide report from the Italian Medicines Agency. J Am Med Dir Assoc. 2016;17(2):168–72.
4. Growdon ME, Gan S, Yaffe K, Steinman MA. Polypharmacy among older adults with dementia compared with those without dementia in the United States. J Am Geriatr Soc. 2021;69(9):2464–75.
5. https://apps.who.int/iris/handle/10665/42682. Accessed 14 Dec 2022.
6. Marengoni A, Monaco A, Costa E, Cherubini A, Prados-Torres A, Muth C, et al. Strategies to improve medication adherence in older persons: consensus statement from the Senior Italia Federanziani Advisory Board. Drugs Aging. 2016;33(9):629–37.

7. Marengoni A, Onder G, Degli Esposti L, Russo P, Sangiorgi D, Buda S, Geriatrics Steering Committee of the Italian Medicines Agency on Behalf of the OsMed Health-DB Network, et al. Adherence to selective serotonin and serotonin–norepinephrine reuptake inhibitor prescriptions affects overall medication adherence in older persons: evidence from the Italian Nationwide OsMed Health-DB Database. J Clin Psychiatry. 2016;77(12):1712–8.
8. Sabatè E. Adherence to long-term therapies: evidence for action. Geneva: World Health Organization. https://apps.who.int/iris/handle/10665/42682; 2003. Accessed 14 Dec 2022
9. https://digital-strategy.ec.europa.eu/en/policies/eip-aha. Accessed 14 Dec 2022.
10. Hogervorst S, Adriaanse M, Brandt H, Vervloet M, van Dijk L, Hugtenburg J. Feasibility study of a digitalized nurse practitioner-led intervention to improve medication adherence in type 2 diabetes patients in Dutch primary care. Pilot Feasibility Stud. 2021;7:152.
11. CDC—TB 101—Directly Observed Therapy—Web Courses—TB [Internet]. https://www.cdc.gov/tb/webcourses/TB101/index.html. Accessed 15 Dec 2022.
12. Andrade SE, Kahler KH, Frech F, Chan KA. Methods for evaluation of medication adherence and persistence using automated databases. Pharmacoepidemiol Drug Saf. 2006;15(8):565–74.
13. Medicines Use Review. NPA. 2015. https://www.npa.co.uk/services-and-support/nhs-services/medicines-use-review/. Accessed 14 Dec 2022.
14. Mardani A, Griffiths P, Vaismoradi M. The role of the nurse in the management of medicines during transitional care: a systematic review. J Multidiscip Healthc. 2020;13:1347–61.
15. Medication Event Monitoring System (MEMS) | NIH. https://clinicalinfo.hiv.gov/en/glossary/medication-event-monitoring-system-mems. Accessed 14 Dec 2022.
16. Nakonezny PA, Byerly MJ, Rush AJ. Electronic monitoring of antipsychotic medication adherence in outpatients with schizophrenia or schizoaffective disorder: an empirical evaluation of its reliability and predictive validity. Psychiatry Res. 2008;157(1):259–63.
17. FDA approves Proteus Digital Health's e-pills for dose monitoring. Engadget. https://www.engadget.com/2012-08-01-fda-approves-ingestible-sensor.html. Accessed 14 Dec 2022.
18. Nguyen T-M-U, Caze AL, Cottrell N. What are validated self-report adherence scales really measuring? A systematic review. Br J Clin Pharmacol. 2014;77(3):427–45.
19. Osterberg L, Blaschke T. Adherence to medication. N Engl J Med. 2005;353(5):487–97.
20. Nieuwlaat R, Wilczynski N, Navarro T, Hobson N, Jeffery R, Keepanasseril A, et al. Interventions for enhancing medication adherence. Cochrane Database Syst Rev. 2014;2014(11):CD000011.
21. Costa E, Giardini A, Savin M, Menditto E, Lehane E, Laosa O, et al. Interventional tools to improve medication adherence: review of literature. Patient Prefer Adherence. 2015;9:1303–14.
22. Campbell NL, Boustani MA, Skopelja EN, Gao S, Unverzagt FW, Murray MD. Medication adherence in older adults with cognitive impairment: a systematic evidence-based review. Am J Geriatr Pharmacother. 2012;10:165–77.
23. Nekui F, Galbraith AA, Briesacher BA, Zhang F, Soumerai SB, Ross-Degnan D, et al. Cost-related medication nonadherence and its risk factors among medicare beneficiaries. Med Care. 2021;59(1):13–21.
24. Golay A. Pharmacoeconomic aspects of poor adherence: can better adherence reduce healthcare costs? J Med Econ. 2011;14(5):594–608.
25. De Geest S, Zullig LL, Dunbar-Jacob J, Helmy R, Hughes DA, Wilson IB, Vrijens B. ESPACOMP medication adherence reporting guideline (EMERGE). Ann Intern Med. 2018;169(1):30–5.
26. Walsh CA, Cahir C, Bennett KE. Longitudinal medication adherence in older adults with multimorbidity and association with health care utilization: results from the Irish longitudinal study on ageing. Ann Pharmacother. 2021;55(1):5–14.
27. Dillon P, Smith SM, Gallagher PJ, Cousins G. Association between gaps in antihypertensive medication adherence and injurious falls in older community-dwelling adults: a prospective cohort study. BMJ Open. 2019;9(3):e022927.

Medication Reconciliation and Review: Theory, Practice and Evidence

8

Tamasine Grimes and Cristin Ryan

8.1 Introduction

As older people age, the complexity of their medication use often increases as does the frequency of healthcare utilisation. The onset of additional age-related morbidity, destabilisation of chronic conditions and increase in frequency of hospitalisation and healthcare utilisation can add to the older person's medication complexity. Previous research shows that at least 10% of hospital admissions in older people are due to adverse drug reactions and that medication error occurs in 50% of cases following hospital discharge [1, 2]. Therefore, strategies are needed to prevent, recognise and manage medication-related problems prevalent in older patients at points of care transition and throughout the clinical care journey. Medication review and medication reconciliation are processes within an overall medication management strategy that address these issues and collectively aim to improve the older person's transitional medication safety (Fig. 8.1). This chapter describes these processes individually and

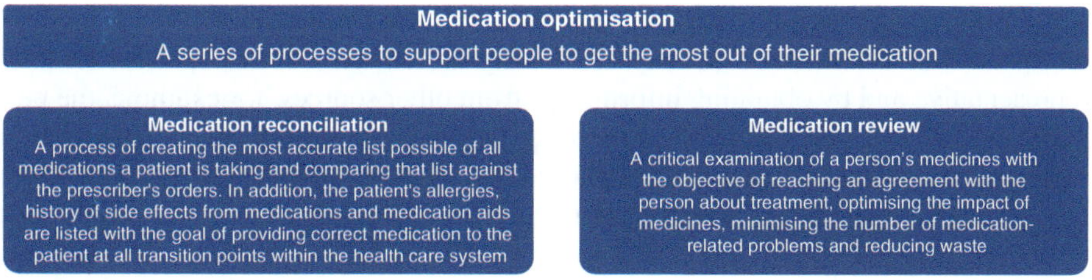

Fig. 8.1 Overview of medication optimisation [3, 4]

T. Grimes (✉) · C. Ryan
School of Pharmacy and Pharmaceutical Sciences, Trinity College Dublin, Dublin, Ireland
e-mail: tagrimes@tcd.ie; Cristin.ryan@tcd.ie

A. Cherubini et al. (eds.), *Optimizing Pharmacotherapy in Older Patients*, Practical Issues in Geriatrics, https://doi.org/10.1007/978-3-031-28061-0_8

collectively within a medication optimisation strategy. It also summarises the evidence regarding effectiveness and implementation and proposes action points for the senior clinician seeking to improve transitional medication safety for older people.

8.2 Medication Reconciliation

8.2.1 Theory

Medication reconciliation is a process intended to increase the integrity of information about a person's medication use that is shared between care providers and settings and across a transition of care, hereon referred to as 'MedRec'. The Delphi consensus definition is presented in Fig. 8.1 [1]. A transition of care is a period in the patient's care when s/he moves from one care setting to another, for example, hospital admission or discharge, or between care providers, for example, transition from one family physician to another. In theory, if a MedRec process is undertaken at a care transition, then information continuity should be achieved, and the likelihood of the patient experiencing medication error or miscommunication should be reduced.

8.2.2 Practice

The MedRec process should ideally be applied at each point of care transition. For example, it should be applied at hospital admission, at internal transfers and then again at hospital discharge (Fig. 8.2). MedRec by itself is quite a transactional process, composed of three steps: (1) collect and create, (2) check by comparing and (3) document and communicate [5].

Step 1: Collect and Create Collect information and create the person's Best Possible Medication History (BPMH). This involves building a comprehensive list of the medications that the person was using immediately prior to the care transition, for example, pre-admission. This is usually created by discussion with the patient or their representative and by obtaining information from other sources, for example, the person's community pharmacist or general practitioner, or an electronic medication record. At least two reference sources should be consulted to build a complete list, one of which is the patient/proxy representative. Importantly, this step should create a list of the medication that the person was actually taking, which can differ from what was prescribed for or dispensed to them. This may uncover potential medication non-adherence; the reader should cross refer to Chap. 7 for information about how to improve adherence.

Step 2: Check by Comparing This is the reconciliation step; it involves either a proactive or a reactive MedRec process (Fig. 8.2). The proactive process sees the BPMH built before the admission orders are made and the *retroactive process* sees the BPMH built after the admission orders are made. In both cases, the BPMH and the post-transition

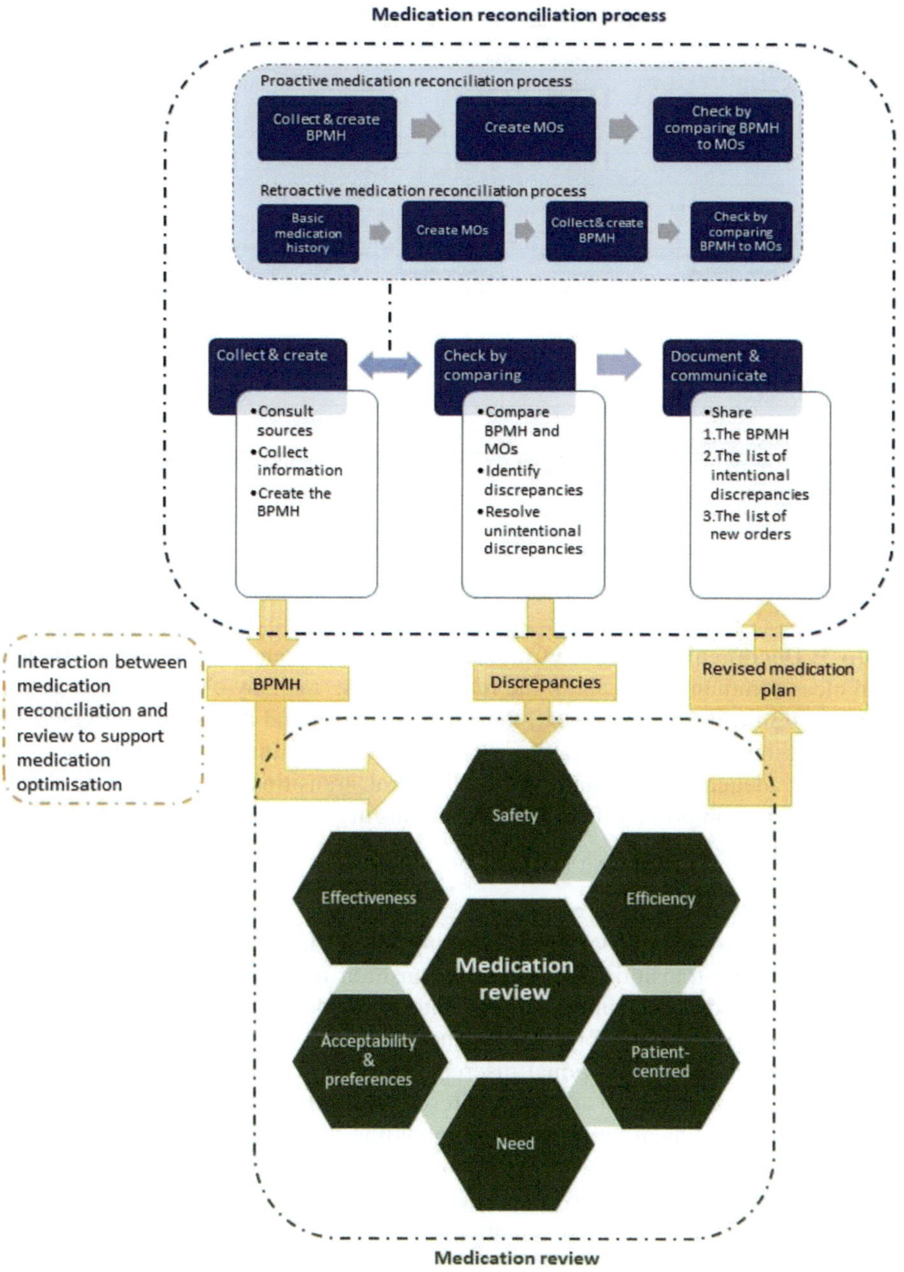

Fig. 8.2 An overview of medication optimisation across care transition. *BPMH* best possible medication history, *MO* medication order

medication orders should be compared to enable identification and resolution of any differences (otherwise called discrepancies) between the two lists. The types of medication discrepancies that are typically identified during MedRec are described below.

A. For use at hospital admission

Healthcare facility identity details				Patient identity details		
Allergy or intolerance information				Vaccination history		
BPMH details (Medication name, dose, frequency, route)		**Medication orders**				
Include all prescribed, over-the-counter, herbal and supplement products	Time/date of last dose	Continue or stop	Discrepancy	Intended	Resolved	Comments
No preadmission medication						

B. For use at hospital discharge

Healthcare facility identity details		Patient identity details		
Allergy or intolerance information		Vaccination history		
List of medication to take after discharge (Medication name, dose, frequency, route, duration)	**Medication reconciliation** Compare discharge list to BPMH and explain any differences			
Include all prescribed, over-the-counter, herbal and supplement products	Unchanged	Changed	New	**Reason for change or addition of medication**
Pre-admission medication stopped in hospital and not to continue after discharge	**Reason for stopping**			

C. For use post-discharge (readmission to the community)

Pre-admission medication list (BPMH) (Medication name, dose, frequency, route)	**Hospital discharge medication list (Medication name, dose, frequency, route, duration)**	**Discrepancy**	**Intended**	**Resolved**	**Comment**

Fig. 8.3 Sample medication reconciliation forms

Step 3: Document and Communicate This step is intended to support complete and clear communication about the medication list, and any changes made across the care transition, to the patient, their representative and the healthcare practitioners contributing to the patient's care following the transition. Sample forms to facilitate adequate communication at several transition points are displayed (Fig. 8.3). It is important that these documents are accessible and readable by lay people (patients/family).

8.2.2.1 Medication Discrepancies

During the MedRec "Check by comparing" step, differences may be identified between the pre-transition and the post-transition medication lists. These differences are termed discrepancies and fall into two broad sub-categories: intentional discrepancies and unintentional discrepancies.

An example of an intentional discrepancy is the omission of a non-steroidal anti-inflammatory drug in a patient presenting to hospital with haematemesis. There is a clear clinical rationale for withholding the medication. Ideally, all people contributing to the person's medication management are aware of that decision, which is typically achieved by documenting in the healthcare record. Studies have identified that undocumented intentional discrepancies can lead to medication error, and therefore, it is helpful to maintain a clear record of prescribing decisions and their rationale. Intentional discrepancies between the pre-transition and post-transition lists are typically the outcome of a medication review and demonstrate the interaction between the two processes to support transitional medication safety.

Unintentional discrepancies are differences between the person's medication list pre-transition and post-transition, which do not have a clinical rationale and are a medication error. For example, omission of long-standing glaucoma eyedrops and respiratory inhalers for a patient admitted with a transient ischaemic attack. The causes of unintentional discrepancies are multi-fold and may relate to the patient, the healthcare professionals, the environment or the organisational care issues.

Medication discrepancies are also categorised by the nature of the difference, the most common being omission of medication, followed by differences in the dosage, frequency, formulation or route of administration, and finally commission of medication, meaning the prescribing or ordering of a medication which the patient is not actually using. Medication discrepancies are a necessary part of medication optimisation and are often a clinically appropriate response to a comprehensive medication review (Fig. 8.2). They become problematic if they are errors (unintentional discrepancies) or if intentional but not documented/communicated (Step 3). Previous studies identified that both unintentional discrepancies and undocumented intentional discrepancies persist across care transitions into the next care setting or episode, potentially exposing the patient to medication-related harm due to incorrect administration or omission of medication.

8.2.3 Evidence

Several systematic reviews have explored the impact of undertaking the MedRec process, few of which have focussed exclusively on older people [6–12]. Most reviews have focussed on the hospital admission and discharge transitions and less on MedRec following hospital discharge or transition to other care settings. Most have investigated the benefit of MedRec as a stand-alone intervention whilst a minority have investigated the benefit of complex transitional care interventions that include MedRec as a component. MedRec interventions have been delivered by a variety of healthcare personnel, most commonly pharmacy, often working interprofessionally, and some studies have investigated electronic solutions.

Medication discrepancy, a process measure, is the most reported outcome in MedRec studies. The available evidence identifies that MedRec alone may reduce the presence of any and sum of medication discrepancies at care transition. However, the certainty of this evidence is low because of the generally poor quality of the available studies. The evidence of a direct benefit of MedRec on clinical outcomes, such as adverse events or healthcare utilisation, is less clear, as is the effect on humanistic outcomes such as quality of life. One systematic review which explored interventions that included activities focussed on medication continuity delivered during hospital stay or following discharge identified that MedRec reduced hospital readmissions [12]. Interventions found to best support older patients' medication continuity and to have the greatest impact on reducing hospital readmission are those that bridge transitions and include patient self-management, telephone follow-up and MedRec activities.

Qualitative research studies, however, enable a broader understanding of the outcomes affected by MedRec at care transitions, for example, the patient's or informal carer's experience, activation, involvement in decision-making, workload around managing medication and knowledge and confidence in medication use at periods around care transitions [13].

8.2.3.1 Optimising Limited Resources

Few studies have undertaken economic analysis of transitional medication safety interventions, providing scant evidence to support investment in scaling up these activities. The MedRec process has been reported to take up to 45 min per patient to complete. Therefore, organisations may not have adequate resources to deliver MedRec to each patient or at each care transition. Decisions may be required about how best to allocate scarce MedRec resources. Risk factors for potentially harmful unintentional medication discrepancy in pre-admission medication have been identified across three domains and may be incorporated into clinical decision support or algorithms to prioritise patients for MedRec at hospital admission [14]:

- Medication-related
  - Increasing number of pre-admission drugs
  - Increasing number of high-risk drugs[a]
  - Class of medication: intake of four of the following classes, gout medication, muscle relaxants, lipid lowering agents, antidepressants and respiratory medication
- Patient-related
  - Age 65+ years is associated with discrepancy compared to younger people, but amongst extremely older (>85) people, advancing age is associated with fewer discrepancies
  - Use of multiple outpatient pharmacies
- Setting-related
  - Lack of availability of a medication list
  - Family member or caregiver consulted as an information source

[a]As defined on the Institute for Safe Medication Practices high-alert or the North Carolina Narrow Therapeutic Index lists

8.2.3.2 Electronic Supports

Studies have explored the benefit of automating all or parts of the MedRec process [10]. Several countries have made national databases of patient's personal medication prescription or dispensing records available for clinical use at care transitions and developed solutions to integrate this information across care settings. Many organisations use electronic medication prescribing and administration systems; some of which include functionality to support the MedRec process. Previous studies have identified a positive benefit of technology-assisted MedRec on medication discrepancies but have also identified challenges with implementing technology at scale and managing human–computer interaction in clinical practice. One review developed a list of ten theories to explain how, why, when, where and for whom personal electronic records of medications (PERMs) are designed, implemented or used in practice at care transitions that impacts on MedRec: (1) Engage stakeholders; (2) Use inclusive design; (3) PERMs should complement existing good practices; (4) Build trust; (5) Tailor training to learners' needs; (6) provide support and deliver on-demand training throughout; (7) Optimise interoperability; (8) Resource investment; (9) Support by legislation or governance to enhance engagement with PERMs; (10) Support patients as users of PERMs [15].

8.2.3.3 The Role of Patients, Family and Informal Carers

Patient and family members contribute meaningfully to the older person's transitional medication safety [13]. For example, they provide critical detail about the patient's medication-taking activities at crucial times, such as patients experiencing acute cognitive changes; they identify and alert the healthcare team to potential medication errors or adverse effects; they participate in decision-making about medication management, and they act as a safety net to mitigate and manage the effects of transitional medication error. Evidence-based opportunities to enhance patient and family involvement in transitional medication optimisation, using the acronym LISTEN, are presented in Table 8.1.

8.2.3.4 Organisational Complexity and Management

Although it appears to be a straightforward process, MedRec has proven to be challenging to implement because it is time consuming and resource intensive. The job of collecting and checking a patient's medication information often spans multiple interpersonal, organisational and temporal boundaries. For example, an older person may be prescribed medication by their family physician and multiple specialist prescribers, s/he may collect medication from one or more community pharmacy(s) and obtain over-the-counter/supplemental medications from multiple retailers. The patient's medication use pattern might change over time, for example, they might be adherent to medication at one moment in time and become non-adherent at another. Therefore, organisations need to invest resources to support MedRec and use those resources efficiently.

Table 8.1 Various ways to engage patients/families in transitional medication safety

L	Listen actively	To patients and families to comprehensively understand the individual patient's complexity, rather than a focus on a single medical condition, to elicit the patient's preferences and aspects of their home situation that may impact on their medication-related needs
I	Involve early	Patients/family early in transition planning and provide opportunity to consider the practical work involved in managing medicines at home, considering who will administer medication; equipment, devices and workforce needed to support this, for example, medication administered via an enteral feeding tube
S	Structure opportunity	To enable patients and families to be actively involved in conversations and decision-making about medication use
T	Timely meetings	Avoid scheduling patient/family meetings at times when patients/family may not be able to engage, for example, the day of discharge
E	Explicit communication	Changes made to a patient's BPMH and the reasoning for them so patients/family can understand and implement these changes when they return to their regular care setting
N	Normalise	Using patients and families during transitions to obtain reliable information about routine medication use

MedRec may be performed by multiple personnel, for example, medical, nursing or pharmacy staff. Studies have examined how accurately different professional groups build the BPMH (the collect and create step), favourably identifying pharmacy and nursing staff, although fewer studies have explored professional roles and responsibilities for the 'check by comparing' and 'document and communicate' steps. In reality, each organisation should assign tasks based on the personnel and resources available to them and ideally should avoid duplication of work, for example, having multiple professionals build a patient's BPMH. All personnel should work to the top of their license, meaning for example, that a pharmacy technician or physician assistant could be tasked with collecting, whilst a pharmacist or physician might be tasked with checking and communicating. Good interprofessional working (teamwork, coordination, collaboration and networking) is essential to MedRec. Opportunities for senior clinicians to support organisational management of MedRec are:

- Assign responsibility for collecting the BPMH to dedicated personnel.
- Employ well-designed forms to support documentation and communication of medication information. This may be electronic or hard-copy.
- Advocate for adequate medical, nursing and pharmacy resource to deliver the MedRec process.
- Measure and monitor MedRec activity and engage in regular audit to assess MedRec performance.
- Encourage training and facilitate competence assessment to support MedRec activities.
- Foster a culture of positive interprofessional working.
- Engineer opportunity to engage and involve patients/family in transitional medication safety activities.

8.3 Medication Review

8.3.1 Theory

A structured clinical medication review is defined as 'a critical examination of a person's medicines with the objective of reaching an agreement with the person about treatment, optimising the impact of medicines, minimising the number of medication-related problems and reducing waste', by the National Institute for Health and Care Excellence in the United Kingdom [3]. The term 'clinical medication review' and linked definition is synonymous with other programmes globally, such as the medication therapy management programme in the United States and the Home Medicines Review in Australia (Table 8.2). The Pharmaceutical Care Network Europe identify that medication review is a step in the pharmaceutical care strategy, that is, it is a component process within a wider medication optimisation system (Figs. 8.1 and 8.2) [16].

Medication reviews, whilst most commonly undertaken by pharmacists, can be undertaken by any healthcare professional in any healthcare setting and are often an

Table 8.2 'Medicines review' and international equivalent terms used defined

Organisation, country	Term used	Definition
Pharmaceutical care network Europe, European-wide	'Medication review'	'A structured evaluation of a patient's medicines with the aim of optimising medicines use and improving health outcomes. This entails detecting drug related problems and recommending interventions'
Pharmaceutical Society of Australia's (PSA), Australia	'Home medicines review'	'Systematic assessment of a consumer's medications and the management of those medications, with the aim of optimising consumer health outcomes and identifying potential medication-related issues within the framework of the quality use of medicines'
National Institute for Health and Care Excellence (NICE, UK), United Kingdom	'Medication review'	'A structured, critical examination of a patient's medicines with the objective of reaching an agreement with the patient about treatment, optimising the impact of medicines, minimising the number of medication related problems and reducing waste'
United States	'Medication therapy management'	'A distinct service or group of services that optimise therapeutic outcomes for individual patients'

interprofessional exercise. When undertaking a medication review, all medicines taken by the patient, that is, prescribed medications and over-the-counter (OTC) medicines, complementary and alternative medicines and supplements should be considered.

The overall aim of undertaking a medication review is to form a partnership with patients to optimise patients' medication regimens and to prevent medication-related problems. Additional aims of a medication review include:

- To enhance patients' knowledge and understanding of their medicines and medical conditions.
- To identify and address any problems that patients' have in adhering to prescribed treatments.
- To identify side effects to prescribed medicines.
- To identify potentially inappropriate prescribing of medicines, including prescribing cascades, drug interactions, therapeutic duplication, suboptimal dosing [i.e. (under and over) and untreated conditions].
- To identify monitoring requirements, for example, cholesterol and undertake appropriate clinical assessments, for example, blood pressure.
- To communicate issues raised during the medication review with the prescriber (if another healthcare professional is undertaking the review).

8.3.2 Practice

A structured medication review should be a collaborative process with the patient/family, facilitating dialogue and shared decision-making, based on the patient's elicited preferences. Skilled questioning is essential to optimise the review by identifying information about preferences, symptoms or signs of adverse effects, achievement of therapeutic goals or evidence of therapeutic failure. There is no single best way to perform a medication review, although tools are available to guide the process, including the Scottish NHS 'seven-step' model and the NO TEARS tool (Table 8.3) [17, 18]. Regardless of the particular approach employed, the review should provide a structured, stepwise approach to developing individualised, patient-centred management plans.

Implementing structured medication review is challenging due to the complexity and consultation time required to manage older patients experiencing (hyper)polypharmacy and multimorbidity. Several tools are available to streamline steps within the medication review process. For example, the 'Stop, sorted, special' approach can help to focus the review by rapidly identifying the medications that should be 'stopped', for example, the condition has resolved or the patient chosen to stop, and those that have already been 'sorted', for example, recently reviewed or no current concerns, thereby maximising the time available to tend to the shortened list of 'special' medications [17]. Additionally, several guidelines and tools exist to support prescribing decisions, including explicit or implicit criteria and mixed or other approaches. The reader is guided to Chaps. 4 and 10 for further detail on this.

A medication-related problem (MRP), also known as a drug-related problem (DRP), is an event or circumstance involving drug therapy that actually or potentially interferes with desired health outcomes. The Pharmaceutical Care Network Europe classifies a DRP as a (potential) problem with (1) treatment effectiveness, (2) treatment safety or (3) other [19]. The (possible) causes for (potential) problems have been categorised (Table 8.3). MRPs have also been classified from the patient perspective into four categories: (1) obtaining medications; (2) taking medications; (3) medication effects, including side effects and concerns over lack of effectiveness and (4) communication and care coordination [14]. The MRPs identified in a

Table 8.3 Sample structured medication review tools and aids

The seven steps medication review	The NO TEARS tool	PCNE DRP causes
Step 1: (Aim) what matters to the patient	**N**eed and indication	Drug selection
Step 2: (Need) identify essential drug therapy	**O**pen questions	Drug form
Step 3: (Need) does the patient take unnecessary drug therapy?	**T**ests and monitoring **E**vidence and guidelines	Dose selection Treatment duration
Step 4: (Effectiveness) are therapeutic objectives being achieved?	**A**dverse events **R**isk reduction or prevention	Dispensing Drug use process
Step 5: (Safety) is the patient at risk of ADRs or suffers actual ADRs?	**S**implification and switches	Patient transfer-related Other
Step 6: (Efficiency) is drug therapy cost-effective?		
Step 7: (Patient-centred) is the patient willing and able to take drug therapy as intended?		

ADR adverse drug reaction, *DRP* drug-related problem, *PCNE* Pharmaceutical Care Network Europe medication review may warrant further intervention at the drug, patient or prescriber level. Such intervention may trigger the need for an additional process such as the management of an interaction (Chap. 3), an inappropriate medication (Chap. 4), a prescribing cascade (Chap. 5), an adverse effect (Chap. 6), adherence (Chap. 7) or deprescribing (Chap. 10), and the reader should consult these chapters for further detail.

8.3.3 Evidence

8.3.3.1 Effectiveness of Medication Review

Systematic reviews have reported the effects of medication review undertaken in multiple settings, including primary care, hospital care and long-term care facilities; some of which included interventions delivered to older people [20–25]. A variety of medication review interventions has been described, including those led by general practice-based pharmacists, hospital pharmacists and pharmacist delivering care to residents of aged care facilities, working independently or collaboratively with prescribers. The findings in general suggest that performing medication review enhances appropriate polypharmacy, supports deprescribing and reduces medication-regimen complexity although the evidence is less clear regarding patient outcomes. Medication review may enhance patient medication adherence, and for certain groups of patients, it may reduce the likelihood of healthcare utilisation (e.g. emergency department visits, hospital (re)admission), patient outcomes (e.g. mortality, adverse drug events, disability), and improve the patient's understanding of and adherence to medication treatment.

8.3.3.2 Optimising Limited Resources

Structured medication review is challenging to implement because it is time consuming and complex. Prioritising medication review for certain patient cohorts of older people using certain classes of medication may enable more efficient use of scarce resources (Table 8.4) [26]. Adverse drug reactions may cause or contribute to hospital admission or may occur during hospital admission. Therefore, medication reviews in secondary care should be targeted at those at risk for or manifesting medication-related harm. There are a number of tools and algorithms available to support this, for example, AT-HARM10 and the DRA Adjudication Guide, and the reader is guided to these and to Chap. 6 to extend learning about this [27, 28].

Table 8.4 Risk patients and risk medications to target for medication review in primary care

Risk medication	Risk patients
Medication increasing risk of falls Anticoagulant medication Blood pressure lowering medication Antidiabetic medication Medication for Parkinson's disease	Frail patients Patients recently discharged from hospital Patients with multimorbidity

8.4 Summary

MedRec, a process to create, check and communicate accurate information about medication use across care settings, should be applied at every care transition including admission to, discharge from and an internal transfer within a healthcare facility. Medication review is a process of critically examining a person's medicines with the objective of reaching an agreement with the person about treatment, optimising the impact of medicines, minimising the number of medication-related problems and reducing waste.

MedRec and medication review may be delivered by medical, nursing or pharmacy staff and often requires patient-centred interprofessional working between these groups. A robust communication infrastructure, electronic or otherwise, is necessary to support both processes, as is workforce planning. MedRec reduces the prevalence and burden of unintentional medication discrepancies and may prevent hospitalisation. Medication review has a positive effect on enhancing the quality of medication use and several patient outcomes, including adherence, the frequency of healthcare utilisation and experiencing medication-related harm.

Patients/family should be facilitated to be actively involved in both MedRec and medication review, and the healthcare professional's interpersonal and interprofessional skills combined with therapeutics expertise are critical to support positive outcomes.

References

1. Alqenae FA, Steinke D, Keers RN. Prevalence and nature of medication errors and medication-related harm following discharge from hospital to community settings: a systematic review. Drug Saf. 2020;43(6):517–37.
2. Oscanoa T, Lizaraso F, Carvajal A. Hospital admissions due to adverse drug reactions in the elderly. A meta-analysis. Eur J Clin Pharmacol. 2017;73(6):759–70.
3. National Institute for Health and Care Excellence. Medicines optimisation: the safe and effective use of medicines to enable the best possible outcomes. NICE Guideline 5. https://www.nice.org.uk/guidance/ng5. Accessed 27 Feb 2022.
4. Penm J, Vaillancourt R, Pouliot A. Defining and identifying concepts of medication reconciliation: an international pharmacy perspective. Res Soc Adm Pharm. 2019;15(6):632–40. https://doi.org/10.1016/j.sapharm.2018.07.020.
5. Institute for Safe Medication Practices Canada. Medication reconciliation in acute care: getting started kit. Canada: Institute for Safe Medication Practices; 2011. https://www.ismp-canada.org/download/MedRec/Medrec_AC_English_GSK_V3.pdf. Accessed 27 Feb 2022
6. Anderson LJ, Schnipper JL, Nuckols TK, Shane R, Le MM, Robbins K, et al. Effect of medication reconciliation interventions on outcomes: a systematic overview of systematic reviews. Am J Health Syst Pharm. 2019;76(24):2028–40. https://doi.org/10.1093/ajhp/zxz236.
7. Guisado-Gil AB, Mejías-Trueba M, Alfaro-Lara ER, Sánchez-Hidalgo M, Ramírez-Duque N, Santos-Rubio MD. Impact of medication reconciliation on health outcomes: an overview of systematic reviews. Res Soc Adm Pharm. 2020;16(8):995–1002. https://doi.org/10.1016/j.sapharm.2019.10.011.
8. Killin L, Hezam A, Anderson KK, Welk B. Advanced medication reconciliation: a systematic review of the impact on medication errors and adverse drug events associated with

transitions of care. Jt Comm J Qual Patient Saf. 2021;47(7):438–51. https://doi.org/10.1016/j.jcjq.2021.03.011.
9. McNab D, Bowie P, Ross A, MacWalter G, Ryan M, Morrison J. Systematic review and meta-analysis of the effectiveness of pharmacist-led medication reconciliation in the community after hospital discharge. BMJ Qual Saf. 2018;27(4):308–20.
10. Mekonnen AB, Abebe TB, McLachlan AJ, Brien JA. Impact of electronic medication reconciliation interventions on medication discrepancies at hospital transitions: a systematic review and meta-analysis. BMC Med Inf Decis Mak. 2016;16:112. https://doi.org/10.1186/s12911-016-0353-9.
11. Redmond P, Grimes TC, McDonnell R, Boland F, Hughes C, Fahey T. Impact of medication reconciliation for improving transitions of care. Cochrane Database Syst Rev. 2018;8:CD010791. https://doi.org/10.1002/14651858.CD010791.pub2.
12. Tomlinson J, Cheong VL, Fylan B, Silcock J, Smith H, Karban K, et al. Successful care transitions for older people: a systematic review and meta-analysis of the effects of interventions that support medication continuity. Age Ageing. 2020;49(4):558–69. https://doi.org/10.1093/ageing/afaa002.
13. Manias E, Bucknall T, Hughes C, Jorm C, Woodward-Kron R. Family involvement in managing medications of older patients across transitions of care: a systematic review. BMC Geriatr. 2019;19(1):95. https://doi.org/10.1186/s12877-019-1102-6.
14. Hias J, Van der Linden L, Spriet I, Vanbrabant P, Willems L, Tournoy J, et al. Predictors for unintentional medication reconciliation discrepancies in preadmission medication: a systematic review. Eur J Clin Pharmacol. 2017;73(11):1355–77.
15. Waldron C, Cahill J, Cromie S, Delaney T, Kennelly SP, Pevnick JM, et al. Personal Electronic Records of Medications (PERMs) for medication reconciliation at care transitions: a rapid realist review. BMC Med Inform Decis Mak. 2021;21(1):1–17. https://doi.org/10.1186/s12911-021-01659-8.
16. Griese-Mammen N, Hersberger KE, Messerli M, Leikola S, Horvat N, van Mil J, et al. PCNE definition of medication review: reaching agreement. Int J Clin Pharm. 2018;40(5):1199–208.
17. Lewis T. A systematic approach to polypharmacy review. BMJ. 2019;364:1034.
18. National Health Service Scotland. The 7-steps medication review. In: Polypharmacy: manage medicines. National Health Service Scotland,, Scotland. 2022. https://managemeds.scot.nhs.uk/for-healthcare-professionals/principles/the-7-steps-medication-review/. Accessed 27 Feb 2022.
19. Pharmaceutical Care Network Europe. PCNE classification for drug-related problems V9.1. Zuidlaren: Pharmaceutical Care Network Europe; 2020. https://www.pcne.org/upload/files/417_PCNE_classification_V9-1_final.pdf. Accessed 27 Feb 2022
20. Christensen M, Lundh A. Medication review in hospitalised patients to reduce morbidity and mortality. Cochrane Database Syst Rev. 2016;2:CD008986. https://doi.org/10.1002/14651858.CD008986.pub3.
21. Hasan Ibrahim AS, Barry HE, Hughes CM. A systematic review of general practice-based pharmacists' services to optimize medicines management in older people with multimorbidity and polypharmacy. Fam Pract. 2021;38(4):509–23. https://doi.org/10.1093/fampra/cmaa146.
22. Jokanovic N, Tan EC, Sudhakaran S, Kirkpatrick CM, Dooley MJ, Ryan-Atwood TE, et al. Pharmacist-led medication review in community settings: an overview of systematic reviews. Res Soc Adm Pharm. 2017;13(4):661–85.
23. Kallio SE, Kiiski A, Airaksinen MS, Mäntylä AT, Kumpusalo-Vauhkonen AE, Järvensivu TP, et al. Community pharmacists' contribution to medication reviews for older adults: a systematic review. J Am Geriatr Soc. 2018;66(8):1613–20.
24. Ming Y, Zecevic AA, Hunter SW, Miao W, Tirona RG. Medication review in preventing older adults' fall-related injury: a systematic review and meta-analysis. Can Geriatr J. 2021;24(3):237–50. https://doi.org/10.5770/cgj.24.478.
25. Thiruchelvam K, Hasan SS, Wong PS, Kairuz T. Residential aged care medication review to improve the quality of medication use: a systematic review. J Am Med Dir Assoc. 2017;18(1):87.e1–e14. https://doi.org/10.1016/j.jamda.2016.10.004.

26. Abrahamsen B, Hansen RN, Rossing C. For which patient subgroups are there positive outcomes from a medication review? A systematic review. Pharm Pract (Granada). 2020;18(4):1976. https://doi.org/10.18549/pharmpract.2020.4.1976.
27. Kempen TG, Hedström M, Olsson H, Johansson A, Ottosson S, Al-Sammak Y, et al. Assessment tool for hospital admissions related to medications: development and validation in older patients. Int J Clin Pharm. 2019;41(1):198–206.
28. Thevelin S, Spinewine A, Beuscart JB, Boland B, Marien S, Vaillant F, et al. Development of a standardized chart review method to identify drug-related hospital admissions in older people. Br J Clin Pharmacol. 2018;84(11):2600–14.

9 The Role of Pharmacists in Optimising Drug Therapy

Anne Spinewine, Stephen Byrne, and Olivia Dalleur

9.1 Pharmaceutical Care at Patient Level

9.1.1 Medication Review

Following a consensus consultative process undertaken in 2018 defined a medication review (MR) "*as a structured evaluation of a patient's medicines with the aim of optimising medicines use and improving health outcomes. This entails detecting drug-related problems and recommending interventions*" [1]. The extensive consultative process included consultation amongst over 200 healthcare professionals (HCPs) across 35 countries and resulted also in a medication review classification, which also took into consideration the available sources of information.

The overarching aim of an MR is to improve the quality, safety and appropriate use of medicines. Such a review can be conducted by multiple HCPs themselves or in collaboration with the prescribing physician [2], and there is a growing body of evidence in the literature that medication reviews result in improved prescribing outcomes such as reduced polypharmacy, inappropriate prescribing and adverse drug effects for patients [3].

The complexity of the medication review is determined by the nature of the patient, their concurrent illnesses and their co-prescribed medications. The depth of the review is also influenced by the level of detailed information available to the

A. Spinewine · O. Dalleur
Université catholique de Louvain, Louvain Drug Research Institute and Faculty of Pharmacy and Biomedical Sciences, Brussels, Belgium
e-mail: anne.spinewine@chuuclnamur.uclouvain.be; anne.spinewine@uclouvain.be; olivia.dalleur@uclouvain.be; olivia.dalleur@saintluc.uclouvain.be

S. Byrne (✉)
Pharmaceutical Care Research Group, School of Pharmacy, University College Cork, Cork, Ireland
e-mail: Stephen.Byrne@ucc.ie

A. Cherubini et al. (eds.), *Optimizing Pharmacotherapy in Older Patients*, Practical Issues in Geriatrics, https://doi.org/10.1007/978-3-031-28061-0_9

HCP at the time of the review. The Pharmaceutical Care Network European (PCNE) group in 2018 also agreed through their consensus process on four subtypes of medication reviews, ranging from those conducted in a community pharmacy, to more comprehensive reviews, which require full access to patient's medical record (e.g. access to medical notes in hospital, long-term care or general practice settings). The subclassification of a medication review is as follows:

- "**PCNE Type 1:** ***Simple MR***: A simple medication review is based on the available medication history in the pharmacy; this type of review occurs routinely during the medication supply/dispensing process, for example, drug–drug interactions, reviewing the appropriateness of a particular medication dosages, potential side effects and medication adherence issues."
- **"PCNE Type 2A:** ***Intermediate MR***: An intermediate medication review can be performed when the patient can be approached for information. Such a review is based on medication history and patient information." Which builds upon a Type 1 review and expands the review to include issues such as drug–food interactions, issues with over-the-counter (OTC) medication and medication effectiveness issues.
- **"PCNE Type 2B: Intermediate MR**: An intermediate medication review can be performed if information from the general practitioner is also available. Such a review is based on medication history and medical information." This type of review builds upon Type 2A by including the identification of potential medicines without a current clinical indication.
- **"PCNE Type 3:** ***Advanced MR***: An advanced medication review is based on medication history, patient information and clinical information. This type of review is the most comprehensive and in-depth review and results in all of the above being addressed with the addition of the identification of an indication without a potential medication being prescribed for its treatment [1].

In addition to strong clinical and technical skills, interprofessional communication and collaboration are central to the effective implementation of medication review services for patients [4].

9.1.2 Continuity of Supply and Care

Continuity of medication supply and continuity of care is essential whenever patients' transition from one setting to another or from one HCP to another takes place. Principles ensuring continuity of care in medication management include: (a) developing processes of care and responsibilities across the caregivers to coordinate the medication discharge plan as early as possible after admission; (b) obtaining an accurate medication history upon admission; (c) evaluating the current medication list as compared to the medication history in order to detect and reconcile discrepancies, to perform medication review and to establish a treatment plan, on admission as well as at discharge; (d) involving the patient in the treatment plan decisions; (e) ensuring the patient has been educated about the discharge treatment plan; (f) dispensing an adequate amount of medication at discharge and (g) communicating to follow-up healthcare [5]. A core concept that is closely related to these principles is medication reconciliation (MedRec) (see Chap. 8). MedRec has been defined as "*the process of identifying the most accurate list of all medications a patient is taking—including name, dosage, frequency, and route—and using this list to provide correct medications for patients anywhere within the health care system*" [6]. MedRec is a safety strategy adopted by most guidelines and health organisations that should be performed at each transition, ideally within 24 h.

MedRec prevents transcribing errors, improves monitoring of prescriptions, facilitates switch from medication taken at home towards formulary medicines upon admission [7]. By improving communication between HCPs and with the patient, MedRec reduces medication discrepancies and potentially harmful medication errors. In older patients specifically, pharmacist-led MedRec reduces medication errors [8]. However, evidence on patient-related clinical outcomes is inconclusive. Nevertheless, a meta-analysis focusing on the effectiveness of pharmacist-led MedRec on patient-related clinical outcomes during the transition to and from hospital settings showed a reduction in drug-related hospital revisits, emergency department visits and in hospital readmissions [9]. Additionally, there is evidence that pharmacist-led MedRec at discharge could be a cost-effective intervention by reducing readmissions [10].

Many pharmaceutical societies provide guidelines, practical tools and educational support for MedRec implementation. Strategies for implementing MedRec include the use of standardised forms, electronic reconciliation tools, collaborative models and patient engagement.

After discharge, many patients might have difficulties with medication management, including delays in filling their medications. Therefore, at discharge, additional pharmacists' interventions complement MedRec to improve continuity of care, often evaluated in the literature in combination: supplying of medications, medication counselling of patients, provision of verbal and written information to the patient, communication between primary and secondary care providers, follow-up phone calls with the patient or the community pharmacist and home visits. These interventions are particularly recommended in older patients and can be performed by both the hospital pharmacist and the community pharmacist.

The written report that all patients and subsequent HCPs receive at discharge, also called discharge plan, contains a detailed list of all medications the patient is currently taking (name and respective indications, strength, form, timing, frequency, duration, date and time of the last dose), identification and explanation about medicines that have been started/stopped, any known adverse reactions and known allergies. This report is in a format suitable and adapted to the patient's and/or carer's health literacy.

9.1.3 Patient Education and Shared Decision-Making

Medication adherence has been defined as "*the process by which patients take their medications as prescribed*" [11]. Several factors influence adherence such as knowledge and skills in managing medications, previous side effects, health literacy, beliefs about the medication and lack of involvement in the treatment decision-making process.

Patient education is a common intervention to improve medication adherence. Pharmacists-led education can be provided in several settings and formats: meeting during hospital stay, consultations, including in community pharmacies, provision of written information, home visits, phone calls and motivational interviewing [12]. Rather than just presenting information about medications, pharmacist discusses it and assesses non-adherence and beliefs about medication. Education to tackle non-adherence should include tailored practical suggestion (e.g. to the type of medicines or regimen, monitoring, use of a pill-box or reminders). Pharmacists also implement patient self-management plans, to support people with chronic conditions who want to be involved in managing of their own medicines. Patient education can be general or specifically focused on oncology medications, anticoagulation, antihypertensive drugs, analgesics, potentially inappropriate medications, fall-risk medications and so forth. Health literacy tools can help pharmacists adapt education and counselling.

Although evidence of pharmacists-led education in older patients on adherence and clinical outcomes is inconsistent, some studies have shown promising results on optimisation of medication in terms of deprescribing of inappropriate medications and benzodiazepines in ambulatory and hospital setting [13, 14].

Most patients, including the older ones, wish to be involved in making decisions about their own medicines. Shared decision-making (SDM) is "*an approach where healthcare professionals and patients share the best available evidence when faced with making decisions regarding healthcare, and where patients are supported to consider options to achieve informed preferences*" [15]. In older patients, SDM and patient involvement are important to reduce inappropriate polypharmacy. Moreover, SDM results in older patient to choose more conservative options (medication reduction or cessation, less initiation of new drugs), which support deprescribing and decrease of treatment burden [16, 17]. Pharmacists should integrate shared decision-making (SDM) with the patient in their medication review and treatment optimisation process. They can also help develop medication decision tools, which will support discussion but not replace it.

9.2 Pharmacists' Role in the Education and Training of Other Healthcare Professionals

Pharmacy teams internationally have played a pivotal role in the education and training of fellow HCPs in both the acute and non-acute settings over several decades. Such education and training sessions take place both in formal, for example, lecture, and/or informal, for example, ward rounds settings, but one thing is clear, if our desire is to improve prescribing amongst older patients, then constant and up-to-date education of all prescribers including non-medical prescribers (e.g. nurse and other HCP prescribers) is crucial. There have been numerous educational interventions published in the literature, which aim to enhance prescribing appropriateness [18, 19].

Several different approaches have been used to deliver these education sessions from traditional lecture sessions with pre-printed materials to more innovative approaches such as massive open online course (MOOC) and academic detailing [20–22]. Interestingly, the majority of reported educational interventions published in the literature examine the impact of an intervention on a single agent of a single drug class, for example, antibiotics [21] and hypnotics [19]. Relatively few educational studies have examined the broader issue of prescribing in an older population. The benefits of such single drug/drug class education interventions are that the prescriber's knowledge of that particular medicine/drug class is enhanced substantially, although broader educational issues, for example, pharmacokinetic and pharmacodynamic alteration in older patients, may be required by the prescriber to prepare them for the complex issues which are routinely present in this population.

In recent years, pharmacists have become increasingly involved in the delivery of educational materials via academic detailing [20]. Academic detailing is a means of delivering continuing education to HCPs by another trained HCP such as a pharmacist, nurse or doctor. The trainer visits the trainee, that is, the prescriber in their practice setting and provides evidence-based information on a selected topic [23]. These outreach educational sessions are interactive in nature and can be tailored to the needs of the trainee. They also facilitate discussion and feedback during the session.

Likewise, pharmacists have embraced the use of online educational platforms. These platforms have facilitated the delivery of materials simultaneous to large audiences via MOOC or E-learning platforms. These online modes of delivery have enabled broader topics such as altered pharmacokinetic and pharmacodynamic principles of an older population to be discussed and delivered to the audience [24, 25]. Both online delivery methods have their advantages and disadvantages, but a key advantage is the ability to deliver tailored materials to large numbers of prescribers simultaneously.

9.3 Models of Pharmacy Practice in Different Settings of Care and Countries

Clinical pharmacy services with a focus on older people (also called "geriatric pharmacy practice") emerged in the mid-1970s, and since then a substantial body of published literature has accumulated, demonstrating patient safety and economic benefits of clinical pharmacy services for older people, including evidence from randomised controlled trials [26]. Clinical pharmacy services have been shown to improve prescribing, prevent adverse drug reactions and medication errors, improve patients' medication knowledge and adherence and, in some populations, reduce the risk of medication-related hospital admissions [26].

This movement of pharmacists' involvement in direct patient care away from the traditional medication-dispensing/supply functions is widespread globally, although there is major inter- and intra-country variability in the practice models and their level of implementation [27, 28]. Below we describe and discuss these models of practice in each type of setting of care.

9.3.1 Ambulatory Care

The availability of MR services provided by pharmacists in ambulatory care is increasing worldwide, although it is varying in content, scope, implementation and level of interprofessional collaboration across countries.

European data show that at least one type of MR service is implemented in community pharmacy in more than half of European countries, either as a project or as an implemented service [29, 30]. Type 2A MR is the more widespread, because it is more convenient to implement in the community pharmacy setting [29]. Four countries (Switzerland, England, The Netherlands and Northern Ireland) had a reimbursed, fully implemented MR (type 2B or type 3) service in the community pharmacy [30]. Such pharmaceutical care service is also available in non-EU countries such as Australia, New Zealand and the United States of America. In Canada, the service is organised on a province level with variability in eligibility criteria and reimbursement of MR services. There is funding for providing specific recommendations to prescribers on various types of drug-related problems. Such pharmaceutical opinions, coupled to sending patients an educational deprescribing brochure, have shown to be effective in discontinuation of inappropriate prescriptions in older people [14].

MR services in the community pharmacy offer significant opportunities to support patients with managing comorbidities and complex medicine regimens, although many challenges remain to be overcome, ranging from poor public awareness and acceptance, organisational constraints, and issues over interprofessional collaboration [31]. As an example, a study of Bulajeva found that only half of intermediate MR services available in Europe incorporated reporting to the physician and a third included multidisciplinary case conferences during the review.

In a few countries, type 3 MR is performed by pharmacists outside the community pharmacy. In England, for example, since 2015, clinical pharmacists can be hired in general practitioner practices and perform, amongst other tasks, MR and medication reconciliation [32]. Evidence from published evaluations suggests that pharmacists in general practice can have a positive impact on clinical outcomes, may reduce medication-related hospitalisations. This model may provide advantages over a community pharmacy service, including (co-)location, access to medical records to inform the quality and appropriateness of recommendations, the potential for formal and informal communication and discussion of the pharmacist's recommendations and reduced fragmentation of care. In Australia, the Home Medicines Review program started in 2001 [4]. This Commonwealth-funded program aims to maximise patient benefit from medicines and prevent drug-related problems through a collaborative process involving both general practitioners and accredited pharmacists. It includes the following steps: the general practitioner identifies and refers the patient for MR; an accredited pharmacist visits the patient at home and obtains a comprehensive medication history, then documents its medication review findings and recommendations in a report for the general practitioner (GP); then based on this, the GP and patient formulate a medication plan [4]. The positive impact has been demonstrated on medication use measures mainly [4].

9.3.2 Acute Care

Drug-related admissions, adverse drug events during hospital stay and after discharge are all frequent in older people with multimorbidity and polypharmacy. The involvement of clinical pharmacists to optimise drug therapy in older inpatients is, therefore, appealing. Various practices for pharmacists' involvement in the care of inpatients exist, ranging from single approaches such as simple or intermediate MR during hospital stay to more comprehensive, multifaceted and collaborative approaches implemented from admission to discharge or even post-discharge. Current evidence to date shows that medication reconciliation, patient education, HCP education and transitional care are essential elements that need to be implemented in addition to medication review to reach an effect on hospital readmissions [33–35]. Even though there has been some progress over the last decade, such comprehensive model of care is not yet widely implemented in hospitals in Europe and beyond. The role of the "ward-based clinical pharmacist," whilst well established in some countries, is still a rarity in others. Lack of capacity, capability and support from managers are the commonly cited reasons for this [36, 37].

In the case of limited resources, pharmacists and hospital managers may decide to have a comprehensive model of practice implemented for a restricted number of older people at highest risk of drug-related problems, or to have a less comprehensive and more diluted approach implemented for a larger population. The former approach is probably preferable, although there are no strong direct comparison data available to date to confirm this.

9.3.3 Long-Term Care

Polypharmacy, together with other factors such as frailty and complexity of the medication use process, makes the safe use of medications for nursing home residents highly challenging, and pharmacists have been involved in many initiatives aiming to optimise the use of medicines in that setting. Pharmacists' contribution to optimise medicines use in the nursing home setting includes (a) practices directed at nursing home residents, often in the form of medication reviews, which can be uni- or multiprofessional, and aimed at specific drugs or the whole regimen and (b) practices directed at HCPs—often educational approaches directed at prescribers [19, 38]. These practices are described further below. Even though most activities performed to date by pharmacists focus on the prescription component, there is wide room for pharmacists' input towards improving administration process—although only limited data are available on the practice models and evidence of effect [38].

In several countries such as the United Kingdom, Australia and the United States, comprehensive MR programs in nursing homes are funded. MRs are generally conducted collaboratively by the resident's general practitioner and a pharmacist who is accredited to conduct MRs (also referred to as consultant pharmacists). As an example, Australian guidelines recommend that a MR (called Residential Medication Management Review—similar to the Home Medicines Review program funded in ambulatory care) is provided as soon as possible after an individual first enters permanent residential care and when clinical circumstances change [4, 39]. Each review identifies an average of 2.7–3.9 medication-related problems per resident receiving the service, with general practitioners accepting 45–84% of pharmacists' recommendations [40]. Targeted MRs for people taking psychotropic drugs is also recommended and encouraged in several countries. There is evidence that such programs lead to more appropriate prescriptions and lower use of sedative and anticholinergics drug use, although certainty of the evidence was found to be low in a Cochrane review [19]. Some recent clinical trials showed positive results of collaborative and innovative approaches towards MR in the nursing home setting, for example, by involving nursing home residents and/or nurses in the process [41, 42]. Wider scale implementation of these approaches has yet to occur.

Pharmacists also contribute to optimised medication use in nursing homes through educational approaches, case conferencing, audit and feedback directed at other HCPs (or sometimes at nursing home residents and their families) [18, 28]. Such practices are less resource intensive—and may, therefore, be encouraged in countries where there is no government-funded MR program. They may contribute to better use of medicines, although probably with lower effect than comprehensive MR. As an example, in Switzerland there is funding for regular meetings (also called quality circles) between pharmacists, physicians and nurses active in a nursing home, with the goal of producing local prescribing consensus to improve drug use [43]. This approach led, in particular, to a reduction in drug costs and improved antibiotics stewardship.

9.3.4 Interprofessional Practice is Desirable But Challenging to Implement

Pharmacists have distinct expertise that can contribute to team knowledge and competence in managing older patients with polypharmacy and multiple chronic conditions. Importantly, evidence shows that globally, interventions developed by a pharmacist within a multidisciplinary team seem to provide greater benefits in terms of clinical outcomes and economic results than those carried out by individual pharmacists [34].

Pharmacists can be members of geriatric evaluation and management (GEM) teams. Such teams provide comprehensive geriatric assessment, which is by nature interdisciplinary. Studies have shown that pharmacists working in geriatric evaluation and management teams have favourable effects on therapeutic, safety, hospitalisation, and adherence outcomes in older adults [27]. This is most easily implemented in the acute care setting with clinical pharmacists.

Interprofessional collaboration in the primary care setting is critical for sustaining high-quality care in the context of the increasing burden on primary healthcare services [44]. Several studies have shown positive effects of working as a team, including better care continuity and coordination, beneficial changes in patient behaviour, improvement of patient symptoms and satisfaction through better response to their needs [45]. However, health providers in primary health care settings—and pharmacists are no exception to this—face enormous ideological, organisational, structural and relational challenges whilst promoting teamwork and interprofessional collaboration [46]. A better understanding of barriers and enablers for effective interprofessional collaboration are essential for adapting services and context, whenever possible. For example, collaboration between general practitioners and community pharmacists is mostly facilitated by an environment with sufficient resources and a close distance between the two professions, clear and regular communication, experience with collaboration and understanding each other's capabilities and roles towards delivering patient care [44]. Although this takes time to evolve, progress is being made in the right direction.

9.3.5 The Prescribing Pharmacist

Traditionally the prescribing role has being a key domain of the medical practitioner, although globally numerous healthcare systems have broadened this authority to other HCPs, for example, nurses, pharmacist, physiotherapist, in the form of supplementary or independent prescribing [47]. The expansion of such authority has demonstrated several benefits in terms of increased patient satisfaction, cost effectiveness [37], concordance with therapeutic regimens [48], increasing continuity of care and increased medication access [49, 50]. This broadening of roles for other HCPs has been in response to changing service needs and increased specialist roles within these professionals [47].

Key drivers resulting in the expansion of prescription authority have been a desire by medical providers to reduce costs whilst simultaneously enhancing patient services, whereas a key barrier for many healthcare professions to take on such roles in the past has been the lack of access to patient's clinical data and medical notes. Without access to such data, it is hard for any professionals to provide clinically appropriate advice pertaining to either prescribing or indeed appropriate advice in relation to deprescribing [25, 47].

The impact of non-medical prescribing upon professional boundaries and relationships is often dependent upon whether supplementary or independent prescribing is legislated. In the former, continued medical authority/responsibility is retained by the physician with supplementary prescribing authority given to the pharmacist by the doctor after they have undertaken the clinical assessment and made the initial diagnosis. This typically involves an agreed clinical management plan/protocol in advance for a given cohort of patient, for example, diabetic treatment plans [47, 51, 52], whereas the independent prescribing model is more self-governing/autonomous allowing the non-medical prescriber to diagnose and prescribe without direct involvement from a medical practitioner [47].

Within the countries where pharmacists have prescribing authorisation either as independent or supplemental prescribers, their scope of practice may vary considerably depending on whether formularies or agreed protocols are in existence [47]. The development of such protocols and formularies in collaboration with medical staff could potentially lead to restrictions being placed upon non-medical prescribers' scope of practice [53].

Generally, the literature has reported that in practice, non-medical prescribing increases effectiveness and independence of the HCP, but it also raises issues concerning confidence, workload and the need for continued specialist training in the form of CPD (continued professional development) [54]. Non-medical prescribers tend also to be aware of their limitations and are known to regularly consult with medical colleagues on complex cases [47].

The role of the pharmacist prescribing continues to grow in various healthcare setting internationally, although differences in legislative procedures/practices by professional bodies and governments has resulted in the implementation of several models of pharmacist prescribing worldwide [47, 54]. Nonetheless, prescribing pharmacists internationally continue to publicise that extending prescribing rights has allowed them to utilise their therapeutics knowledge, gain increased professional recognition and demonstrate enhanced patient care [47].

9.4 Conclusions and Perspectives

Pharmacists have specific knowledge and skills that are essential to optimising medication use in older people. At the patient individual level, pharmacists' activities most frequently encompass medication review, medication reconciliation and patient education. Several models of care have been implemented in different settings of care (ambulatory, acute and long-term care) in many countries, although there remains a large variability in the existence and implementation for such services worldwide. More comprehensive, patient-centred and interprofessional approaches seem to provide greater benefit, although there are more challenges to implementing these approaches, especially in the ambulatory setting. Standardisation and enhanced coverage/implementation of geriatric pharmacist practice are important challenges for the future.

Pharmacists also make an important contribution to optimising medication use in older people by educating other HCPs. This can happen through different approaches, from traditional lecture sessions to more innovative approaches such as massive open online course and academic detailing.

Finally, and even though this was not specifically addressed in the current chapter, the role of pharmacists as researchers—to measure the quality of medication use, understand the barriers and enablers, and design and evaluate the effect of optimisation approaches—is also an important contribution towards optimising pharmacotherapy in older patients.

References

1. Griese-Mammen N, Hersberger KE, Messerli M, Leikola S, Horvat N, van Mil JWF, et al. PCNE definition of medication review: reaching agreement. Int J Clin Pharm. 2018;40(5):1199–208.
2. Blenkinsopp A, Bond C, Raynor DK. Medication reviews. Br J Clin Pharmacol. 2012;74(4):573–80.
3. O'Mahony D, Gudmundsson A, Soiza RL, Petrovic M, Jose Cruz-Jentoft A, Cherubini A, et al. Prevention of adverse drug reactions in hospitalized older patients with multi-morbidity and polypharmacy: the SENATOR* randomized controlled clinical trial. Age Ageing. 2020;49(4):605–14.
4. Chen TF. Pharmacist-led home medicines review and residential medication management review: the Australian model. Drugs Aging. 2016;33(3):199–204.
5. Australian Pharmaceutical Advisory Council. National guidelines to achieve the continuum of quality use of medicines between hospital and community. Canberra: Commonwealth Department of Health and Family Services; 1998.
6. review I-IfHIMr. http://www.ihi.org:80/resources/Pages/Tools/MedicationReconciliationReview.aspx.
7. Redmond P, Grimes TC, McDonnell R, Boland F, Hughes C, Fahey T. Impact of medication reconciliation for improving transitions of care. Cochrane Database Syst Rev. 2018;8:CD010791.
8. Cameli D, Francis M, Francois VE, Medder NR, Von Eden L, Truglio-Londrigan M. A systematic review of medication reconciliation strategies to reduce medication errors in community dwelling older adults. JBI Libr Syst Rev. 2012;10(42 Suppl):1–18.
9. Mekonnen AB, McLachlan AJ, Brien JA. Effectiveness of pharmacist-led medication reconciliation programmes on clinical outcomes at hospital transitions: a systematic review and meta-analysis. BMJ Open. 2016;6(2):e010003.
10. Najafzadeh M, Schnipper JL, Shrank WH, Kymes S, Brennan TA, Choudhry NK. Economic value of pharmacist-led medication reconciliation for reducing medication errors after hospital discharge. Am J Manag Care. 2016;22(10):654–61.
11. Vrijens B, De Geest S, Hughes DA, Przemyslaw K, Demonceau J, Ruppar T, et al. A new taxonomy for describing and defining adherence to medications. Br J Clin Pharmacol. 2012;73(5):691–705.
12. Kini V, Ho PM. Interventions to improve medication adherence: a review. JAMA. 2018;320(23):2461–73.
13. Marcum ZA, Hanlon JT, Murray MD. Improving medication adherence and health outcomes in older adults: an evidence-based review of randomized controlled trials. Drugs Aging. 2017;34(3):191–201.
14. Martin P, Tamblyn R, Benedetti A, Ahmed S, Tannenbaum C. Effect of a pharmacist-led educational intervention on inappropriate medication prescriptions in older adults: the D-PRESCRIBE randomized clinical trial. JAMA. 2018;320(18):1889–98.
15. Joseph-Williams N, Lloyd A, Edwards A, Stobbart L, Tomson D, Macphail S, et al. Implementing shared decision making in the NHS: lessons from the MAGIC programme. BMJ. 2017;357:j1744.
16. Jansen J, Naganathan V, Carter SM, McLachlan AJ, Nickel B, Irwig L, et al. Too much medicine in older people? Deprescribing through shared decision making. BMJ. 2016;353:i2893.
17. Tinetti ME, Naik AD, Dindo L, Costello DM, Esterson J, Geda M, et al. Association of patient priorities-aligned decision-making with patient outcomes and ambulatory health care burden among older adults with multiple chronic conditions: a nonrandomized clinical trial. JAMA Intern Med. 2019;179(12):1688–97.

18. Loganathan M, Singh S, Franklin BD, Bottle A, Majeed A. Interventions to optimise prescribing in care homes: systematic review. Age Ageing. 2011;40(2):150–62.
19. Alldred DP, Kennedy MC, Hughes C, Chen TF, Miller P. Interventions to optimise prescribing for older people in care homes. Cochrane Database Syst Rev. 2016;2:CD009095.
20. Duckett A, Cuoco T, Pride P, Wiley K, Iverson PJ, Marsden J, et al. Academic detailing to teach aging and geriatrics. Gerontol Geriatr Educ. 2015;36(4):331–42.
21. Lutters M, Harbarth S, Janssens JP, Freudiger H, Herrmann F, Michel JP, et al. Effect of a comprehensive, multidisciplinary, educational program on the use of antibiotics in a geriatric university hospital. J Am Geriatr Soc. 2004;52(1):112–6.
22. Nicolas C, Balardy L, Antoine V, Albarede J, Azria D, Cristol L, et al. Spreading geriatric oncology culture through professional caregivers: results of a French massive open online course (MOOC). J Geriatr Oncol. 2021;13(1):94–9.
23. O'Brien MA, Rogers S, Jamtvedt G, Oxman AD, Odgaard-Jensen J, Kristoffersen DT, et al. Educational outreach visits: effects on professional practice and health care outcomes. Cochrane Database Syst Rev. 2007;4:CD000409.
24. Cullinan S, O'Mahony D, Byrne S. Use of an e-learning educational module to better equip doctors to prescribe for older patients: a randomised controlled trial. Drugs Aging. 2017;34(5):367–74.
25. Rankin A, Cadogan CA, Patterson SM, Kerse N, Cardwell CR, Bradley MC, et al. Interventions to improve the appropriate use of polypharmacy for older people. Cochrane Database Syst Rev. 2018;9:CD008165.
26. Elliott RA. Geriatric medicine and pharmacy practice: a historical perspective. J Pharm Pract Res. 2016;46:9.
27. Lee JK, Slack MK, Martin J, Ehrman C, Chisholm-Burns M. Geriatric patient care by U.S. pharmacists in healthcare teams: systematic review and meta-analyses. J Am Geriatr Soc. 2013;61(7):1119–27.
28. Spinewine A, Fialova D, Byrne S. The role of the pharmacist in optimizing pharmacotherapy in older people. Drugs Aging. 2012;29(6):495–510.
29. Imfeld-Isenegger TL, Soares IB, Makovec UN, Horvat N, Kos M, van Mil F, et al. Community pharmacist-led medication review procedures across Europe: characterization, implementation and remuneration. Res Soc Adm Pharm. 2020;16(8):1057–66.
30. Soares IB, Imfeld-Isenegger TL, Makovec UN, Horvat N, Kos M, Arnet I, et al. A survey to assess the availability, implementation rate and remuneration of pharmacist-led cognitive services throughout Europe. Res Soc Adm Pharm. 2020;16(1):41–7.
31. Latif A. Community pharmacy medicines use review: current challenges. Integr Pharm Res Pract. 2017;7:83–92.
32. Alshehri AA, Cheema E, Yahyouche A, Haque MS, Jalal Z. Evaluating the role and integration of general practice pharmacists in England: a cross-sectional study. Int J Clin Pharm. 2021;43(6):1609–18.
33. Dautzenberg L, Bretagne L, Koek HL, Tsokani S, Zevgiti S, Rodondi N, et al. Medication review interventions to reduce hospital readmissions in older people. J Am Geriatr Soc. 2021;69(6):1646–58.
34. Delgado-Silveira E, Velez-Diaz-Pallares M, Munoz-Garcia M, Correa-Perez A, Alvarez-Diaz AM, Cruz-Jentoft AJ. Effects of hospital pharmacist interventions on health outcomes in older polymedicated inpatients: a scoping review. Eur Geriatr Med. 2021;12(3):509–44.
35. Van der Linden L, Hias J, Walgraeve K, Flamaing J, Tournoy J, Spriet I. Clinical pharmacy services in older inpatients: an evidence-based review. Drugs Aging. 2020;37(3):161–74.
36. European Association of Hospital Pharmacists aKU, Center for Medicines Optimisation. European Statements of Hospital Pharmacy survey results 2018: statements sections 1, 3, 4. Brussels: EAHP; 2018–2019.
37. Dalton K, Byrne S. Role of the pharmacist in reducing healthcare costs: current insights. Integr Pharm Res Pract. 2017;6:37–46.
38. Spinewine A, Evrard P, Hughes C. Interventions to optimize medication use in nursing homes: a narrative review. Eur Geriatr Med. 2021;12(3):551–67.

39. Sluggett JK, Bell JS, Lang C, Corlis M, Whitehead C, Wesselingh SL, et al. Variation in provision of collaborative medication reviews on entry to long-term care facilities. J Am Med Dir Assoc. 2021;22(1):148–55 e1.
40. Chen EYH, Wang KN, Sluggett JK, Ilomaki J, Hilmer SN, Corlis M, et al. Process, impact and outcomes of medication review in Australian residential aged care facilities: a systematic review. Australas J Ageing. 2019;38(Suppl 2):9–25.
41. Strauven G, Anrys P, Vandael E, Henrard S, De Lepeleire J, Spinewine A, et al. Cluster-controlled trial of an intervention to improve prescribing in nursing homes study. J Am Med Dir Assoc. 2019;20(11):1404–11.
42. Wouters H, Scheper J, Koning H, Brouwer C, Twisk JW, van der Meer H, et al. Discontinuing inappropriate medication use in nursing home residents: a cluster randomized controlled trial. Ann Intern Med. 2017;167(9):609–17.
43. Cateau D, Ballabeni P, Niquille A. Effects of an interprofessional quality circle-deprescribing module (QC-DeMo) in Swiss nursing homes: a randomised controlled trial. BMC Geriatr. 2021;21(1):289.
44. Bollen A, Harrison R, Aslani P, van Haastregt JCM. Factors influencing interprofessional collaboration between community pharmacists and general practitioners—a systematic review. Health Soc Care Community. 2019;27(4):e189–212.
45. Rawlinson C, Carron T, Cohidon C, Arditi C, Hong QN, Pluye P, et al. An overview of reviews on interprofessional collaboration in primary care: barriers and facilitators. Int J Integr Care. 2021;21(2):32.
46. Sangaleti C, Schveitzer MC, Peduzzi M, Zoboli E, Soares CB. Experiences and shared meaning of teamwork and interprofessional collaboration among health care professionals in primary health care settings: a systematic review. JBI Database System Rev Implement Rep. 2017;15(11):2723–88.
47. Weeks G, George J, Maclure K, Stewart D. Non-medical prescribing versus medical prescribing for acute and chronic disease management in primary and secondary care. Cochrane Database Syst Rev. 2016;11:CD011227.
48. Berry D, Bradlow A, Courtenay M. Patients' attitudes towards, and information needs in relation to, nurse prescribing in rheumatology. J Clin Nurs. 2008;17(2):266–73.
49. Cooper R, Anderson C, Avery T, Bissell P, Guillaume L, Hutchinson A, et al. Stakeholders' views of UK nurse and pharmacist supplementary prescribing. J Health Serv Res Policy. 2008;13(4):215–21.
50. Emmerton L, Marriott J, Bessell T, Nissen L, Dean L. Pharmacists and prescribing rights: review of international developments. J Pharm Pharm Sci. 2005;8(2):217–25.
51. Cooper RJ, Bissell P, Ward P, Murphy E, Anderson C, Avery T, et al. Further challenges to medical dominance? The case of nurse and pharmacist supplementary prescribing. Health (London). 2012;16(2):115–33.
52. Iqbal MZ, Khan AH, Iqbal MS, Syed Sulaiman SA. A review of pharmacist-led interventions on diabetes outcomes: an observational analysis to explore diabetes care opportunities for pharmacists. J Pharm Bioallied Sci. 2019;11(4):299–309.
53. Kroezen M, Francke AL, Groenewegen PP, van Dijk L. Nurse prescribing of medicines in Western European and Anglo-Saxon countries: a survey on forces, conditions and jurisdictional control. Int J Nurs Stud. 2012;49(8):1002–12.
54. Jebara T, Cunningham S, MacLure K, Awaisu A, Pallivalapila A, Stewart D. Stakeholders' views and experiences of pharmacist prescribing: a systematic review. Br J Clin Pharmacol. 2018;84(9):1883–905.

Deprescribing: Evidence Base and Implementation

10

Denis Curtin and Denis O'Mahony

10.1 Introduction

Older people in their final years are commonly prescribed multiple medications to manage their chronic diseases. These medications may ameliorate symptoms, prevent future adverse health events and extend life. However, the use of multiple medications is also associated with an increased risk of adverse side effects, drug interactions and medication adherence problems. Furthermore, as older people become increasingly frail, the use of multiple medications may be considered burdensome or even futile. For frailer older patients taking multiple medications, when does the balance shift from net benefit to net harm? If declining health and death are unavoidable, it follows logically that there must come a point in time when patients no longer benefit from certain chronic disease drug therapies.

Chapter 4 discussed the process of deprescribing in the context of potentially inappropriate medication (PIM) use where the goal is to minimize the adverse consequences of inappropriate prescribing that is, adverse drug reactions (ADRs) and adverse drug events (ADEs). The present chapter will focus on older people with more advanced degrees of frailty and the discontinuation of medications that may, ordinarily, be therapeutically useful and appropriate but of less clinical value or possibly futile in the patient who is likely to be approaching end-of-life. In this context, the key question for the clinician is how to separate essential medications from those that are non-essential.

D. Curtin · D. O'Mahony (✉)
Department of Medicine (Geriatrics), University College Cork, Cork, Ireland

Department of Geriatric Medicine, Cork University Hospital, Cork, Ireland
e-mail: denis.omahony@ucc.ie

A. Cherubini et al. (eds.), *Optimizing Pharmacotherapy in Older Patients*, Practical Issues in Geriatrics, https://doi.org/10.1007/978-3-031-28061-0_10

10.2 Definition of Deprescribing

The term 'deprescribing' is a relatively new term and first appeared in the English language literature in 2003 [1]. In the first review of the subject, Woodward outlined the principals of deprescribing. These included:

(a) Reviewing all current medications.
(b) Identifying medications to be discontinued, substituted or reduced.
(c) Planning a deprescribing regimen in partnership with the patient.
(d) Frequently reviewing and supporting the patient [1].

Since then, several new definitions have been proposed [2–4]. A 2015 systematic review of the literature by Reeve et al. was conducted to determine whether a standardized definition of deprescribing could be reached to inform future research on the subject [5]. The most common characteristics of the various definitions were used by the authors to develop a new definition: 'Deprescribing is the process of withdrawal of an inappropriate medication, supervised by a health care professional with the goal of managing polypharmacy and improving outcomes'.

10.2.1 Evidence Base for Deprescribing

Several recent systematic reviews have examined the impact of deprescribing interventions on prescribing and clinical outcomes [6–8]. Thillainadesan et al. [6] focused on older hospitalized patients (i.e. ≥65 years); Dills et al. [7] included adult patients aged ≥18 years in outpatient, assisted living, nursing home and acute care settings; while Shrestha et al. [8] specifically examined the impact of deprescribing interventions on older patients with life-limiting illnesses and reduced life expectancy. In Thillainadesan's and Dills' reviews, only randomized controlled trials (RCTs) were included, whereas Shrestha included both randomized and non-randomized studies. Heterogeneity in design and outcome measurement as well as small sample sizes in included studies were limitations reported by authors in each review. All three reviews concluded that deprescribing interventions can reduce potentially inappropriate prescribing, but evidence of a positive impact on important clinical outcomes such as ADRs, falls, re-hospitalization, quality of life and mortality was currently weak or of low quality. Nevertheless, it is generally agreed among specialists in geriatric medicine and clinical pharmacology that discontinuation of excessive or unnecessary medication in frailer older people is generally desirable.

10.3 Operationalizing Deprescribing for Older People Approaching End-of-Life

10.3.1 Prognostication of Survival

An assessment of survival prognosis is central to the decision to discontinue an otherwise appropriate medication in a frail older person. Prognostic estimates may be formulated subjectively (i.e. clinician prediction) or objectively (i.e. using prognostic models). Clinician prediction has the advantage of being instantaneous and convenient, and while it may incorporate known prognostic factors in its determination, accuracy will undoubtedly vary depending on the knowledge, experience and insight into the particular case on the part of the clinician. Most studies have found that clinicians generally give optimistic estimations of life expectancy [9–11]. Christakis and Lamont described clinicians' prognostic accuracy in terminally ill patients [10]. In their study, 343 doctors provided survival estimates for 468 terminally ill patients at the time of hospice referral. Only 20% of survival predictions were accurate (i.e. predicted survival rate within ±33% of actual survival), and overall, doctors overestimated survival by an average factor of 5.3 times that of actual survival. The most experienced clinicians tended to be most accurate, whereas the longer the duration of the doctor–patient relationship, the greater the likelihood of an inaccurate prediction [10].

Prognostic models synthesize clinical and demographic data to produce a mortality risk estimate for a specified time period. In a similar manner, frailty scales utilize clinical data to predict risk of a range of adverse health outcomes (e.g. falls, dependency, institutionalization, complications related to invasive procedures etc.) in addition to death. The clinical data included are generally taken at a fixed timepoint, and therefore, the predicted risk may vary depending on whether the patient is in the acute or recovery phase of illness. Multiple prognostic models and frailty scales have been developed in the last two decades but lack the support of validation and impact studies to be recommended for use as mortality prediction tools [12, 13]. Predication models, even when very accurate, indicate the likely outcome in an average patient with a given set of risk factors under average conditions. Therefore, while prediction models and frailty scales may be useful to identify *groups* of patients with shared characteristics who may benefit from a particular care pathway, it is questionable whether they should influence important decisions about *individual* patient care.

For now, prognostic certainty seems unattainable and clinical judgement is likely to be the physician's best tool. Clinical judgement may be improved by posing the prognostic question slightly differently: rather than asking 'How long is this patient likely to live?' which is associated with overly optimistic predictions, the clinician could ask, 'Would I be surprised if this patient were to die within the next 12 months?' [14]. The answer to the 'surprise question' is binary (yes or no) and essentially functions as a method of separating those with an intermediate-to-high probability of dying (the clinician answers that he/she would *not* be surprised if the patient died within the specified time period i.e. surprise question positive [SQ+])

from those with a low probability of dying (the clinician *would be* surprised, i.e. surprise question negative [SQ−]). Recent systematic reviews of the 'surprise question' indicate that while it leads to the detection of many false positives, the method appears to be very effective at excluding patients with longer survival times (negative predictive value >90% in both reviews) [15, 16]. Clinical judgement may also be improved by considering the illness and disability trajectory of the patient. Most older people experience loss of functional capabilities in the last year of life and very often this decline coincides with acute illness requiring hospitalization [15, 16]. One large Scottish study indicates that more than one in four patients aged ≥65 years admitted to hospital will be deceased in the prospective 12 months [17]. An acute hospital admission, therefore, is often a sentinel event for an older person, especially if associated with new or additional disability, and may be an appropriate trigger for discussions around goals of care medication rationalization.

10.3.2 Identifying Medications to be Deprescribed

A logical approach to deprescribing would involve examining the likelihood of a drug-conferring benefit within the remaining life expectancy of the patient. Holmes et al. have suggested that number needed to treat (NNT), time to benefit (TTB) and time to harm (TTH; see Table 10.1 for definitions) data from drug trials could be balanced against an estimate of remaining life expectancy in order to determine an accurate evaluation of net benefit (or net harm) of a particular drug [18]. This approach has problems however: first, drug data are derived from trials that generally exclude older patients approaching end-of-life and therefore may have limited applicability [19]; second, as discussed, estimates of remaining life expectancy are commonly inaccurate [9–11]; third, the approach is likely to be time-consuming and, therefore, impractical in a routine clinical setting.

Approaches to deprescribing through multidisciplinary team consensus and pharmacist- and physician-led interventions have been described in the literature. The reproducibility of these methods is uncertain. Several tools have been developed in recent years to support clinicians to make systematic deprescribing decisions in older people approaching end-of-life. Many of these tools were examined in a recent systematic review by Thompson et al. [20] This chapter focuses

Table 10.1 Definitions of number needed to treat (NNT), time to benefit (TTB) and time to harm (TTH)

	Definition
Number needed to treat (NNT)	The number of patients that need to be treated for one patient to benefit
Time to benefit (TTB)	The time taken for a statistically significant benefit to be observed in trials of people receiving a particular medication or therapy compared to the control group
Time to harm (TTH)	The time period until a statistically significant adverse effect is observed in a trial within the treatment group compared to the control group

primarily on the two most widely used deprescribing tools that have been tested as interventions in well-designed clinical trials, that is, Scott's deprescribing algorithm and STOPPFrail criteria.

The algorithm proposed by Scott et al. (Fig. 10.1) requires the user to answer a series of questions about each individual medication in the patient's regimen [21]. Although comprehensive and patient-centred, the outcome is likely to depend on the knowledge, experience and attitudes of the user. Nuanced clinical judgement is

STOPPFrail is a list of potentially inappropriate prescribing indicators designed to assist physicians with deprescribing decisions. It is intended for <u>older people with limited life expectancy for whom the goal of care is to optimize quality of life and minimize the risk of drug-related morbidity</u>. Goals of care should be clearly defined and, where possible, medication changes should be discussed and agreed with patient and/or family. Appropriate candidates for STOPPFrail-guided deprescribing typically meet ALL of the following criteria:

1. **ADL dependency (i.e. assistance with dressing, washing, transferring, walking) <u>and/or</u> severe chronic disease <u>and/or</u> terminal illness**
2. **Severe irreversible frailty i.e. high risk of acute medical complications and clinical deterioration**
3. **Physician overseeing care of patient would not be surprised if the patient died in the next 12 months**

Section A: General	i. Any drug that the patient persistently fails to take or tolerate despite adequate education and consideration of all appropriate formulations. ii. Any drug without a clear clinical indication iii. Any drug for symptoms which have now resolved (e.g. pain, nausea, vertigo, pruritis)
Section B: Cardiology system	i. **Lipid lowering therapies (statins, ezetimibe, bile acid sequestrants, fibrates, nicotinic acid, lomitapide, andacipimox)** ii. **Antihypertensive therapies:** Carefully reduce or discontinue these drugs in patients with systolic blood pressure (SBP) persistently <130mmHg. An appropriate SBP target in frail older people is 130 -160mmHg. Before stopping, consider whether the drug is treating additional conditions (e.g. beta-blocker for rate control in atrial fibrillation, diuretics for ymptomatic heart failure) iii. **Anti-anginal therapy (specifically: nitrates, nicorandil, ranolazine):** None of these anti-anginal drugs havebeen proven to reduce cardiovascular mortality or the rate of myocardial infarction. Aim to carefully reduce and discontinue these drugs in patients who have had no reported anginal symptoms in the previous 12 months AND who have no proven or objective evidence of coronary artery disease.
Section C: Coagulation system	i. **Anti-platelets:** No evidence of benefit forprimary (as distinct from secondary) cardiovascular prevention. ii. **Aspirin for stroke prevention in atrial fibrillation:** Aspirin has little or no role for stroke prevention in frail older people who are not candidates for anticoagulation therapy and may significantly increase bleeding risk.
Section D: Central Nervous System	i. **Neuroleptic antipsychotics in patients with dementia:** Aim to reduce dose and discontinue these drugs in patients taking them for longer than 12 weeks if there are no current clinical features of behavioural and psychiatric symptoms of dementia (BPSD). ii. **Memantine:** Discontinue and monitor in patients with moderate to severe dementia, unless memantine has clearly improved BPSD
Section E: Gastrointestinal System	i. **Proton Pump Inhibitors:** Reduce dose of Proton Pump Inhibitors when used at full therapeutic dose ≥ 8 weeks, unless persistent dyspeptic symptoms at lower maintenance dose. ii. **H2 receptor antagonist:** Reduce dose of H2 receptor antagonists when used at full therapeutic dose for ≥ 8 weeks, unless persistent dyspeptic symptoms at lower maintenance dose.
Section F: Respiratory System	i. **Theophylline and aminophylline:** These drugs have a narrow therapeutic index,have doubtful therapeutic benefit andrequire monitoring of serum levels and interact with other commonly prescribed drugs putting patients at an increased risk of ADEs. ii. **Leukotriene antagonists (Montelukast, Zafirlukast):** These drugs have no proven role in COPD, they are indicated only in asthma.
Section G: Musculoskeletal System	i. **Calcium supplements:** Unlikely to be of any benefitin short-termunless proven, symptomatic hypocalcaemia. ii. **Vitamin D (ergocalciferol and colecalciferol):** Lack of clearevidence to support the use of vitamin D to prevent falls and fractures, cardiovascular events, or cancer. iii. **Anti-resorptive/bone anabolic drugs**<u>*FOR OSTEOPOROSIS*</u> **(bisphosphonates, strontium, teriparatide, denosumab)** iv. **Long-term oral NSAIDs:** Increased risk of side effects (e.g. peptic ulcer disease, bleeding, worsening heart failure) when taken regularly for ≥ 2 months. v. **Long-term oral corticosteroids:** Increased risk of major side effects (e.g. fragility fractures, proximal myopathy, peptic ulcer disease) when taken regularly for ≥ 2 months. Consider careful dose reduction and discontinuation.
Section H: Urogenital System	i. **Drugs for benign prostatic hyperplasia (5-alpha reductase inhibitors and alpha-blockers) in catheterized male patients:** No benefit with longtermbladder catheterisation. ii. **Drugs for overactive bladder (muscarinic antagonists and mirabegron):** No benefit in patients with persistent, irreversible urinary incontinenceunless clear history ofpainful detrusor hyperactivity.
Section I: Endocrine System	i. **Anti-diabetic drugs:** De-intensify therapy. Avoid HbA1c targets (HbA1C <7.5% [58 mmol/mol] associated with net harm in this population). Goal of care is to minimize symptoms related to hyperglycaemia(e.g. excessive thirst, polyuria).
Section J: Miscellaneous	i. **Multi-vitamin combination supplements:** Discontinue when prescribed for prophylaxis rather than treatmentof hypovitaminosis. ii. **Folic acid:** Discontinue when treatment course completed. Usual treatment duration 1-4 months unless malabsorption, malnutrition or concomitant methotrexate use. iii. **Nutritional supplements:**Discontinue when prescribed for prophylaxis rather than treatment of malnutrition.

Fig. 10.1 STOPPFrail version 2 deprescribing criteria [24]

required, the user is not provided with resources or decision aids to estimate treatment benefit–harm trade-offs in individual patients. The use of implicit medication assessment tools is, in general, time-consuming and is likely to result in variations in practice between physicians, and for these reasons, integration into routine clinical practice has been limited [22]. Serial considerations for deprescribing according to the CEASE algorithm of Scott et al. [21] comes in the form of four key questions relating to any medication that the patient is taking. If the answer to these four questions in series is 'No', the drug may be continued. If there is a 'Yes' answer to any of the four questions, deprescribing should be considered. The four questions are as follows:

1. Does a drug provide no current patient benefit?
2. Does a drug present greater harm than benefit?
3. Are disease symptoms stable or non-existent?
4. If a drug is prescribed for disease prevention, is the patient's life expectancy too short to realize benefit from that drug?

STOPPFrail (Screening Tool of Older Persons Prescriptions in Frail adults with limited life expectancy; Fig. 10.1) Criteria were first published in 2017 and updated in 2020 [23, 24]. The updated criteria include a method for identifying patients approaching end-of-life and comprise 25 predominantly explicit indicators to assist physicians with deprescribing decisions [24]. The criteria were created following a literature appraisal and Delphi validation process involving clinicians with expertise geriatric medicine, clinical pharmacology, palliative medicine, general practice and psychiatry. Substantial inter-rater reliability has been demonstrated between users of different clinical disciplines and STOPPFrail-guiding deprescribing recommendations have been shown to generally align with gold-standard deprescribing decisions [25, 26].

Scott's deprescribing algorithm and STOPPFrail have been evaluated individually as interventions in randomized controlled trials involving older people with advanced frailty. These trials are summarized in Table 10.2. While both methods resulted in reduced numbers of prescribed medications compared with usual pharmaceutical care, neither trial was sufficiently powered to detect significant changes in secondary patient-related end points.

Table 10.2 Randomized controlled trials using Scott's algorithm and STOPPFrail

Study	Intervention	Design	Population	Outcomes measured	Results
Potter et al. (2016) [27]	Scott's algorithm	RCT Follow-up: 1 year	Nursing home residents 95 patients (47 intervention patients; 48 control patients) Mean age (SD): 84.3 (6.9)	Primary: change in number of medications Secondary: mortality, falls, fractures, unplanned hospital presentations, cognitive status, functional status, QOL, sleep	Mean change in number of medications −1.9 ± 4.1 in intervention group compared with +0.1 ± 3.5 in control group ($p = 0.04$). No statistically significant differences between groups for secondary outcomes.
Curtin et al. (2020) [28]	STOPPFrail version 1	RCT Follow-up: 3 months	Hospitalized patients with advanced frailty undergoing transition to nursing home care. 130 patients (65 intervention patients and 65 control patients) Mean age (SD): 85.1 (5.7)	Primary: change in number of medications Secondary: mortality, acute hospital presentations, unscheduled medical reviews, falls, non-vertebral fractures, medication costs, QOL, prescription of antipsychotic medications	Mean change in number of medications −2.6 ± 2.73 in intervention group compared with −0.36 ± 2.60 in control group ($p < 0.001$). Reduction in medication costs 28% in intervention group vs 5% in control group ($p < 0.02$). No statistically significant differences between groups for other secondary outcomes.

10.4 Shared Decision-Making

Patient involvement in healthcare decisions is a key component of patient-centred care [29]. Qualitative studies indicate that clinicians are often reluctant to initiate discussions about deprescribing with older people, believing that they would resist having their medications discontinued or that they would interpret deprescribing as withdrawal of care or 'giving up' on active treatment [30, 31]. These perceptions, however, have not been borne out in patient-focussed research [32, 33]. Reeve et al. recently examined attitudes of older people towards deprescribing in a nationally representative sample of Medicare beneficiaries in the United States [32]. In that study, 92% of people indicated a willingness to discontinue one or more of their medications if their physician said it was possible, and 66% reported a desire to reduce the number of medications that they were taking. The greatest predictor of willingness to deprescribe was the consumption of six or more daily medications [32]. The results are important and suggest that physicians can be reassured that broaching the topic of deprescribing with their older patients is generally acceptable to them.

Decisions about medications represent just one aspect of many considerations that patients and their physicians face when they discuss goals of care, and sometimes other aspects of the discussion may take priority. For this reason, a focus on the patient's values, such as whether the patient favours a primary focus on extending life or on symptom palliation, may be more worthwhile than concentrating on the merits of individual therapies. Once a shared understanding of the patient's values is established, prescribed medications can be aligned with the goals of care. Some patients may desire more detailed information, and, in general, the discussion should be adapted to the patient's information preferences. Although withdrawal of certain treatments may be recommended, commitment to supporting patients through their illness should be re-emphasized.

10.5 Conclusion

Larger, multi-centre, randomized trials with extended follow-up times are required to provide further clarification on the impact of deprescribing interventions on patient-related outcomes such as hospital admissions, quality of life and mortality. Expectation that deprescribing interventions will improve these outcomes may be overreaching. Deprescribing involves the *withdrawal* of a medical intervention, and, therefore, demonstrating that patient's symptoms do not subsequently deteriorate and that quality of life is maintained may be enough to justify the process.

The goal of deprescribing is to minimize drug-related morbidity and medication burden for older people approaching end-of-life. Central to this goal is the recognition that clinicians have prescribing responsibilities beyond the restoration and maintenance of health. Increasing dependency and, ultimately, death do not necessarily represent a failure of medical care but are natural processes for which science has no ultimate remedy. In this context, clinicians need to support their older frailer patients approaching end of life with personalized care that prioritizes symptom control rather than survival extension.

Finally, deprescribing is generally acceptable to older patients and their carers [33]. Recent evidence also indicates that deprescribing in older people is cost-effective [34].

References

1. Woodward M. Deprescribing: achieving better health outcomes for older people through reducing medications. J Pharm Pract Res. 2003;33:323–8.
2. Scott I, Jayathissa S. Quality of drug prescribing in older patients: is there a problem and can we improve it? Intern Med J. 2010;40:7–18.
3. Hardy JE, Hilmer SN. Deprescribing in the last year of life. J Pharm Pract Res. 2011;41:146–51.
4. Thompson W, Farrell B. Deprescribing: what is it and what does the evidence tell us? Can J Hosp Pharm. 2013;66:201.
5. Reeve E, Gnjidic D, Long J, Hilmer S. A systematic review of the emerging definition of 'deprescribing' with network analysis: implications for future research and clinical practice. Br J Clin Pharmacol. 2015;80(6):1254–68.
6. Thillainadesan J, Gnjidic D, Green S, Hilmer SN. Impact of deprescribing interventions in older hospitalised patients on prescribing and clinical outcomes: a systematic review of randomised trials. Drugs Aging. 2018;35(4):303–19.
7. Dills H, Shah K, Messinger-Rapport B, Bradford K, Syed Q. Deprescribing medications for chronic diseases management in primary care settings: a systematic review of randomized controlled trials. J Am Med Dir Assoc. 2018;19(11):923–935.e2.
8. Shrestha S, Poudel A, Steadman K, Nissen L. Outcomes of deprescribing interventions in older patients with life-limiting illness and limited life expectancy: a systematic review. Br J Clin Pharmacol. 2019;86(10):1931–45. https://doi.org/10.1111/bcp.14113.
9. Parkes CM. Accuracy of predictions of survival in later stages of cancer. BMJ. 1972;2:29–31.
10. Christakis N, Lamont E. Extent and determinants of error in doctors' prognoses. BMJ. 2000;320:469–73.
11. Vigano A, Dorgan M, Buckingham J, Bruera E, Suarez-Alzamor ME. Survival prediction in terminal cancer patients: a systematic review of the medical literature. Palliat Med. 2000;14:363–74.
12. Yourman LC, Lee SJ, Schonberg MA, Widera EW, Smith AK. Prognostic indices for older adults: a systematic review. JAMA. 2012;307(2):182–92.
13. Curtin D, Dahly D, Van Smeden M, et al. Predicting 1-year mortality in older hospitalized patients: external validation of the HOMR model. J Am Geriatr Soc. 2019;67(7):1478–83. https://doi.org/10.1111/jgs.15958.
14. Lynn J. Living long in fragile health: the new demographics shape end of life care. Hast Cent Rep. 2005;35(7):s14–8.
15. Downar J, Goldman R, Pinto R, Englesakis M, Adhikari NK. The "surprise question" for predicting death in seriously ill patients: a systematic review and meta-analysis. CMAJ. 2017;189(13):E484–93.
16. White N, Kupeli N, Vickerstaff V, Stone P. How accurate is the 'surprise question' at identifying patients at the end of life? A systematic review and meta-analysis. BMC Med. 2017;15:139.
17. Clark D, Armstrong M, Allen A, et al. Imminence of death among hospital inpatients: prevalent cohort study. Palliat Med. 2014;28(6):274–9.
18. Holmes HM, Min LC, Yee M, et al. Rationalizing prescribing for older patients with multimorbidity: considering time to benefit. Drugs Aging. 2013;30(9):655–66.

19. Fortin M, Dionne J, Pinho G, Gignac J, Almirall J, Lapointe L. Randomized controlled trials: do they have external validity for patients with multiple co-morbidities? Ann Fam Med. 2006;4:104–8.
20. Thompson W, Lundby C, Graabaek T, et al. Tools for deprescribing in frail older persons and those with limited life expectancy: a systematic review. J Am Geriatr Soc. 2019;67(1):172–80. https://doi.org/10.1111/jgs.15616.
21. Scott IA, Hilmer SN, Reeve E, et al. Reducing inappropriate polypharmacy: the process of deprescribing. JAMA Intern Med. 2015;175(5):827–34.
22. Spinewine A, Schmader KE, Barber N, et al. Appropriate prescribing in elderly people: how well can it be measured and optimised? Lancet. 2007;370(9582):173–84.
23. Lavan AH, Gallagher P, Parsons C, O'Mahony D. STOPPFrail (screening tool of older persons prescriptions in frail adults with limited life expectancy): consensus validation. Age Ageing. 2017;46(4):600–7.
24. Curtin D, Gallagher P, O'Mahony D. Deprescribing in older people approaching end-of-life: development and validation of STOPPFrail version 2. Age Ageing. 2021;50(2):465–71.
25. Lavan AH, Gallagher P, O'Mahony D. Inter-rater reliability of STOPPFrail [screening tool of older persons prescriptions in frail adults with limited life expectancy] criteria amongst 12 physicians. Eur J Clin Pharmacol. 2018;74(3):331–8.
26. Curtin D, Dukelow T, James K, O'Donnell D, O'Mahony D, Gallagher P. Deprescribing in multi-morbid older people with polypharmacy: agreement between STOPPFrail explicit criteria and gold standard deprescribing using 100 standardized clinical cases. Eur J Clin Pharmacol. 2019;75(3):427–32.
27. Potter K, Flicker L, Page A, Etherton-Beer CD. Deprescribing in frail older people: a randomised controlled trial. PLoS One. 2016;11:e0149984.
28. Curtin D, Jennings E, Daunt R, et al. Deprescribing in older people approaching end of life: a randomized controlled trial using STOPPFrail criteria. J Am Geriatr Soc. 2020;68(4):762–9.
29. Charles C, Gafni A, Whelan T. Shared decision-making in the medical encounter: what does it mean? (Or it takes at least two to tango). Soc Sci Med. 1997;44(5):681–92.
30. Schuling J, Gebben H, Veehof LJ, Haaijer-Ruskamp FM. Deprescribing medication in very elderly patients with multimorbidity: the view of Dutch GPs. A qualitative study. BMC Fam Pract. 2012;13:56.
31. Anthierens S, Tansens A, Petrovic M, Christiaens T. Qualitative insights into general practitioners views on polypharmacy. BMC Fam Pract. 2010;11:65.
32. Reeve E, Wolff JL, Skehan M, Bayliss EA, Hilmer SN, Boyd CM. Assessment of attitudes toward deprescribing in older medicare beneficiaries in the United States. JAMA Intern Med. 2018;178(12):1673–80.
33. Seewoodharry M, Khunti K, Davies MJ, Gillies C, Seidu S. Attitudes of older adults and their carers towards de-prescribing: a systematic review. Diabet Med. 2022;39(7):e14801.
34. Romano S, Figueira D, Teixeira I, Perelman J. Deprescribing interventions among community-dwelling older adults: a systematic review of economic evaluations. PharmacoEconomics. 2022;40(3):269–95.

Part II

Geriatric Syndromes and Common Chronic Conditions

General Principles of Management of Patients with Multimorbidity and Frailty

11

Camilla Cocchi, Graziano Onder,
and Maria Beatrice Zazzara

11.1 Multimorbidity, Frailty and Their Interconnection

The progressive ageing of the population has led to a new health scenario, where frailty and multimorbidity are extremely common. Although both are strongly associated with poor quality of life, increased risk of disability, hospitalization, institutionalization and higher mortality, multimorbidity and frailty should be considered as different entities.

11.1.1 Multimorbidity

Multimorbidity is usually described as the coexistence of two or more chronic diseases in the same individual. This condition should be considered as an entity by itself and not just the co-occurrence of multiple diseases. It is in fact a synergy of different clinical conditions associated with worse health outcomes and a more complex clinical management.

In high-income countries, 20% of the population before the age of 40, and almost 70% of those above 60, have two or more chronic diseases, making multimorbidity itself 'the most common chronic condition'[1]. Low- and middle-income countries are expected to present similar figures in few decades. Onset and severity of multimorbidity are influenced by behavioural, clinical and social factors and lifestyle during the entire lifespan. The clinical picture of multimorbidity is heterogeneous across individuals, and it is characterized by a great complexity, which impacts on quality

C. Cocchi (✉)
Università Cattolica del Sacro Cuore, Rome, Italy

Fondazione Universitaria Policlinico Gemelli, IRCCS, Rome, Italy
e-mail: camilla.cocchi01@icatt.it

G. Onder · M. B. Zazzara
Fondazione Universitaria Policlinico Gemelli, IRCCS, Rome, Italy

A. Cherubini et al. (eds.), *Optimizing Pharmacotherapy in Older Patients*,
Practical Issues in Geriatrics, https://doi.org/10.1007/978-3-031-28061-0_11

of life, frequency of healthcare use, level of required assistance and survival, with a consequent challenging medical and care management.

Multimorbidity should not be confused with comorbidity, which refers to the presence of one or more additional conditions co-occurring with a primary condition. The difference between the two is important, because it implies a different clinical approach. In fact, whereas *multimorbidity* suggests a holistic assessment that takes into consideration the individual's clinical complexity, equally weighting all diseases, *comorbidity* implies the presence of a prevailing clinical condition requiring attention. To put it simple, multimorbidity refers to a patient-centred vision, while comorbidity is more disease-centred.

Even though multimorbidity as a concept is now well known and established, it is not free from limitations. In particular, multimorbidity suggests that diseases are equally weighted, whereas the impact on the individual's health is greater than the mere sum of the singular clinical effects of every disease [1, 2].

11.1.2 Polypharmacy

One of the most problematic consequences of multimorbidity is polypharmacy, which is defined as the concurrent use of multiple drugs in the same individual. This phenomenon is greatly spread in the older population, and its prevalence varies between 10 and 90% depending on the country or setting. The simultaneous use of a large number of drugs in the context of an ageing organism, characterized by reduced kidney and liver function and an altered volume of drug distribution, increases the likelihood of adverse drug reactions, including drug–drug interactions and drug–disease interactions. Polypharmacy has been associated with a high number of adverse outcomes, including adverse drug reactions, hospitalizations related to adverse drug events, an increased risk of falling, a higher incidence of disability and increased mortality. To date, there is agreement on considering the correct management of polypharmacy as one of the key strategies for treating patients with multimorbidity [3].

11.1.3 Frailty

Frailty is a condition of extreme vulnerability of the individual to endogenous and exogenous stressors. It is determined by the age-related exhaustion of the body's homeostatic reserves and involves an increased risk of adverse events. Even minor stressors can lead to rapid changes in health status. Frailty is common in older adults, with a prevalence between 8 and 16% in community-dwelling older adults and up to 85% among nursing home residents. Frailty is associated with shorter survival, poor quality of life and increased risk of disability, hospitalization, and institutionalization.

Chronic diseases play a crucial role in the onset of frailty. According to the widely used frailty phenotype construct proposed by Fried et al., the presence of chronic diseases has a central role in initiating or worsening frailty. In addition, the frailty index proposed by Rockwood et al., which is based on a combination of different deficits, primarily includes chronic diseases as a criterion [4, 5]. In a recent meta-analysis, the prevalence of multimorbidity in frail individuals was 72%, and the prevalence of frailty among multimorbid individuals was 16%. This means that most frail individuals are also multimorbid, whereas very few people with multimorbidity are also frail. In the general adult population, only 6% are both frail and multimorbid [1].

As chronic diseases and multimorbidity have such a strong role in determining frailty, it could be hypothesized that treating these conditions may counteract the development of frailty, eventually reducing any associated negative consequences. However, the hypothesis that intensive treatment of chronic diseases might reduce the progression of frailty is poorly supported by existing studies. In contrast, some evidence suggests that intensive treatment of chronic diseases may increase negative health outcomes in frail older adults. For example, polypharmacy, anticholinergic and psychotropic medications have been associated with incident frailty and pre-frailty over 2 to 5-year follow-up periods [6].

The clinical picture of patients with chronic diseases is strongly influenced by the presence of frailty features (see Table 11.1): presence of chronic disease might represent a limited part of the complexity of frail patients that usually present with multiple impairments in systems and organs, and this complexity might influence the approach to pharmacological treatment.

Table 11.1 Clinical picture of frail and non-frail patients with chronic conditions[a]

Characteristic/ Domain	Non-frail	Frail
Chronic diseases	Diabetes, hypertension	Diabetes, hypertension
Symptoms	None	Present (i.e. pain, dyspnoea, dizziness)
Functional status	Physically active Independent in instrumental activities of daily, including managing finances and/or medications, use of transportation, housework, shopping, walking outside alone, preparing meals	Slow walking speed Need help in instrumental activities of daily living, including managing finances and/or medications, use of transportation, housework, shopping, walking outside alone, preparing meals
Cognition	Not impaired	Mild to moderate impairment
Social function	Availability social support (i.e. lives with spouse or relatives)	Poor social support (i.e. lives alone, limited support available from relatives or friends)
Continence	Continent	Urinary incontinence
Nutrition	Normal nutritional status	Obesity or malnutrition, recent weight loss
Mood	Normal	Depressive symptoms, sad or depressed

[a] Tables 1 and 2 inspired by Onder G. (coauthor of this work), Vetrano DL et al. "Accounting for frailty when treating chronic diseases". Consent obtained by other coauthors via email

Whereas multimorbidity offers a nosological risk profile, frailty studies focus on the individual in a more exhaustive manner through a comprehensive assessment that also consider social determinants of health (i.e. environment, social entourage etc.), thus facilitating the implementation of tailored interventions. With this regard, frailty might be used to identify multimorbid patients who need a comprehensive and integrated intervention, instead of a traditional disease-oriented approach [1, 7, 8].

11.2 Management of Multimorbidity

With increasing multimorbidity and frailty, the world of healthcare must reinvent itself to find effective ways of dealing with complexity. As of today, medicine is still single-disease oriented, an approach that appears obsolete when confronted with today's reality.

One of the main problems for multimorbid patients is represented by the fragmentation of care. Patients are often subjected to a large number of specialist visits and treated with a large number of drugs. The models of care must be modified to cope with this new type of patient. A new clinical approach is needed, and it must be multidisciplinary-centred and focused on promoting individual's independence.

The complexity and heterogeneity of patients with multimorbidity and polypharmacy make traditional guidelines often inadequate and not supportive in decision-making. An increasing number of studies have pointed out that disease-specific guidelines are difficult to apply in multimorbid patients. This difficulty arises primarily from how these guidelines are developed. Indeed, disease-specific guidelines are developed on data collected with randomized clinical trials that exclude fragile individuals a priori, to avoid confounding factors. Second, these guidelines often do not account for other coexisting chronic diseases: drug–drug or drug–disease interactions may easily occur in persons suffering from multiple chronic conditions.

New guidelines have recently been developed (i.e. Ariadne principles, NICE, JA-CHRODIS) for the management of the multimorbid patient. The first purpose of these guidelines is to maximize the quality of life, focusing not on the symptom nor the disease but on the individual as a whole. Those guidelines present several commonalities. First, they try to identify a target population that can benefit from the application of these principles (e.g. fragile individuals). In addition, they support the flexible use of existing guidelines on individual diseases, focusing on treatment burden. Moreover, they theorize the importance of coordinating all the different specialists involved in patient care, often via the specialized figure of the case manager, who acts as facilitator. Those guidelines also focus on a shared decision-making with the patient, in order to agree on an individualized care plan. Lastly, they emphasize on patient and caregivers' education to improve self-management and self-efficacy. Below, we will analyze in more detail the main points of the recent guidelines on the management of the multimorbid patient [6, 9].

11.2.1 Target Population

Patients with multimorbidity are heterogeneous, and their global health status and risk of negative outcomes may vary largely. Furthermore, the consequences of multimorbidity cannot be linearly estimated on the basis of the number of clinical conditions. In order to develop the best care plan for each individual patient, it is important to be able to identify different care needs. Indeed, there are older adults who, despite the presence of multiple coexisting chronic conditions, are in good health and have a good life expectancy, so they must receive the standard level of assistance, including preventive programs and appropriate diagnostic-therapeutic interventions. On the other hand, there are patients who are more at risk of developing negative events and who, therefore, need specific treatment plans.

In the population with multimorbidity, stratification strategies carried out on the basis of patterns of different diseases, presence of symptoms, and physical, cognitive, and socio-economic status help to identify the most demanding and complex-to-treat groups—those that might benefit most from individualized and integrated healthcare plans. In this context, the assessment of frailty with appropriate instruments (i.e. Frailty index, Clinical Frailty Scale, physical performance measures) can be used to identify the most care-demanding groups that might benefit most from individualized and integrated approaches. Both guidelines from the National Institute for Health and Care Excellence on multimorbidity and Italian Guidelines on Multimorbidity and Polypharmacy suggest to assess frailty status to identify people with multimorbidity who are susceptible and at risk of negative health outcomes, thus more likely to benefit from a patient-centred approach [3, 10, 11].

11.2.2 Assessing of Interacting Conditions and Treatments

The therapeutic management of the multimorbid patient can be extremely complex and requires a holistic approach, which considers the individual in his/her entirety. In multimorbid patients, who naturally take multiple prescriptions, various interactions between disease and therapies can occur, which can lead to the onset of numerous adverse events, including worsening of clinical conditions and the onset of new symptoms that can complicate the patient's therapeutic management. In this context, the so-called *cascades-effect*—when additional medications are prescribed to counteract side effects of other drugs—can take place and increase the burden of pharmacological treatment.

Therefore, once the target population has been identified, it would be advisable to make a multidimensional assessment of the patient, studying different aspects of the patient's life, including clinical conditions, adherence to medication, social context and psychological status. In particular, the following aspects seem important to develop an individualized approach to multimorbidity:

- Diseases and health problems, including clinical and functional status, cognition, geriatric syndromes, life expectancy, presence of any symptoms, their severity and their impact on quality of life

- Psychosocial context
- Treatment burden (pharmacological and nonpharmacological): evaluating potential interactions or adverse effect, adherence or underuse and treatment burden

All of these elements should be reviewed regularly, with special attention for signs and symptoms of cognitive impairment and psychological or social problems, since they could modify our intervention [3, 6, 10–13].

11.2.3 Incorporate Patient Preferences and Goal Setting

Since the management of the multimorbid patient is complex and challenging, the identification of health priorities, shared between patients and care provider, represents a relevant step to provide individualized, patient-centred care. Decisions about the patient's health must be made in full agreement with patient and caregivers. It is necessary to explain the purpose of the therapeutic approach and the realistically achievable goals so that the patient can express his/her preferences based on personal values and priorities. When suggesting a treatment, the person's prognosis should always be taken into consideration, as well as the patient's attitude towards the treatment, his expectations and objectives. Monitoring and re-discussing priorities is fundamental, as they can change overtime [3, 6, 10, 11].

11.2.4 Individualized Management

After performing a comprehensive assessment and identifying shared and achievable goals together, it is necessary to develop an individualized treatment plan with the patient and the caregiver. Once a care plan has been discussed, it is necessary to choose therapies that optimize benefits, minimize potential harms and enhance quality of life. It is also important to consider treatment burden and all possible interaction, considering not only other medications but also food and food supplements as well.

Finding balance between the treatment of chronic disease and drug-related harm is a key goal of drug prescribing but has proven difficult to achieve in clinical practice. In fact, multimorbidity can modify the patient's risks, harms or even the potential treatment benefit. In addition, complex medications regimens are difficult to comply with, so when planning a treatment, it is advisable to consider also the patient's/caregiver's ability to adhere to it. The prescribing process should be individualized and flexible, and it should be based upon using effective drugs, at the minimum effective dose, with the lowest number of dosage units per day and daily administrations. These interventions must be targeted health priorities identified with the patient during the multidimensional assessment. The use of IT support tools for the prescription can provide a valuable support to evaluate cumulative drug toxicity, risk of interactions and adverse drug reactions and risk of fall [3, 6, 10, 11].

11.2.5 Self-management

Multimorbid patients are the major users of healthcare resources, and their involvement in disease management is a goal to be pursued. Self-management of chronic diseases is a treatment process characterized by the responsible and proactive participation of the patient himself, allowing the patient to be aware of his own health condition and empowering his/her involvement in the therapeutic decision-making process. Self-management represents a fundamental lever for the effectiveness and efficiency of the health system. On the assumption that knowledgeable and expert patients are able to manage their quality of life to the fullest of their potential, educational programs are useful to enable patients to acquire a central role in the management of his own health. Many patients who have lived with chronic diseases for years can be trained to manage the disease and take active responsibility of both non pharmaceutical (i.e. diet, physical exercises) and pharmaceutical (i.e. use of medications) management [3, 6, 10, 11].

11.2.6 Monitoring and Follow-Up

Patients with multimorbidity often receive disjointed care, which leads to inefficient, ineffective and possibly harmful clinical interventions. Ideally, care for patients with multimorbidity should involve numerous healthcare professionals, include various dimensions (clinical, functional and social), and be based on solid evidence. A careful coordination by a case manager of the various healthcare professionals is therefore essential.

Care plans for multimorbid patients are not static, but they can often change due to a change in the patient's priorities, to the onset of new problems or as a result of co-occurring events. This is why it is important to re-evaluate the patient, especially after hospitalizations or the prescription of new drugs [3, 6, 10, 11].

11.3 Treatment of Chronic Diseases and Multimoridity in Frail Patients

As mentioned earlier, the identification of frailty is a key step to stratify the population with multimorbidity and to identify patients that need an individualized care approach. In particular, the use of symptomatic and preventive drugs in persons with frailty should be evaluated carefully based on several considerations.

11.3.1 Symptomatic Treatment of Diseases in Frailty

Symptoms related to chronic diseases might have a relevant role in the onset or worsening of frailty status, and the treatment of these symptoms might potentially reverse frailty. For example, pain is a strong determinant of frailty in patients with osteoarthritis and it could be considered as a component of the frailty phenotype. Pain impacts on walking ability, speed, and strength and consequently cause a reduction in physical activity levels. These parameters are all criteria used to assess Fried's phenotype and can contribute to the development of frailty. In addition, pain increases the risk of falls, causes depression, reducing the individual's quality of life and consequently precipitating the onset of frailty. Therefore, the pharmacological treatment of pain could virtually reverse the frailty status.

Similarly, Parkinson's disease is often associated with frailty, and its symptomatic treatment (e.g. levodopa) might have an impact on frailty status. Medications used for symptomatic treatment of Parkinson's disease impact on the motor symptoms, improving walking ability and speed and potentially reducing the risk of exhaustion and falls, with great benefit in persons with frailty.

Another example is dyspnoea. This condition could lead to physical inactivity, loss of skeletal muscle strength, mobility problems (including walking deficits) and ultimately frailty. For this reason, an optimized treatment of dyspnoea might reduce frailty progression.

Despite a beneficial effect of treatment of pain, motor symptoms of Parkinson's disease and dyspnoea on frailty seem clinically obvious, studies providing evidence on this association are currently lacking [14].

11.3.2 Preventive Treatment of Diseases in Frailty

Treatment of chronic diseases might have an impact on the onset of frailty by preventing the occurrence of negative health events. For example, it would be reasonable to hypothesize that pharmacological treatment of frail persons who experienced a bone fracture may prevent the onset of new fractures and reduce the risk of frailty and disability. However, evidence has suggested lack of benefit from treatment with bisphosphonates on fractures and mortality in frail women in nursing home. Similarly, possible benefits related to preventive pharmacological treatment of hypertension on frailty onset are still being discussed. In observational studies, hypertension does not seem to have an impact on frailty, and the negative effects of antihypertensive treatment seem to be more pronounced in patients with frailty. In addition, the negative effects of hypertension on health outcomes might be reduced in the presence of frailty, suggesting a reverse epidemiology phenomenon in patients with frailty.

The example of hypertension could also apply to other chronic diseases, where the pros and the cons of intensive pharmacological treatment in frailty are still debated, and any possible positive effects might be counterbalanced by an increased risk of negative effects. Indeed, treatment of chronic diseases in frail individuals may raise several concerns that might alter the risk/benefit ratio of a given treatment (Table 11.2).

Table 11.2 Factors challenging pharmacological treatment of chronic diseases in the presence of frailty[a]

Problem	Consequences	Potential solutions
Exclusion of frail persons from studies	Uncertainties about the efficacy and safety of treatment in frail persons	Inclusion of frail patients in RCTs; Evidence from observational studies
Reduced life expectancy in frail persons	Reduced/absent beneficial effects	Assess life expectancy; Evaluate risk-benefit ratio of treatments
Increased susceptibility to iatrogenic events due to intensive treatment	Higher rate of adverse drug events	Periodic therapeutic review and reconciliation; Evaluate risk-benefit ratio of treatments; Focus treatment on specific goals
Functional deficits associated with frailty	Poor medication adherence; Medication errors	Assess the capacity of patients to self-manage their medication regimen; Focus treatment on health priorities; Adjust communication strategies; Use of tools to improve adherence; Reduce number medications and medication regimen complexity (frequency of medication administrations, use of appropriate dose forms)

[a] Tables 1 and 2 inspired by Onder G. (coauthor of this work), Vetrano DL et al. “Accounting for frailty when treating chronic diseases”. Consent obtained by other coauthors via email

Exclusion from studies. Frail older people are often excluded from randomized clinical trials assessing the effects of treatments for chronic diseases. Practical limitation—difficulties in reaching the research centre—or and higher mortality rates that prevent having appropriate follow-up times may in part justify this exclusion. However, this limits the generalizability of clinical trial findings and estimation of the efficacy and safety of treatments for chronic diseases in persons with frailty.

Limited life expectancy. Frailty is associated with limited life expectancy; estimates from the SHARE study suggests that life expectancy for frail individuals at age of 70 years ranges between 0.1 and 1.8 years in men and between 0.4 and 5.5 years in women. This suggests that several preventive treatments for chronic disease might have limited benefits in persons with frailty, given that the *time-until-benefit* might exceed the actual life expectancy in frail individuals. In frail populations, it is essential to assess life expectancy, evaluate the risk/benefit ratio of treatments and consider discontinuing medications aimed at prolonging life or preventing adverse clinical events if the time needed to obtain the expected benefits is longer than the estimated life expectancy and when they do not offer symptomatic benefits.

Increased risk of negative outcomes from intensive treatment. Frailty is associated with an increased risk of negative events associated with pharmacological treatments. Some of the current guidelines for the treatment of chronic diseases acknowledge this increased risk of negative events. For example, guidelines for treatment of type II diabetes supports the adoption of less strict blood glucose targets in frail patients, given the increased risk of hypoglycaemia without accruing meaningful benefit for frail older adults.

Ability to adhere. Functional deficits related to frailty might be associated with unintentional non-adherence through reduced ability to manage pill containers, open child-resistant containers and/or split tablets. Functional impairment may reduce the ability to adhere to a complex medication regimen and in case of polypharmacy, increase the risk of medication errors and limit the capacity to self-report adverse drug events. Treatment of chronic diseases in frailty should be simplified and focused on clinical priorities, established by the patient and his/her physician. Communication strategies should be implemented to empower and educate frail patients and their caregivers on how to properly take a medication, discussing with patients and caregivers about the importance of medication adherence, providing information about health and associated treatments and suggesting the use of aids (i.e. pill boxes) to improve adherence. Medication regimen complexity can often be reduced through consolidating the number of dose times and using long-acting formulations where appropriate [14].

11.4 Treatment of Multimorbidity and Frailty in the Precision Medicine Era

Precision medicine, as suggested by the Precision Medicine Initiative, is an innovative approach to provide personalized care focused on individual characteristics and deliver the most appropriate one by taking into consideration individual variability in genes, environment and lifestyle. This is opposed to the more common "one-size-fits-all" approach, whereby treatment and prevention strategies are developed for an average person. The precision medicine approach could represent an epochal change in the field of chronic diseases and a breakthrough in research and clinical trials performed in the last 30 years that assess the average effect of a given treatment with little consideration for individual differences. However, so far this approach has been poorly implemented in the multimorbidity field for several reasons.

First, precision medicine approach has been successfully applied in the treatment of mono-factorial diseases, in which it is easier to identify a single, potentially targetable, predictor of the disease. This may explain the wide application of precision medicine for the treatment of some diseases, especially cancer, and possible difficulties in implementing this approach to the care of multifactorial conditions, such as multimorbidity. Second, there is lack of a clear understanding of risk factors contributing to the onset and evolution of multimorbidity. A personalized approach to multimorbidity prevention and treatment would require the presence of reliable biomarkers and a systematic investigation of potential risk factors. Third, precision medicine is mainly focused on understanding genetic aspects of diseases, undermining other characteristics that are important to define profiles of frail multimorbid individuals. Such clinical and non-clinical characteristics (i.e. function and living environment, education and social capital, lifestyle) represent key elements of care in the approach to multimorbidity and can influence treatment adherence and success. This approach focuses on identifying multiple targetable risk factors of multimorbidity and individual pathways that could drive effective interventions and tailored management of the persons with multimorbidity, in line with the principles of precision medicine.

At the same time, however, numerous different individual pathways may lead to the development of different multimorbidity phenotypes, characterized by several combinations of individual factors. A clear understanding interplay and interaction between these factors might be extremely complex, making the definition of individual and personalized interventions challenging. Given multimorbidity heterogeneity, a possible solution to simplify the application of precision medicine to this condition is to reduce the dimensionality of its complexity and to find homogeneous patterns that may work as effective targets of preventive and therapeutic strategies. Focusing on clusters of chronic diseases could represent a useful strategy aiming to identify diseases that co-occur in the same person beyond chance. Diseases tend to cluster together because they share common risk factors and pathophysiological mechanisms or because one disease is the direct cause of another. Knowing how and why diseases cluster together can lead to the development of preventive and therapeutic strategies targeting specific but common pathways. At the time of writing, applying precision medicine to specific clusters of diseases remains a work in progress that requires further research including the analyses of large epidemiological and biological datasets investigating the interplay between genetic disease predisposition and personal and environmental determinants of multimorbidity such as gender, social and living factors, performance status, education and lifestyles. More information is needed to identify specific factor or combination of factors that need to be systematically assessed in individuals with specific clusters of diseases and understand how these factors also interact at an individual level. This approach could help define interventions that might comprehensively target multimorbidity [15].

References

1. Vetrano DL, Palmer K, Marengoni A, Marzetti E, Lattanzio F, Roller-Wirnsberger R, et al. Frailty and multimorbidity: a systematic review and meta-analysis. J Gerontol A Biol Sci Med Sci [Internet]. 2019 [cited 2022 Mar 15];74(5):659–666. https://pubmed.ncbi.nlm.nih.gov/29726918/.
2. Cesari M, Pérez-Zepeda MU, Marzetti E. Frailty and multimorbidity: different ways of thinking about geriatrics. J Am Med Dir Assoc [Internet]. 2017 [cited 2022 Mar 16];18(4):361–4. http://www.jamda.com/article/S1525861017300348/fulltext.
3. Onder G, Vetrano DL, Palmer K, Trevisan C, Amato L, Berti F, Campomori A, Catalano L, Corsonello A, Kruger P, Medea G, Nobili A, Trifirò G, Vecchi S, Veronese N, Marengoni A. Italian guidelines on management of persons with multimorbidity and polypharmacy. [Internet]. Aging Clin Exp Res. 2022. [cited 2022 Mar 15]. https://www.sigg.it/news/linea-guida-inter-societaria-per-la-gestione-della-multimorbilita-e-polifarmacoterapia-2021/.

4. Buta BJ, Walston JD, Godino JG, Park M, Kalyani RR, Xue QL, et al. Frailty assessment instruments: systematic characterization of the uses and contexts of highly-cited instruments. Ageing Res Rev [Internet]. 2016 [cited 2022 Mar 16];26:53. /pmc/articles/PMC4806795/.
5. Clegg A, Young J, Iliffe S, Rikkert MO, Rockwood K. Frailty in elderly people. Lancet [Internet]. 2013 [cited 2022 Mar 16];381(9868):752–62. http://www.thelancet.com/article/S0140673612621679/fulltext.
6. Muth C, Blom JW, Smith SM, Johnell K, Gonzalez-Gonzalez AI, Nguyen TS, et al. Evidence supporting the best clinical management of patients with multimorbidity and polypharmacy: a systematic guideline review and expert consensus. J Intern Med [Internet]. 2019 [cited 2022 Mar 15];285(3):272–88. https://onlinelibrary.wiley.com/doi/full/10.1111/joim.12842.
7. Villacampa-Fernández P, Navarro-Pardo E, Tarín JJ, Cano A. Frailty and multimorbidity: two related yet different concepts. Maturitas [Internet]. 2017 [cited 2022 Mar 15];95:31–5. https://pubmed.ncbi.nlm.nih.gov/27889050/.
8. Zucchelli A, Vetrano DL, Marengoni A, Grande G, Romanelli G, Calderón-Larrañaga A, et al. Frailty predicts short-term survival even in older adults without multimorbidity. Eur J Intern Med [Internet]. 2018 [cited 2022 Mar 15];56:53–6. http://www.ejinme.com/article/S0953620518302620/fulltext.
9. Yarnall AJ, Sayer AA, Clegg A, Rockwood K, Parker S, Hindle JV. New horizons in multimorbidity in older adults. Age Ageing [Internet]. 2017 [cited 2022 Mar 15];46(6):882–8. https://academic.oup.com/ageing/article/46/6/882/4103436.
10. Overview | Multimorbidity: clinical assessment and management | Guidance | NICE [Internet]. [cited 2022 Mar 19]. https://www.nice.org.uk/guidance/ng56.
11. Muth C, van den Akker M, Blom JW, Mallen CD, Rochon J, Schellevis FG, et al. The Ariadne principles: how to handle multimorbidity in primary care consultations. BMC Med [Internet]. 2014 [cited 2022 Mar 19];12(1):1–11. https://bmcmedicine.biomedcentral.com/articles/10.1186/s12916-014-0223-1
12. Boyd C, Smith CD, Masoudi FA, Blaum CS, Dodson JA, Green AR, et al. Decision making for older adults with multiple chronic conditions: executive summary for the American Geriatrics Society guiding principles on the care of older adults with multimorbidity. J Am Geriatr Soc [Internet]. 2019 [cited 2022 Mar 19];67(4):665–73. https://onlinelibrary.wiley.com/doi/full/10.1111/jgs.15809.
13. Mazya AL, Garvin P, Ekdahl AW. Outpatient comprehensive geriatric assessment: effects on frailty and mortality in old people with multimorbidity and high health care utilization. Aging Clin Exp Res [Internet]. 2019 [cited 2022 Mar 15];31(4):519–25. https://pubmed.ncbi.nlm.nih.gov/30039453/.
14. Onder G, Vetrano DL, Marengoni A, Bell JS, Johnell K, Palmer K. Accounting for frailty when treating chronic diseases. Eur J Intern Med [Internet]. 2018 [cited 2022 Mar 15];56:49–52. http://www.ejinme.com/article/S0953620518300815/fulltext.
15. Onder G, Bernabei R, Vetrano DL, Palmer K, Marengoni A. Facing multimorbidity in the precision medicine era. Mech Ageing Dev. 2020;190:111287.

12 Frailty and Drug Therapy

Annette Eidam, Matteo Cesari, and Jürgen M. Bauer

12.1 The Concept of Frailty

Frailty is a complex, multidimensional geriatric syndrome [1]. The theoretical concept of frailty was formally defined in 2013 by an international group of experts as "A medical syndrome with multiple causes and contributors that is characterized by diminished strength, endurance, and reduced physiologic function that increases an individual's vulnerability for developing increased dependency and/or death" [2]. This theoretical framework embraces different operational models that have been proposed over the years, especially since the beginning of this century. These models try to determine the main characteristics of the frailty condition, paving the way for its assessment in the clinical and research settings through the development of ad hoc instruments. The most widely known and adopted models of frailty are [3]:

- The physical phenotype model. Proposed in 2001 by Fried and colleagues [4], this model is based on the evaluation of five signs/symptoms (i.e., exhaustion, slowness, muscle weakness, involuntary weight loss, sedentary behavior) phenotypically describing the frail individual. Older adults who are negative for all these criteria are considered robust, those who are positive for one or two are considered prefrail, and those who are positive for three or more are considered frail.
- The accumulation of health deficit model. This model was proposed by Mitnitski and colleagues in 2001 [5]. It stems from the observation that the aging process

A. Eidam (✉) · J. M. Bauer
Center for Geriatric Medicine, Heidelberg University Hospital, Agaplesion Bethanien Hospital, Heidelberg, Germany
e-mail: Annette.Eidam@agaplesion.de

M. Cesari
Department of Clinical Sciences and Community Health, University of Milan, Milan, Italy

A. Cherubini et al. (eds.), *Optimizing Pharmacotherapy in Older Patients*, Practical Issues in Geriatrics, https://doi.org/10.1007/978-3-031-28061-0_12

is associated with an accumulation of health deficits (i.e., signs, symptoms, diseases, disabilities, laboratory abnormalities). The so-called Frailty Index is quantitatively computed by the ratio between the deficits the person presents and the number of potential deficits evaluated during a comprehensive assessment. It estimates the biological age and the proximity of death (due to the unsustainability of the deficits accumulation with life).

However, there is still an ongoing discussion on the best method for diagnosing frailty, in clinical practice and in research as well [6]. Besides the physical phenotype and the Frailty Index, a large number of other instruments to assess frailty have been developed and are used, with the exception of the Clinical Frailty Scale mostly in research settings. Examples include the Edmonton Frail Scale and the Groningen Frailty Indicator [7].

Independently of the preferred model for its operationalization, frailty has been acknowledged by the scientific community not only as a clinically relevant condition associated with major adverse health outcomes (e.g., hospitalization, institutionalization, disability, falls, death [8]) but also as a valuable approach that can improve the care of older persons [9]. In fact, it has become evident that chronological age does not adequately capture the heterogeneity of the biological, clinical, and social background of older persons [10]. Furthermore, a preference of chronological age over biological age in the clinical decisional process may increase ageism in medicine by excluding older persons from preventive and therapeutic options. In other words, frailty may represent an alternative approach for measuring the individual's biological age.

The detection of frailty and the exploration of its underlying causes are critical for the proper management of the older person. It means understanding whether the individual, regardless of his/her age, is biologically fit to sustain and benefit from standard interventions or whether an adapted approach with potentially different treatment strategies and objectives should be put in place. The adapted approach may include the design of a personalized plan aimed at solving potentially reversible barriers to restore (at least, partially) robustness to allocate the highest standards of care. Such an adapted approach should also acknowledge the particular vulnerabilities of the frail older patient.

In this context, the evaluation and management of frailty play an important role in the drugs prescription. The holistic approach needed to identify the underlying causes of frailty (i.e., the comprehensive geriatric assessment) allows to measure the priorities, needs, and resources of the individual [8]. This approach supports the clinician in the therapeutical choice by allowing a more informed evaluation of the risk–benefit profile of their frail patient. However, it cannot be overlooked that frail older persons are often excluded from randomized controlled trials given their complexity [11]. For this reason, the conduction of evidence-based medicine and prescribing in this population are frequently challenging. Frailty may, thus, become a condition to weigh the endogenous and exogenous factors potentially interfering with the "one-fits-all" approach typical of traditional medicine, supporting the delivery of a person-centered model of care and pharmacotherapy.

12.2 Influence of Frailty on Pharmacokinetics

As outlined above, frailty may be regarded as a proxy estimate of individual biological age [12]. Therefore, age-related changes in pharmacokinetics (Chap. 1) are likely to be more distinct in frail than in robust older adults [13], which may put frail older patients at a higher risk for inappropriate dosing and adverse drug reactions [14]. However, evidence from studies that compared pharmacokinetics in robust and frail older adults is still sparse [15].

Pathophysiological changes associated with frailty may affect pharmacokinetic processes, including the absorption, distribution, metabolism, and elimination of drugs [13]. Physical frailty has a pronounced overlap with sarcopenia (Chap. 13) [16]. Sarcopenia has been defined as a geriatric syndrome characterized by low muscle strength in combination with low quantity and quality of skeletal muscle [16]. In addition, it may be associated with an increase in fat mass [17]. These changes in body composition may alter the volume of distribution of both lipophilic and hydrophilic drugs. In this context, the volume of distribution of lipophilic drugs would be expected to increase, whereas the volume of distribution of hydrophilic drugs would be expected to decrease [13]. However, empirical data describing the pharmacokinetics of hydrophilic drugs in frailty have been inconsistent. Using the Reported Edmonton Frail Scale to define frailty, Hilmer and colleagues reported that the volume of distribution of gentamicin did not differ between frail and non-frail older participants [18]. On the other hand, Bendayan and colleagues found that lower appendicular lean mass was associated with supratherapeutic apixaban or rivaroxaban peak and trough concentrations in older adults. The authors attributed this increase in plasma concentrations to a decreased volume of distribution of the hydrophilic direct oral anticoagulants in frail individuals with reduced skeletal muscle mass [19].

Age-related physiological changes that could affect hepatic metabolism, such as the reduction in liver size and hepatic blood flow, might be more pronounced in frailty [13]. In addition, frailty is associated with a state of chronic inflammation [20]. Because inflammatory markers such as interleukin-6 may reduce the expression of certain cytochrome P450 (CYP) enzymes [21], phase I drug metabolism via these enzymes could be inhibited in frailty. However, two studies examining the activity of CYP3A and CYP2D6 in frail versus robust older adults failed to demonstrate a reduced CYP activity in their frail participants [22, 23]. On the other hand, Hubbard and colleagues found that the activity of different drug metabolizing plasma esterases was reduced in individuals with frailty, probably because of the underlying chronic inflammatory state [24].

Renal failure is highly prevalent in frail older persons [25]. Because of the accelerated decrease in muscle mass in frail persons, estimations of glomerular filtration rate (GFR) based on creatinine are likely to underestimate the degree of renal failure in this population compared to estimations based on cystatin C [25, 26]. There has been emerging evidence that the difference between estimated GFR based on cystatin C and estimated GFR based on creatinine might suggest the presence of frailty [27, 28]. Given the high number of renally eliminated drugs used by frail older patients, careful dose adaptation appears to be particularly relevant in this population [13, 25].

To date, only a limited number of pharmacokinetic studies have used validated frailty assessments to characterize their study populations [15]. So far, Fried and colleagues' physical phenotype of frailty [22–24] and variants of the Edmonton Frail Scale [18, 26, 29, 30] remain the most frequently used assessment instruments in this context. A small number of studies have used disease-specific assessments (International Myeloma Working Group Frailty Score [31]) or functional parameters (grip strength [26]) to evaluate the presence of frailty. Applying a standardized assessment to measure frailty would be essential for future pharmacokinetic studies, as this approach would facilitate the comparison across studies [15]. At present, many instruments are used to diagnose frailty, which differ significantly in their components and consecutively in the populations that are interpreted as being frail [7, 32]. It remains to be identified which frailty criteria would be particularly relevant to pharmacokinetics in older persons and could support optimized dosing schemes in this patient group.

12.3 Frail Populations in Clinical Trials

Age-sensitive eligibility criteria often exclude older adults from clinical drug trials [33]. A recent evaluation found that almost 80 % of adults with elevated blood pressure aged ≥ 80 years met at least one exclusion criterion of two major clinical trials that informed guideline recommendations for arterial hypertension [34]. Frail older adults are particularly underrepresented in clinical trials [35]. Moreover, trials that include a relevant number of older adults usually do not assess and report on the participants' frailty status [35]. As frailty is associated with both mortality [36] and adverse drug reactions [14], the therapeutic outcome and especially the risk–benefit ratio of drug therapy might differ significantly in frail compared to robust older persons. Therefore, it is essential to include older adults in clinical drug trials and characterize older study populations regarding their functionality, including frailty.

In the absence of standardized baseline frailty assessments of clinical trial populations, several research groups have attempted to identify frail study participants retrospectively. By including a 26-item frailty index in a pooled analysis of 14 multicenter trials of primarily cardiovascular medicines, Farooqi and colleagues found that frail participants had a higher risk of cardiovascular events, cardiovascular mortality, and all-cause mortality than non-frail participants [37]. Using a 40-item frailty index, Hanlon and colleagues reported that mild to moderate frailty was unexpectedly common in phase 3/4 trials of drug therapies for rheumatoid arthritis, type 2 diabetes mellitus, and chronic obstructive pulmonary disease [38]. Brefka and colleagues proposed a categorization for the retrospective identification of older study participants with functional impairments [39]. Including 51 assessments of physical frailty and functionality in their analysis, the authors defined specific cut-offs for four levels of functional impairment, which were designated as "independent," "slightly impaired," "significantly impaired," and "severely impaired/disabled/dependent" [39]. The application of this retrospective categorization may help compare treatment evidence between studies that used different instruments to assess frailty and functional status in general [39].

Applying the classification by Brefka and colleagues, two systematic reviews revealed evidence gaps in the pharmacological treatment of two common chronic diseases in frail older persons: hypertension and type 2 diabetes mellitus [40, 41]. The authors could not identify a single randomized clinical trial (RCT) that had assessed the effectiveness and safety of antihyperglycemic drug therapy in frail older adults [41]. Concerning antihypertensive treatment, they identified two RCTs that assessed functional status and two RCTs that applied validated frailty assessments [40]. Warwick and colleagues reported that the positive effects of antihypertensive treatment with indapamide ± perindopril on the risk of stroke, cardiovascular events, and total mortality were preserved in a separate analysis of frail individuals that participated in the "HYpertension in the Very Elderly Trial" (HYVET) study [42]. In an exploratory secondary analysis in participants aged ≥ 75 years of the "Systolic Blood Pressure Intervention Trial" (SPRINT), absolute event rates of cardiovascular and mortality outcomes were lower in the intensive treatment group in both slow and normal walkers and all frailty index groups compared with the standard treatment group [43].

There are emerging efforts from regulatory agencies to provide guidance on how to address frailty in clinical trials. For example, in 2018, the European Medicines Agency (EMA) published a "Reflection paper on physical frailty" [44]. In this paper, EMA recommended the "Short Physical Performance Battery" (SPPB) for baseline characterization of older adults in clinical trials or other clinical investigations [44]. The SPPB takes 10–15 min when applied in an older individual, and it measures lower extremity performance with three subtests: standing balance, gait speed, and chair rise test [45]. If the complete SPPB is not feasible, EMA encourages the isolated use of gait speed as an alternative to assess baseline physical function [44].

Up to now, the assessment of frailty is still uncommon in ongoing clinical drug trials, and if it is included, different assessment instruments might be chosen, thereby complicating the comparison of results. The "PRagmatic EValuation of evENTs And Benefits of Lipid-lowering in oldEr Adults" (PREVENTABLE) trial (https://clinicaltrials.gov/ct2/show/NCT04262206) examines the benefit of atorvastatin 40 mg for reducing the risk of dementia and chronic disability in community-dwelling adults aged ≥ 75 years. In this trial, the SPPB is applied for baseline characterization of the study population. The "Switching anticoagulant management from a VKA to a NOAC-based treatment strategy in frail elderly patients with atrial fibrillation" (FRAIL-AF) study (https://www.clinicaltrialsregister.eu/ctr-search/trial/2017-000393-11/NL) assesses the safety of switching from a vitamin K antagonist to a direct oral anticoagulant in adults aged ≥ 75 years with atrial fibrillation and a score ≥ 3 on the Groningen Frailty Indicator [46]. Few studies focus on frailty as an outcome parameter of drug therapy. The phase 2 trial "Metformin for Preventing Frailty in High-risk Older Adults" (https://clinicaltrials.gov/ct2/show/NCT02570672) investigates whether regular intake of metformin could prevent the progression of frailty status in robust and prefrail older adults with prediabetes [47]. In this trial, Fried and colleagues' physical phenotype is used.

12.4 Measuring Frailty in Healthcare Databases

In the absence of sufficient evidence from randomized controlled trials, researchers have turned to routine healthcare databases, for example, administrative claims data, to analyze outcomes of drug therapy in frail older patients. Routine healthcare databases offer real-world longitudinal data from large populations that include individuals with frailty [48]. However, as clinicians in most countries do not routinely assess and encode frailty, surrogate measures are needed to identify frailty in healthcare databases [48]. Several research groups have developed frailty indicators that each include a set of proxy variables for frailty, such as codes for frailty-related diagnoses and procedures and demographic variables such as age [48]. The Johns Hopkins claims-based frailty indicator was validated against the physical phenotype of frailty. It predicts adverse outcomes such as death and nursing home admission [49]. The claims-based frailty index by Kim and colleagues is based on the deficit-accumulation concept of frailty [50]. It has been validated in a Medicare data sample against physical performance measures (grip strength, gait speed) and several adverse health outcomes [50]. The electronic frailty index is also based on the frailty model of deficit accumulation. It has been developed and validated using two large primary care databases in the United Kingdom [51]. Since 2017, the National Health Service England has mandated that general practitioner's offices screen patients for frailty via the application of the electronic frailty index or other validated frailty measures [52] with the final aim of allocating ad hoc preventive strategies (including medication reviews and possible deprescribing).

Direct oral anticoagulants (DOAC) may serve as an example that illustrates how analyses of healthcare databases provide relevant evidence on outcomes of drug therapy in frail older patients. Both the Johns Hopkins claims-based frailty indicator and the claims-based frailty index have been used to generate data on the effectiveness and safety of treatment with direct oral anticoagulants in older patients with frailty and atrial fibrillation [53–56]. In a large 1:1 propensity score-matched analysis in Medicare beneficiaries aged ≥ 65 years, Kim and colleagues found that frailty levels affected the association of DOAC versus warfarin therapy with the composite primary endpoint (death, ischemic stroke, or major bleeding) [56]. Whereas hazard ratios in the dabigatran and rivaroxaban groups were lower compared to warfarin in the non-frail but not in the prefrail and frail older patients, therapy with apixaban showed consistent relative reductions across all three frailty levels [56].

12.5 The Complex Relationship of Frailty and Polypharmacy

Polypharmacy is highly prevalent in prefrail and frail older individuals [57]. Although there has been no universally accepted definition of polypharmacy, it is most commonly defined as the chronic intake of five or more medicines [58]. Some authors use the added term hyperpolypharmacy, usually defined as the regular intake of 10 or more medicines [58]. Polypharmacy has been linked to several adverse outcomes in older patients, including hospitalization and inappropriate prescribing [59]. There is an ongoing debate whether polypharmacy might also contribute to the development of frailty. While there is a strong association between frailty and polypharmacy in cross-sectional analyses, only a limited number of longitudinal studies have examined the relationship of polypharmacy with incident frailty [57]. In a cohort of community-dwelling adults, participants with polypharmacy or hyperpolypharmacy at baseline were at a higher risk of developing frailty within 3 years [60]. This finding was independent of the number and the severity of the participants' comorbidities [60]. In a meta-analysis of three longitudinal studies that used identical criteria for defining frailty (Fried physical phenotype) and polypharmacy ($\geq$ 5 drugs), robust individuals with baseline polypharmacy had a significantly higher risk of prefrailty at follow-up [57].

Considering the limited evidence resulting from longitudinal studies, the causal relationship between frailty and polypharmacy may still be regarded as undetermined. It has also been described as a "chicken and egg" scenario [61]. Most authors have assumed a bidirectional relationship between both entities [57, 61–63]. Frail older individuals are more likely to suffer from multiple chronic conditions than their robust counterparts [64], and multimorbidity itself may lead to polypharmacy [65]. Yet, there are several mechanisms through which medicines and polypharmacy may interfere with the pathogenesis of frailty. Polypharmacy and specific drug classes might cause malnutrition and weight loss [66]. Certain drugs increase the risk of experiencing a fall [67], and falls and fall-related injuries could precipitate a decline in functionality and overall physical activity in older adults [68]. Several drug classes, for example, anticholinergics and benzodiazepines, could negatively affect cognitive performance in older adults [69, 70], while cognitive impairment may be considered an element of the frailty concept [71].

However, the positive association between frailty and polypharmacy or hyperpolyharmacy may not apply to every setting. Cross-sectional studies found that polypharmacy was less common in frail older nursing home residents than in nonfrail residents [72], or they failed to find an association between both variables in this population [73]. This observation may reflect both inappropriate underprescription and an appropriate shift of focus from preventive to primarily symptomatic drug prescribing in this population [72, 73].

12.6 Adverse Drug Reactions and the Development of Frailty

As indicated in the previous paragraph, polypharmacy is associated with inappropriate prescribing [59], and adverse drug reactions due to low-quality prescribing might contribute to the development of frailty in patients with polypharmacy. Several drug classes have been implicated in the development of frailty. Most research in this area has focused on medicines with potentially unfavorable adverse effects in older adults, the so-called "Potentially Inappropriate Medications", such as anticholinergics and sedatives.

In a cross-sectional analysis in older community-dwelling veterans, frailty was associated with both past and current exposure to strong anticholinergic drugs as defined by the Anticholinergic Cognitive Burden Scale [74]. In a cross-sectional analysis of the Australian Longitudinal Study of Aging, users of anticholinergics and sedatives had higher odds for frailty and components of frailty such as slower walking speed [75]. After adjusting for polypharmacy, the prescription of anticholinergics was found to be the only potentially inappropriate medication significantly associated with frailty in a French cross-sectional analysis [76].

Longitudinal data focusing on a possible causal relationship between certain medicines and frailty are again limited. In an Australian cohort study in community-dwelling men aged $\geq$ 70 years, the Drug Burden Index was used to measure exposure to medicines with anticholinergic and sedative properties. Drug Burden Index exposure at baseline increased the risk of developing frailty within 2 years. Every unit increase in the Drug Burden Index was associated with an increased risk of transitioning from the robust state to prefrailty [77, 78]. In a prospective population-based cohort study in community-dwelling older adults from Germany, use of specific drug classes from the 2015 Beers criteria (anticholinergics, benzodiazepines, z-substances, and antipsychotics) was significantly associated with prevalent frailty and showed a nonsignificant association with incident frailty [79]. In a French longitudinal study in community-dwelling older adults, prescription drug use to manage pain and insomnia was associated with incident frailty [80].

Trials on the effect of deprescribing might further examine the relationship between frailty and high risk prescribing and polypharmacy [60, 78]. Deprescribing is the supervised withdrawal of an inappropriate medication to manage polypharmacy and improve outcomes [81]. Mach and colleagues realized an interesting preclinical study that may contribute to the current discussion on frailty and drug therapy, examining deprescribing in a mouse model of polypharmacy [82]. The authors found that in male mice, polypharmacy significantly increased frailty only in combination with a high Drug Burden Index exposure. With deprescribing, the authors observed a significant reduction in the animals' frailty score compared to continued treatment [82].

12.7 Frailty and Medication Management

12.7.1 Deprescribing

There has been a growing interest in the concept of deprescribing and in withdrawing potentially harmful and/or unnecessary medicines in older adults, particularly in those with frailty. Current research focuses on the question, whether deprescribing might be feasible without causing a negative impact on favorable health outcomes and whether it might reduce adverse drug reactions that contribute to frailty.

Several instruments have been developed to address deprescribing in frail older adults [83]. Such instruments may offer a framework for targeting deprescribing, a deprescribing approach for the patient's entire medication list, or guidance on deprescribing specific medications [83]. Some deprescribing instruments have been developed for a particular subgroup within the frail population. For example, in 2017, Lavan and colleagues published the Screening Tool of Older Persons Prescriptions in Frail adults with limited life expectancy (STOPPFrail) [84]. They later provided an updated version of this tool [85]. STOPPFrail has been designed to support physicians with deprescribing medications in older patients living with severe frailty who approach the end of their lives. This tool, therefore, only applies to this specific group of frail individuals. It does not apply to all frail patients and especially not to prefrail individuals. The tool was validated using the Delphi consensus methodology [84, 85], and currently includes 25 deprescribing criteria [85].

The evidence from empirical studies examining the practicality and the benefits and harms of deprescribing in older patients with frailty is still limited, and comparison of deprescribing studies in frail older individuals is complicated due to heterogeneity in interventions, outcome measures, and frailty criteria [86]. Nevertheless, though still incomplete, existing research indicates that deprescribing in this patient group might be both feasible and safe as well as beneficial [86].

12.7.2 Medication Underuse

Frailty is not only associated with polypharmacy and the prescription of potentially harmful medicines but also with potential prescribing omissions and underprescription of potentially beneficial medicines. The individual frailty status may affect the decision whether to start or to withhold anticoagulation therapy in older adults with atrial fibrillation [87, 88]. A retrospective cohort study found that between 2009 and 2018, the prescription of anticoagulants had increased in patients with nonvalvular atrial fibrillation who met guideline indications for anticoagulation [89]. However, this increase was less pronounced in the frail population [89]. Initiation of statin treatment after acute coronary syndrome was inversely correlated to the degree of frailty in older patients [90]. In a prospective population-based cohort study in older adults, underuse of preventive cardiovascular medicines was significantly associated with frailty [91].

Medication underuse in frail older individuals could reflect a degree of ageism and indicate true undertreatment [73]. On the other hand, underuse might also be rational and result from a patient-centered prescribing process that considers expected time-to-benefit, individual risk profiles, and a shift in therapeutic goals [73].

12.7.3 Medication Optimization

In the absence of robust evidence on the impact of medication optimization on frailty and favorable health outcomes in frail older adults [92, 93], there is currently no standardized approach to optimal medication management for this group of patients. Under these circumstances, recommendations derived from expert group discussions may serve as guiding principles. The Optimizing Geriatric Pharmacotherapy through Pharmacoepidemiology Network published a list of international consensus principles for medication management in frail older adults [94]. Key recommendations for medication management in clinical practice call on providers to (1) **reconcile the patient's medications**, resulting possibly from different prescribers, and to keep an up-to-date medication list, (2) **consider the patient's capacity for self-management of their medication**, and (3) guarantee **appropriate prescribing and deprescribing** [94]. Medication regimen complexity is known to increase with the degree of frailty [95], and clinicians should (4) consider **simplifying a frail patient's medication regimen** [94]. Because common symptoms in older adults could be drug-related, healthcare professionals should (5) pay **vigilance to the contribution of medicines in the development of geriatric syndromes**, such as delirium and incontinence [94].

Given the lack of evidence from randomized controlled trials and because of potential trade-offs between competing health outcomes, individuals with multiple chronic conditions, polypharmacy, and frailty usually face several preference-sensitive decisions concerning their medication. Although data specifically focusing on older patients with frailty are lacking, evidence from studies in older adults with multiple chronic conditions and/or polypharmacy suggests that preference-based prescribing could reduce treatment burden and the number of health complaints affecting daily life as well as improve health-related quality of life [96, 97]. Clinicians are asked to (6) **regularly repeat medication reviews** and adapt the patients' medication to their changing goals of care, and (7) **promote multidisciplinary communication** and include patients, caregivers, and other healthcare professionals in the medication management process [94].

12.8 Knowledge Gaps

Although frailty is a highly relevant geriatric syndrome, evidence on drug therapy in frail older adults is still limited. In addition to providing critical recommendations for practical medication management in individuals with frailty (Sect. 12.7.3), the Optimizing Geriatric Pharmacotherapy through Pharmacoepidemiology

Network has named international consensus principles for research activities in this context. The authors emphasize the need to include frail older adults in randomized controlled trials and identify strategies that would improve recruitment and reduce dropout rates in this population [94]. Research studies should include outcome measures that reflect the priorities of frail older patients by focusing both on physical health and on social well-being, such as physical and cognitive function as well as functional independence [94]. Moreover, the authors encourage research in the nursing home setting, which has been particularly underrepresented in clinical studies despite the fact that nursing home residents carry a notably high medication burden [94].

Frailty might be a better predictor of an individual's response to drug therapy than chronological age, and frailty is likely to modify the effect and risk–benefit profile of medicines [94, 98]. However, reflecting the lack of an international consensus on the diagnostic criteria of frailty, it is still unclear which frailty assessment could be best suited for application in drug trials and for evaluating the effects of polypharmacy in the older population. Although different frailty measures correlate significantly with each other, different frail populations are identified by the various assessment tools [99, 100]. However, the best choice might differ between study settings, as the physical, cognitive, emotional, or social domains of the frailty construct are likely to be of varying relevance to pharmacokinetic studies, randomized controlled drug trials, or studies examining medication management strategies. Furthermore, the choice of the instrument for the detection of frailty should also be made considering the intervention and resources that will be allocated if the screening result is positive.

Frail older adults carry an exceptionally high medication burden. Without comprehensive evidence on the benefits and the risks of drug therapy in this patient group, prescribing in frail older individuals is likely to be inadequate and potentially harmful. Academic researchers and regulatory authorities are called upon to design feasible strategies to recruit and characterize frail older individuals in pharmacological research, and all clinicians involved in the medical care of older patients need to acknowledge the demands of this important population during the prescribing process.

References

1. Chen X, Mao G, Leng SX. Frailty syndrome: an overview. Clin Interv Aging. 2014;9:433–41. https://doi.org/10.2147/CIA.S45300.
2. Morley JE, Vellas B, van Kan GA, Anker SD, Bauer JM, Bernabei R, et al. Frailty consensus: a call to action. J Am Med Dir Assoc. 2013;14(6):392–7. https://doi.org/10.1016/j.jamda.2013.03.022.
3. Cesari M, Gambassi G, van Kan GA, Vellas B. The frailty phenotype and the frailty index: different instruments for different purposes. Age Ageing. 2014;43(1):10–2. https://doi.org/10.1093/ageing/aft160.
4. Fried LP, Tangen CM, Walston J, Newman AB, Hirsch C, Gottdiener J, et al. Frailty in older adults: evidence for a phenotype. J Gerontol A Biol Sci Med Sci. 2001;56(3):M146–56. https://doi.org/10.1093/gerona/56.3.m146.

5. Mitnitski AB, Mogilner AJ, Rockwood K. Accumulation of deficits as a proxy measure of aging. ScientificWorldJournal. 2001;1:323–36. https://doi.org/10.1100/tsw.2001.58.
6. Buta BJ, Walston JD, Godino JG, Park M, Kalyani RR, Xue QL, et al. Frailty assessment instruments: systematic characterization of the uses and contexts of highly-cited instruments. Ageing Res Rev. 2016;26:53–61. https://doi.org/10.1016/j.arr.2015.12.003.
7. Dent E, Martin FC, Bergman H, Woo J, Romero-Ortuno R, Walston JD. Management of frailty: opportunities, challenges, and future directions. Lancet. 2019;394(10206):1376–86. https://doi.org/10.1016/S0140-6736(19)31785-4.
8. Ellis G, Gardner M, Tsiachristas A, Langhorne P, Burke O, Harwood RH, et al. Comprehensive geriatric assessment for older adults admitted to hospital. Cochrane Database Syst Rev. 2017;9:CD006211. https://doi.org/10.1002/14651858.CD006211.pub3.
9. Cesari M, Prince M, Thiyagarajan JA, De Carvalho IA, Bernabei R, Chan P, et al. Frailty: an emerging public health priority. J Am Med Dir Assoc. 2016;17(3):188–92. https://doi.org/10.1016/j.jamda.2015.12.016.
10. Clegg A, Young J, Iliffe S, Rikkert MO, Rockwood K. Frailty in elderly people. Lancet. 2013;381(9868):752–62. https://doi.org/10.1016/S0140-6736(12)62167-9.
11. Cherubini A, Corsonello A, Lattanzio F. Underprescription of beneficial medicines in older people: causes, consequences and prevention. Drugs Aging. 2012;29(6):463–75. https://doi.org/10.2165/11631750-000000000-00000.
12. Diebel LWM, Rockwood K. Determination of biological age: geriatric assessment vs biological biomarkers. Curr Oncol Rep. 2021;23(9):104. https://doi.org/10.1007/s11912-021-01097-9.
13. Hilmer SN, Wu H, Zhang M. Biology of frailty: implications for clinical pharmacology and drug therapy in frail older people. Mech Ageing Dev. 2019;181:22–8. https://doi.org/10.1016/j.mad.2019.111119.
14. Maher D, Ailabouni N, Mangoni AA, Wiese MD, Reeve E. Alterations in drug disposition in older adults: a focus on geriatric syndromes. Expert Opin Drug Metab Toxicol. 2021;17(1):41–52. https://doi.org/10.1080/17425255.2021.1839413.
15. Hilmer SN, Kirkpatrick CMJ. New horizons in the impact of frailty on pharmacokinetics: latest developments. Age Ageing. 2021;50(4):1054–63. https://doi.org/10.1093/ageing/afab003.
16. Cruz-Jentoft AJ, Bahat G, Bauer J, Boirie Y, Bruyere O, Cederholm T, et al. Sarcopenia: revised European consensus on definition and diagnosis. Age Ageing. 2019;48(1):16–31. https://doi.org/10.1093/ageing/afy169.
17. Bauer JM, Cruz-Jentoft AJ, Fielding RA, Kanis JA, Reginster JY, Bruyere O, et al. Is there enough evidence for osteosarcopenic obesity as a distinct entity? A critical literature review. Calcif Tissue Int. 2019;105(2):109–24. https://doi.org/10.1007/s00223-019-00561-w.
18. Hilmer SN, Tran K, Rubie P, Wright J, Gnjidic D, Mitchell SJ, et al. Gentamicin pharmacokinetics in old age and frailty. Br J Clin Pharmacol. 2011;71(2):224–31. https://doi.org/10.1111/j.1365-2125.2010.03825.x.
19. Bendayan M, Mardigyan V, Williamson D, Chen-Tournoux A, Eintracht S, Rudski L, et al. Muscle mass and direct oral anticoagulant activity in older adults with atrial fibrillation. J Am Geriatr Soc. 2021;69(4):1012–8. https://doi.org/10.1111/jgs.16992.
20. Soysal P, Stubbs B, Lucato P, Luchini C, Solmi M, Peluso R, et al. Inflammation and frailty in the elderly: a systematic review and meta-analysis. Ageing Res Rev. 2016;31:1–8. https://doi.org/10.1016/j.arr.2016.08.006.
21. de Jong LM, Jiskoot W, Swen JJ, Manson ML. Distinct effects of inflammation on cytochrome P450 regulation and drug metabolism: lessons from experimental models and a potential role for pharmacogenetics. Genes (Basel). 2020;11(12):1509. https://doi.org/10.3390/genes11121509.
22. Schwartz JB. Erythromycin breath test results in elderly, very elderly, and frail elderly persons. Clin Pharmacol Ther. 2006;79(5):440–8. https://doi.org/10.1016/j.clpt.2006.01.006.
23. Opdam FL, Modak AS, Mooijaart SP, Louwerens M, de Waal MW, Gelderblom H, et al. CYP2D6 metabolism in frail elderly compared to non-frail elderly: a pilot feasibility study. Drugs Aging. 2015;32(12):1019–27. https://doi.org/10.1007/s40266-015-0319-0.

24. Hubbard RE, O'Mahony MS, Calver BL, Woodhouse KW. Plasma esterases and inflammation in ageing and frailty. Eur J Clin Pharmacol. 2008;64(9):895–900. https://doi.org/10.1007/s00228-008-0499-1.
25. Ballew SH, Chen Y, Daya NR, Godino JG, Windham BG, McAdams-DeMarco M, et al. Frailty, kidney function, and polypharmacy: the atherosclerosis risk in communities (ARIC) study. Am J Kidney Dis. 2017;69(2):228–36. https://doi.org/10.1053/j.ajkd.2016.08.034.
26. Tan SJ, Cockcroft M, Page-Sharp M, Arendts G, Davis TME, Moore BR, et al. Population pharmacokinetic study of ceftriaxone in elderly patients, using cystatin C-based estimates of renal function to account for frailty. Antimicrob Agents Chemother. 2020;64(10):e00874–20. https://doi.org/10.1128/AAC.00874-20.
27. Potok OA, Ix JH, Shlipak MG, Katz R, Hawfield AT, Rocco MV, et al. The difference between cystatin C- and creatinine-based estimated GFR and associations with frailty and adverse outcomes: a cohort analysis of the systolic blood pressure intervention trial (SPRINT). Am J Kidney Dis. 2020;76(6):765–74. https://doi.org/10.1053/j.ajkd.2020.05.017.
28. Potok OA, Katz R, Bansal N, Siscovick DS, Odden MC, Ix JH, et al. The difference between cystatin C- and creatinine-based estimated GFR and incident frailty: an analysis of the cardiovascular health study (CHS). Am J Kidney Dis. 2020;76(6):896–8. https://doi.org/10.1053/j.ajkd.2020.05.018.
29. Johnston C, Hilmer SN, McLachlan AJ, Matthews ST, Carroll PR, Kirkpatrick CM. The impact of frailty on pharmacokinetics in older people: using gentamicin population pharmacokinetic modeling to investigate changes in renal drug clearance by glomerular filtration. Eur J Clin Pharmacol. 2014;70(5):549–55. https://doi.org/10.1007/s00228-014-1652-7.
30. Hias J, Van der Linden L, Walgraeve K, Gijsen M, Mian P, Koch BCP, et al. Pharmacokinetics of 2 oral paracetamol formulations in hospitalized octogenarians. Br J Clin Pharmacol. 2022;88:1020–30. https://doi.org/10.1111/bcp.15049.
31. Nampoothiri RV, Kasudhan KS, Patil AN, Malhotra P, Khadwal A, Prakash G, et al. Impact of frailty, melphalan pharmacokinetics, and pharmacogenetics on outcomes post autologous hematopoietic cell transplantation for multiple myeloma. Bone Marrow Transplant. 2019;54(12):2088–95. https://doi.org/10.1038/s41409-019-0631-0.
32. Faller JW, Pereira DDN, de Souza S, Nampo FK, Orlandi FS, Matumoto S. Instruments for the detection of frailty syndrome in older adults: a systematic review. PLoS One. 2019;14(4):e0216166. https://doi.org/10.1371/journal.pone.0216166.
33. Beers E, Moerkerken DC, Leufkens HG, Egberts TC, Jansen PA. Participation of older people in preauthorization trials of recently approved medicines. J Am Geriatr Soc. 2014;62(10):1883–90. https://doi.org/10.1111/jgs.13067.
34. Anderson TS, Odden MC, Penko J, Kazi DS, Bellows BK, Bibbins-Domingo K. Characteristics of populations excluded from clinical trials supporting intensive blood pressure control guidelines. J Am Heart Assoc. 2021;10(7):e019707. https://doi.org/10.1161/JAHA.120.019707.
35. Cerreta F, Padrao A, Skibicka-Stepien I, Strampelli A, de Orbe Izquierdo MS. Medicines for older people: assessment and transparency at the European Medicines Agency regarding cardiovascular and antithrombotic medicinal products. Eur Geriatr Med. 2018;9(4):415–8. https://doi.org/10.1007/s41999-018-0071-1.
36. Ekram A, Woods RL, Britt C, Espinoza S, Ernst ME, Ryan J. The association between frailty and all-cause mortality in community-dwelling older individuals: an umbrella review. J Frailty Aging. 2021;10(4):320–6. https://doi.org/10.14283/jfa.2021.20.
37. Farooqi MAM, Gerstein H, Yusuf S, Leong DP. Accumulation of deficits as a key risk factor for cardiovascular morbidity and mortality: a pooled analysis of 154 000 individuals. J Am Heart Assoc. 2020;9(3):e014686. https://doi.org/10.1161/JAHA.119.014686.
38. Hanlon P, Butterly E, Lewsey J, Siebert S, Mair FS, McAllister DA. Identifying frailty in trials: an analysis of individual participant data from trials of novel pharmacological interventions. BMC Med. 2020;18(1):309. https://doi.org/10.1186/s12916-020-01752-1.
39. Brefka S, Dallmeier D, Muhlbauer V, von Arnim CAF, Bollig C, Onder G, et al. A proposal for the retrospective identification and categorization of older people with functional

impairments in scientific studies-recommendations of the Medication and Quality of Life in Frail Older Persons (MedQoL) Research Group. J Am Med Dir Assoc. 2019;20(2):138–46. https://doi.org/10.1016/j.jamda.2018.11.008.
40. Muhlbauer V, Dallmeier D, Brefka S, Bollig C, Voigt-Radloff S, Denkinger M. The pharmacological treatment of arterial hypertension in frail, older patients-a systematic review. Dtsch Arztebl Int. 2019;116(3):23–30. https://doi.org/10.3238/arztebl.2019.0023.
41. Bollig C, Torbahn G, Bauer J, Brefka S, Dallmeier D, Denkinger M, et al. Evidence gap on antihyperglycemic pharmacotherapy in frail older adults: a systematic review. Z Gerontol Geriatr. 2021;54(3):278–84. https://doi.org/10.1007/s00391-020-01724-3.
42. Warwick J, Falaschetti E, Rockwood K, Mitnitski A, Thijs L, Beckett N, et al. No evidence that frailty modifies the positive impact of antihypertensive treatment in very elderly people: an investigation of the impact of frailty upon treatment effect in the HYpertension in the Very Elderly Trial (HYVET) study, a double-blind, placebo-controlled study of antihypertensives in people with hypertension aged 80 and over. BMC Med. 2015;13:78. https://doi.org/10.1186/s12916-015-0328-1.
43. Williamson JD, Supiano MA, Applegate WB, Berlowitz DR, Campbell RC, Chertow GM, et al. Intensive vs standard blood pressure control and cardiovascular disease outcomes in adults aged >/=75 years: a randomized clinical trial. JAMA. 2016;315(24):2673–82. https://doi.org/10.1001/jama.2016.7050.
44. European Medicines Agency. Reflection paper on physical frailty: instruments for baseline characterisation of older populations in clinical trials. https://www.ema.europa.eu/en/documents/scientific-guideline/reflection-paper-physical-frailty-instruments-baseline-characterisation-older-populations-clinical_en.pdf. Accessed 25 Oct 2021.
45. Guralnik JM, Simonsick EM, Ferrucci L, Glynn RJ, Berkman LF, Blazer DG, et al. A short physical performance battery assessing lower extremity function: association with self-reported disability and prediction of mortality and nursing home admission. J Gerontol. 1994;49(2):M85–94. https://doi.org/10.1093/geronj/49.2.m85.
46. Joosten LPT, van Doorn S, Hoes AW, Nierman MC, Wiersma NM, Koek HL, et al. Safety of switching from vitamin K antagonist to non-vitamin K antagonist oral anticoagulant in frail elderly with atrial fibrillation: rationale and design of the FRAIL-AF randomised controlled trial. BMJ Open. 2019;9(12):e032488. https://doi.org/10.1136/bmjopen-2019-032488.
47. Espinoza SE, Musi N, Wang CP, Michalek J, Orsak B, Romo T, et al. Rationale and study design of a randomized clinical trial of metformin to prevent frailty in older adults with prediabetes. J Gerontol A Biol Sci Med Sci. 2020;75(1):102–9. https://doi.org/10.1093/gerona/glz078.
48. Kim DH, Patorno E, Pawar A, Lee H, Schneeweiss S, Glynn RJ. Measuring frailty in administrative claims data: comparative performance of four claims-based frailty measures in the U.S. Medicare data. J Gerontol A Biol Sci Med Sci. 2020;75(6):1120–5. https://doi.org/10.1093/gerona/glz224.
49. Segal JB, Chang HY, Du Y, Walston JD, Carlson MC, Varadhan R. Development of a claims-based frailty indicator anchored to a well-established frailty phenotype. Med Care. 2017;55(7):716–22. https://doi.org/10.1097/MLR.0000000000000729.
50. Kim DH, Glynn RJ, Avorn J, Lipsitz LA, Rockwood K, Pawar A, et al. Validation of a claims-based frailty index against physical performance and adverse health outcomes in the health and retirement study. J Gerontol A Biol Sci Med Sci. 2019;74(8):1271–6. https://doi.org/10.1093/gerona/gly197.
51. Clegg A, Bates C, Young J, Ryan R, Nichols L, Ann Teale E, et al. Development and validation of an electronic frailty index using routine primary care electronic health record data. Age Ageing. 2016;45(3):353–60. https://doi.org/10.1093/ageing/afw039.
52. Attwood D, Stevens K, Jones L, Harris L, Roberts F. Home visits: a new screening tool for frailty? A retrospective exploratory study. J Family Med Prim Care. 2018;7(5):1007–11. https://doi.org/10.4103/jfmpc.jfmpc_159_18.
53. Grymonprez M, Steurbaut S, De Backer TL, Petrovic M, Lahousse L. Effectiveness and safety of oral anticoagulants in older patients with atrial fibrillation: a systematic

review and meta-analysis. Front Pharmacol. 2020;11:583311. https://doi.org/10.3389/fphar.2020.583311.
54. Martinez BK, Sood NA, Bunz TJ, Coleman CI. Effectiveness and safety of apixaban, dabigatran, and rivaroxaban versus warfarin in frail patients with nonvalvular atrial fibrillation. J Am Heart Assoc. 2018;7(8):e008643. https://doi.org/10.1161/JAHA.118.008643.
55. Hohmann C, Hohnloser SH, Jacob J, Walker J, Baldus S, Pfister R. Non-vitamin K oral anticoagulants in comparison to phenprocoumon in geriatric and non-geriatric patients with non-valvular atrial fibrillation. Thromb Haemost. 2019;119(6):971–80. https://doi.org/10.1055/s-0039-1683422.
56. Kim DH, Pawar A, Gagne JJ, Bessette LG, Lee H, Glynn RJ, et al. Frailty and clinical outcomes of direct oral anticoagulants versus warfarin in older adults with atrial fibrillation: a cohort study. Ann Intern Med. 2021;174(9):1214–23. https://doi.org/10.7326/M20-7141.
57. Palmer K, Villani ER, Vetrano DL, Cherubini A, Cruz-Jentoft AJ, Curtin D, et al. Association of polypharmacy and hyperpolypharmacy with frailty states: a systematic review and meta-analysis. Eur Geriatr Med. 2019;10(1):9–36. https://doi.org/10.1007/s41999-018-0124-5.
58. Masnoon N, Shakib S, Kalisch-Ellett L, Caughey GE. What is polypharmacy? A systematic review of definitions. BMC Geriatr. 2017;17(1):230. https://doi.org/10.1186/s12877-017-0621-2.
59. Davies LE, Spiers G, Kingston A, Todd A, Adamson J, Hanratty B. Adverse outcomes of polypharmacy in older people: systematic review of reviews. J Am Med Dir Assoc. 2020;21(2):181–7. https://doi.org/10.1016/j.jamda.2019.10.022.
60. Saum KU, Schottker B, Meid AD, Holleczek B, Haefeli WE, Hauer K, et al. Is polypharmacy associated with frailty in older people? Results from the ESTHER cohort study. J Am Geriatr Soc. 2017;65(2):e27–e32. https://doi.org/10.1111/jgs.14718.
61. Rochon PA, Stall NM, Holmes HM. Drug therapy and frailty: chicken or the egg? J Am Geriatr Soc. 2019;67(12):2441–3. https://doi.org/10.1111/jgs.16213.
62. Gutierrez-Valencia M, Izquierdo M, Cesari M, Casas-Herrero A, Inzitari M, Martinez-Velilla N. The relationship between frailty and polypharmacy in older people: a systematic review. Br J Clin Pharmacol. 2018;84(7):1432–44. https://doi.org/10.1111/bcp.13590.
63. Cesari M. How polypharmacy affects frailty. Expert Rev Clin Pharmacol. 2020;13(11):1179–81. https://doi.org/10.1080/17512433.2020.1829467.
64. Vetrano DL, Palmer K, Marengoni A, Marzetti E, Lattanzio F, Roller-Wirnsberger R, et al. Frailty and multimorbidity: a systematic review and meta-analysis. J Gerontol A Biol Sci Med Sci. 2019;74(5):659–66. https://doi.org/10.1093/gerona/gly110.
65. Nobili A, Marengoni A, Tettamanti M, Salerno F, Pasina L, Franchi C, et al. Association between clusters of diseases and polypharmacy in hospitalized elderly patients: results from the REPOSI study. Eur J Intern Med. 2011;22(6):597–602. https://doi.org/10.1016/j.ejim.2011.08.029.
66. Jyrkka J, Mursu J, Enlund H, Lonnroos E. Polypharmacy and nutritional status in elderly people. Curr Opin Clin Nutr Metab Care. 2012;15(1):1–6. https://doi.org/10.1097/MCO.0b013e32834d155a.
67. Seppala LJ, Wermelink A, de Vries M, Ploegmakers KJ, van de Glind EMM, Daams JG, et al. Fall-risk-increasing drugs: a systematic review and meta-analysis: II. Psychotropics. J Am Med Dir Assoc. 2018;19(4):371.e11–7. https://doi.org/10.1016/j.jamda.2017.12.098.
68. Tinetti ME, Williams CS. The effect of falls and fall injuries on functioning in community-dwelling older persons. J Gerontol A Biol Sci Med Sci. 1998;53(2):M112–9. https://doi.org/10.1093/gerona/53a.2.m112.
69. Risacher SL, McDonald BC, Tallman EF, West JD, Farlow MR, Unverzagt FW, et al. Association between anticholinergic medication use and cognition, brain metabolism, and brain atrophy in cognitively normal older adults. JAMA Neurol. 2016;73(6):721–32. https://doi.org/10.1001/jamaneurol.2016.0580.
70. Nafti M, Sirois C, Kroger E, Carmichael PH, Laurin D. Is benzodiazepine use associated with the risk of dementia and cognitive impairment-not dementia in older persons? The

Canadian Study of Health and Aging. Ann Pharmacother. 2020;54(3):219–25. https://doi.org/10.1177/1060028019882037.
71. Kelaiditi E, Cesari M, Canevelli M, van Kan GA, Ousset PJ, Gillette-Guyonnet S, et al. Cognitive frailty: rational and definition from an (I.A.N.A./I.A.G.G.) international consensus group. J Nutr Health Aging. 2013;17(9):726–34. https://doi.org/10.1007/s12603-013-0367-2.
72. Villani ER, Vetrano DL, Liperoti R, Palmer K, Denkinger M, van der Roest HG, et al. Relationship between frailty and drug use among nursing homes residents: results from the SHELTER study. Aging Clin Exp Res. 2021;33(10):2839–47. https://doi.org/10.1007/s40520-021-01797-z.
73. Gutierrez-Valencia M, Izquierdo M, Lacalle-Fabo E, Marin-Epelde I, Ramon-Espinoza MF, Domene-Domene T, et al. Relationship between frailty, polypharmacy, and underprescription in older adults living in nursing homes. Eur J Clin Pharmacol. 2018;74(7):961–70. https://doi.org/10.1007/s00228-018-2452-2.
74. Ruiz SJ, Cevallos V, Baskaran D, Mintzer MJ, Ruiz JG. The cross-sectional association of frailty with past and current exposure to strong anticholinergic drugs. Aging Clin Exp Res. 2021;33(8):2283–9. https://doi.org/10.1007/s40520-020-01742-6.
75. Lim R, Kalisch Ellett LM, Widagdo IS, Pratt NL, Roughead EE. Analysis of anticholinergic and sedative medicine effects on physical function, cognitive function, appetite and frailty: a cross-sectional study in Australia. BMJ Open. 2019;9(9):e029221. https://doi.org/10.1136/bmjopen-2019-029221.
76. Herr M, Sirven N, Grondin H, Pichetti S, Sermet C. Frailty, polypharmacy, and potentially inappropriate medications in old people: findings in a representative sample of the French population. Eur J Clin Pharmacol. 2017;73(9):1165–72. https://doi.org/10.1007/s00228-017-2276-5.
77. Gnjidic D, Hilmer SN, Blyth FM, Naganathan V, Cumming RG, Handelsman DJ, et al. High-risk prescribing and incidence of frailty among older community-dwelling men. Clin Pharmacol Ther. 2012;91(3):521–8. https://doi.org/10.1038/clpt.2011.258.
78. Jamsen KM, Bell JS, Hilmer SN, Kirkpatrick CM, Ilomaki J, Le Couteur D, et al. Effects of changes in number of medications and drug burden index exposure on transitions between frailty states and death: the Concord Health and Ageing in Men Project Cohort Study. J Am Geriatr Soc. 2016;64(1):89–95. https://doi.org/10.1111/jgs.13877.
79. Muhlack DC, Hoppe LK, Saum KU, Haefeli WE, Brenner H, Schottker B. Investigation of a possible association of potentially inappropriate medication for older adults and frailty in a prospective cohort study from Germany. Age Ageing. 2019;49(1):20–5. https://doi.org/10.1093/ageing/afz127.
80. Cil G, Park J, Bergen AW. Self-reported prescription drug use for pain and for sleep and incident frailty. J Am Geriatr Soc. 2019;67(12):2474–81. https://doi.org/10.1111/jgs.16214.
81. Reeve E, Gnjidic D, Long J, Hilmer S. A systematic review of the emerging definition of 'deprescribing' with network analysis: implications for future research and clinical practice. Br J Clin Pharmacol. 2015;80(6):1254–68. https://doi.org/10.1111/bcp.12732.
82. Mach J, Gemikonakli G, Logan C, Vander Wyk B, Allore H, Ekambareshwar S, et al. Chronic polypharmacy with increasing Drug Burden Index exacerbates frailty and impairs physical function, with effects attenuated by deprescribing, in aged mice. J Gerontol A Biol Sci Med Sci. 2021;76(6):1010–8. https://doi.org/10.1093/gerona/glaa060.
83. Thompson W, Lundby C, Graabaek T, Nielsen DS, Ryg J, Sondergaard J, et al. Tools for deprescribing in frail older persons and those with limited life expectancy: a systematic review. J Am Geriatr Soc. 2019;67(1):172–80. https://doi.org/10.1111/jgs.15616.
84. Lavan AH, Gallagher P, Parsons C, O'Mahony D. STOPPFrail (Screening Tool of Older Persons Prescriptions in Frail adults with limited life expectancy): consensus validation. Age Ageing. 2017;46(4):600–7. https://doi.org/10.1093/ageing/afx005.
85. Curtin D, Gallagher P, O'Mahony D. Deprescribing in older people approaching end-of-life: development and validation of STOPPFrail version 2. Age Ageing. 2021;50(2):465–71. https://doi.org/10.1093/ageing/afaa159.

86. Ibrahim K, Cox NJ, Stevenson JM, Lim S, Fraser SDS, Roberts HC. A systematic review of the evidence for deprescribing interventions among older people living with frailty. BMC Geriatr. 2021;21(1):258. https://doi.org/10.1186/s12877-021-02208-8.
87. Papakonstantinou PE, Asimakopoulou NI, Papadakis JA, Leventis D, Panousieris M, Mentzantonakis G, et al. Frailty status affects the decision for long-term anticoagulation therapy in elderly patients with atrial fibrillation. Drugs Aging. 2018;35(10):897–905. https://doi.org/10.1007/s40266-018-0587-6.
88. Sanghai SR, Liu W, Wang W, Rongali S, Orkaby AR, Saczynski JS, et al. Prevalence of frailty and associations with oral anticoagulant prescribing in atrial fibrillation. J Gen Intern Med. 2022;37(4):730–6. https://doi.org/10.1007/s11606-021-06834-1.
89. Orlandi M, Dover DC, Sandhu RK, Hawkins NM, Kaul P, McAlister FA. The introduction of direct oral anticoagulants has not resolved treatment gaps for frail patients with nonvalvular atrial fibrillation. Can J Cardiol. 2022;38(1):77–84. https://doi.org/10.1016/j.cjca.2021.09.021.
90. Lopez D, Nedkoff L, Briffa T, Preen DB, Etherton-Beer C, Flicker L, et al. Effect of frailty on initiation of statins following incident acute coronary syndromes in patients aged >/=75 years. Maturitas. 2021;153:13–8. https://doi.org/10.1016/j.maturitas.2021.07.006.
91. Meid AD, Quinzler R, Freigofas J, Saum KU, Schottker B, Holleczek B, et al. Medication underuse in aging outpatients with cardiovascular disease: prevalence, determinants, and outcomes in a prospective cohort study. PLoS One. 2015;10(8):e0136339. https://doi.org/10.1371/journal.pone.0136339.
92. Pazan F, Petrovic M, Cherubini A, Onder G, Cruz-Jentoft AJ, Denkinger M, et al. Current evidence on the impact of medication optimization or pharmacological interventions on frailty or aspects of frailty: a systematic review of randomized controlled trials. Eur J Clin Pharmacol. 2021;77(1):1–12. https://doi.org/10.1007/s00228-020-02951-8.
93. Saeed D, Carter G, Parsons C. Interventions to improve medicines optimisation in frail older patients in secondary and acute care settings: a systematic review of randomised controlled trials and non-randomised studies. Int J Clin Pharm. 2022;44(1):15–26. https://doi.org/10.1007/s11096-021-01354-8.
94. Liau SJ, Lalic S, Sluggett JK, Cesari M, Onder G, Vetrano DL, et al. Medication management in frail older people: consensus principles for clinical practice, research, and education. J Am Med Dir Assoc. 2021;22(1):43–9. https://doi.org/10.1016/j.jamda.2020.05.004.
95. Chen EY, Bell JS, Ilomaki J, Keen C, Corlis M, Hogan M, et al. Medication regimen complexity in 8 Australian residential aged care facilities: impact of age, length of stay, comorbidity, frailty, and dependence in activities of daily living. Clin Interv Aging. 2019;14:1783–95. https://doi.org/10.2147/CIA.S216705.
96. Tinetti ME, Naik AD, Dindo L, Costello DM, Esterson J, Geda M, et al. Association of patient priorities-aligned decision-making with patient outcomes and ambulatory health care burden among older adults with multiple chronic conditions: a nonrandomized clinical trial. JAMA Intern Med. 2019;179(12):1688–97. https://doi.org/10.1001/jamainternmed.2019.4235.
97. Verdoorn S, Kwint HF, Blom JW, Gussekloo J, Bouvy ML. Effects of a clinical medication review focused on personal goals, quality of life, and health problems in older persons with polypharmacy: a randomised controlled trial (DREAMeR-study). PLoS Med. 2019;16(5):e1002798. https://doi.org/10.1371/journal.pmed.1002798.
98. Tan ECK, Sluggett JK, Johnell K, Onder G, Elseviers M, Morin L, et al. Research priorities for optimizing geriatric pharmacotherapy: an international consensus. J Am Med Dir Assoc. 2018;19(3):193–9. https://doi.org/10.1016/j.jamda.2017.12.002.
99. Rockwood K, Andrew M, Mitnitski A. A comparison of two approaches to measuring frailty in elderly people. J Gerontol A Biol Sci Med Sci. 2007;62(7):738–43. https://doi.org/10.1093/gerona/62.7.738.
100. Roppolo M, Mulasso A, Gobbens RJ, Mosso CO, Rabaglietti E. A comparison between uni- and multidimensional frailty measures: prevalence, functional status, and relationships with disability. Clin Interv Aging. 2015;10:1669–78. https://doi.org/10.2147/CIA.S92328.

Falls and Impaired Mobility

13

Lotta Seppala and Nathalie van der Velde

13.1 Impact of Falls

Falls are a significant and rapidly growing global public health problem. A third of people aged 65 years and older fall at least once per year [1]. In long-term care, falls are even more common. Approximately, half of the nursing home residents will experience one or more falls yearly [2]. Furthermore, in adult inpatients, falls are the most frequently reported safety incident [3]. For example, the rate of falls has been estimated to range from 3.3 to 11.5 falls per 1000 patient days in US hospitals [4]. Falls have substantial impact on both mortality and morbidity. More than 684,000 people die as the result of a fall every year globally [5]. Older people are at highest risk of dying as a result of a fall and this risk grows with advancing age [5]. Falls can have both physical and mental consequences. Over 60% of those who experienced a fall in the past year report being injured [6]. It has been estimated that annually, 172 million are left with short or long-term disability globally [5]. The main physical consequences in older persons include hip fracture, other fractures, traumatic brain injury, damage to intrathoracic and intra-abdominal organs, spinal and nerve injuries, joint distortion and dislocation, soft-tissue damage, and bruises and cuts [5]. Fear of falling (FOF) is common among older fallers, and FOF is linked to impaired mobility and decreased functional status [1]. Negative mental health effects in older persons include social withdrawal, symptom of anxiety and depression [1]. Also, due to all negative health-related effects, falls place a

L. Seppala (✉) · N. van der Velde
Internal Medicine, Section of Geriatric Medicine, Amsterdam UMC Location University of Amsterdam, Amsterdam, The Netherlands

Amsterdam Public Health Research Institute, Amsterdam, The Netherlands
e-mail: l.j.seppala@amsterdamumc.nl; n.vandervelde@amsterdamumc.nl

A. Cherubini et al. (eds.), *Optimizing Pharmacotherapy in Older Patients*, Practical Issues in Geriatrics, https://doi.org/10.1007/978-3-031-28061-0_13

significant burden on healthcare expenditure. Around 0.85–1.5% of the total healthcare expenditure are fall-related costs in Western countries [7].

13.2 Risk Factors for Falls

Mostly falls result from several interacting risk factors [8], of which medication use and mobility, both modifiable key risk factors, will be discussed in detail in this chapter. Fall risk factors have been intensively studied during the past decades. In general, fall risk factors can be classified into intrinsic (such as medical conditions) and extrinsic risk factors (such as home hazards) [8]. Perhaps the most important risk factors in terms of predictive power are older age and history of past falls [5]. Some of the other key risk factors are first of all as earlier mentioned the use of certain medications and mobility disorders as well as poor balance, visual impairment, cognitive impairment and Parkinson's disease, arthritis, and/or depression [5]. The risk factors for falls in long-term care or in hospital differ somewhat from the risk factors among community-dwellers [5].

13.3 Mobility and Risk of Falling

Impaired mobility is a key risk factor for falls and includes impairments in muscle strength, balance and/or gait [5]. In a systematic review by Deandrea et al., gait problems doubled the odds of falling [9]. Also, quantitative performance measures of gait including gait variability and gait speed have been shown to be robust predictors of fall risk [10]. Gait disorders are believed to occur among a third of older adults aged 70 years or older [11]. The origins of gait disorders include orthopedic problems (e.g., osteoarthritis and skeletal deformities), neurological conditions (e.g., sensory or motor impairments), and medical conditions (e.g., respiratory insufficiency, heart failure, peripheral arterial occlusive disease, and obesity) [12], and also certain medication use is linked to reduced gait speed [13]. With advancing age, gait disorders usually have multiple origins [12]. Also, balance disorders are one of the most significant reasons resulting in falls [5]. Sensory, motor, and central processing mediate balance activity, and impairment in any of these three systems can lead to a deficit in balance control [14]. Sensory inputs are integrated by the central nervous system, and the central nervous system created the motor commands [14]. The impairments can be due to the progressive decline of function in the course of normal aging or due to specific pathology including use of certain medications [14]. The prevalence of balance impairment has been estimated to vary between 20 and 50% [14]. Last, muscle weakness (in particular lower extremity weakness) is a major risk factor for falls [15]. Muscle strength is an essential component of preserved mobility. The rate of muscle loss has been estimated to vary from 1 to 2% past the age of 50 years [16]. Aging and inactivity or disuse is associated with a decline in strength, muscle mass, and structure [16]. Use of certain medications can negatively affect either muscle strength or mass or both.

13.4 Falls and Impaired Mobility, Common Adverse Drug Events

In general, several medication classes belonging to cardiovascular and psychotropic medication groups have been considered to increase fall risk. FRIDs are commonly prescribed to older people. According to recent literature review, the use of FRIDs is ranging from 65 to 93% in older adults with a fall-related injury [17]. In addition, almost 90% of older adults visiting their general practitioner due to dizziness are using at least one FRID [18]. The prescriptions of the FRIDs in general have been increasing in the past decades [19]. Shaver et al. found that the percentage of older persons who were prescribed a FRID increased to 94% in 2017, a significant leap from 57% in 1999 [19]. Antihypertensives were the most often prescribed FRIDs [19]. However, there was also a major rise in the prescriptions of antidepressants from 1999 to 2017 as the amount prescriptions was more than fourfold [19]. Data on FRIDs is mostly based on observational studies, as regrettably fall incidents are not standardly assessed as adverse events in drug trials to date [20]. Data on observational studies have been summarized in several systematic reviews and meta-analyses during past decades. For example, in the meta-analyses by the European Geriatric Medicine Society (EuGMS) Task and Finish Group on FRIDs, a significant association for falls was found for the following medication classes: antidepressants [selective serotonin reuptake inhibitors, tricyclic antidepressants], antipsychotics, benzodiazepines, loop diuretics, antiepileptics, opioids, and polypharmacy (four or more medications) [21–23]. Furthermore, it was concluded that digitalis may increase fall risk [21]. In addition, inconsistent associations were observed for antiarrhythmics, antihypertensives, diuretics, anticholinergics, NSAIDs, analgesics, antiplatelets, and laxatives [21, 22]. However, these kinds of systematic reviews and meta-analysis are confined to evaluation of commonly prescribed medication classes and to addressing the average risk in the older population instead of individual risk [24]. To overcome these shortcomings, the STOPPFall (Screening Tool of Older Persons Prescriptions in older adults with high fall risk) was developed and published in 2020 [24].This is the first European expert consensus FRID list of 14 medication groups [24]. The European consensus list of FRIDs is presented in Table 13.1 [24]. In addition to STOPPFall, in other general (de)prescribing tools, several medication classes are listed as potentially inappropriate among fallers. The medication classes included in the STOPP/START version 2 and 2019 updated Beers Criteria are presented in Table 13.2 [41, 42]. FRIDs can induce fall risk through different mechanisms (cardiovascular, central nervous system, or motoric) including, for example, orthostatic hypotension, sedation, dizziness, and muscle weakness [24]. The possible pathways leading to falls of STOPPFall medication classes are shown in Table 13.1. Most of these adverse effects are reversible after deprescribing [43, 44]. One of the key pathways to increased fall risk due to FRID use is motoric mechanisms. Drugs with sedative properties have been consistently associated with reduced gait speed [13]. In contrast, statin use has not been consistently associated with reduced gait speed [13]. In addition, the evidence for other drug classes is mixed, and other quantitative gait parameters have not been sufficiently investigated [13]. Most of the research regarding FRIDs and falls have

Table 13.1 Fall risk-increasing drugs according to Delphi consensus effort [24] and their possible mechanisms leading to falls

• **Benzodiazepines and benzodiazepine-related drugs**
– Muscular weakness, ataxia, sedation, extrapyramidal symptoms, imbalance and/or dizziness, visual disorders, delirium, possibly orthostatic hypotension [25, 26]
• **Antipsychotics**
– Sedation, drowsiness or somnolence, dizziness or vertigo, orthostatic hypotension, extrapyramidal side effects, cardiac effects (QTc prolongation and tachycardia), anticholinergic effects (e.g., blurred vision), delirium, confusion, hyponatremia [27, 28]
• **Antidepressants**
– Sedation, impaired balance/reaction time, orthostatic hypotension, cardiac conduction and rhythm disorders, visual impairment, hyponatremia, delirium, and drug-induced movement disorders [29]
• **Diuretics**
– Orthostatic hypotension, hypotension, electrolyte disturbances [30]
• **Alpha-blockers used as antihypertensives**
– Orthostatic hypotension, hypotension, dizziness, asthenia, and syncope [31]
• **Centrally acting antihypertensives**
– Orthostatic hypotension, hypotension, weakness and sedation [32]
• **Vasodilators used in cardiac diseases**
– Hypotension, orthostatic hypotension, dizziness, syncope [33]
• **Opioids**
– Orthostatic hypotension, drowsiness, sedation, confusion, delirium, eye disorders, muscle problems (e.g., rigidity) [34]
• **Antiepileptics**
– Drowsiness, fatigue, dizziness, unsteadiness, vertigo, imbalance, ataxia, diplopia, cognitive impairment, and hyponatraemia [35]
• **Anticholinergics**
– Effects on central nervous system (sedation, confusion, delirium, dizziness, cognitive impairment, impaired concentration) and blurred vision, tachycardia [36]
• **Alpha-blockers used for prostate hyperplasia**
– Orthostatic hypotension, hypotension, dizziness, somnolence, visual impairment, and syncope [37, 38]
• **Overactive bladder and incontinence medications**
– Dizziness or vertigo, somnolence, delirium, visual impairment [38, 39]
• **Antihistamines**
– Central nervous system side effects (e.g., sedation, drowsiness, somnolence, fatigue, cognitive decline), anticholinergic effects, cardiovascular toxicities (e.g., arrhythmias, prolongation of the QT interval, and postural hypotension) [40]

focused on commonly prescribed overarching medication classes (such as beta-blockers), and little is known regarding the differences of fall risk-increasing properties between pharmacological subclasses (such as selective versus nonselective beta-blockers). In STOPPFall, these differences between subclasses were explored based on expert opinion [24]. The differences between subclasses that reached consensus are presented in Table 13.3. In addition to risk differences within pharmacological groups, there are other medication-related issues such as initiation or duration of use and dosage, which all appear to play a role in medication-related falls. Higher dosages of psychotropics have been associated with increased fall risk [23]. The higher blood and tissue concentrations related to higher dosages might explain this dose-dependent relationship. In addition, the fall risk related to certain medication use appears to be highest when starting the medication use. For example, the risk of

Table 13.2 Fall-related potentially inappropriate medication in older persons: STOPP/START version 2 and Beers Criteria

STOPP/START Version 2: Drugs That Increase the Risk of Falls in Older People [41]
• Benzodiazepines
• Neuroleptic drugs
• Vasodilator drugs with persistent postural hypotension, i.e., recurrent drop in systolic blood pressure ≥ 20 mmHg
• Hypnotic Z-drugs
2019 Updated AGS Beers Criteria®: Potentially Inappropriate Medication Use in Case of History of Falls or Fractures [42]
• Antiepileptics
• Antipsychotics
• Benzodiazepines
• Hypnotic Z-drugs
• Antidepressants
• Opioids

Table 13.3 The differences of fall risk-increasing properties between pharmacological subclasses according to STOPPFall

Antipsychotics: agents with strong (1) sedative, (2) anticholinergic, and (3) alpha-receptor properties
Opioids: strong opioids[a]
Antidepressants: tricyclic antidepressants (TCAs), agents with strong (1) sedative effects, (2) propensity to cause orthostatic hypotension, and (3) anticholinergic activity
Anticholinergics: agents high anticholinergic activity
Antiepileptics: older generation antiepileptics, agents with strong sedative effects
Diuretics: loop diuretics
Alpha-blockers for benign prostatic hyperplasia: nonselective alpha-blockers
Antihistamines: first-generation antihistamines, agents with strong (1) sedative effects and (2) anticholinergic activity
Medications for overactive bladder and urge incontinence: agents with strong anticholinergic activity
Oral hypoglycemics: agents that can cause hypoglycemia

[a] A low dose of a more potent opioid, e.g., morphine, may be better tolerated than weak opioids at a higher dose

benzodiazepine related falls has been found to be highest after starting the therapy [45, 46], and the association between thiazide prescription and falls was found to be strongest in the 3 weeks after prescription [47]. The role of drug-drug interactions in medication-related falls is still unclear [20]. But potentially, drug-drug interactions can cause additive pharmacological effects and lead to cytochrome P-450 interactions possibly resulting in increased drug efficacy and toxicity [48]. Furthermore, some patient characteristics appear to be of importance when defining the medication-related fall risk of an individual. Tinetti et al. reported that antihypertensive use was associated with an increased risk of serious fall injuries especially among those with history of injurious falls, which could be a marker, for example, for multimorbidity or frailty [49]. Ham et al. showed that individuals using benzodiazepines and having reduced CYP2C9 enzyme activity, on the basis of their genotype, had an increased fall risk [50]. Nevertheless in general the majority of studies have focused on general risk related to medication use instead of personalized medication optimization.

13.5 Prevention of (Medication-Related) Falls: Background and Evidence

The new world guidelines for fall prevention and management exist to guide professionals regarding fall prevention in clinical practice [51]. According to the guidelines, all older adults should be advised on fall prevention and physical activity [51], and those considered at high risk should be offered a comprehensive multifactorial fall risk assessment with a view to codesign and implement personalized multidomain interventions [51]. One of the standard domains to be included in the intervention is medication review [51]. This is supported by among others the recent network meta-analysis showing that basic fall risk assessment including a medication review is one the effective components of multifactorial fall prevention intervention [52].

There is however uncertainty regarding the effectiveness of deprescribing as a *single* intervention in fall prevention in the literature. The meta-analysis by Lee et al. showed no effect of pure FRID deprescribing on any of the fall outcomes as a single intervention [53]. In addition, Cameron et al. reported that a medication review, as a single intervention, may make little or no difference to risk of falling or rate of falls in long-term care facilities [54]. Nevertheless, in a meta-analysis of the FRID working group of the "World Falls Guidelines for the Prevention and Management of Falls in Older Adults" investigating the effect of medication reviews, a trend for a lower number of fallers in long-term care was seen [55]. This suggests that in a frailer subgroup of older adults (e.g., in case of severe frailty, advanced dementia, long-term care residents), deprescribing might be effective also as a single intervention. Thus, as recommended by the World Falls Guidelines Task Force, in long-term care residents, the fall prevention strategy should always include rational deprescribing of fall risk-increasing drugs [51]. However, given the multifactorial nature of falls, deprescribing interventions are recommended to be implemented as a part of multimodal strategy rather than a stand-alone strategy [55], and multifactorial fall prevention intervention has consistently shown to reduce falls rate [56]. Common components of multiple interventions significantly associated with a reduction in number of fallers and falls rate are exercise, assistive technology, quality improvement strategies, environmental assessment and modifications, and basic fall risk assessment (including a medication review) as mentioned above [52]. Nevertheless, in current clinical practice, deprescribing FRIDs after a fall incident is not frequently conducted. According to a recent review, FRID use was not reduced at 1 and 6 months following the fall-related healthcare contact in observational studies [17]. In addition, when implementing fall preventive strategies among primary care providers, majority of patients with high fall risk received most of recommended interventions and assessments, except medication modification. The reluctance can be partly explained by the general overestimation of the benefits of the medication and underestimation of the potential harms by both physicians and patients [20]. In additions, many physicians perceive the uncertainty related to the consequences of withdrawing FRIDs as uncomfortable and challenging [20]. Nevertheless, in general, deprescribing of FRIDs can be conducted safely [57]. Few adverse withdrawal effects occur, and if symptoms reoccur, they can be treated safely by reintroducing the stopped medication or if possible a safer alternative [57]. To increase the implementation uptake of a complex intervention such as medication review, education and engagement of both healthcare professionals and patients are essential [58]. Given the complexity of the intervention, supporting structured tools accompanied with appropriate training are warranted [24, 59]. In addition, allocation of sufficient time and resources is necessary to optimize the uptake and effectiveness.

13.6 Effect of Deprescribing of FRIDs on Impaired Mobility and Other Adverse Effects

As described above, FRIDs have mostly cardiovascular, motoric, and central nervous system related adverse effects which can lead to falls, and most of these adverse effects are reversible after deprescribing [43, 44]. In terms of mobility outcomes, van der Velde et al. found that withdrawal of FRIDs among geriatric outpatients improved Timed Up and Go Test and the walking time on the 10-m walking test in a follow-up (mean, 6.7 months) and reduced occurrence of orthostatic hypotension [43, 44]. In addition, Tsunoda et al. found that benzodiazepine withdrawal improved the stability of the body and a recovery of cognitive functions [60]. In a study by Nurminen et al., benzodiazepine withdrawal was found to improve muscle strength and balance rapidly [61].

13.7 How to Perform Medication Management of FRIDs

The first step in reducing the risk of falls caused by FRIDs is to prevent their inappropriate use in the older population (primary prevention) [20]. Therefore, as recommended by the World Falls Guideline Task Force, a history of falls and risk of falling should be checked before prescribing FRIDs, and the risks and benefits should be weighted for older persons [51]. In addition, possible safer alternatives should be considered. Furthermore, medication review (including FRIDs review) should be performed regularly (at least annually in older persons). In frail older adults, a medication review should be done minimally every 6 months [62–64]. In a medication review of risks for developing adverse drug events (ADEs), the safety and effectiveness of each drug and compliance are assessed, and views of patients and carers are being considered [65]. FRID review is an essential part of the regular medication review as falls are important ADEs. The regularity of these reviews will help to keep the exposure to FRIDs as short as possible and potentially reduce associated fall risk. It is recommended to use a validated, structured screening and assessment tool (such as STOPPFall) to identify FRIDs when performing medication review [51]. As described earlier, studies have shown that the effect of FRIDs on fall risk appears to be dependent on characteristics [49]. Thus, these characteristics, including polypharmacy, frailty status, comorbidities, patient's preferences, and other geriatric syndromes, should be taken into account when performing a medication review [65]. To succeed in this, the medication review is optimally embedded in a holistic assessment to enable personalized medication strategy. Furthermore, it is important to realize that in practice, when deprescribing of FRIDs is initiated, compliance is notoriously poor, especially for psychotropic medications

[66]. Thus, a single one-time advice does not suffice. For the long-term success of deprescribing provision of support, monitoring, and documentation are essential [67]. Monitoring should be arranged on individual basis [24]. Finally, about 10–15% of falls result in fractures, and therefore, in the medication review, the known drugs to affect skeletal fragility should also be considered [20].

The generic steps of medication management of older fallers are shown in Fig. 13.1 [20]. Further practical guidance regarding deprescribing of FRIDs is

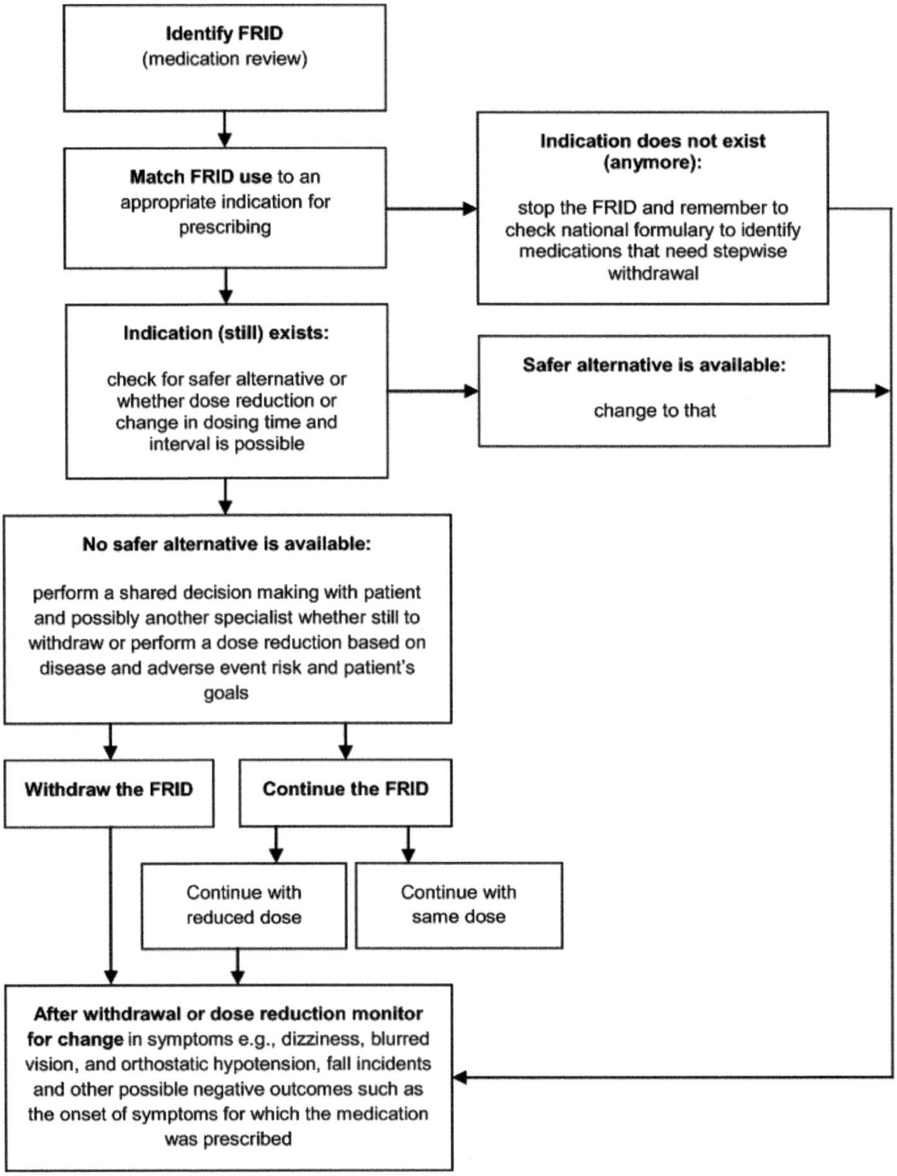

Fig. 13.1 Generic steps of medication management in older fallers [20]

provided in the STOPPFall deprescribing tool [24]. The tool is a freely available online decision support tool which works in a stepwise manner containing all the steps of the decision tree of the Fig. 13.1 separately for each STOPPFall medication class [68]. For example, for antidepressants, it states that at least in the following cases deprescribing should be considered: (1) hyponatremia, orthostatic hypotension, dizziness, sedative symptoms, or tachycardia/arrhythmia; (2) if given for sleep disorder; and (3) if given for depression, but this is dependent on symptom-free time and history of symptoms [24]. Furthermore, the tool indicates that stepwise deprescribing is needed and after deprescribing at least the following symptoms should be monitored: recurrence of depression, anxiety, irritability, and insomnia [24]. Also a paper version is available in the Appendix of the publication [24].

13.8 Conclusion

Falls have a major impact on both individual and societal level. Mostly falls tend to occur due to several interacting risk factors in an individual. Some of the key risk factors are older age, past falls, mobility, and certain medication use (fall risk-increasing drugs). Several psychotropic medications (benzodiazepines and related drugs, antidepressants, antipsychotics), anticholinergics (such as overactive bladder and incontinence medications and antihistamines), opioids, alpha-blockers, and other cardiovascular medications (diuretics and centrally acting antihypertensives) are considered to induce increased fall risk. FRIDs have cardiovascular, motoric, and central nervous system related adverse effects which can lead to falls. Medication review with the aim of FRID deprescribing as a part of multifactorial fall prevention strategy is effective in fall prevention. This medication review should be a holistic assessment including the evaluation of characteristics such as frailty and patient goals to produce a personalized medication optimization plan. Regular medication reviews will help to keep the exposure to FRIDs as short as possible. Structured tools (such as STOPPFall) can aid with FRID deprescribing.

References

1. Berry SD, Miller RR. Falls: epidemiology, pathophysiology, and relationship to fracture. Curr Osteoporos Rep. 2008;6(4):149–54.
2. Montero-Odasso M, van der Velde N, Alexander NB, Becker C, Blain H, Camicioli R, et al. New horizons in falls prevention and management for older adults: a global initiative. Age Ageing. 2021;50(5):1499–507.
3. Morris R, O'Riordan S. Prevention of falls in hospital. Clin Med (Lond). 2017;17(4):360–2.
4. Bouldin EL, Andresen EM, Dunton NE, Simon M, Waters TM, Liu M, et al. Falls among adult patients hospitalized in the United States: prevalence and trends. J Patient Saf. 2013;9(1):13–7.
5. Step safely: strategies for preventing and managing falls across the life-course. Geneva: World Health Organization; 2021. Licence: CC BY-NC-SA 3.0 IGO.
6. Milat AJ, Watson WL, Monger C, Barr M, Giffin M, Reid M. Prevalence, circumstances and consequences of falls among community-dwelling older people: results of the 2009 NSW falls prevention baseline survey. N S W Public Health Bull. 2011;22(3–4):43–8.
7. Heinrich S, Rapp K, Rissmann U, Becker C, König H-H. Cost of falls in old age: a systematic review. Osteoporos Int. 2010;21(6):891–902.

8. Ganz DA, Latham NK. Prevention of falls in community-dwelling older adults. N Engl J Med. 2020;382(8):734–43.
9. Deandrea S, Lucenteforte E, Bravi F, Foschi R, La Vecchia C, Negri E. Risk factors for falls in community-dwelling older people: a systematic review and meta-analysis. Epidemiology. 2010;21(5):658–68.
10. Kyrdalen IL, Thingstad P, Sandvik L, Ormstad H. Associations between gait speed and well-known fall risk factors among community-dwelling older adults. Physiother Res Int. 2019;24(1):e1743.
11. Verghese J, LeValley A, Hall CB, Katz MJ, Ambrose AF, Lipton RB. Epidemiology of gait disorders in community-residing older adults. J Am Geriatr Soc. 2006;54(2):255–61.
12. Pirker W, Katzenschlager R. Gait disorders in adults and the elderly : a clinical guide. Wien Klin Wochenschr. 2017;129(3–4):81–95.
13. Osman A, Kamkar N, Speechley M, Ali S, Montero-Odasso M. Fall risk-increasing drugs and gait performance in community-dwelling older adults: a systematic review. Ageing Res Rev. 2022;77:101599.
14. Nnodim JO, Yung RL. Balance and its clinical assessment in older adults—A review. J Geriatr Med Gerontol. 2015;1(1):003.
15. Moreland JD, Richardson JA, Goldsmith CH, Clase CM. Muscle weakness and falls in older adults: a systematic review and meta-analysis. J Am Geriatr Soc. 2004;52(7):1121–9.
16. Seene T, Kaasik P. Muscle weakness in the elderly: role of sarcopenia, dynapenia, and possibilities for rehabilitation. Eur Rev Aging Phys Act. 2012;9(2):109–17.
17. Hart LA, Phelan EA, Yi JY, Marcum ZA, Gray SL. Use of fall risk-increasing drugs around a fall-related injury in older adults: a systematic review. J Am Geriatr Soc. 2020;68(6):1334–43.
18. Stam H, Harting T, van der Sluijs M, van Marum R, van der Horst H, van der Wouden JC, et al. Usual care and management of fall risk increasing drugs in older dizzy patients in Dutch general practice. Scand J Prim Health Care. 2016;34(2):164–70.
19. Shaver AL, Clark CM, Hejna M, Feuerstein S, Wahler RG Jr, Jacobs DM. Trends in fall-related mortality and fall risk increasing drugs among older individuals in the United States,1999–2017. Pharmacoepidemiol Drug Saf. 2021;30(8):1049–56.
20. Seppala LJ, van der Velde N, Masud T, Blain H, Petrovic M, van der Cammen TJ, et al. EuGMS Task and Finish group on Fall-Risk-Increasing Drugs (FRIDs): position on knowledge dissemination, management, and future research. Drugs Aging. 2019;36(4):299–307.
21. de Vries M, Seppala LJ, Daams JG, van de Glind EMM, Masud T, van der Velde N. Fall-risk-increasing drugs: a systematic review and meta-analysis: I. Cardiovascular drugs. J Am Med Dir Assoc. 2018;19(4):371.e1–9.
22. Seppala LJ, van de Glind EMM, Daams JG, Ploegmakers KJ, de Vries M, Wermelink A, et al. Fall-risk-increasing drugs: a systematic review and meta-analysis: III. Others. J Am Med Dir Assoc. 2018;19(4):372.e1–8.
23. Seppala LJ, Wermelink A, de Vries M, Ploegmakers KJ, van de Glind EMM, Daams JG, et al. Fall-risk-increasing drugs: a systematic review and meta-analysis: II. Psychotropics. J Am Med Dir Assoc. 2018;19(4):371.e11–7.
24. Seppala LJ, Petrovic M, Ryg J, Bahat G, Topinkova E, Szczerbińska K, et al. STOPPFall (Screening Tool of Older Persons Prescriptions in older adults with high fall risk): a Delphi study by the EuGMS Task and Finish Group on Fall-Risk-Increasing Drugs. Age Ageing. 2020;50:1189.
25. Rivasi G, Kenny RA, Ungar A, Romero-Ortuno R. Effects of benzodiazepines on orthostatic blood pressure in older people. Eur J Intern Med. 2020;72:73–8.
26. Capiau A, Huys L, van Poelgeest E, van der Velde N, Petrovic M, Somers A. Therapeutic dilemmas with benzodiazepines and Z-drugs: insomnia and anxiety disorders versus increased fall risk—a clinical review. Eur Geriatr Med. 2022.
27. Stroup TS, Gray N. Management of common adverse effects of antipsychotic medications. World Psychiatry. 2018;17(3):341–56.

28. Korkatti-Puoskari N, Tiihonen M, Caballero-Mora MA, Topinkova E, Szczerbińska K, Hartikainen S. Therapeutic dilemma's: antipsychotics and risk of falling in older adults: a clinical review. Under review.
29. van Poelgeest EP, Pronk AC, Rhebergen D, van der Velde N. Depression, antidepressants and fall risk: therapeutic dilemmas—a clinical review. Eur Geriatr Med. 2021;12(3):585–96.
30. Weinberger MH. Diuretics and their side effects. Dilemma in the treatment of hypertension. Hypertension. 1988;11(3 Pt 2):II16–20.
31. Carruthers SG. Adverse effects of α1-adrenergic blocking drugs. Drug Saf. 1994;11(1):12–20.
32. Sica DA. Centrally acting antihypertensive agents: an update. J Clin Hypertens (Greenwich). 2007;9(5):399–405.
33. Thadani U, Rodgers T. Side effects of using nitrates to treat angina. Expert Opin Drug Saf. 2006;5(5):667–74.
34. Virnes RE, Tiihonen M, Karttunen N, van Poelgeest EP, van der Velde N, Hartikainen S. Opioids and falls risk in older adults: a narrative review. Drugs Aging. 2022;39(3):199–207.
35. Perucca P, Gilliam FG. Adverse effects of antiepileptic drugs. Lancet Neurol. 2012;11(9):792–802.
36. Nishtala PS, Salahudeen MS, Hilmer SN. Anticholinergics: theoretical and clinical overview. Expert Opin Drug Saf. 2016;15(6):753–68.
37. Chapple CR. A comparison of varying alpha-blockers and other pharmacotherapy options for lower urinary tract symptoms. Rev Urol. 2005;7 Suppl 4(Suppl 4):S22–30.
38. Ilhan B, Erdoğan T, Topinkova E, Bahat G. Management of commonly used urinary incontinence and benign prostatic hyperplasia drugs in older adults at risk of falls: a clinical review. Under review.
39. Lam S, Hilas O. Pharmacologic management of overactive bladder. Clin Interv Aging. 2007;2(3):337–45.
40. Kaliner MA. H1-antihistamines in the elderly. Clin Allergy Immunol. 2002;17:465–81.
41. O'Mahony D, O'Sullivan D, Byrne S, O'Connor MN, Ryan C, Gallagher P. STOPP/START criteria for potentially inappropriate prescribing in older people: version 2. Age Ageing. 2015;44(2):213–8.
42. American Geriatrics Society 2019 updated AGS beers criteria® for potentially inappropriate medication use in older adults. J Am Geriatr Soc. 2019;67(4):674–94.
43. van der Velde N, van den Meiracker AH, Pols HA, Stricker BH, van der Cammen TJ. Withdrawal of fall-risk-increasing drugs in older persons: effect on tilt table test outcomes. J Am Geriatr Soc. 2007;55(5):734–9.
44. van der Velde N, Stricker BH, Pols HA, van der Cammen TJ. Withdrawal of fall-risk-increasing drugs in older persons: effect on mobility test outcomes. Drugs Aging. 2007;24(8):691–9.
45. Neutel CI, Hirdes JP, Maxwell CJ, Patten SB. New evidence on benzodiazepine use and falls: the time factor. Age Ageing. 1996;25(4):273–8.
46. Ray WA, Thapa PB, Gideon P. Benzodiazepines and the risk of falls in nursing home residents. J Am Geriatr Soc. 2000;48(6):682–5.
47. Gribbin J, Hubbard R, Gladman J, Smith C, Lewis S. Risk of falls associated with antihypertensive medication: self-controlled case series. Pharmacoepidemiol Drug Saf. 2011;20(8):879–84.
48. Zazzara MB, Palmer K, Vetrano DL, Carfì A, Graziano O. Adverse drug reactions in older adults: a narrative review of the literature. Eur Geriatr Med. 2021;12(3):463–73.
49. Tinetti ME, Han L, Lee DS, McAvay GJ, Peduzzi P, Gross CP, et al. Antihypertensive medications and serious fall injuries in a nationally representative sample of older adults. JAMA Intern Med. 2014;174(4):588–95.
50. Ham AC, Ziere G, Broer L, Swart KM, Enneman AW, van Dijk SC, et al. CYP2C9 genotypes modify benzodiazepine-related fall risk: original results from three studies with meta-analysis. J Am Med Dir Assoc. 2017;18(1):88.e1–88.e15.
51. Montero-Odasso M, van der Velde N, Martin FC, Petrovic M, Tan MP, Ryg J, et al. World guidelines for falls prevention and management for older adults: a global initiative. Age Ageing. 2022;51(9):afac205.

52. Dautzenberg L, Beglinger S, Tsokani S, Zevgiti S, Raijmann R, Rodondi N, et al. Interventions for preventing falls and fall-related fractures in community-dwelling older adults: a systematic review and network meta-analysis. J Am Geriatr Soc. 2021;69:2973.
53. Lee J, Negm A, Peters R, Wong EKC, Holbrook A. Deprescribing fall-risk increasing drugs (FRIDs) for the prevention of falls and fall-related complications: a systematic review and meta-analysis. BMJ Open. 2021;11(2):e035978.
54. Cameron ID, Dyer SM, Panagoda CE, Murray GR, Hill KD, Cumming RG, et al. Interventions for preventing falls in older people in care facilities and hospitals. Cochrane Database Syst Rev. 2018;9(9):CD005465.
55. Seppala LJ, Kamkar N, van Poelgeest EP, Thomsen K, Daams JG, Ryg J, et al. Medication reviews and deprescribing as a single intervention in falls prevention: a systematic review and meta-analysis. Age Ageing. 2022;51(9):afac191.
56. Hopewell S, Copsey B, Nicolson P, Adedire B, Boniface G, Lamb S. Multifactorial interventions for preventing falls in older people living in the community: a systematic review and meta-analysis of 41 trials and almost 20 000 participants. Br J Sports Med. 2020;54(22):1340–50.
57. Iyer S, Naganathan V, McLachlan AJ, Le Conteur DG. Medication withdrawal trials in people aged 65 years and older. Drugs Aging. 2008;25(12):1021–31.
58. Sawan M, Reeve E, Turner J, Todd A, Steinman MA, Petrovic M, et al. A systems approach to identifying the challenges of implementing deprescribing in older adults across different health-care settings and countries: a narrative review. Expert Rev Clin Pharmacol. 2020;13(3):233–45.
59. Tinetti ME, Gordon C, Sogolow E, Lapin P, Bradley EH. Fall-risk evaluation and management: challenges in adopting geriatric care practices. Gerontologist. 2006;46(6):717–25.
60. Tsunoda K, Uchida H, Suzuki T, Watanabe K, Yamashima T, Kashima H. Effects of discontinuing benzodiazepine-derivative hypnotics on postural sway and cognitive functions in the elderly. Int J Geriatr Psychiatry. 2010;25(12):1259–65.
61. Nurminen J, Puustinen J, Lähteenmäki R, Vahlberg T, Lyles A, Partinen M, et al. Handgrip strength and balance in older adults following withdrawal from long-term use of temazepam, zopiclone or zolpidem as hypnotics. BMC Geriatr. 2014;14(1):121.
62. Shrank WH, Polinski JM, Avorn J. Quality indicators for medication use in vulnerable elders. J Am Geriatr Soc. 2007;55(s2):S373–S82.
63. Medicines and older people: implementing medicines related aspects of the National Service Framework for older people. London: DoH: Department of Health; 2001.
64. NICE. Medicines management in care homes. Quality standard [QS85].
65. Beuscart JB, Pelayo S, Robert L, Thevelin S, Marien S, Dalleur O. Medication review and reconciliation in older adults. Eur Geriatr Med. 2021;12:499.
66. Boye ND, van der Velde N, de Vries OJ, van Lieshout EM, Hartholt KA, Mattace-Raso FU, et al. Effectiveness of medication withdrawal in older fallers: results from the Improving Medication Prescribing to reduce Risk Of FALLs (IMPROveFALL) trial. Age Ageing. 2017;46(1):142–6.
67. Reeve E, Shakib S, Hendrix I, Roberts MS, Wiese MD. Review of deprescribing processes and development of an evidence-based, patient-centred deprescribing process. Br J Clin Pharmacol. 2014;78(4):738–47.
68. EuGMS. Task & Finish Groups. FRID—Fall Risk Increasing Drugs. https://www.eugms.org/research-cooperation/task-finish-groups/frid-fall-risk-increasing-drugs.html.

Optimizing Pharmacotherapy in Older Patients: Delirium

14

Giuseppe Bellelli and Alessandro Morandi

14.1 Introduction

Delirium is a complex neuropsychiatric syndrome characterized by acute onset of fluctuating inattention, altered arousal, cognitive, and behavioral disorders [1]. It is common in older people across various settings of care, but mainly in acute hospitalized patients [2].

Delirium can be regarded as a healthcare priority since it is associated with several negative outcomes, including patient's increased risk of mortality, institutionalization, cognitive and functional worsening [3–7], as well as increased patients' and caregiver's emotional burden [8, 9]. Furthermore, delirium is associated with increased healthcare expenditure [10].

Historically, a relatively short list of medications, such as barbiturates, analgesic, and alkaloids of the morphine groups [11], has been associated with delirium in the older people. However, in the recent years, it has become clear that almost all drugs are causal or contributing factors for delirium if used in individuals vulnerable, such as those with dementia and/or frailty. Knowing the potential danger of these drugs in terms of delirium development is key, given the impact of delirium on healthcare outcomes.

This article provides an approach for clinicians to recognize delirium potentially induced by drugs and reviews the current evidence regarding the mechanisms of drug-induced delirium, the existing tools to evaluate the contribution of drugs to

G. Bellelli (✉)
School of Medicine and Surgery, University of Milano-Bicocca, Monza, Italy

IRCCS San Gerardo Hospital Monza, Acute Geriatrics Unit, Monza, Italy
e-mail: giuseppe.bellelli@unimib.it

A. Morandi
REFiT Barcelona Research Group, Parc Sanitari Pere Virgili and Vall d'Hebron Institut de Recerca (VHIR), Barcelona, Spain

A. Cherubini et al. (eds.), *Optimizing Pharmacotherapy in Older Patients*, Practical Issues in Geriatrics, https://doi.org/10.1007/978-3-031-28061-0_14

delirium development, and the prevention and treatment of delirium using the pharmacological approaches in older patients outside of intensive care settings.

14.2 Mechanisms of Medications-Induced Delirium

There is general agreement that delirium represents an altered reaction of the central nervous system (CNS) to the effect of one or more precipitating factors that interplay with one or more predisposing factors of delirium [12]. Drugs, in this context, may represent either a precipitating or a predisposing factor (or both).

The exact mechanisms of drug-induced delirium are yet to be completely understood. However, neurotransmitter imbalances involving acetylcholine, dopamine, and gamma aminobutyric acid (GABA) traversing the cortical and subcortical nervous system pathways have been observed in drug-induced delirium [13]. It is hypothesized that delirium may develop as the result of an alteration of function of the ascending arousal system directly provoked by an effect of GABAergic sedatives, anesthetics, and antihistamine drugs [14]. GABA acting at GABA-A receptors inhibits the release of dopamine GABA antagonist [15], or a sudden withdrawal from a GABA agonist may increase the risk of a hyperdopaminergic state, which in turn facilitates the action of glutamate at N-methyl-D-aspartate (NMDA) receptors [16]. This can explain why an abrupt benzodiazepine withdrawal may precipitate delirium. In addition, this can explain why an imbalance of the brain cholinergic and dopaminergic activity, which can be induced by a broad list of drugs with muscarinic antagonist activity, is also involved in delirium onset [14, 17–19]. Indeed, drugs acting on GABA and NMDA receptors or with dopaminergic activity, such as digoxin, quinolone antibiotics, morphine, and histamine (H2) receptor blockers, are well-known causes of delirium [20].

Importantly, the receptor distribution of cholinergic and dopaminergic neurotransmitters among layers of prefrontal cortex and temporal lobe indirectly suggests that neurons of these areas could interact with each other during delirium [18]. It follows that a drug prescribed, for instance, to calm an agitated patient may lead to a completely different effect in specific circumstances and patients, depending on the receptor subtype which is more prevalent in those cortical areas. Older adults are particularly sensitive to anticholinergic medication adverse effects because of increased permeability of the blood-brain barrier, heightened sensitivity of cholinergic receptors, deficient drug metabolism/elimination, and deficits in central cholinergic transmission. Anticholinergic activity has also been associated with an increased severity of delirium [21].

The incidence of drug-induced delirium is particularly high even among older individuals with multimorbidity and polypharmacy. Multimorbidity refers to a coexistence of two or more chronic conditions in the same individual, and polypharmacy is commonly defined as the chronic use of five or more prescribed drugs [22, 23]. Patients with multimorbidity have an increased odd of assuming multiple medications and are thus at risk of polypharmacy prescription [24]. In addition, they commonly have other co-occurring conditions, such as malnutrition, muscle mass reduction, and low albumin serum levels, which leads to alterations in distribution, with water-soluble drugs having a reduced volume of distribution and lipophilic drugs having increased volume of distribution [25].

Aloisi and colleagues evaluated the association between polypharmacy and delirium in a cohort of 4133 older inpatients, of which 23.4% had delirium [26]. The authors found that polypharmacy was higher in patients with delirium, but the association was statistically significant only in surgical but not medical units. A possible explanation was that in surgical settings, where the healthcare professionals were not trained in geriatric care, older individuals were relatively overtreated with psychoactive drugs. Indeed, patients with delirium in these units had higher prescription of benzodiazepines and antipsychotics [26]. However, another study including 410 consecutive patients admitted to an acute geriatric ward, of whom 25% developed delirium, found that polypharmacy was an independent risk factor for delirium, after adjusting for covariates [27].

In addition to polypharmacy, Catic identified the following risk factors that placed elders at increased risk of delirium: >9 chronic medications, >12 doses of medication per day, >6 concurrent chronic diagnoses, prior adverse drug reaction, low body weight, estimated creatinine clearance <50 mL/min, and age >85 years [20].

14.3 Scales to Assess Patient's Drug Burden of Delirium

The observation that neurotransmitter dysfunctions are implicated in delirium pathophysiology gave the impulse to the development of scales to assess the contribution of this dysfunction on the onset of delirium. One of the obvious targets was the anticholinergic drug load. A recent systematic literature search reviewed the existing scales that are commonly used to evaluate the anticholinergic drug burden (ADB) and are potentially associated with delirium [28]. In the 16 studies included in the qualitative analysis of this systematic review, ADB was measured with 6 different scales, namely, the Anticholinergic Risk Scale (ARS) [29, 30], the Anticholinergic Cognitive Burden Scale (ACB) [19, 31, 32], the list of Chew [33], the Anticholinergic Drug Scale (ADS) [21, 34, 35], a modified version of the ARS [36], and a modified version of the ACB [37]. The ARS is a tool for estimating the extent to which a patient may be at risk of anticholinergic adverse effects leading to cognitive dysfunction and delirium. The ARS ranks a list of 500 drugs for anticholinergic potential on a three-point scale (0, no or low risk; 3, high anticholinergic potential), and the ARS score is given by the sum of points for the patient's number of medications [30]. The ACB was developed by Boustani [38] and includes a list of 88 drugs with known anticholinergic activities. A multidisciplinary panel assessed individual drugs to have none, possible, or definite anticholinergic properties with a score ranging from 0 to 3. The ADS was developed by Carnahan et al., based on expert consensus, and ranks medicines with anticholinergic properties in an ordinal fashion from 0 to 3, with 0 indicating no known anticholinergic activity and 3 indicating definite/high anticholinergic activity [39].

Overall, the systematic review found that ARS was the only scale which was consistently associated with delirium and thus supports its use. On the contrary, when ADB was assessed with other scales, the findings were inconclusive.

However, delirium can be precipitated also by drugs which have not relevant anticholinergic properties, such as opioids, steroids, and sedatives [4]. Therefore, other researchers have developed other scales to assess a patient's drug burden of delirium. The Delirium Drug Scale (DDS) is a tool evaluation scale developed to this aim [40, 41]. A rank of 1 or 2 is attributed to each member of the DDS drug list, and to calculate the DDS score, the patient's medication list is compared to the DDS. The rank attributed to the drug is multiplied by the dosage factor to give a weighted rank. The dosage factor is the result of the administered daily dose taken divided by the sum of the administered daily dose and the minimal daily geriatric dose (as reported by the *Geriatric Dosage Handbook*). The DDS score is the sum of all weighted rank present in the patient's drug list [40]. In an observational retrospective study on 1205 older individuals, Nguyen and colleagues found that the DDS was associated with an increased risk of delirium incidence [41]. Importantly, the risk of delirium increased as the DDS score rises from low to high exposure, independently of risk and precipitating factors for delirium. The authors concluded that the DDS could act as a decision tool for physicians when a new medication is added to a patient's drug therapy [41]. However, further research is required to confirm their results.

In addition, it is also important to highlight those other causal mechanisms, unrelated to drugs, can interfere with neurotransmission. For instance, during a sepsis, a brain neuroinflammatory response triggered by inflammatory cytokines is commonly seen, leading to endothelial damage, disruption of the blood-brain barrier, impaired blood flow, and neuronal apoptosis. Neuroinflammation can lead to microglial overactivation, resulting in a neurotoxic response with further neuronal injury. In these conditions, weighting the contribution of a specific drug to delirium development might not always be possible, since the different inflammatory factors and neurotransmitters are closely intertwined [42].

14.4 The Recommendations of the Scientific Societies on the Medications with Potential Impact on Delirium

The American Geriatrics Society (AGS) Beers Criteria are an explicit list of potentially inappropriate medications that, under specific situations, should be avoided in older adults. The AGS Beers Criteria are updated on a 3-year cycle by an interdisciplinary expert panel that periodically reviews the evidence published since the last update and then releases their recommendations [43, 44]. In the last update (i.e., 2019), the list of drugs that should be avoided in people with delirium includes the H2-receptor antagonists, the benzodiazepine (short, intermediate, and long acting), the benzodiazepine receptor agonist hypnotics (i.e., the "Z drugs": zolpidem, eszopiclone, and zaleplon), first (conventional) and second (atypical) generation antipsychotics, and some pain medications, such as meperidine. In addition, the AGS Beers

Criteria recommend that all drugs acting on the central nervous system should be avoided in older adults at high risk of delirium because of their potential to precipitate delirium. In general, it is recommended that antipsychotics should not be prescribed for behavioral problems of dementia and/or delirium unless nonpharmacological options have failed or are not possible and the older adult is threatening substantial harm to self or others [45].

The STOPP/START (Screening Tool of Older People's Prescriptions and Screening Tool to Alert to Right Treatment) criteria include a list of both potential inappropriate medications and potential prescribing omissions in older people [46, 47], which was developed by a panel of European experts. There are not explicit recommendations to avoid the use of medications for preventing delirium; however, it is recommended to avoid tricyclic antidepressants in individuals with dementia, the long-term use of long-acting benzodiazepines (e.g., chlordiazepoxide, flurazepam, nitrazepam, chlorazepate, and diazepam), and the long-term use of neuroleptics as hypnotics, especially in those with parkinsonism, as well as anticholinergics to treat extrapyramidal side effects of neuroleptic medications.

14.5 Medication Candidates for Delirium Prevention

In 1999, Inouye and colleagues proposed firstly the Hospital Elder Life Program (HELP), a model of care tailored for older patients and specifically oriented to prevent delirium during the hospital stay, including cognitive stimulation, sleep enhancement, promotion of mobility, and avoidance of dehydration and sensory impairments (i.e., visual and hearing impairments) [48]. Since then, several studies, systematic reviews, and meta-analysis have confirmed the effectiveness of nonpharmacological, multicomponent, and multidisciplinary interventions in delirium prevention [49, 50]. The most recently updated delirium guidelines support such approach as the first step for delirium prevention [51], leading to a reduction of delirium incidence by almost 43%.

On the contrary, there is insufficient evidence to recommend the use of specific medications for delirium prevention [52]. Fok and colleagues reported a possible role on the use of antipsychotics to reduce the incidence of postoperative delirium, mainly in orthopedic settings and in those patients at higher risk of delirium [53]. However, a subsequent systematic review investigating the possible effect of haloperidol vs. placebo in adult patients reported a limited evidence of a small dose of haloperidol in delirium reduction among surgical patients [54]. Therefore, guidelines suggest that the pharmacological risk reduction should occur only by acting on three specific areas of intervention: (a) medication reconciliation with a thorough review of medication including over-the-counter and herbal medications; (b) the physiological changes related to aging and their effects on medication metabolism; and (c) considering the risk of delirium related to the introduction of a new drug [52].

Recent studies have claimed potential applications for some medications. For example, there is emerging evidence that dexmedetomidine—a highly selective α2-adrenergic agonist—alone or in combination with other sedatives may reduce postoperative delirium [55]. This type of medication has been widely studied in critically ill patients admitted to intensive care units (ICU) [56], and its potential use outside the ICU needs to be further investigated.

Given that sleep-cycle alterations are often present in patients with delirium and especially in delirium superimposed on dementia, there has been an increasing interest on the effect of melatonin and melatonin receptor agonist (i.e., ramelteon) for delirium prevention. A recent meta-analysis showed that both melatonin and ramelteon are effective in reducing delirium incidence in hospitalized patients, but this effect was found significant in surgical patients and not in medical patients [57]. Furthermore, in a recent multicenter randomized placebo-controlled trial, Hatta et al. showed that suvorexant (an orexin inhibitor used in the treatment of insomnia) significantly reduced the occurrence of delirium compared to the administration of placebo [58]. A meta-analysis that included seven studies conducted in patients undergoing this treatment compared with controls showed that delirium incidence could be reduced in the treatment groups compared to controls [59]. However, further larger studies are required.

14.6 Medications to Treat Delirium

As for the prevention of delirium, even for delirium treatment, it is important to provide a timely non-pharmacological approach and identify and treat the underlying causes of delirium[52]. Different acronyms are available to help clinicians systematically reminding the possible causes of delirium [60].

Several studies investigated the possibility to treat delirious patients with antipsychotics. However, one meta-analysis showed that antipsychotic medications are not effective to reduce delirium duration or severity in adult surgical and medical patients [61]. Two Cochrane reviews confirmed these findings both in non-ICU patients and ICU patients [62], and two other systematic reviews found that the routine use of haloperidol or second-generation antipsychotics is not useful to treat delirium in adult inpatients [63, 64].

It is also interesting to report that a relatively recent large randomized clinical trial found that palliative care patients treated with haloperidol or risperidone compared with placebo had worse delirium symptom scores [65]. However, one study on patients affected by advanced cancer in the last weeks or days of their life showed a reduction in agitated behavior by adding a single 3 mg dose of lorazepam intravenously to haloperidol, when compared with placebo [66].

Other medications have been investigated for their possible role in delirium treatment. One systematic review found no efficacy of acetylcholinesterase inhibitors (i.e., donepezil or rivastigmine) compared to placebo on delirium duration and severity [67], and one trial investigating the effect of the adjunct of rivastigmine to usual care based on haloperidol on delirium duration in critically ill patients was halted because of increased mortality in the rivastigmine group compared to placebo [68]. Finally, a systematic review, including only two studies outside the ICU, reported that there is not enough evidence to determine whether benzodiazepines are effective when used to treat patients with delirium [69].

According to the current evidence, antipsychotics should therefore be prescribed only in patients with disturbing psychotic symptoms (e.g., delusions, hallucinations) and when the patients' safety or the safety of those around them was compromised [52]. The prescription and dosages should be reviewed on a daily basis for the medication tapering and discontinuation.

14.7 Conclusions

Drug-induced delirium is often encountered in clinical practice, especially in older people who are frail or have dementia. It is therefore important that all clinicians should be aware of the impact of specific medications in inducing delirium, to avoid their use and/or rapidly detect them as a potential cause of delirium. A conceptual framework and an algorithm to guide clinicians in managing medications to prevent and treat delirium are provided in Fig. 14.1. The first step includes drug reconciliation, keeping in mind the physiological changes related to aging and their effects on metabolism. Adjusting drug doses considering the pharmacokinetic changes and the potential interactions between drugs will reduce the risk of drug-induced delirium. Furthermore, before initiating a new medication, it is appropriate to consider all the factors that placed elders at increased risk of delirium, including dementia, multimorbidity, frailty, polypharmacy, prior adverse drug reaction, malnutrition, and chronic renal failure. Then, it should be chosen the tool to measure the anticholinergic drug burden. There are several scales that can be used to this aim. Finally, specific drugs can be used to prevent (i.e., drugs acting on the sleep-wake rhythm) or to treat delirium. It's important to recognize that the use of antipsychotics is allowed only when patients are suffering psychotic symptoms (e.g., delusions, hallucinations) or when the safety around them is compromised. Heightening the awareness of drug-induced delirium among clinicians will encourage them to use more conservatively and closely monitor the drugs at highest risk.

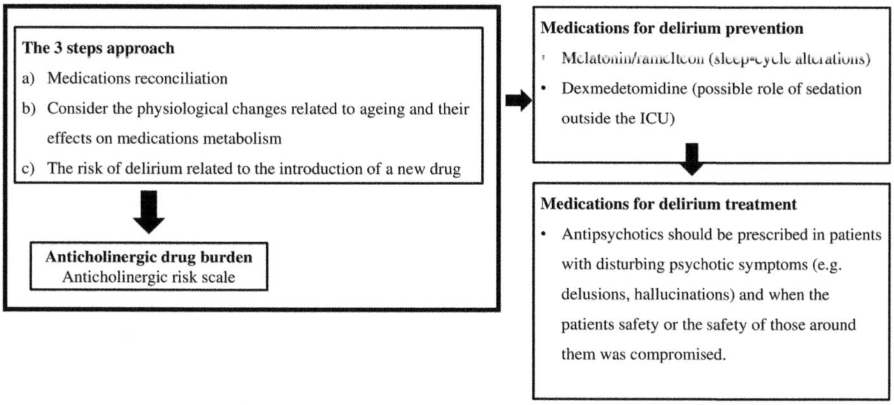

Fig. 14.1 Medication management and delirium

This is a very important area of research that promises to provide exciting news for clinicians and opportunities for the patients.

References

1. American Psychiatric Association. Diagnostic and statistical manual of mental disorders. 5th ed. Arlington: American Psychiatric Association; 2013.
2. Bellelli G, Morandi A, Di Santo SG, et al. "Delirium Day": a nationwide point prevalence study of delirium in older hospitalized patients using an easy standardized diagnostic tool. BMC Med. 2016;14(1):106. https://doi.org/10.1186/s12916-016-0649-8.
3. Morandi A, Di Santo SG, Zambon A, et al. Delirium, dementia and in-hospital mortality: the results from the Italian Delirium Day 2016, a national multicenter study. J Gerontol A Biol Sci Med Sci. 2019, 74(6):910–6. https://doi.org/10.1093/gerona/gly154.
4. Inouye SK, Westendorp RG, Saczynski JS. Delirium in elderly people. Lancet. 2014;383(9920):911–22. https://doi.org/10.1016/S0140-6736(13)60688-1.
5. Morandi A, Davis D, Fick D, et al. Delirium superimposed on dementia strongly predicts worse outcomes in older rehabilitation inpatients. J Am Med Dir Assoc. 2014;15(5):349–54. https://doi.org/10.1016/j.jamda.2013.12.084.
6. Wilcox ME, Girard TD, Hough CL. Delirium and long term cognition in critically ill patients. BMJ. 2021;373:n1007. https://doi.org/10.1136/bmj.n1007.
7. Pereira JV, Aung Thein MZ, Nitchingham A, Caplan GA. Delirium in older adults is associated with development of new dementia: a systematic review and meta-analysis. Int J Geriatr Psychiatry. 2021;36(7):993–1003. https://doi.org/10.1002/gps.5508.
8. Morandi A, Lucchi E, Turco R, et al. Delirium superimposed on dementia: a quantitative and qualitative evaluation of informal caregivers and health care staff experience. J Psychosom Res. 2015;79(4):272–80. https://doi.org/10.1016/j.jpsychores.2015.06.012.
9. Morandi A, Lucchi E, Turco R, et al. Delirium superimposed on dementia: a quantitative and qualitative evaluation of patient experience. J Psychosom Res. 2015;79(4):281–7. https://doi.org/10.1016/j.jpsychores.2015.07.010.
10. Leslie DL, Marcantonio ER, Zhang Y, Leo-Summers L, Inouye SK. One-year health care costs associated with delirium in the elderly population. Arch Intern Med. 2008;168(1):27–32. https://doi.org/10.1001/archinternmed.2007.4.
11. Gould J, Lond BS. Treatment of delirium, psychosis, and coma due to drugs. Lancet. 1953;1(6760):570–3. https://doi.org/10.1016/s0140-6736(53)91696-1.
12. Inouye SK, Charpentier PA. Precipitating factors for delirium in hospitalized elderly persons. Predictive model and interrelationship with baseline vulnerability. JAMA. 1996;275(11):852–7.
13. Alagiakrishnan K, Wiens CA. An approach to drug induced delirium in the elderly. Postgrad Med J. 2004;80(945):388–93. https://doi.org/10.1136/pgmj.2003.017236.
14. Wilson JE, Mart MF, Cunningham C, et al. Delirium. Nat Rev Dis Primers. 2020;6(1):90. https://doi.org/10.1038/s41572-020-00223-4.
15. Hauber W. Involvement of basal ganglia transmitter systems in movement initiation. Prog Neurobiol. 1998;56(5):507–40. https://doi.org/10.1016/s0301-0082(98)00041-0.
16. Cepeda C, Levine MS. Dopamine and N-methyl-D-aspartate receptor interactions in the neostriatum. Dev Neurosci. 1998;20(1):1–18. https://doi.org/10.1159/000017294.
17. Trzepacz PT. The neuropathogenesis of delirium. A need to focus our research. Psychosomatics. 1994;35(4):374–91. https://doi.org/10.1016/S0033-3182(94)71759-X.
18. Trzepacz PT. Is there a final common neural pathway in delirium? Focus on acetylcholine and dopamine. Semin Clin Neuropsychiatry 2000;5(2):132–148. https://doi.org/10.153/SCNP00500132.
19. Pasina L, Colzani L, Cortesi L, et al. Relation between delirium and anticholinergic drug burden in a cohort of hospitalized older patients: an observational study. Drugs Aging. 2018;36:85–91. https://doi.org/10.1007/s40266-018-0612-9.

20. Catic AG. Identification and management of in-hospital drug-induced delirium in older patients. Drugs Aging. 2011;28(9):737–48. https://doi.org/10.2165/11592240-000000000-00000.
21. Han L, McCusker J, Cole M, Abrahamowicz M, Primeau F, Elie M. Use of medications with anticholinergic effect predicts clinical severity of delirium symptoms in older medical inpatients. Arch Intern Med. 2001;161(8):1099–105. https://doi.org/10.1001/archinte.161.8.1099.
22. Saum KU, Schöttker B, Meid AD, et al. Is polypharmacy associated with frailty in older people? Results from the ESTHER cohort study. J Am Geriatr Soc. 2017;65(2):e27–32. https://doi.org/10.1111/jgs.14718.
23. Marengoni A, Rizzuto D, Wang HX, Winblad B, Fratiglioni L. Patterns of chronic multimorbidity in the elderly population. J Am Geriatr Soc. 2009;57(2):225–30. https://doi.org/10.1111/j.1532-5415.2008.02109.x.
24. Rawle MJ, Richards M, Davis D, Kuh D. The prevalence and determinants of polypharmacy at age 69: a British birth cohort study. BMC Geriatr. 2018;18(1):118. https://doi.org/10.1186/s12877-018-0795-2.
25. Drenth-van Maanen AC, Wilting I, Jansen PAF. Prescribing medicines to older people-how to consider the impact of ageing on human organ and body functions. Br J Clin Pharmacol. 2020;86(10):1921–30. https://doi.org/10.1111/bcp.14094.
26. Aloisi G, Marengoni A, Morandi A, et al. Drug prescription and delirium in older inpatients: results from the Nationwide multicenter Italian delirium day 2015-2016. J Clin Psychiatry. 2019;80(2):18m12430. https://doi.org/10.4088/JCP.18m12430.
27. Hein C, Forgues A, Piau A, Sommet A, Vellas B, Nourhashémi F. Impact of polypharmacy on occurrence of delirium in elderly emergency patients. J Am Med Dir Assoc. 2014;15(11):850.e11–5. https://doi.org/10.1016/j.jamda.2014.08.012.
28. Egberts A, Moreno-Gonzalez R, Alan H, Ziere G, Mattace-Raso FUS. Anticholinergic drug burden and delirium: a systematic review. J Am Med Dir Assoc. 2021;22(1):65–73.e4. https://doi.org/10.1016/j.jamda.2020.04.019.
29. Landi F, Dell'Aquila G, Collamati A, et al. Anticholinergic drug use and negative outcomes among the frail elderly population living in a nursing home. J Am Med Dir Assoc. 2014;15(11):825–9. https://doi.org/10.1016/j.jamda.2014.08.002.
30. Egberts A, van der Craats ST, van Wijk MD, Alkilabe S, van den Bemt PMLA, Mattace-Raso FUS. Anticholinergic drug exposure is associated with delirium and postdischarge institutionalization in acutely ill hospitalized older patients. Pharmacol Res Perspect. 2017;5(3):e00310. https://doi.org/10.1002/prp2.310.
31. Campbell N, Perkins A, Hui S, Khan B, Boustani M. Association between prescribing of anticholinergic medications and incident delirium: a cohort study. J Am Geriatr Soc. 2011;59(Suppl 2):S277–81. https://doi.org/10.1111/j.1532-5415.2011.03676.x.
32. Rigor J, Rueff Rato I, Ferreira PM, et al. Prehospital anticholinergic burden is associated with delirium but not with mortality in a population of acutely ill medical patients. J Am Med Dir Assoc. 2020;21(4):481–5. https://doi.org/10.1016/j.jamda.2019.12.018.
33. Chew ML, Mulsant BH, Pollock BG, et al. Anticholinergic activity of 107 medications commonly used by older adults. J Am Geriatr Soc. 2008;56(7):1333–41. https://doi.org/10.1111/j.1532-5415.2008.01737.x.
34. Mueller A, Spies CD, Eckardt R, et al. Anticholinergic burden of long-term medication is an independent risk factor for the development of postoperative delirium: a clinical trial. J Clin Anesth. 2020;61:109632. https://doi.org/10.1016/j.jclinane.2019.109632.
35. Moorey HC, Zaidman S, Jackson TA. Delirium is not associated with anticholinergic burden or polypharmacy in older patients on admission to an acute hospital: an observational case control study. BMC Geriatr. 2016;16(1):162. https://doi.org/10.1186/s12877-016-0336-9.
36. Hwang S, Jun K, Ah YM, Han E, Chung JE, Lee JY. Impact of anticholinergic burden on emergency department visits among older adults in Korea: a national population cohort study. Arch Gerontol Geriatr. 2019;85:103912. https://doi.org/10.1016/j.archger.2019.103912.
37. Ah YM, Suh Y, Jun K, Hwang S, Lee JY. Effect of anticholinergic burden on treatment modification, delirium and mortality in newly diagnosed dementia patients starting a cholinesterase

inhibitor: a population-based study. Basic Clin Pharmacol Toxicol. 2019;124(6):741–8. https://doi.org/10.1111/bcpt.13184.
38. Boustani M, Campbell N, Munger S, et al. Impact of anticholinergics on the aging brain: a review and practical application. Aging Health. 2008;4:311–20.
39. Carnahan RM, Lund BC, Perry PJ, Pollock BG, Culp KR. The anticholinergic drug scale as a measure of drug-related anticholinergic burden: associations with serum anticholinergic activity. J Clin Pharmacol. 2006;46(12):1481–6. https://doi.org/10.1177/0091270006292126.
40. Nguyen P, Pelletier L, Payot I, Latour J. Drug Delirium Scale (DDS): a tool to evaluate drugs as a risk factor for delirium. Int J Innov Res Med Sci. 2016;1(6):232–7.
41. Nguyen PV, Pelletier L, Payot I, Latour J. The Delirium Drug Scale is associated to delirium incidence in the emergency department. Int Psychogeriatr. 2018;30(4):503–10. https://doi.org/10.1017/S1041610217002538.
42. van Gool WA, van de Beek D, Eikelenboom P. Systemic infection and delirium: when cytokines and acetylcholine collide. Lancet. 2010;375(9716):773–5. https://doi.org/10.1016/S0140-6736(09)61158-2.
43. American Geriatrics Society, Beers Criteria Update Expert Panel. Updated Beers criteria for potentially inappropriate medication use in older adults. J Am Geriatr Soc. 2012;60(4):616–31. https://doi.org/10.1111/j.1532-5415.2012.03923.x.
44. American Geriatrics Society, Beers Criteria Update Expert Panel. Updated Beers criteria for potentially inappropriate medication use in older adults. J Am Geriatr Soc. 2015;63(11):2227–46. https://doi.org/10.1111/jgs.13702.
45. AGS Choosing Wisely Workgroup. American Geriatrics Society identifies another five things that healthcare providers and patients should question. J Am Geriatr Soc. 2014;62:950–60.
46. Gallagher P, O'Mahony D. STOPP (Screening Tool of Older Persons' potentially inappropriate prescriptions): application to acutely ill elderly patients and comparison with Beers' criteria. Age Ageing. 2008;37(6):673–9. https://doi.org/10.1093/ageing/afn197.
47. O'Mahony D, O'Sullivan D, Byrne S, O'Connor MN, Ryan C, Gallagher P. STOPP/START criteria for potentially inappropriate prescribing in older people: version 2. Age Ageing. 2015;44(2):213–8. https://doi.org/10.1093/ageing/afu145.
48. Inouye SK, Bogardus ST Jr, Charpentier PA, et al. A multicomponent intervention to prevent delirium in hospitalized older patients. Clinical trial comparative study controlled clinical trial research support, non-U.S. Gov't research support, U.S. Gov't, P.H.S. N Engl J Med. 1999;340(9):669–76. https://doi.org/10.1056/NEJM199903043400901.
49. Hshieh TT, Yue J, Oh E, et al. Effectiveness of multicomponent nonpharmacological delirium interventions: a meta-analysis. JAMA Intern Med. 2015;175(4):512–20. https://doi.org/10.1001/jamainternmed.2014.7779.
50. Hshieh TT, Yang T, Gartaganis SL, Yue J, Inouye SK. Hospital elder life program: systematic review and meta-analysis of effectiveness. Am J Geriatr Psychiatry. 2018;26(10):1015–33. https://doi.org/10.1016/j.jagp.2018.06.007.
51. Burton JK, Craig LE, Yong SQ, et al. Non-pharmacological interventions for preventing delirium in hospitalised non-ICU patients. Cochrane Database Syst Rev. 2021;7:CD013307. https://doi.org/10.1002/14651858.CD013307.pub2.
52. Scottish Imtercollegiate Group Network (SIGN). Risk reduction and management of delirium. A national clinical guideline. 2019. SIGN. http://www.sign.ac.uk.
53. Fok MC, Sepehry AA, Frisch L, et al. Do antipsychotics prevent postoperative delirium? A systematic review and meta-analysis. Int J Geriatr Psychiatry. 2015;30(4):333–44. https://doi.org/10.1002/gps.4240.
54. Shen YZ, Peng K, Zhang J, Meng XW, Ji FH. Effects of haloperidol on delirium in adult patients: a systematic review and meta-analysis. Med Princ Pract. 2018;27(3):250–9. https://doi.org/10.1159/000488243.
55. Lee JM, Cho YJ, Ahn EJ, Choi GJ, Kang H. Pharmacological strategies to prevent postoperative delirium: a systematic review and network meta-analysis. Anesth Pain Med (Seoul). 2021;16(1):28–48. https://doi.org/10.17085/apm.20079.

56. Burry LD, Cheng W, Williamson DR, et al. Pharmacological and non-pharmacological interventions to prevent delirium in critically ill patients: a systematic review and network meta-analysis. Intensive Care Med. 2021;47(9):943–60. https://doi.org/10.1007/s00134-021-06490-3.
57. Khaing K, Nair BR. Melatonin for delirium prevention in hospitalized patients: a systematic review and meta-analysis. J Psychiatr Res. 2021;133:181–90. https://doi.org/10.1016/j.jpsychires.2020.12.020.
58. Hatta K, Kishi Y, Wada K, et al. Preventive effects of Suvorexant on delirium: a randomized placebo-controlled trial. J Clin Psychiatry. 2017;78(8):e970–9. https://doi.org/10.4088/JCP.16m11194.
59. Xu S, Cui Y, Shen J, Wang P. Suvorexant for the prevention of delirium: a meta-analysis. Medicine (Baltimore). 2020;99(30):e21043. https://doi.org/10.1097/MD.0000000000021043.
60. Flaherty JH, Tariq SH, Raghavan S, Bakshi S, Moinuddin A, Morley JE. A model for managing delirious older inpatients. Research Support, U.S. Gov't, P.H.S. J Am Geriatr Soc. 2003;51(7):1031–5.
61. Neufeld KJ, Yue J, Robinson TN, Inouye SK, Needham DM. Antipsychotic medication for prevention and treatment of delirium in hospitalized adults: a systematic review and meta-analysis. Meta-Analysis Research Support, N.I.H., Extramural Research Support, Non--U.S. Gov't Review. J Am Geriatr Soc. 2016;64(4):705–14. https://doi.org/10.1111/jgs.14076.
62. Burry L, Mehta S, Perreault MM, et al. Antipsychotics for treatment of delirium in hospitalised non-ICU patients. Cochrane Database Syst Rev. 2018;6:CD005594. https://doi.org/10.1002/14651858.CD005594.pub3.
63. Nikooie R, Neufeld KJ, Oh ES, et al. Antipsychotics for treating delirium in hospitalized adults: a systematic review. Ann Intern Med. 2019;171(7):485–95. https://doi.org/10.7326/M19-1860.
64. Barbateskovic M, Krauss SR, Collet MO, et al. Haloperidol for the treatment of delirium in critically ill patients: a systematic review with meta-analysis and trial sequential analysis. Acta Anaesthesiol Scand. 2020;64(2):254–66. https://doi.org/10.1111/aas.13501.
65. Agar MR, Lawlor PG, Quinn S, et al. Efficacy of oral risperidone, haloperidol, or placebo for symptoms of delirium among patients in palliative care: a randomized clinical trial. JAMA Intern Med. 2017;177(1):34–42. https://doi.org/10.1001/jamainternmed.2016.7491.
66. Hui D, Frisbee-Hume S, Wilson A, et al. Effect of lorazepam with haloperidol vs haloperidol alone on agitated delirium in patients with advanced cancer receiving palliative care: a randomized clinical trial. JAMA. 2017;318(11):1047–56. https://doi.org/10.1001/jama.2017.11468.
67. Tampi RR, Tampi DJ, Ghori AK. Acetylcholinesterase inhibitors for delirium in older adults. Am J Alzheimers Dis Other Dement. 2016;31(4):305–10. https://doi.org/10.1177/1533317515619034.
68. van Eijk MM, Roes KC, Honing ML, et al. Effect of rivastigmine as an adjunct to usual care with haloperidol on duration of delirium and mortality in critically ill patients: a multicentre, double-blind, placebo-controlled randomised trial. Lancet. 2010;376(9755):1829–37. https://doi.org/10.1016/S0140-6736(10)61855-7.
69. Li Y, Ma J, Jin Y, et al. Benzodiazepines for treatment of patients with delirium excluding those who are cared for in an intensive care unit. Cochrane Database Syst Rev. 2020;2:CD012670. https://doi.org/10.1002/14651858.CD012670.pub2.

Optimizing Pharmacotherapy in Older Adults: Urinary Incontinence

15

Antoine Vella and Claudio Pedone

15.1 Introduction

Urinary incontinence (UI) in older persons is common and increases with age, affecting around 70% of older persons over 85 years of age. It can have a major adverse impact on their quality of life and is one of the reasons why older persons end up in long-term care. Unfortunately, it is frequently underdiagnosed and often not treated even though it is potentially reversible.

Management of patients suffering from UI requires not only a focused history, examination, and investigations for an accurate diagnosis to be made but also a comprehensive geriatric assessment that usually requires the involvement of a multidisciplinary team. Treatment options usually include lifestyle changes, behavioral interventions, often pharmacotherapy, and less commonly surgical interventions besides the use of appropriate devices and absorbent aids.

Pharmacotherapy in the incontinence setting must have a two-pronged approach. Before considering specific pharmacotherapy targeting the incontinence, a comprehensive review of all ongoing medications, including those over-the-counter, must be undertaken. This is because there are several drugs that, directly or indirectly, can

A. Vella (✉)
Department of Geriatric Medicine, St. Vincent De Paul Hospital, Luqa, Malta
e-mail: antoine.b.vella@gov.mt

C. Pedone
Department of Medicine and Surgery, Research Unit of Geriatrics, Università Campus Bio-Medico di Roma, Rome, Italy

Fondazione Policlinico Universitario Campus Bio-Medico, Rome, Italy
e-mail: C.Pedone@policlinicocampus.it

A. Cherubini et al. (eds.), *Optimizing Pharmacotherapy in Older Patients*, Practical Issues in Geriatrics, https://doi.org/10.1007/978-3-031-28061-0_15

impact negatively on the patient's continence status. This shall be discussed separately below. The second aspect of the pharmacotherapeutic management can then be directed more specifically at the patient's continence problem.

Pharmacotherapy for incontinence should form part of a holistic approach and must take the patients' comorbidities, desires, and quality of life into account. Treatment must be carefully monitored with special vigilance for side effects of medications. The value of team management, preferably with a continence outreach service, cannot be overstressed.

The mode of actions and effects that medications have on micturition, whether they are medications that the patient is on or pharmacotherapy for incontinence, can only be understood when the basis of the complex micturition process is comprehended.

The lower urinary tract consists essentially of two units: the bladder which acts as a reservoir and the outlet unit which consists of the bladder neck, the urethra, and the external urethral sphincter (EUS). The bladder and bladder neck, including the internal urethral sphincter (IUS), consist of smooth muscle, while the EUS consists of striated muscle. The bladder has two modes of action—storage and elimination—and works in a switch on/off pattern which is under voluntary control. The mechanisms that underlie the control of micturition consist of complex neural pathways that function at the levels of the brain, spinal cord, and peripheral nerves that are mediated via multiple neurotransmitters at all levels. A complex description of this is beyond the scope of the chapter, but a very simplified version of the efferent neural pathways and neurotransmitter mechanisms that regulate the lower urinary tract (LUT) will be summarized in Fig. 15.1.

The LUT has three main nerve supplies: the sympathetic, parasympathetic, and somatic systems [1].

The sympathetic system via the hypogastric nerve is inhibitory to the detrusor muscle and motor to the IUS. Sympathetic postganglionic neurons release noradrenaline (NA) which activates the following:

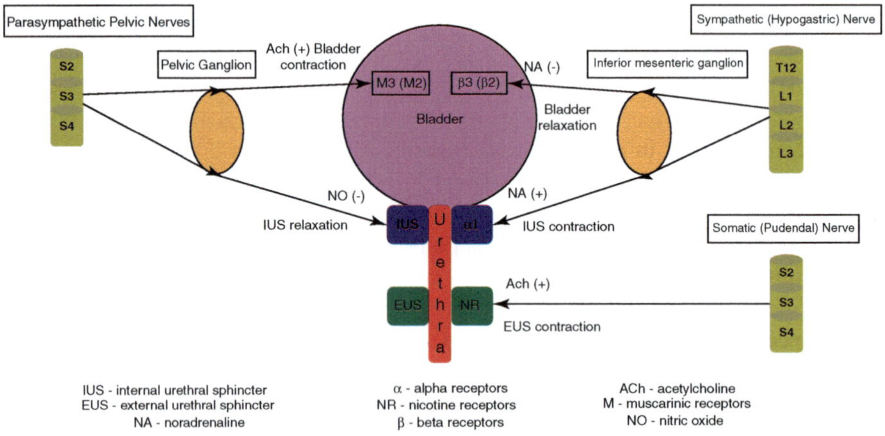

Fig. 15.1 Lower urinary tract: efferent innervation and neurotransmitter–receptor mechanisms

- Beta adrenergic inhibitory (−ve) receptors in the detrusor muscle resulting in bladder relaxation
- Alpha-adrenergic excitatory (+ve) receptors in the bladder neck and urethra resulting in contraction

The parasympathetic system via the pelvic nerve plexus is motor to the detrusor muscle and inhibitory to the IUS. When the bladder fills to beyond 300 mL, stretch mechanoreceptors in the bladder wall relay via pelvic splanchnic nerves to the spinal cord. Efferent parasympathetic nerves synapse with postganglionic nerves in the bladder wall and IUS via acetylcholine (ACh) acting on muscarinic receptors (M). This results in the following:

- Bladder contraction
- Relaxation of the IUS

The somatic system via the pudendal nerve is motor to the EUS which is under voluntary control and is always contracted except during micturition when the EUS is inhibited. The somatic axons release acetylcholine which via nicotinic receptors (NR) result in the following:

- EUS contraction

The majority of the pharmacotherapeutic agents used to manage incontinence act on one or more of the above systems (Fig. 15.2); however, the control of micturition is far more complex than as described above and includes spinal, pontine, and cortical centers. The spinal center results in reflex incomplete bladder evacuation, the

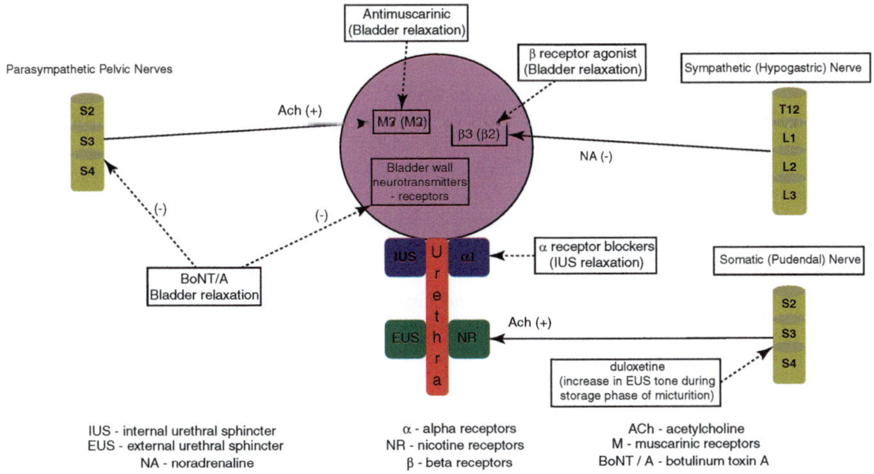

Fig. 15.2 Mechanisms of action of therapeutic agents on the lower urinary tract

pontine center synchronizes and maintains sustained bladder contractions, and the cortical center inhibits the pontine center until a suitable time and place for micturition is available. These centers are regulated by several neurotransmitters which can be affected by disease processes a well as medications that the patients are taking.

15.2 Medications Review

An important part of the comprehensive geriatric assessment (CGA) in the management of UI is a careful evaluation of the medications that the patient is on. There are several medications (Table 15.1) that could precipitate or worsen LUTS through a direct or an indirect effect on the LUT. Sometimes even a simple over-the-counter medication such as a pseudoephedrine-containing common cold preparation can give rise to obstructive symptoms in men with consequent urinary retention with overflow incontinence.

This list is not exhaustive, and a possible medication-induced effect on the lower urinary tract (LUT) should be suspected if the symptoms of UI develop soon after the introduction of a new agent. Lower urinary tract symptoms (LUTS) secondary to medications are particularly common in patients with polypharmacy, those who have been recently hospitalized and the frail. If possible, when one or more medications are suspected to be the cause of incontinence/LUTS, the particular medication should be changed to that of another class, e.g., using an ARB instead of an ACEI; the dose or time of administration adjusted (e.g., in the case of diuretics) or the

Table 15.1 Medications as causative or predisposing factors for UI [2]

Medication	Effects on lower urinary tract
ACE inhibitors	Cough, stress urinary incontinence
Calcium channel inhibitors	Frequency, nocturia, and obstructive symptoms (especially in males)
Diuretics	Polyuria
Lithium	Polyuria
Alpha-adrenergic agonists	Stimulate the IUS, urinary retention
Antihistamines	Retention of urine, delirium
Acetylcholinesterase inhibitors	Increased detrusor contractility, urge incontinence
Opiates	Urinary retention, constipation with overflow incontinence
Alpha-adrenergic inhibitors	Reduction in urethral/IUS tone, stress urinary incontinence
Benzodiazepines	Delirium, stress urinary incontinence (relaxation of EUS), impaired mobility (functional incontinence)
Gabapentin	Nocturnal polyuria, delirium
NSAIDs	Nocturnal polyuria
SSRIs	Increased detrusor contractility (cholinergic effect), urge incontinence
Anticholinergic medications	Retention of urine with overflow incontinence, delirium
Antipsychotics	Anticholinergic effects, sedation, immobility, delirium

suspected medication should be stopped, e.g., in the case of an acetylcholinesterase inhibitor.

15.3 Evaluation of Bowel Function

Attention to bowel care is an integral part of a workup for urinary incontinence since constipation can have a profound effect on bladder function particularly in the frail older person and severe constipation can result in retention of urine with overflow incontinence. This is especially common in hospitalized patients where all too often bowel and bladder care is not given due importance. Older persons with moderate to severe dementia and patients who are recovering from surgery, e.g., fracture of the neck of femur (often on opiates), are particularly prone to constipation and its consequences on the LUT. Their treatment must be reviewed and accurate stool charting encouraged.

15.4 Pharmacological Treatment for Urinary Incontinence

Pharmacological treatment for UI is usually commenced after a trial of conservative treatment (Table 15.2) has not proven to be adequately effective. However, the conservative measures should still be pursued after the initiation of pharmacological treatment since they have a complementary effect.

Most pharmacological interventions for UI are for use in urge UI and bladder outflow obstruction (BOO), while a few agents have been used in stress UI (SUI).

The agents used for urge UI and SUI have a moderate efficacy when used for the correct indication but unfortunately are not without adverse effects to a greater or lesser extent. These factors result in a relatively poor perseverance and a high dropout

Table 15.2 Conservative management of urinary incontinence [2]

Lifestyle interventions	
No specific data in the frail elderly	
Weight reduction	May be inappropriate in the frail older patient
Fluid intake	Only modify if excessive; avoid caffeine and carbonated beverages
Constipation	Chronic constipation should be addressed
Smoking	Smoking cessation is recommended
Behavioural interventions	
Continuous incorporation into daily routine is essential	
Motivation of patient and/or caregiver is required	
Timed voiding	Applicable in older patients with or without cognitive impairment
Prompted voiding	Gold standard in care dependent older patients in nursing homes
Pelvic floor muscle training	Advised in stress incontinence Could be implemented to decrease bladder contractions in OAB Must be continued to maintain beneficial effect
Bladder training	Can be applied for any type of UI Sufficient motivation is required

rate from treatment. Adverse effects can be short term, e.g., nausea with duloxetine for SUI, but can also be long term, e.g., worsening of cognitive impairment with antimuscarinic agents in predisposed older patients. Treatment for BOO is usually better tolerated, but long-term adverse effects such as erectile dysfunction can be a problem.

One must therefore carefully weigh the risk of adverse effects, taking into consideration the particular patient's comorbidities, quality of life, and wishes, before embarking on treatment. Evidence of efficacy of these medications in the frail older person is scant, and patients that started on these medications should be monitored vigilantly for adverse effects.

15.5 Drug Management of Overactive Bladder/Urge Incontinence

15.5.1 Antimuscarinic Drugs

Antimuscarinic drugs are the mainstay of the drug therapy for overactive bladder (OAB), with or without urinary urge incontinence (UUI). These drugs seem to be effective in the short term, while data on long-term efficacy are scant [3]. Overall, the effect on incontinence itself is limited (about 20% reduction of incontinence episodes), but the effect on quality of life seems to be more substantial. Evidence pertaining to efficacy in older and frail people is limited. Side effects due to systemic anticholinergic action are common and frequently lead to therapy discontinuation. In older people, negative effects on cognition are of some concern, and these drugs should be avoided in patients with cognitive impairment.

15.5.1.1 Mechanism of Action

All anticholinergic drugs used for OAB and UUI exert their action by blocking the M2 and M3 muscarinic receptor that are expressed in several tissues including the detrusor muscle. The M3 receptor is primarily involved in detrusor contraction, while the M2 receptor stimulation induces an increase in detrusor muscle tone. The selectivity of antimuscarinic drugs for these receptors varies: only solifenacin and darifenacin are selective for the M3 receptor, while all other compounds bind also to other antimuscarinic receptor, including M1 that is abundantly expressed in the central nervous system. The propensity of nonselective antimuscarinic drugs to cause cognitive side effects (e.g., confusion) is a function not only of their receptor affinity but also of their lipophilicity and capacity of penetrating the blood-brain barrier. Oxybutynin is a nonselective antimuscarinic, and being small and highly lipophilic can easily cross the blood-brain barrier, and consequently it is the drug with the highest risk for cognitive side effects. Other nonselective antimuscarinics are much larger and in normal conditions do not cross the blood-brain barrier, with lower risk for cognitive side effects. It must be kept in mind, however, that several conditions such as diabetes or neurodegenerative disorders (Alzheimer's disease, Parkinson's disease) can disrupt the integrity of the blood-brain barrier, increasing the risk of central side effects even for drugs that normally do not enter the central nervous system.

15.5.1.2 Evidence

In older people, antimuscarinic drugs improve the severity of urinary incontinence, although the effect size is generally small and no data are available on their long-term efficacy. No evidence is available, however, in older people with multiple morbidities and polypharmacotherapy. Side effects are common and related to systemic anticholinergic activity: dry mouth, constipation, blurred vision, and dizziness. These side effects have a sizable impact on persistence on treatment: about 40% of patients discontinue these drugs within 3 months of therapy.

15.5.1.3 Clinical Use

Oxybutynin is currently not frequently used because of the less favorable risk/benefit ratio compared to other available agents, and extended-release formulations are preferred. With respect to other available drugs (tolterodine, solifenacin, darifenacin, propiverine, trospium), there is no clear-cut indication that one drug may be preferable over another in older people. Given the high prevalence of polypharmacy in older people, attention to possible drug-drug interaction is warranted. Most of these drugs are metabolized by CYP3A4 and must be used with caution in patients taking potent inhibitors of this enzyme.

Inherent to the mechanism of action of these drugs is the risk for urinary retention that is especially high in men with severe prostatic hyperplasia: in this situation, antimuscarinic drugs may be contraindicated.

15.5.2 β3 Receptor Agonists

β3 receptor agonists (mirabegron and vibegron) are generally considered safe, but data specific for older people is scant. In particular, their effect on the QT interval in people also taking drugs known to cause QT prolongation is unknown.

15.5.2.1 Mechanism of Action

These drugs cause an increase of cAMP concentration in bladder smooth muscle cells with muscle relaxation and consequent improvement in filling capacity. It does not impair voiding pressure because the activation of M2 muscarinic receptor that triggers muscular contraction also inhibits the cAMP signaling.

15.5.2.2 Evidence

A meta-analysis of head-to-head studies has shown that mirabegron is as effective as solifenacin in reducing the burden of OAB/UUI, with comparable rates of adverse events [4].

15.5.2.3 Clinical Use

They are recommended as a stand-alone or add-on pharmacological therapy in patients with UUI. In people taking a combination of β3 receptor agonists and antimuscarinic drugs, special attention must be paid to the risk of urinary retention. These drugs are metabolized by CYP3A, and dose adjustment may be required in patients with renal or liver function impairment also taking potent inhibitors of this cytochrome. Furthermore, they should not be used in patients with poorly controlled arterial hypertension.

15.5.3 Botulinum Toxin

Botulinum toxin A (BoNT/A) could be offered to patients with UUI who are refractory to treatment with antimuscarinics or beta 3 receptor agonists. This therapy is not without side effects, and patients need to be counseled before embarking on this treatment. Evidence in frail older persons is limited.

15.5.3.1 Mechanism of Action

BoNT/A seems to have an effect on three neural pathways [5]. Firstly, it inhibits the fusion of neurosecretory vesicles and blocks acetylcholine release from the presynaptic nerve terminals. This affects both the afferent suburothelial and the efferent (motor) nerve endings, thereby inhibiting bladder contraction in response to increase in the intravesical pressure. Secondly BoNT/A exerts complex inhibitory effects on bladder neurotransmitters, neuropeptides, and receptors involved with neurotransmission. It was shown that patients with detrusor overactivity had an increased expression of capsaicin and purinergic receptors, and intravesical infiltration of BoNT/A resulted in a decrease of these sensory receptors. Thirdly, evidence suggests that this agent could act centrally by an effect on the lumbosacral cord causing peripheral desensitization as well.

15.5.3.2 Evidence

BoNT/A infiltration for UUI has been shown to decrease the number of micturitions and episodes of UI per day and increase bladder filling capacity and the volume of urine per voiding episode. In a meta-analysis comparing BoNT/A treatment to placebo, 30% of the patients were cured against 7% in the placebo arm. Quality of life at 6 months was higher in the treatment group. A study comparing BoNT/A to antimuscarinics showed similar rates of improvement in the first 6 months, but the cure rate was higher in the BoNT/A arm [6]. However, there were higher rates of urinary tract infections (UTIs) and retention of urine than with the antimuscarinics. These side effects as well as the need for this treatment to be repeated at 5–9-month intervals result in a high dropout rate from treatment which has been shown to be 60% at 5-year follow-up [7].

15.5.3.3 Clinical Use

Onabotulinum toxin A has been licensed for use to treat OAB or treatment refractory UUI in Europe. The intravesical injection can be performed under both local and general anesthesia, and the trigone area is usually spared to reduce the potential complication of vesicoureteral reflux.

Although side effects are mainly limited to the urinary tract, patients should be counseled before starting therapy about the need for repeated treatment sessions and the possible side effects of retention of urine (5%) requiring clean intermittent catheterization (CIC) as well as UTIs (30%). Risk factors for adverse effects include age over 61 years as well as a low maximal flow rate, low voiding efficiency, and a high PVR baseline prior to starting treatment. Evidence for use in the frail older person is limited, and CIC in this patient group can prove difficult to perform safely.

15.6 Pharmacotherapeutic Management of Stress Urinary Incontinence

15.6.1 Duloxetine

Duloxetine is the main pharmacotherapeutic agent available for the management of stress urinary incontinence (SUI) in both females and males. It is not a cure for UI but provides temporary relief of symptoms. It is usually commenced after a trial of conservative treatment with pelvic floor muscle training (PFMT) has not proven to be adequately effective. However, PMFT should be anyway continued when starting duloxetine since it has been shown that clinical improvement as well as improvement in quality of life (QoL) is more significant when duloxetine is combined with PFMT. Unfortunately, this treatment is associated with a high withdrawal rate because of side effects. There is very scant data on its efficacy in the older and frail older persons.

15.6.1.1 Mechanism of Action

Duloxetine is a dual norepinephrine (NE) and serotonin (5HT) reuptake inhibitor. NE and 5HT receptors are abundantly present in the sacral areas of the spinal cord particularly in the region of Onuf's nucleus [8]. NE and 5HT stimulate the motor neurons (via the pudendal nerve) that results in increased resting tone and contraction of the external urethral sphincter (EUS). However, this effect depends on a descending neurotransmitter from the brain (thought to be glutamate) that acts as an on-off switch for micturition to occur. In the presence of glutamate, in the storage phase of micturition, NE and 5HT enhance EUS contraction but in the voiding phase, in the absence of glutamate, this enhancing effect is lost [9]. Duloxetine therefore preferentially works during the storage phase with no significant effect on the voiding phase, in this way not affecting voiding function and not resulting in retention of urine.

15.6.1.2 Evidence

Duloxetine improves SUI, mixed urinary incontinence (MUI), and to a lesser extent UUI in women. It can improve SUI in males and has also been shown to decrease post-prostatectomy leakage [6].

It is more effective than PFMT alone in reducing leakage although a trial of PFMT is usually recommended prior to commencing the medication. However, PFMT works synergistically with duloxetine, and the effect of the latter on quality of life (QoL) is better when combined with PFMT.

Unfortunately, duloxetine is associated with a high patient withdrawal rate of 20–40% in the short term and up to 90% in the long term. Side effects include poor appetite, dry mouth, nausea and vomiting, constipation, headache, dizziness, falls, sleep disturbance, tremor, palpitations, and sexual dysfunction. The option of effective minimally invasive surgical procedures in the younger elderly women, which offers a more definitive form of treatment, could be a contributing factor to the high withdrawal rate in the long term.

There is no clear data in older persons regarding the duration of usage and whether the efficacy of duloxetine is sustainable in the long term.

15.6.1.3 Clinical Use

Duloxetine can be used in patients suffering from SUI, MUI, and in women UUI. Ideally it should be combined with PFMT and bladder training. It should be explained to the patient that this treatment will not result in a permanent cure for the UI but can provide temporary relief of their symptoms.

In older persons, it should ideally be started at 20 mg twice daily for 2 weeks and then increased to 40 mg twice daily which is the recommended therapeutic dose [10]. Patients should be assessed for benefit and tolerability after 2–4 weeks on the therapeutic dose.

Duloxetine is eliminated primarily in the urine (one-half life of 12 h) after extensive hepatic metabolism. It can cause some inhibition of CYP2D6 and should not be used in combination with CYP1A2 inhibitors or nonselective irreversible monoamine oxidase inhibitors. Caution must be taken for interactions including possible serotonergic effects with several antidepressants. Ciprofloxacin inhibits metabolism of duloxetine and should therefore be avoided. Also, duloxetine could inhibit metabolism of tamoxifen to its active metabolites.

Because of its side effects and paucity of evidence in the frail older person, in certain situations such as a high level of dependence and advanced cognitive impairment, the use of appropriate absorbent aids could be a valuable alternative.

15.6.2 Desmopressin

Desmopressin, a synthetic analog of vasopressin (antidiuretic hormone), is primarily used in the treatment of diabetes insipidus but has also been used to treat nocturia. However, it is not licensed for the treatment of UI and is associated with hyponatraemia.

15.6.2.1 Mechanism of Action

Desmopressin acts as a selective agonist on receptors present throughout the collecting ducts and distal convoluted tubules of the kidneys, and it increases the amount of solute-free water that is reabsorbed into the circulation from the filtrate in this way concentrating the urine and decreasing its volume.

15.6.2.2 Evidence

Although it has been shown to be beneficial in the treatment of nocturia, there is no evidence to support its use in UI. Two RCTs have shown some decrease in daytime incontinence in the 4-h period following its administration; however, this effect was not sustained thereafter. Its long-term use does not improve UI in men and women.

15.6.2.3 Clinical Use

Desmopressin should not be used to manage UI in older patients. Hyponatremia is a relatively common and serious risk when using this medication, and, in several cases, patients required hospitalization [11]. This risk increases with age and with a baseline hyponatremia.

15.7 Topical Estrogen Therapy

Vaginal estrogen therapy can be used to treat incontinence in postmenopausal women. It has been shown to improve quality of life and can improve continence especially UUI, but there is no consistent data of its effect on SUI.

15.7.1 Mechanism of Action

Estrogen receptors have been found in the pelvic floor muscles, urogenital ligaments, the epithelial tissue of the bladder, urethra and trigone, detrusor muscle, and vagina.

Estrogens produce a trophic effect on the epithelial mucosa in the vagina, urethra, and bladder in this way enhancing the "mucosal sphincter" effect as well as increasing the periurethral vascularization which is important in regulating the urethral closing pressure [12]. They also increase the ratio of alpha to beta adrenergic receptors favoring increased urethral tonicity. Some of the perceived improvement in lower urinary tract symptoms might be because of their estrogenic effect of decreasing vaginal discomfort associated with vaginal atrophy.

The effects of estrogens on incontinence comes about from the fact that estrogen receptors are ubiquitous in the LUT and therefore maintain a stable balance between tissues that confers improvement in postmenopausal UI.

15.7.2 Evidence

Vaginal estrogen therapy improves UI in postmenopausal women particularly those with symptoms of vulvovaginal atrophy. It is most effective in urge urinary incontinence. There is no consistent evidence on its effect in SUI, but in some studies, it has been shown to improve symptoms and quality of life. Evidence on their use in frail older patients is mainly related to prophylaxis of urinary tract infections rather than for UI.

Oral or any other non-vaginal routes of administration do not improve UI and can actually worsen it [13].

15.7.3 Clinical Use

Vaginal estrogen therapy can be administered as estradiol, estriol, or conjugated equine estrogen in various forms that include creams, vaginal pessaries, and impregnated vaginal rings. There is no significant difference between these modes of delivery, and this might have to be adapted to the patient's ability to apply these preparations. Commoner side effects include abdominal pain, vaginal hemorrhage, and vulvovaginal disorders.

It has been shown that there is a degree of systemic absorption of these topical preparations, and one should anyway be vigilant for side effects. The ideal duration of treatment and the long-term side effects in older persons are uncertain, and this treatment should be used at the smallest effective dose to minimize systemic effects. Patients should be reviewed at least annually with special considerations given to any symptoms of endometrial hyperplasia.

They are contraindicated in patients with breast cancer taking aromatase inhibitors since they could counteract the therapeutic benefit of the chemotherapy.

15.8 Drugs for Benign Prostatic Hypertrophy (BPH)

In men, one of the most common causes of overactive bladder and urge incontinence is benign prostatic hypertrophy (BPH). In people with this condition, the association of drugs for BPH and antimuscarinic/mirabegron may be used, although the latter must be avoided in the presence of severe obstruction. Among drugs used for BPH, both 5-alpha-reductase inhibitors (including *Serenoa repens*) and alpha-adrenergic antagonists are effective in reducing overactive bladder symptoms. In the older people, however, alpha-adrenergic antagonists are associated with increased risk of hypotension and falls, and while the risk is smaller with prostate-specific drugs, it is still significant. *Serenoa repens* is also used to treat symptoms. Phosphodiesterase inhibitors such as tadalafil may also be used as adjuvant therapy in selected subset of patients.

15.8.1 Mechanism of Action

5-Alpha-reductase inhibitors block the conversion of testosterone to 5-alpha-dihydrotestosterone (DIT) that has higher affinity for the androgen receptor and therefore reduce the androgen stimulation on the prostate. Alpha-adrenergic blockers act by relaxing smooth muscle both within the prostatic gland and the bladder neck; phosphodiesterase inhibitors also act on prostatic smooth muscle cells. However, the effects of these drugs are at least in part independent on their effects on bladder outlet obstruction.

15.8.2 Evidence

5-Alpha-reductase inhibitors, even in monotherapy, can reduce lower urinary tract symptoms, although the effect of alpha-blockers is more evident [14]. These drugs, however, may be less tolerated by older patients because of the risk of orthostatic hypotension. Evidence on the effect of *Serenoa repens* are conflicting.

15.8.3 Clinical Use

5-Alpha-reductase inhibitors are the first-line medical therapy in the treatment of BPH. They are generally well tolerated but may mask an increase of prostate-specific antigen (PSA) in people with prostate cancer. It is recommended to obtain the PSA serum concentration before starting the therapy with these drugs and then to repeat the assessment after the beginning of the therapy to have a baseline for prostate cancer screening (when indicated). Alpha-receptor blockers may be used when rapid symptom control is desired, but the risk for falls due to orthostatic hypotension must be weighed against the potential benefits.

15.9 Conclusions

Drug therapy is to be considered a second-line option in the management of UI in older people. Currently, options are available especially for overactive bladder/urge incontinence. These drugs seem to be effective, especially in the short term, and the risk for serious drug-related adverse events is low. Nonetheless, evidence on very old and frail people is scant, and the very low rate of persistence on drug therapy indicates that the overall benefit may not offset the untoward effects of these drugs. Currently, new drug targets are being investigated, and a selective norepinephrine reuptake inhibitor has shown promising results in a phase II clinical trial.

In conclusion, drug therapy may be an option in the treatment of UI, but patients' expectations and risk profile (e.g., low cognitive reserve) must be weighed against a realistic evaluation of efficacy.

References

1. Fowler CJ, Griffiths D, de Groat WC. The neural control of micturition. Nat Rev Neurosci. 2008;9:453–66.
2. Aharony L, De Cock J, Nuotio M, Pedone C, Vande Walle N, Velge A, Vella A, Verdejo BC. Consensus document on the management of urinary incontinence in older persons. Eur Geriatr Med. 2017;8:202–9.
3. Nabi G, Cody JD, Ellis G, Hay-Smith J, Herbison GP. Anticholinergic drugs versus placebo for overactive bladder syndrome in adults. Cochrane Database Syst Rev. 2006;4:CD003781.
4. Wang J, Zhou J, Cui Y, Li Y, Yuan H, Gao Z, Zhu Z, Wu J. Meta-analysis of the efficacy and safety of mirabegron and solifenacin monotherapy for overactive bladder. Neurourol Urodyn. 2019;38:22–30.
5. Hsieh PF, Hung-Chieh C, Chao-Hsiang C, Chieh-Lung CE. Botulinum toxin A for the treatment of overactive bladder. Toxins. 2016;8:59. https://doi.org/10.3390/toxins8030059.
6. Lucas MG, Bedretdinova D, Berghmans LC, Bosch JLHR, Burhard FC, Cruz F et al. Guidelines on urinary incontinence—partial update. 2015 European Association of Urology.
7. Mohee A, Khan A, Harris N, Eardley I. BJU Int. 2012;111:106–13. https://doi.org/10.1111/j.1464-410x.2012.11282.x.

8. Abreu-Mendes P, Silva J, Cruz F. Pharmacology of the lower urinary tract: update on LUTS treatment. Ther Adv Urol. 2020;12:1–16. https://doi.org/10.1177/1756287220922425.
9. Schuessler B. What do we know about Duloxetine's mode of action? BJOG. 2006;113(Suppl 1):5–9. https://doi.org/10.1111/j.1471-0528.2006.00877.x.
10. Jinhang L, Yang L, Chunxiao P, Tana Y, Haichao Y, Han P. The role of duloxetine in stress urinary incontinence: a systematic review and meta-analysis. Int Urol Nephrol. 2013;45:679–86. https://doi.org/10.1007/s11255-013-0410-6.
11. Weatherall M. The risk of hyponatremia in older adults using desmopressin for nocturia: a systematic review and meta-analysis. Neurourol Urodyn. 2004;23:302–5.
12. Legendre G, Ringa V, Fauconnier A, Fritel X. Menopause, hormone treatment and urinary incontinence at mid-life. Maturitas. 2013;74:26–30.
13. Weber MA, Lim V, Oryszcyn J, te West N, Soujet J, Jeffrey S, Roovers JP, Moore KH. The effect of vaginal oestriol cream on subjective and objective symptoms of stress urinary incontinence and vaginal atrophy: an international multi-centre pilot study. Gynecol Obstet Invest. 2017;82:15–21. https://doi.org/10.1159/000445074.
14. McConnell JD, Roehrborn CG, Bautista OM, Andriole GL Jr, Dixon CM, Kusek JW, Lepor H, McVary KT, Nyberg LM Jr, Clarke HS, Crawford ED, Diokno A. The long-term effect of doxazosin, finasteride, and combination therapy on the clinical progression of benign prostatic hyperplasia. N Engl J Med. 2003;349:2387–98.
15. Takahashi S, Kato K, Takei M, Yokoyama O, Gotoh M. Efficacy and safety of the noradrenaline reuptake inhibitor, TAS-303, in women with stress urinary incontinence: results of a double-blind, randomized, placebo-controlled, early phase II trial. Int J Urol. 2021;28(1):82–90. https://doi.org/10.1111/iju.14411.

Constipation

16

Giammarco Fava

Constipation is a common clinical manifestation in older adults. The prevalence of constipation increases with age and differs among settings with ranges in the elderly from 24 to 50% [1–7]. The correct etiology of constipation in the elderly is required to establish the best management. In fact, constipation may be chronic functional or secondary to other etiologic factors [8]. Primary colorectal dysfunction consists of three overlapping subtypes: slow transit constipation, dyssynergic defecation, and irritable bowel syndrome with constipation. Secondary causes of constipation should be excluded by history, physical examination, and medical history followed by diagnostic testing [8]. The treatment of secondary constipation is beyond the aim of this chapter. The first step for the treatment of chronic functional constipation is modification of lifestyle and diet behavior.

16.1 Lifestyle

General measures such as increased fluid intake and exercise are suggested to manage constipation (Fig. 16.1). Even if poor evidences support this advice [9], it is suggested increasing water intake to 1.5–2 L daily to enhance the effects of fiber in constipated patients [10] (Fig. 16.1). Patients with a normal bowel transit usually empty stools at approximately the same time daily [11, 12], and defecation is partially a conditioned reflex. Colonic motor activity is more active after waking and after a meal [13]; thus, the optimal time for defecation is usually within the first 2 h after waking and after breakfast. For this reason, there is a rationale in educating patients to attempt a bowel movement at least twice a day, usually 30 min after meals, and to strain for no more than 5 min [14].

G. Fava (✉)
Gastroenterology and Digestive Endoscopy Unit, Italian National Research Center on Aging (IRCCS-INRCA), Ancona, Italy
e-mail: g.fava@inrca.it

A. Cherubini et al. (eds.), *Optimizing Pharmacotherapy in Older Patients*, Practical Issues in Geriatrics, https://doi.org/10.1007/978-3-031-28061-0_16

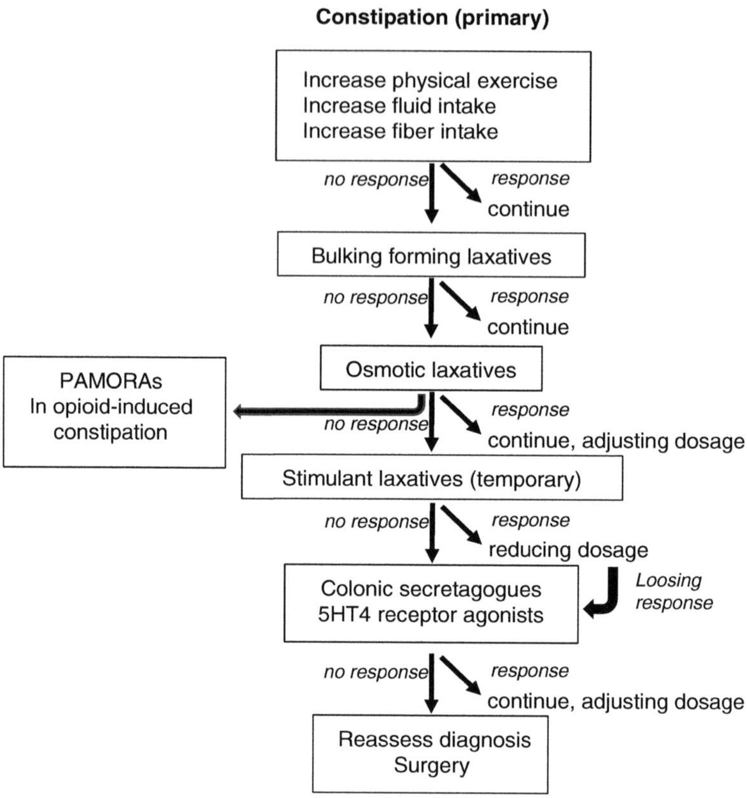

Fig. 16.1 Algorithm for the choice of laxative

16.2 Diet and Fiber

Fiber increases stool bulk, which causes colonic distention and promotes stool propulsion. Fiber is obtained primarily from grains and bran cereals [12]. There is a weak evidence for the effectiveness of fiber consumption as treatment of constipation in older people. One study demonstrates that higher fiber intake was associated with lower laxative use among older women [15], but another work shows that higher intake of bran was associated with no reduction in constipation symptoms and greater fecal loading in the colon [5]. In practical terms, a daily fiber intake of 20–30 g/day is generally recommended to improve bowel transit (Fig. 16.1). The effects of fiber on bowel movements may take several weeks. Bloating, flatulence, and cramps are a common problem with increased fiber intake, especially bran fiber [16].

16.3 Pharmacologic Treatment

Laxatives are prescribed in patients with constipation not responding to lifestyle and dietary modification. Many studies comparing laxative effects in older people are of poor quality and limited by unclear definitions for constipation, inconsistent outcome measurement, and underreporting of potential confounding factors during the trial period (e.g., fiber intake) [17–26]. Laxatives are used daily by 10–18% of community dwelling older adults and 74% of nursing home residents [4, 27, 28]. These data suggest that sometimes these drugs are empirically prescribed to older patients [29, 30]. However, osmotic salts, sugars and sugar alcohols, polyethylene glycol (PEG), anthraquinones, diphenolic laxatives, and diphenylmethanes generally have been shown efficacy and safety [17, 29, 30].

16.4 Bulk Forming Laxatives

Bulk forming laxatives include psyllium husk, methylcellulose, calcium polycarbophil, and wheat dextrin. They are natural, synthetic polysaccharides or cellulose derivatives that primarily exert their laxative effect by absorbing water and swelling in the small and large intestine to form soft and bulky stool [17]. These drugs increase the frequency and reduce the consistency of stool with a minimum of adverse effects. They may be used alone or in combination with an increase in dietary fiber and require an adequate amount of fluid intake (Fig. 16.1); otherwise, they may worsen constipation [17]. Despite anecdotal clinical experience indicating benefit for bulk forming laxatives, clear evidence regarding the effectiveness is inconsistent. A systematic review found evidence that psyllium increases stool frequency in patients with chronic constipation but found insufficient evidence for benefit of other forms of fiber including calcium polycarbophil, methylcellulose, and bran [18]. On the contrary, another review shows efficacy and safety of calcium polycarbophil instead of psyllium and methylcellulose [19]. No statistically significant differences in adverse events were identified between any bulking agent and an active comparator or placebo. Task force members noted that large quantities of psyllium may be associated with bloating. Also, mechanical obstruction of the esophagus and colon has been rarely reported with bulking agents, and anaphylactic reactions have been reported with psyllium [18].

16.5 Osmotic Laxatives

Osmotic laxatives should be used in patients not responding to bulk forming laxatives [20] (Fig. 16.1). Osmotic laxatives increase fecal volume and reduce stool consistency by creating an intraluminal osmotic gradient that leads to secretion of water and electrolytes into the intestinal lumen [17]. They are divided into three categories: poorly absorbed ions, nonabsorbable carbohydrates, and polyethylene glycol.

16.5.1 Poorly Absorbed Ions

Magnesium, sulfate, and phosphate ions are partly absorbed by the intestine, thus creating a hyperosmolar intraluminal environment. This leads to an osmotic mechanism, even if they have other possible effects with unclear consequences, such as increase of prostaglandin concentrations in the stool [21]. Magnesium hydroxide typically induces a bowel movement within 6 h (Table 16.1). Moreover, magnesium sulfate is a potent laxative that produces a large volume of liquid stool and often leads to abdominal distention and sudden passage of a foul-smelling liquid stool. However, the assumption of magnesium, particularly in older adults, needs to be limited since it could cause adverse effects such as flatulence, abdominal cramps, and volume overload. A small amount of magnesium is actively absorbed in the small intestine, while the remainder draws water into the intestine by an osmotic gradient [22]. Hypermagnesemia can develop particularly in patients with kidney diseases and in children, and hypermagnesemia-induced paralytic ileus was described as a rare complication [23]. Absorption of magnesium can cause electrolyte and volume overload in patients with kidney failure or cardiac dysfunction. Also, in case of dehydration, excessive use of magnesium based laxatives can develop these complications even in healthy patients.

Phosphate is mostly absorbed by the small intestine; thus, a large quantity needs to be ingested to produce an osmotic laxative effect, and this is not ideal for routine use [17]. Rare but serious reports of acute phosphate nephropathy have been described in patients treated with oral sodium phosphate products for colon cleansing prior to colonoscopy. Some patients have resulted in permanent damage of renal function and required long-term dialysis. While some cases have occurred in patients with normal baseline renal function, risk factors of acute phosphate nephropathy include advanced age, hypovolemia, increased bowel transit time (such as bowel obstruction), active colitis, kidney disease, and use of medicines that affect renal perfusion or function such as diuretics, angiotensin-converting enzyme [ACE] inhibitors, angiotensin receptor blockers, and possibly nonsteroidal anti-inflammatory drugs [NSAIDs]. Patients should be advised to split dosage regimen and warning about the importance of adequate hydration before, during, and after use of oral sodium phosphate products. Additional sodium phosphate-based purgative or enema products should be avoided [24].

16.5.2 Nonabsorbable Carbohydrates

Lactulose. Lactulose is a nonabsorbable synthetic disaccharide constituted by galactose and fructose linked by a bond resistant to lactase. Lactulose is not absorbed by

Table 16.1 Summary of more common laxatives

		Osmotic laxatives													
		Poorly absorbed ions		Nonabsorbable carbohydrates	Metabolically inert	Stimulant laxatives		Colonic secretagogues		Serotoninergics	Stool softener	Enemas		Suppositories	
Drugs (generic name)	Bulking agents (psyllium, methylcellulose, polycarbophil)	Magnesium hydroxide	Sodium phosphate	Lactulose	PEG	Senna	Bisacodyl	Lubiprostone	Linaclotide	Prucalopride	Docusate sodium	Phosphate enema	Bisacodyl	Bisacodyl	Glycerin
Recommended dose (daily)	4–20 g	15–30 mL once or twice	20 mL once	15–30 mL once or twice	17–34 g once or twice	5–20 mL once; 7.5–15 mg once	10–30 mg once	24 µg twice	290 µg once	2 mg once	100 mg twice	120 mL once	10 mg once	10 mg once	60 g once
Side effects	Bloating, intestinal obstruction, allergic reactions (rare)	Bloating, abdominal cramps, volume overload (in pts. with kidney disease or cardiac dysfunction), hypermagnesemia	Acute phosphate nephropathy (during bowel preparation)	Bloating, diarrhea, nausea, hyperglycemia in diabetics	Bloating, cramps, flatulence, electrolyte imbalance, allergic reaction, Mallory Weiss tears (rare, during bowel prep)	Cramps, diarrhea, nausea, vomiting, melanosis coli	Cramps, nausea, electrolyte imbalance, vomiting	Headache, nausea, diarrhea	Diarrhea, bloating	Nausea, headache, diarrhea	*Efficacy not well defined*	Rectal mucosa injury, hyperphosphatemia	Rectal mucosa irritation	Rectal mucosa irritation	Rectal mucosa irritation

the small intestine and is transformed in the colon to yield short-chain fatty acids, hydrogen, and carbon dioxide, with consequent pulling water out from the body and into the colon and lowering of the fecal pH. If lactulose is administered at dosage of 20 g (30 mL) daily, the sugar is not detectable in the stool. Indeed, in larger doses, some drug passes through the colon unchanged; thus, it should be used with caution in diabetic patients because of the risk of increasing glycemia. The recommended dose of lactulose in adults is 15–30 mL once or twice daily. The time to onset of action is longer than that of other osmotic laxatives since 2 or 3 days are required for lactulose to achieve an effect. Some patients report that lactulose is effective initially but then gradually loses its effect, possibly due to alteration in the intestinal flora in response to the medication [25]. Side effects related to lactulose include abdominal distention or discomfort, presumably as a result of colonic gas production, diarrhea, and nausea. Cases of lactulose-induced megacolon have been also reported [25].

The osmotic laxatives are consistently better than placebo for improving the symptoms of constipation [26, 31]. Four studies compared osmotic laxative with placebo, and three studies compared two osmotic laxatives. In two RCTs, lactulose significantly increased the defecation frequency in respect with placebo and significantly decreased the need for laxative use [32, 33]. Lactitol also significantly increased the number of defecations, improved stool consistency, and decreased laxative use compared with placebo [34].

Sorbitol and Mannitol. Sorbitol is widely used in the food industry as an artificial sweetener but is rarely used in clinical practice. Ingestion of 5 g sorbitol causes a rise in breath hydrogen, and 20 g produces diarrhea in about half of normal subjects [35]. Sorbitol is as effective as lactulose and less expensive. A randomized double-blind crossover trial of lactulose (20 g/day) and sorbitol (21 g/day) in ambulatory older men with chronic constipation showed no difference between the two compounds with regard to frequency or normality of bowel movements or patient preference [36]. The frequency of side effects was similar except for nausea, which was more common with lactulose. Mannitol is another sugar alcohol that can be used as a laxative. Like sorbitol, it is rarely used for clinical management of constipation.

16.5.3 Polyethylene Glycol

Polyethylene glycol (PEG) is an isosmotic and metabolically inert laxative able to bind water molecules, thereby increasing intraluminal water retention [37]. PEG is not metabolized by colonic bacteria and is excreted mostly unaltered into the feces leading to an increase in stool volume and softer stools, which may become liquid depending to the volume of PEG ingested. Electrolytes are added to PEG solutions used for colonic preparation before colonoscopy to avoid the potential adverse effects associated with diarrhea, such as dehydration and electrolyte imbalance. PEG-3350 without electrolytes is available as an over-the-counter powder and is mixed in smaller doses with water for regular use to treat constipation. The most common adverse events of PEG, especially if used at high dosage (34 g/day), include abdominal bloating, cramps, and flatulence [37, 38] (Table 16.1). In addition, the most commonly reported side effects of PEG used for colonoscopy preparation include electrolyte imbalances, allergic reactions, and Mallory-Weiss tears [39] (Table 16.1). Cases of fulminant pulmonary edema have been reported after administration of PEG solution by nasogastric tube, with one fatality [40, 41]. In each case, the patient had emesis, suggesting aspiration of PEG. PEG also may delay gastric emptying [42]. The strongest evidence for clinical benefit exists for PEG, which has been evaluated in 19 trials, mostly compared to placebo, followed by lactulose and tegaserod [31, 43]. In the largest study (304 patients treated for 6 months), patients given PEG had more bowel movements per week than patients of placebo group [44]. In a retrospective series study, its efficacy was maintained for up to 24 months [44, 45]. Patients prefer PEG preparations without electrolyte supplements [46], which are necessary when a large volume is required [47].

16.6 Stimulant Laxatives

Stimulant laxatives are generally used as a rescue in case of no response to osmotic laxatives (Fig. 16.1), especially if patients have not defecated for 2–3 days [48]. These compounds accelerate intestinal motility and secretion of water, electrolytes, and prostaglandin into the lumen of colon [49], thus accelerating transit [50]. Their effect starts within hours after assumption, and it is often accompanied by abdominal cramps. Stimulant laxatives include anthraquinone derivatives (e.g., cascara, aloe, senna) and diphenylmethane derivatives (e.g., bisacodyl, sodium picosulfate, phenolphthalein). Castor oil is used less commonly because of its side-effect profile. The effect of these stimulant laxatives is dose dependent. Low doses prevent absorption of water and sodium, whereas high doses stimulate secretion of sodium, followed by water, into the colonic lumen [17]. Stimulant laxatives are sometimes abused, especially in patients with an eating disorder even though at high doses they have only a modest effect on calorie absorption [51]. Stimulant laxatives can produce normal, soft, formed stools in some patients but are often associated with abdominal cramps and diarrhea even in standard doses (Table 16.1). They act rapidly and are particularly suitable for use in a single dose for temporary constipation [17]. Most clinicians are cautious about recommending daily dosing of stimulant laxatives indefinitely for chronic constipation. Stimulant laxatives vary widely in clinical effectiveness, and some patients with severe constipation are nonresponder [17].

16.6.1 Anthraquinone Derivatives

Anthraquinones (e.g., cascara, senna, aloe, frangula) are obtained by a variety of plants [17]. They are constituted by inactive glycosides which pass unabsorbed and unchanged through the small intestine. These drugs are hydrolyzed into the colon by bacterial glycosidases to active metabolites able to increase the transport of electrolytes into the lumen and stimulate myenteric plexuses to induce intestinal motility. The anthraquinones typically permit defecation 6–8 h after ingestion [51] (Table 16.1). Senna has been shown to soften stools [52] and increase stool frequency and weight. Anthraquinones cause apoptosis of colonic epithelial cells, which are then phagocytosed by macrophages and appear as a lipofuscin-like pigment that darkens the colonic mucosa, a condition termed *Melanosis coli* [53] (Table 16.1). Moreover, these laxatives don't induce significant adverse functional or structural changes in the intestine. Animal studies have shown neither damage to the myenteric plexus after long-term administration of sennosides [54] nor a functional defect in motility [55].

16.6.2 Diphenylmethane Derivatives

Diphenylmethane compounds include bisacodyl and sodium picosulfate. After oral ingestion, bisacodyl and sodium picosulfate are hydrolyzed to the same active metabolite, but the mode of hydrolysis differs since the first is hydrolyzed by intestinal enzymes, thus acting in the small and large intestines, and the second is hydrolyzed by colonic bacteria [17]. Like anthraquinones, the action of sodium picosulfate is confined to the colon, and its activity depends by the bacterial flora. The effects of bisacodyl, and presumably sodium picosulfate, on the colon are similar to those of the anthraquinone laxatives [17]. When applied to the colonic mucosa, bisacodyl induces an almost immediate, powerful, propulsive motor activity in healthy and constipated subjects, although the effect is sometimes reduced in the latter [56]. These laxatives also stimulate colonic secretion. Similarly to the anthraquinone laxatives, bisacodyl leads to apoptosis of colonic epithelial cells, the remnants of which accumulate in phagocytic macrophages, but these cellular remnants are not pigmented [57]. Bisacodyl is a useful and predictable laxative, especially suitable for single-dose use in patients with temporary constipation. Bisacodyl was evaluated in a randomized, double-blind, placebo-controlled, parallel-group study in which patients were randomized to bisacodyl (10 mg) or placebo for 4 weeks. The mean number of complete spontaneous bowel movements (CSBMs) per week, the number of spontaneous bowel movements (SBMs), constipation-associated symptoms, and quality of life were significantly improved in the bisacodyl group compared to placebo [58]. Treatment with bisacodyl was also well tolerated (Table 16.1). However, the long-term safety of stimulant laxatives has not been established.

Sodium picosulfate is available as part of a colonoscopy preparation. In a randomized, double-blind, placebo-controlled study conducted in Germany, 233 patients with chronic constipation were randomized to sodium picosulfate (10 mg drops) or placebo once daily for 4 weeks. Patients of the sodium picosulfate group reported a greater number of CSBM per week during the treatment period compared with those in the placebo group (0.9 ± 0.1 at baseline increased to 3.4 ± 0.2 in the sodium picosulfate group and 1.1 ± 0.1 at baseline increased to 1.7 ± 0.1 in the placebo group). Patients who received sodium picosulfate reported improvement in straining, incomplete evacuation, a feeling of anal obstruction, and improvement in stool form and had increased quality-of-life scores compared with those who received placebo. Diarrhea was reported by 32% of patients who received the sodium picosulfate [59] (Table 16.1).

A systematic review and meta-analysis of pharmacotherapies for chronic constipation showed that bisacodyl and sodium picosulfate met the primary endpoints of responder analysis with greater than or equal to 3 CSBM per week and an increase over baseline of greater than or equal to 1 CSBM per week [60]. However, bisacodyl may be superior to other prescription drugs in secondary endpoints, including an increase from baseline in the number of spontaneous bowel movements (SBM) per week and in the number of CSBM per week [17]. No studies have compared bisacodyl to placebo in elderly patients with constipation [26].

16.6.3 Castor Oil

Castor oil is obtained from the castor bean. After oral ingestion, it is hydrolyzed by lipase in the small intestine to ricinoleic acid, which inhibits intestinal water absorption and stimulates intestinal motor function by damaging mucosal cells and releasing neurotransmitters [61]. Cramping is frequent, and consequently castor oil is not commonly used in clinical practice.

16.7 Other Therapies for Chronic Constipation

Several agents have been studied or are undergoing further studies for the treatment of chronic constipation. These include colonic secretagogues, opioid antagonists, and $5HT_4$ receptor agonists (Fig. 16.1 and Table 16.1).

16.8 Colonic Secretagogues

Lubiprostone is an oral bicyclic fatty acid that activates the type 2 chloride channels on the intestinal epithelial cells, thus secreting chloride and water into the intestinal lumen [14]. In two phase III studies of 4 weeks' duration, lubiprostone 24 μg twice daily significantly enhanced bowel movement frequency and relieved other constipation-related symptoms compared with placebo [62]. In a subgroup analysis, lubiprostone also demonstrated efficacy in older patients. It is best reserved for patients with severe constipation in whom other approaches have been unsuccessful [8]. Nausea was the most common reported adverse event, occurring in up to 31.7% of patients and leading to discontinuation in 5% [63] (Table 16.1). Lubiprostone is also approved in the USA for the treatment of opioid-induced constipation as well as for women with IBS with constipation at a dose of 8 μg twice daily [17].

Linaclotide and plecanatide are guanylate cyclase C receptor (GCC) agonists that stimulate intestinal fluid secretion and transit [64]. Linaclotide is a minimally absorbed 14-amino-acid peptide that activates the guanylate cyclase C receptor on the luminal surface of the intestinal epithelium, resulting in increased levels of cyclic guanosine monophosphate and increased secretion of chloride and bicarbonate into the intestinal lumen. In animal models, cyclic guanosine monophosphate also appears to reduce firing of afferent nerves in the bowel [65].

In two large phase III trials of patients with chronic constipation, the linaclotide-treated groups (both 145 μg and 290 μg) had significantly higher rates of three or more complete spontaneous bowel movements (CSBM) per week and an increase in one or more CSBMs from baseline during at least 9 out of 12 weeks as compared with placebo (145 μg: 21 and 16%; 290 μg: 19 and 21%; placebo: 3 and 6%) [66]. Linaclotide also increased stool frequency, improved stool consistency, and reduced straining, abdominal bloating, and discomfort as compared with placebo [66]. The most common dose-related adverse event was diarrhea that led to discontinuation of treatment in 4% of patients in both linaclotide-treated groups [66].

16.9 Opioid Antagonists

Opioids are a drug family largely used to manage chronic pain in clinical practice. Opioid-induced constipation (OIC) results from the agonist actions of opioid medications at μ-opioid receptors, which are abundant throughout the gastrointestinal tract. This adverse event is often underrecognized and undertreated in the elderly [67]. In elderly patients with OIC and chronic pain who do not respond to lifestyle interventions or laxatives, treatment of symptoms of constipation may be obtained using peripherally acting μ-opioid receptor antagonists (PAMORAs), such as alvimopan, methylnaltrexone, naloxegol, naldemedine, or alvimopan for paralytic ileus [68]. These opioid receptor antagonists act peripherally and do not cross the blood-brain barrier, thus decreasing the constipating effects of opioids without impairing their analgesic effects [69]. The availability of the new pharmacologic agents methylnaltrexone, naloxegol, and lubiprostone may offer more specific and effective treatment options for elderly patients with OIC and noncancer pain. Moreover, healthcare providers should consider that methylnaltrexone [70] and naloxegol [71], because of their peripheral mechanism of action, do not interfere with opioid-induced, centrally mediated analgesia when administered to patients with noncancer pain and OIC [67]. The complex multifactorial nature of constipation and its potentially negative impact in elderly patients with OIC and chronic pain, coupled with the availability of newer pharmacologic agents that target the underlying mechanisms of constipation (i.e., PAMORAs), and the locally acting secretagogue lubiprostone, provide an opportunity for healthcare providers to better manage their elderly patients with OIC and chronic pain without change in pain medications [67].

16.10 Serotonergic Laxatives

Serotonin (5HT) is a key regulator of gastrointestinal motility. Stimulation of the 5-HT_4 receptor on afferent nerves in the wall of the GI tract stimulates peristaltic contraction of the intestine. Several 5-HT_4 agonists have been tested for treating constipation. Among them, cisapride, was widely used and clinically effective [72] but was withdrawn from the commercial market in July 2000 for inducing potentially lethal cardiac dysrhythmias. Similarly, tegaserod, another partial 5-HT_4 agonist, was also withdrawn in 2007 because of its potential cardiovascular effects.

Prucalopride, a selective high affinity 5HT_4 receptor agonist, is a benzofuran derivative that accelerates colonic transit in healthy humans and patients with chronic constipation [73]. In a dose of 1 and 4 mg once daily, prucalopride has been shown to be superior to placebo in 4- and 12-week trials and safe and well tolerated in patients aged 65 years or older [74, 75]. In clinical trials, prucalopride 2 mg provided comparable efficacy to 4 mg, and it is therefore the widely used dosage in clinical practice. The dose of prucalopride can be titrated up based on clinical response [8]. The most frequent adverse effects were headaches, nausea, and diarrhea (Table 16.1). No cardiovascular side effects have been observed to date with prucalopride, nor any electrocardiographic abnormalities been reported. In addition, in a study of elderly constipated patients in nursing homes, no differences in vital signs, electrocardiograph parameters, or Holter-monitoring results were found in patients receiving prucalopride and placebo. Approximately 88% of the patients had a history of cardiovascular disease [76].

16.11 Enemas and Suppositories

Enemas and suppositories should be used only as needed for constipation in the older adult, i.e., after several days of constipation, in order to prevent fecal impaction. Both stimulate evacuation by distention or chemical action toward the rectal walls, or soften hard stools, or both [17]. Enemas, in particular, need to be used with caution since the extravasation of the solution into the submucosa can induce serious damage to the rectal wall [17].

16.11.1 Phosphate Enemas

Hypertonic sodium phosphate enemas cause distention and stimulation of the rectum. Meisel et al. showed that in normal subjects, a single hypertonic phosphate enema caused disruption of the surface epithelium in 17 of 21 biopsy specimens [77]. The damage was evident by scanning electron microscopy, showing patchy denudation of the surface epithelium, exposure of the lamina propria, and absence of goblet cells. In every case, the mucosa was endoscopically pathological but returned to normal within 1 week [77]. Phosphate enemas are widely used, although studies documenting their efficacy are lacking. The use of sodium phosphate enemas for the treatment of constipation in older adults is contraindicated. In a retrospective series, the use of sodium phosphate enemas in this setting of patients (mean age, 80 years) was followed by complications including hypotension and volume depletion, hyperphosphatemia, hypo- or hyperkalemia, metabolic acidosis, severe hypocalcemia, renal failure, and electrocardiogram changes (prolonged QT interval) [78]. In January 2014, the US Food and Drug Administration (FDA) issued a safety warning regarding electrolyte abnormalities and severe dehydration caused by a single dose of over-the-counter sodium phosphate that was larger than recommended or with more than one dose in 24 h [79]. The FDA stated that individuals at higher risk for potential adverse effects when the recommended dose is exceeded include individuals older than 55 years; patients with dehydration, bowel obstruction, or inflammation; and patients with kidney disease or on medication that may affect renal function [80].

16.11.2 Saline, Tap Water, and Soapsuds Enemas

Saline, tap water, or soapsuds enemas exert their action by distending the rectum and softening feces. Stool evacuation typically occurs 2–5 min following administration. If utilized with small volume, they usually don't induce damage; however, large volumes can be accompanied by serious effects such as water intoxication hyperphosphatemia and other electrolyte disturbances in case of enema retention. Soapsuds enemas can cause rectal mucosal damage and necrosis [17] (Table 16.1).

16.11.3 Stimulant Suppositories and Enemas

Glycerin or bisacodyl suppositories can be used in institutionalized older adults with dyssynergic defecation to favor evacuation by stimulating the rectum through an osmotic effect. The effect of glycerin on the rectal mucosa is unknown, while bisacodyl 10 mg acts topically by stimulating enteric neurons [81] (Table 16.1). A study showed that in normal subjects, a single bisacodyl suppository or an enema containing 19 mg of bisacodyl in 100 or 200 mL of water produced marked changes in 23 of 25 rectal mucosal biopsy specimens. The epithelium of the surface and within the crypts was altered; with use of the enema, the surface epithelium was absent [77]. Regular use of bisacodyl suppositories, therefore, is contraindicated.

16.11.4 Dioctyl Sulfosuccinate (Docusate)

Dioctyl sulfosuccinate, commonly named docusate (calcium or sodium), is a stool softener acting as an anionic surfactant able to stimulate fluid secretion in the small and large intestines [82, 83]. Findings from systematic reviews involving hospitalized patients indicate that docusate does not prevent or improve symptoms of constipation [19] and was less effective than psyllium for treating chronic idiopathic constipation [84]. The clinical practice guideline in the diagnosis, assessment, and management of constipation in advanced cancer from the European Society for Medical Oncology lists docusate as a medication not recommended in the treatment of constipation in patients with advanced malignancies [82]. Thus, for older adults and patients at risk for constipation, the adverse effects of inappropriate prescribing of docusate are of concern. A recent investigation suggests to remove docusate from all standardized order sets and/or hospital [85].

16.12 Mineral Oils

Mineral oils alter the stool by undergoing emulsification into the stool mass and facilitating lubrication for stool passage. Long-term use can cause intestinal malabsorption of fat-soluble vitamins, anal seepage, and lipoid pneumonia in patients predisposed to aspiration of liquids [17].

16.13 Probiotics

A recent review of the literature showed that probiotic supplementation decreases intestinal time, thus significantly improving constipation and increasing defecation frequency in elderly individuals by 10–40% compared to placebo controls. The strain of bacteria most commonly tested was *Bifidobacterium longum* [86]. In addition, a more recent Japanese observational study [87] demonstrated that almost daily consumption of *Lactobacillus casei* strain Shirota (LcS)-containing fermented milk products could benefit older people who tend to be constipated by increasing the intestinal population of beneficial microbes (*Lactobacillus* species) and raising the intestinal level of metabolites of microbial fermentation (lactic acids), thus stimulating intestinal peristalsis/motility [88, 89]. However, caution is needed when interpreting these reports because of the heterogeneity of the original study designs, populations, and the risk of bias. Therefore, further placebo-controlled trials are necessary to determine the most efficient strains, doses, and the optimal treatment duration.

16.14 Conclusion

In older adults, constipation is a very common clinical problem with challenging treatment. Laxative prescription should be individualized according to the patient's history (cardiac and kidney diseases), drug interactions, cost, side effects, and other considerations (e.g., chewing/swallowing disorders). Although laxatives are a first-line treatment option and considered generally well tolerated, sometimes evidence is lacking to support their effectiveness. Healthcare providers should take a stepwise approach (Fig. 16.1) when considering the various treatment options for constipation in the elderly.

References

1. Talley NJ, O'Keefe EA, Zinsmeister AR, Melton LJ 3rd. Prevalence of gastrointestinal symptoms in the elderly: a population-based study. Gastroenterology. 1992;102:895.
2. Talley NJ, Fleming KC, Evans JM, et al. Constipation in an elderly community: a study of prevalence and potential risk factors. Am J Gastroenterol. 1996;91:19.
3. Everhart JE, Go VL, Johannes RS, et al. A longitudinal survey of self-reported bowel habits in the United States. Dig Dis Sci. 1989;34:1153.

4. Whitehead WE, Drinkwater D, Cheskin LJ, et al. Constipation in the elderly living at home. Definition, prevalence, and relationship to lifestyle and health status. J Am Geriatr Soc. 1989;37:423.
5. Donald IP, Smith RG, Cruikshank JG, et al. A study of constipation in the elderly living at home. Gerontology. 1985;31:112.
6. Harari D, Gurwitz JH, Avorn J, et al. Bowel habit in relation to age and gender. Findings from the National Health Interview Survey and clinical implications. Arch Intern Med. 1996;156:315.
7. Choung RS, Locke GR 3rd, Schleck CD, et al. Cumulative incidence of chronic constipation: a population-based study 1988-2003. Aliment Pharmacol Ther. 2007;26:1521.
8. Rao SSC. Constipation in the older adult. Up to date literature review current through: Jan 2022. This topic last updated: May 20, 2020.
9. Lindeman RD, Romero LJ, Liang HC, et al. Do elderly persons need to be encouraged to drink more fluids? J Gerontol A Biol Sci Med Sci. 2000;55:M361.
10. Anti M, Pignataro G, Armuzzi A, et al. Water supplementation enhances the effect of high-fiber diet on stool frequency and laxative consumption in adult patients with functional constipation. Hepatogastroenterology. 1998;45:727–32.
11. Heaton EA. The call to stool and its relationship to constipation: a community study. Eur J Gastroenterol Hepatol. 1994;6:145.
12. Harari D. Constipation and fecal incontinence in old age. Brocklehurst's textbook of geriatric medicine and gerontology, 8th edition. 2017;105, 877–894.e5.
13. Rao SS, Kavelock R, Beaty J, et al. Effects of fat and carbohydrate meals on colonic motor response. Gut. 2000;46:205.
14. Rao SS, Go JT. Update on the management of constipation in the elderly: new treatment options. Clin Interv Aging. 2010;5:163.
15. Johnson CK, Kolasa K, Chenoweth W, et al. Health, laxation and food habit influences on fiber intake of older women. J Am Diet Assoc. 1980;77:551–7.
16. Gallagher P, O'Mahony D. Constipation in old age. Best Pract Res Clin Gastroenterol. 2009;23:875.
17. Iturrino JC, Lembo AJ. Chapter 19. Constipation. In: Sleisenger and Fordtran's gastrointestinal and liver disease. 2020. p. 250–275.e8.
18. American College of Gastroenterology Chronic Constipation Task Force. An evidence- based approach to the management of chronic constipation in North America. Am J Gastroenterol. 2005;100(Suppl 1):S1.
19. Ramkumar D, Rao SS. Efficacy and safety of traditional medical therapies for chronic constipation: systematic review. Am J Gastroenterol. 2005;100:936.
20. Locke GR 3rd, Pemberton JH, Phillips SF. American Gastroenterological Association medical position statement: guidelines on constipation. Gastroenterology. 2000;119:1761.
21. Donowitz M, Rood RP. Magnesium hydroxide: new insights into the mechanism of its laxative effect and the potential involvement of prostaglandin E2. J Clin Gastroenterol. 1992;14:20–6.
22. Saris NE, Mervaala E, Karppanen H, et al. Magnesium. An update on physiological, clinical and analytical aspects. Clin Chim Acta. 2000;294:1–26.
23. Izdes S, Kesimci E, Kanbak O. Paralytic ileus as a complication of iatrogenic hypermagnesaemia without renal dysfunction. Anaesth Intensive Care. 2008;36:124.
24. Phosphate, potassium and sodium. Source Lexycomp®.
25. Wright RA. Lactulose-induced megacolon. Gastrointest Endosc. 1988;34:489–90.
26. Kang SJ, Cho YS, Lee TH, Kim SE, Ryu HS, Kim JW, Park SY, Lee YJ, Shin JE, Constipation Research Group of the Korean Society of Neurogastroenterology and Motility. Medical management of constipation in the elderly patients: systematic review. J Neurogastroenterol Motil. 2021;27(4):495–512.
27. Ruby CM, Fillenbaum GG, Kuchibhatla MN, Hanlon JT. Laxative use in the community-dwelling elderly. Am J Geriatr Pharmacother. 2003;1:11.
28. Harari D, Gurwitz JH, Avorn J, et al. Constipation: assessment and management in an institutionalized elderly population. J Am Geriatr Soc. 1994;42:947.

29. Petticrew M, Watt I, Sheldon T. Systematic review of the effectiveness of laxatives in the elderly. Health Technol Assess. 1997;1:i–iv, 1–52.
30. Fleming V, Wade WE. A review of laxative therapies for treatment of chronic constipation in older adults. Am J Geriatr Pharmacother. 2010;8:514–50.
31. Ford A, Suares N. Effect of laxatives and pharmacological therapies in chronic idiopathic constipation: systematic review and meta-analysis. Gut. 2011;60:209–18. [PubMed: 21205879].
32. Wesselius-De Casparis A, Braadbaart S, Bergh-Bohlken GE, Mimica M. Treatment of chronic constipation with lactulose syrup: results of a double-blind study. Gut. 1968;9:84–6.
33. Sanders JF. Lactulose syrup assessed in a double-blind study of elderly constipated patients. J Am Geriatr Soc. 1978;26:236–9.
34. Vanderdonckt J, Coulon J, Denys W, Ravelli GP. Study of the laxative effect of lactitol (importalr) in an elderly institutionalized, but not bedridden, population suffering from chronic constipation. J Clin Exp Gerontol. 1990;12:171–89.
35. Hyams JS. Sorbitol intolerance: an unappreciated cause of functional gastrointestinal complaints. Gastroenterology. 1983;84:30–3.
36. Lederle FA, Busch DL, Mattox KM, et al. Cost-effective treatment of constipation in the elderly: a randomized double-blind comparison of sorbitol and lactulose. Am J Med. 1990;89:597–601.
37. Corazziari E, Badiali D, Habib FI, et al. Small volume isosmotic polyethylene glycol electrolyte balanced solution (PMF-100) in treatment of chronic nonorganic constipation. Dig Dis Sci. 1996;41:1636–42.
38. Garlehner G, Jonas DE, Morgan LC, et al. Drug class review on constipation drugs. Portland: Oregon Health & Science University; 2007.
39. Belsey J, Epstein O, Heresbach D. Systematic review: adverse event reports for oral sodium phosphate and polyethylene glycol. Aliment Pharmacol Ther. 2009;29:15–28.
40. Argent A, Hatherill M, Reynolds L, Purves L. Fulminant pulmonary oedema after administration of a balanced electrolyte polyethylene glycol solution. Arch Dis Child. 2002;86:209.
41. Marschall HU, Bartels F. Life-threatening complications of nasogastric administration of polyethylene glycol-electrolyte solutions (Go-lytely) for bowel cleansing. Gastrointest Endosc. 1998;47:408–10.
42. Coremans G, Vos R, Margaritis V, et al. Small doses of the unabsorbable substance polyethylene glycol 3350 accelerate oro-caecal transit, but slow gastric emptying in healthy subjects. Dig Liver Dis. 2005;37:97–101.
43. Pare P, Fedorak RN. Systematic review of stimulant and nonstimulant laxatives for the treatment of functional constipation. Can J Gastroenterol Hepatol. 2014;28:549–57.
44. DiPalma JA, Cleveland MV, McGowan J, et al. A randomized, multicenter, placebo-controlled trial of polyethylene glycol laxative for chronic treatment of chronic constipation. Am J Gastroenterol. 2007;102:1436–41.
45. Migeon-Duballet I, Chabin M, Gautier A, et al. Long-term efficacy and cost-effectiveness of polyethylene glycol 3350 plus electrolytes in chronic constipation: a retrospective study in a disabled population. Curr Med Res Opin. 2006;22:1227–35.
46. Szojda MM, Mulder CJJ, Felt-Bersma RJF. Differences in taste between two polyethylene glycol preparations. J Gastrointest Liver Dis. 2007;16:379–81.
47. DiPalma JA, Smith JR, Cleveland MV. Overnight efficacy of polyethylene glycol laxative. Am J Gastroenterol. 2002;97:1776–9.
48. Bharucha AE, Lacy BE. Mechanisms, evaluation, and management of chronic constipation. Gastroenterology. 2020;158(5):1232–1249.e3.
49. Ikarashi N, Baba K, Ushiki T, et al. The laxative effect of bisacodyl is attributable to decreased aquaporin-3 expression in the colon induced by increased PGE2 secretion from macrophages. Am J Physiol Gastrointest Liver Physiol. 2011;301:G887–95.
50. Manabe N, Cremonini F, Camilleri M, et al. Effects of bisacodyl on ascending colon emptying and overall colonic transit in healthy volunteers. Aliment Pharmacol Ther. 2009;30:930–6.
51. Neims DM, McNeill J, Giles TR, Todd F. Incidence of laxative abuse in community and bulimic populations: a descriptive review. Int J Eat Disord. 1995;17:211–28.

52. Exton-Smith AN, Bendall MJ, Kent F. A new technique for measuring the consistency of faeces: a report on its application to the assessment of Senokotot therapy in the elderly. Age Ageing. 1975;4:58–62.
53. Badiali D, Marcheggiano A, Pallone F, et al. Melanosis of the rectum in patients with chronic constipation. Dis Colon Rectum. 1985;28:241–5.
54. Rudolph RL, Mengs U. Electron microscopical studies on rat intestine after long-term treatment with sennosides. Pharmacology. 1988;36(Suppl. 1):188–93.
55. Fioramonti J, Dupuy C, Buéno L. In vivo motility of rat colon chronically pretreated with sennosides. Pharmacology. 1993;47(Suppl. 1):155–61.
56. Kamm MA, Lennard-Jones JE, Thompson DG, et al. Dynamic scanning defines a colonic defect in severe idiopathic constipation. Gut. 1988;29:1085–92.
57. Mengs U, Rudolph RL. Light and electron-microscopic changes in the colon of the Guinea pig after treatment with anthranoid and non-anthranoid laxatives. Pharmacology. 1993;47(Suppl. 1):172–7.
58. Kamm MA, Mueller-Lissner S, Wald A, Richter E, Swallow R, Gessner U. Oral bisacodyl is effective and well-tolerated in patients with chronic constipation. Clin Gastroenterol Hepatol. 2011;9(7):577. Epub 2011 Mar 25.
59. Mueller-Lissner S, Kamm MA, Wald A, et al. Multicenter, 4-week, double-blind, randomized, placebo-controlled trial of sodium picosulfate in patients with chronic constipation. Am J Gastroenterol. 2010;105:897–903.
60. Nelson AD, Camilleri M, Chirapongsathorn S, et al. Comparison of efficacy of pharmacological treatments for chronic idiopathic constipation: a systematic review and network meta-analysis. Gut. 2017;66:1611–22.
61. van Gorkom BA, de Vries EG, Karrenbeld A, Kleibeuker JH. Review article: anthranoid laxatives and their potential carcinogenic effects. Aliment Pharmacol Ther. 1999;13:443–52.
62. Johanson JF, Morton D, Geenen J, Ueno R. Multicenter, 4-week, double-blind, randomized, placebo-controlled trial of lubiprostone, a locally-acting type-2 chloride channel activator, in patients with chronic constipation. Am J Gastroenterol. 2008;103(1):170. Epub 2007 Oct 4.
63. Rohack JJ, Mehta BR, Subramanyam K. Hyperphosphatemia and hypocalcemic coma associated with phosphate enema. South Med J. 1985;78:1241–2.
64. Lembo AJ, Kurtz CB, Macdougall JE, Lavins BJ, Currie MG, Fitch DA, Jeglinski BI, Johnston JM. Efficacy of linaclotide for patients with chronic constipation. Gastroenterology. 2010;138(3):886. Epub 2010 Jan 4.
65. Eutamene H, Bradesi S, Larauche M, et al. Guanylate cyclase C-mediated antinociceptive effects of linaclotide in rodent models of visceral pain. Neurogastroenterol Motil. 2010;22:312–e84.
66. Schoenfeld P, Lacy BE, Chey WD, Lembo AJ, Kurtz CB, Reasner DS, Bochenek W, Tripp K, Currie MG, Fox SM, Blakesley RE, O'Dea CR, Omniewski ND, Hall ML. Low-dose Linaclotide (72 μg) for chronic idiopathic constipation: a 12-week, randomized, double-blind, placebo-controlled trial. Am J Gastroenterol. 2018;113(1):105. Epub 2017 Aug 22.
67. Chokhavatia S, John ES, Bridgeman MB, Dixit D. Constipation in elderly patients with noncancer pain: focus on opioid-induced constipation. Drugs Aging. 2016;33:557–74. https://doi.org/10.1007/s40266-016-0381-2.
68. Crockett SD, Greer KB, Heidelbaugh JJ, Falck-Ytter Y, Hanson BJ, Sultan S, American Gastroenterological Association Institute Clinical Guidelines Committee. American Gastroenterological Association Institute guideline on the medical management of opioid-induced constipation. Gastroenterology. 2019;156(1):218. Epub 2018 Oct 16.
69. Nelson AD, Camilleri M. Chronic opioid induced constipation in patients with nonmalignant pain: challenges and opportunities. Ther Adv Gastroenterol. 2015;8:206–20.
70. Thomas J, Karver S, Cooney GA, et al. Methylnaltrexone for opioid-induced constipation in advanced illness. N Engl J Med. 2008;358:2332–43.
71. Chey WD, Webster L, Sostek M, et al. Naloxegol for opioid-induced constipation in patients with noncancer pain. N Engl J Med. 2014;370:2387–96.

72. Müller-Lissner SA. Treatment of chronic constipation with cisapride and placebo. Gut. 1987;28:1033–8.
73. Bouras EP, Camilleri M, Burton DD, et al. Prucalopride accelerates gastrointestinal and colonic transit in patients with constipation without a rectal evacuation disorder. Gastroenterology. 2001;120:354–60.
74. Quigley EM, Vandeplassche L, Kerstens R, Ausma J. Clinical trial: the efficacy, impact on quality of life, and safety and tolerability of prucalopride in severe chronic constipation—a 12-week, randomized, double-blind, placebo-controlled study. Aliment Pharmacol Ther. 2009;29(3):315. Epub 2008 Nov 8.
75. Müller-Lissner S, Rykx A, Kerstens R, Vandeplassche L. A double-blind, placebo-controlled study of prucalopride in elderly patients with chronic constipation. Neurogastroenterol Motil. 2010;22(9):991.
76. Camilleri M, Beyens G, Kerstens R, et al. Safety assessment of prucalopride in elderly patients with constipation: a double-blind, placebo-controlled study. Neurogastroenterol Motil. 2009;21:1256–e117.
77. Meisel JL, Bergman D, Graney D, et al. Human rectal mucosa: proctoscopic and morphological changes caused by laxatives. Gastroenterology. 1977;72:1274–9.
78. Ori Y, Rozen-Zvi B, Chagnac A, Herman M, Zingerman B, Atar E, Gafter U, Korzets A. Fatalities and severe metabolic disorders associated with the use of sodium phosphate enemas: a single center's experience. Arch Intern Med. 2012;172(3):263.
79. FDA warns of possible harm from exceeding recommended dose of over-the-counter sodium phosphate products to treat constipation. http://www.fda.gov/Drugs/DrugSafety/ucm380757.htm. Accessed 8 Jan 2014.
80. Mendoza J, Legido J, Rubio S, Gisbert JP. Systematic review: the adverse effects of sodium phosphate enema. Aliment Pharmacol Ther. 2007;26(1):9.
81. Flig E, Hermann TW, Zabel M. Is bisacodyl absorbed at all from suppositories in man? Int J Pharm. 2000;196:11–20.
82. Larkin PJ, Cherny NI, La Carpia D, et al. Diagnosis, assessment and management of constipation in advanced cancer: ESMO clinical practice guidelines. Ann Oncol. 2018;29 Suppl 4(Suppl 4):iv111–25.
83. Gandell D, Straus SE, Bundookwala M, Tsui V, Alibhai SMH. Treatment of constipation in older people. CMAJ. 2013;185(8):663–70.
84. McRorie JW, Daggy BP, Morel JG, et al. Psyllium is superior to docusate sodium for treatment of chronic constipation. Aliment Pharmacol Ther. 1998;12:491–7.
85. von Maltzahn M, Tanzini RM, Leu R, Wong CL. When less may be more: discontinuing docusate from a standardized hospital order set. J Geriatr Oncol. 2022;13:111–3.
86. Martínez-Martínez MI, Calabuig-Tolsá R, Cauli O. The effect of probiotics as a treatment for constipation in elderly people: a systematic review. Arch Gerontol Geriatr. 2017;71:142–9.
87. Aoyagi Y, et al. Independent and interactive effects of habitually ingesting fermented milk products containing *Lactobacillus casei* strain Shirota and of engaging in moderate habitual daily physical activity on the intestinal health of older people. Front Microbiol. 2019;10:1477.
88. Matsumoto K. Modification of gastrointestinal function: improvement of diarrhea and constipation. In: Lactobacillus casei strain Shirota—intestinal microbiota and human health: new advances—Supplementary Edition, ed. Yakult Central Institute for Microbiological Research Tokyo: Yakult Honsha Co., Ltd. 2013. p. 41–51.
89. Mai TT, Hop DV, Anh TTV, Lam NT. Recovery of Lactobacillus casei strain Shirota (LcS) from the intestine of healthy Vietnamese adults after intake of fermented milk. Asia Pac J Clin Nutr. 2017;26:72–7.

Pain

17

Sophie Pautex, Monica Escher, and Petra Vayne-Bossert

17.1 Introduction

The International Association for the Study of Pain (IASP) definition states that pain is an unpleasant sensory and emotional experience associated with actual or potential tissue damage or described in terms of such damage. Although aging and especially neurocognitive disorders are associated with structural, biochemical, and functional changes in the nervous system, there are no arguments that these changes have a clear and important influence on the perception of pain in the older patient population [1]. Chronic pain, i.e. pain present for more than 3–6 months, affects 25–76% of home-dwelling people over 65 years and up to 93% of older people in nursing homes [2, 3]. Most common causes are musculoskeletal pain (up to 83% of patients) such as joint pain and low back pain due to osteoarthritis, pain from previous fractures, and peripheral neuropathies. Older adults have often multiple pain-associated conditions that likely reflect multiple physiological mechanisms for pain. Linking pain qualities with other associated pain characteristics serve to develop a multidimensional approach to geriatric pain assessment [4]. In most studies, about 60% of pain is of pure nociceptive origin resulting from an actual or threatened damage to nonneural tissue and is due to the activation of nociceptors located in somatic (e.g., skin, musculoskeletal tissues) or visceral tissues. Secondly, pain can be caused by a lesion or disease of the nervous system which is called neuropathic pain. Pure neuropathic pain is present in about 10% of the older population, while combined nociceptive and neuropathic pain is found in about 1 out of 3 older persons. Persistent pain has a significant impact on all levels of functioning and on quality of life. Inadequate treatment is associated with various adverse outcomes in older people, including functional impairment, falls, slow rehabilitation, mood

S. Pautex (✉) · M. Escher · P. Vayne-Bossert
Palliative Medicine Division, University Hospital Geneva and University of Geneva, Geneva, Switzerland
e-mail: Sophie.pautex@hcuge.ch; monica.escher@hcuge.ch; petra.vayne-bossert@hcuge.ch

A. Cherubini et al. (eds.), *Optimizing Pharmacotherapy in Older Patients*, Practical Issues in Geriatrics, https://doi.org/10.1007/978-3-031-28061-0_17

changes (depression and anxiety), decreased socialization, sleep and appetite disturbance, and greater healthcare use and costs [5, 6]. The management of this persistent pain should be more multidimensional than for acute pain, in particular in this population.

Pain management includes nonpharmacologic and pharmacologic approaches, and shared decision making is essential to balance their benefits and burdens. Pain management goals should be determined with patients before the initiation of any treatment, and there must be ongoing monitoring of treatment efficacy and adverse effects over time. Interventions should generally be targeted at improvements in pain-related disability rather than pain intensity, because improvements in disability are more tangible outcomes among persons with persistent pain [7, 8].

17.2 Practical Recommendations for the Use of Analgesics in Older Patients

17.2.1 Paracetamol

Paracetamol is indicated for the management of mild to moderate pain. It is often considered as the first-line therapy for acute and chronic pain in the older population, and regular use has been shown to increase over the years among community-dwelling older persons, from 2% in 1999 to 11% in 2019 [9]. Paracetamol does not exhibit significant anti-inflammatory or antiplatelet effects because it does not inhibit thromboxane. Taken at recommended doses, it is considered safe although decreased clearance is observed in frail older people, which might change its safety in this population [10]. Malnutrition, a common finding in older people, and an acute fasting state such that which occurs after surgery, may expose older patients to an increased risk of liver toxicity, notably because of diminished stores of glutathione, an antioxidant that neutralizes N-acetyl-p-benzoquinone-imine (NAPQI), a toxic metabolite of paracetamol [11]. Furthermore, acute liver toxicity due to inadvertent overdose can happen when patients unknowingly consume multiple paracetamol-containing products simultaneously [12]. One meta-analysis of seven randomized controlled trials showed superior efficacy of paracetamol compared to placebo in reducing moderate pain but inferior to NSAIDs for both pain reduction and physical functioning [13].

17.2.2 Nonsteroidal Anti-inflammatory Drugs

NSAIDs are particularly helpful in treating an inflammatory type of pain where paracetamol has limited efficacy. However, the American Geriatric Society recommends great caution while using NSAID therapy in older patients due to its established gastrointestinal, renal, and cardiovascular side effects and recommends giving NSAIDs preferably for only short periods of time during episodic flares. A study on drug reactions leading to hospitalizations in the older population showed

NSAID-related side effects as the cause for hospitalization in 23.5% of patients [14, 15]. Gastrointestinal toxicity due to NSAIDs is dose dependent, increases with age and the concomitant use of cardioprotective doses of aspirin, which is a common medication in this group. Use of NSAIDs can also lead to renal impairment through sodium and water retention, electrolyte imbalances, prerenal azotemia, and reduced blood flow to the kidneys. The concomitant use of NSAIDS and several medications commonly prescribed in older adults (i.e., anticoagulants, aspirin, and selective serotonin reuptake inhibitors) increases the risk of bleeding.

Topical NSAIDs are often used for knee or hand osteoarthritis (OA)-related pain. Evidence from a recent randomized controlled trial showed the comparable efficacy of topical diclofenac sodium and oral NSAIDs in the treatment of knee osteoarthritis with fewer adverse effects [16]. The mechanism is thought to be an increased delivery of the drug to the adjacent synovium without significant systemic absorption.

17.2.3 Opioids

Opioid analgesics are considered for managing severe pain or failed response to other treatments in older patients. Although the short-term efficacy of opioid analgesics in chronic pain in this group is established, limited evidence is available regarding the long-term efficacy because of the discontinuation of opioid therapy due to various poorly tolerated side effects. A prerequisite before initiation of opioid therapy is the evaluation of risk versus benefit. While taking into account the adverse outcomes, mandatory efforts should be made to reduce the risks. Administration of opioids in the older patient is done on a trial basis to titrate the effective dose reaching the therapeutic goal with minimal adverse effects, starting with the lowest possible dose and continuing with gradual titration. Patients with moderate to severe pain and diminished pain-related quality of life should be considered for opioid therapy (low quality of evidence, strong recommendation) [17]. Studies comparing the efficacy and tolerability of opioids, such as transdermal fentanyl, oral morphine, and sublingual or transdermal buprenorphine in the older population and other populations have shown that older people respond to opioid treatment as well as, or even better than, younger age groups [18–20]. The "start low and go slow" approach is essential when dosing opioids. Patients who report severe pain or those who have experienced uncontrolled pain for prolonged periods of time will likely require ongoing titration of opioid therapy to balance pain relief with adverse effects. Opioids should be started at 25–50% of the recommended dose for younger adults [21].

The decreased volume of distribution that occurs owing to decreased total body water with aging may also result in increased plasma levels of more hydrophilic opioids (e.g., morphine) compared with levels observed in younger persons. In general, oral bioavailability does not seem to be affected by age, and although first-pass metabolism may be affected, dosage adjustments are not routinely necessary beyond the 25–50% dose reduction recommended at opioid initiation [22, 23]. Decrements in renal function may decrease the excretion of some neurotoxic opioid-related metabolites. This caution is particularly true for codeine, morphine, hydromorphone, and oxycodone, and dose adjustments with even low doses of these agents should be made accordingly, along with close monitoring for toxicity (e.g., myoclonus [24, 25]).

17.2.3.1 Side Effects of Opioids

Nausea develops in about one-third of patients initiated on opioids and occurs because these agents slow down the motility of the gastrointestinal (GI) tract, stimulate the chemoreceptor trigger zone, and sensitize the vestibular apparatus. If severe nausea occurs, low-dose haloperidol (0.5 mg), metoclopramide (10 mg), or ondansetron (4 mg) scheduled or "as needed" typically manage nausea until it resolves over the first week of therapy.

Constipation is common in older persons with serious illnesses and nearly universal in patients taking an opioid. It is often cited by older adults as a reason to refuse opioid therapy. Constipation results from binding to the mu-receptors in the GI tract, resulting in slower transit time and subsequent increased water resorption. Prevention is the cornerstone of constipation management with a bowel stimulant of senna or bisacodyl scheduled daily at initiation and increased to twice daily if needed [26]. Osmotic agents, such as polyethylene glycol or milk of magnesia, as monotherapy generally lack sufficient action to counteract opioid GI effects but can be helpful in conjunction with stimulant laxatives when needed. Bulk-forming agents such as psyllium are ineffective and can worsen symptoms if patients do not ingest an adequate amount of fluid.

Falls: The relationship between pain, falls, and opioids is complex and not completely understood. Cohort studies support that pain interference is associated with an increased risk of falls among community-dwelling older adults. The use of opioids in older patients with arthritis may increase the likelihood of falls compared with patients treated with an NSAID. The risk seems to be higher with short-acting opioids and at treatment initiation or shortly after [27, 28]. A limitation of published studies examining the relationship between analgesic use and falls is the lack of adjustment for the starting opioid dose. Older patients with multiple comorbidities are more likely to be prescribed opioids for pain. This confounder was addressed in a study determining the safety of various classes of analgesics in older patients. Opioids were found to be significantly associated with an increased risk of fracture compared with NSAIDS and highly selective cox-2 inhibitors (coxibs) [29].

Cognition impairment: The relationship among pain, cognition, and opioids also remains inconclusive. Undertreated pain may predispose to an increased risk of confusion, particularly in the hospital. For example, a study of hospitalized hip fracture patients found that patients taking higher opioid doses had a lower delirium risk compared with patients taking low-dose or no opioid [30].

Recommendations from The European Association of Palliative Care (EAPC) Research Network for management of opioid side effects include the following: dose reduction, symptomatic management of the adverse effects using drugs targeting the symptoms, opioid rotation, and switching the route of administration [31, 32].

Misuse or abuse: In recent years, the abuse or misuse of opioids has steadily gone up, especially in the USA [33]. The older population is also concerned although much less than the younger adults. Nevertheless, clinicians must remain vigilant about the possibility of misuse or abuse of opioid agents in older adults and apply the abovementioned precautions while prescribing and initiating these agents in patients with non-cancer pain [34].

Respiratory depression is more frequent (although still rare) in patients who are opioid naive, receive the agent intravenously, and have increased their doses rapidly. Furthermore, patients receiving drugs with variable pharmacokinetics such as methadone, patients with concomitant use of central nervous system depressing drugs such as benzodiazepines or barbiturates, or patients who develop sudden acute kidney failure are more at risk for this adverse event.

17.2.3.2 Examples of Opioids Frequently Used for Pain Management (See Table 17.1)

Tramadol

Tramadol, a weak mu-opioid agonist with additional serotonin and norepinephrine reuptake inhibition, is not routinely recommended for older adults with moderate to severe pain but is commonly used. Importantly, its mu-opioid receptor activity results in a similar side effect profile as other opioids and requires similar cautions described herein. Nausea, dizziness, and tiredness seem particularly common [35]. In addition, tramadol increases seizure risk, particularly at doses higher than 300 mg/day, the maximum daily dose recommended in an older adult. Lastly, the development of serotonin syndrome may occur with the use of tramadol, particularly with concomitant use of serotonergic drugs. Tramadol is activated to its opioid metabolite by CYP2D6. Patients should be closely monitored to detect a potential clinical impact—either decreased efficacy or increased side effects—due to drug-drug interactions or to modified metabolism in ultrarapid and poor metabolizers. Tramadol should be initiated at 25 mg three or four times daily and increased in 25 mg increments every 2–3 days to an initial goal of 100 mg–200 mg/day.

Tapentadol

Tapentadol is a weak opioid that acts on the mu receptor and on neuronal reuptake of noradrenaline. Unlike tramadol, it has only weak effects on serotonin reuptake. It has no active metabolites and does not need to be activated to exert its analgesic opioid effect [36]. There are no sufficient data to support the use of newer drug tapentadol over other opioids.

Morphine

Morphine has been used to treat malignant pain for many years and has been the subject of a large number of trials, generally involving small numbers of patients. Morphine is metabolized in the liver by glucuronidation. Morphine-6-glucuronide (M6G) is a potent analgesic, and morphine-3-glucuronide (M3G) may cause neuro-excitatory effects [37]. Renal excretion accounts for about 90% of the elimination

Table 17.1 Opioids commonly used in older patients

Medication	Route of admin	Onset of action	Duration of action	Recommended and maximal doses		Comments
Tramadol	p.o immediate release p.o. extended release s.c., i.m. i.v.			IR: 25–50 mg every 6–8 h ER: 50–100 mg every 12 h	75 mg every 6 h 150 mg every 12 h	Often in association with paracetamol Reduces the seizure threshold Risk of serotoninergic syndrome in combination with other serotoninergic drugs Drug-drug interaction (in particular CYP2D6)
Tapentadol	p.o. immediate release p.o. extended release			IR: 25 mg every 4–6 h ER: 50 mg every 12 h	150 mg every 6 h 300 mg every 12 h	Low potential for drug interactions Because of a lack of evidence, not recommended in frail older people
Morphine	p.o. immediate release p.o. extended release s.c., i.m. i.v.	30–60 min 3 h 15 min 15 min	4 h 8–12 h 4 h 4 h	IR: 2.5–5 mg every 4–6 h ER: 10 mg every 12 h	NA	M6G contributes to the overall analgesic effect; M3G passes the blood-brain barrier and may cause neurotoxic effects. Decreased glomerular filtration rate causes accumulation of those metabolites causing even more severe side effects

Table 17.1 (continued)

Medication	Route of admin	Onset of action	Duration of action	Recommended and maximal doses		Comments
Oxycodone	p.o. immediate release p.o. extended release	15–30 min 3–4 h	4 h 12 h	IR: 2.5 mg every 4–6 h ER: 5–10 mg every 12 h	See comment	Daily maximal dose for extended release oxycodone combined with naloxone: 160 mg/80 mg Active opioid metabolite (CYP2D6)
Fentanyl	i.v., s.cut. Transdermic	5 min 30 min 12–14 h	30–60 min 6–12 h 72 h 2–3 h	12 mcg/h patch every 72 h	NA	Avoid starting in opioid naïve patients No dose adaptations necessary in renal failure patients
Buprenorphine	Sublingual i.v., s. cut. Transdermic**	45–60 min 20–40 min 12–24 h	6–8 h 6–8 h 72 h	17.5 mcg/h patch every 72–96 h	NA	No dose adaptations necessary in renal failure patients
Hydromorphone	p.o. immediate release p.o. extended release s.c. i.v.	30–60 min 3 h 15 min 15 min	4 h 12 h 4 h 4 h	IR: 1 mg every 4–6 h ER: 4 mg every 12 h	NA	

of morphine and its metabolites. Therefore, accumulation of the metabolites in patients with renal impairment can occur and cause side effects requiring dose adjustment or switching to an alternative opioid [38]. Older adults are more sensitive to the analgesic and side effects of morphine than younger subjects, which warrants low starting doses and careful monitoring.

Fentanyl

Fentanyl, a phenylpiperidine derivative, is chemically related to pethidine. It is a pure fat-soluble μ-opioid agonist. Its volume of distribution increases in older patients because of the increased fat-to-lean body mass ratio that accompanies aging, hence prolonging its effective half-life. Fentanyl can be used in renal failure. It makes it an interesting alternative to morphine as renal function is altered with age and older patients are more likely to experiment acute renal failure in case of dehydration or nephrotoxic drugs use.

Buprenorphine

Buprenorphine is a semisynthetic, partial μ-opioid agonist. It also weakly binds as an antagonist at kappa and delta receptors. It has high affinity for μ-receptors and is not readily reversed by naloxone. Buprenorphine is excreted primarily in the feces unchanged and is considered safe in persons with renal impairment [39]. Because of significant first-pass effect, it is available in sublingual form or transdermal patch. The sublingual formulation is of limited utility in patients with cognitive impairment or dry mouth since the tablet must be kept under the tongue until it is dissolved completely.

Methadone

Methadone is a synthetic lipophilic opioid analgesic. It is extensively metabolized by CYP450 enzymes (CYP3A4, CYP2B6, CYP2C19, CYP2C9, and CYP2D6) into inactive metabolites, and it is considered safe for use in persons with renal impairment. However, equianalgesic ratios between morphine and methadone are dose dependent, the half-life is highly variable, and numerous drug interactions must be considered. Therefore, methadone should be used only by practitioners experienced with this agent [40].

17.2.4 Adjuvant Drugs and Treatment of Neuropathic Pain

Neuropathic pain: Co-analgesics such as antidepressants and anticonvulsants are often recommended and especially beneficial for neuropathic pain in older people. If acute rescue therapy is needed, the addition of a weak (tramadol) or a strong opioid can be considered [41].

The two anticonvulsants most commonly used for neuropathic pain, gabapentin and pregabalin, both presynaptically bind to the a2d subunit on voltage-dependent calcium channels, modulating calcium influx and reducing overall excitatory neurotransmitter release. The difference between the agents is that pregabalin has increased binding affinity to the subunit and has predictable linear absorption compared to gabapentin. Both medications have few drug interactions [42]. They are excreted renally as unchanged drug, and dose reduction with renal insufficiency is necessary. Dizziness, sedation, and peripheral edema are the most common side effects and are more common in older adults. Anticonvulsants, including gabapentin and pregabalin, have been associated with increased rates of falls in several studies of older patients in the community and in nursing homes. Additionally, inhibition of serotonin reuptake in platelets may lead to a reduction in serotonin-induced platelet aggregation. Evidence for the efficacy of other anticonvulsants in neuropathic pain is either lacking (e.g., clonazepam) or negative (e.g., lamotrigine, oxcarbazepine, topiramate). Benzodiazepines, which have muscle relaxant effects, are associated with sedation and increased risk of falls. Furthermore, when a benzodiazepine is combined with an opioid, the risk for potentially fatal opioid-induced respiratory depression increases [43].

Serotonin-norepinephrine reuptake inhibitors (SNRIs) such as venlafaxine and duloxetine can be used for neuropathic pain in older adults. SNRIs are generally well tolerated. Side effects include hyponatremia, giddiness, nausea, and abdominal pain. Venlafaxine is given at a daily starting dose of 37.5 mg, which can be increased up to 300 mg particularly in patients with associated depression. Its use in the older patient population is still debated and may be limited by the occurrence of hypertensive episodes. Duloxetine has no cardiovascular effects, and it showed a 50% reduction in diabetic neuropathic pain compared to placebo [44]. Although tricyclic antidepressants may be useful in treating neuropathic pain, anticholinergic and cardiovascular side effects limit their use in older patients [45, 46].

17.2.5 Cannabinoids

The efficacy and safety profile of cannabinoids are not established in this population. Common side effects include euphoria, anxiety, psychosis, sedation, dizziness, cognitive effects, tachycardia, palpitations, and postural hypotension. Due to a narrow therapeutic index, older patients are at higher risk of dysphoric effects of cannabinoids [47].

In conclusion, as the quality of research is weak, and few older patients have been enrolled in cannabinoid studies, dedicated research is needed to determine the efficiency and safety of cannabinoids in older patients.

References

1. Gibson SJ, Farrell M. A review of age differences in the neurophysiology of nociception and the perceptual experience of pain. Clin J Pain. 2004;20(4):227–39.
2. American Geriatrics Society Panel on Pharmacological Management of Persistent Pain in Older Persons. Pharmacological management of persistent pain in older persons. J Am Geriatr Soc. 2009;57(8):1331–46.
3. AGS Panel on Persistent Pain in Older Persons. The management of persistent pain in older persons. J Am Geriatr Soc. 2002;50(6 Suppl):S205–24.
4. Thakral M, Shi L, Foust JB, Patel KV, Shmerling RH, Bean JF, et al. Pain quality descriptors in community-dwelling older adults with nonmalignant pain. Pain. 2016;157(12):2834–42.
5. Sawyer P, Bodner EV, Ritchie CS, Allman RM. Pain and pain medication use in community-dwelling older adults. Am J Geriatr Pharmacother. 2006;4(4):316–24.
6. Won AB, Lapane KL, Vallow S, Schein J, Morris JN, Lipsitz LA. Persistent nonmalignant pain and analgesic prescribing patterns in elderly nursing home residents. J Am Geriatr Soc. 2004;52(6):867–74.
7. Bernabei R, Gambassi G, Lapane K, Landi F, Gatsonis C, Dunlop R, et al. Management of pain in elderly patients with cancer. SAGE Study Group. Systematic assessment of geriatric drug use via epidemiology. JAMA. 1998;279(23):1877–82.

8. Landi F, Onder G, Cesari M, Gambassi G, Steel K, Russo A, et al. Pain management in frail, community-living elderly patients. Arch Intern Med. 2001;161(22):2721–4.
9. Lehti TE, Rinkinen MO, Aalto U, Roitto HM, Knuutila M, Ohman H, et al. Prevalence of musculoskeletal pain and analgesic treatment among community-dwelling older adults: changes from 1999 to 2019. Drugs Aging. 2021;38(10):931–7.
10. Mian P, Allegaert K, Spriet I, Tibboel D, Petrovic M. Paracetamol in older people: towards evidence-based dosing? Drugs Aging. 2018;35(7):603–24.
11. Pickering G, Schneider E, Papet I, Pujos-Guillot E, Pereira B, Simen E, et al. N metabolism after major surgery: a greater challenge with increasing age. Clin Pharmacol Ther. 2011;90(5):707–11.
12. Graham GG, Davies MJ, Day RO, Mohamudally A, Scott KF. The modern pharmacology of paracetamol: therapeutic actions, mechanism of action, metabolism, toxicity and recent pharmacological findings. Inflammopharmacology. 2013;21(3):201–32.
13. da Costa BR, Reichenbach S, Keller N, Nartey L, Wandel S, Jüni P, et al. Effectiveness of non-steroidal anti-inflammatory drugs for the treatment of pain in knee and hip osteoarthritis: a network meta-analysis. Lancet. 2017;390(10090):e21–33.
14. Trelle S, Reichenbach S, Wandel S, Hildebrand P, Tschannen B, Villiger PM, et al. Cardiovascular safety of non-steroidal anti-inflammatory drugs: network meta-analysis. BMJ. 2011;342:c7086.
15. Wegman A, van der Windt D, van Tulder M, Stalman W, de Vries T. Nonsteroidal antiinflammatory drugs or acetaminophen for osteoarthritis of the hip or knee? A systematic review of evidence and guidelines. J Rheumatol. 2004;31(2):344–54.
16. Tugwell PS, Wells GA, Shainhouse JZ. Equivalence study of a topical diclofenac solution (pennsaid) compared with oral diclofenac in symptomatic treatment of osteoarthritis of the knee: a randomized controlled trial. J Rheumatol. 2004;31(10):2002–12.
17. Kaye AD, Baluch A, Scott JT. Pain management in the elderly population: a review. Ochsner J. 2010;10(3):179–87.
18. Kaiko RF. Age and morphine analgesia in cancer patients with postoperative pain. Clin Pharmacol Ther. 1980;28(6):823–6.
19. Menten J, Desmedt M, Lossignol D, Mullie A. Longitudinal follow-up of TTS-fentanyl use in patients with cancer-related pain: results of a compassionate-use study with special focus on elderly patients. Curr Med Res Opin. 2002;18(8):488–98.
20. Nasar MA, McLeavy MA, Knox J. An open study of sub-lingual buprenorphine in the treatment of chronic pain in the elderly. Curr Med Res Opin. 1986;10(4):251–5.
21. Mercadante S, Giarratano A. Assessing age and gender in studies of breakthrough pain medications. Curr Med Res Opin. 2014;30(7):1353–6.
22. Tegeder I, Geisslinger G, Lotsch J. [Therapy with opioids in liver or renal failure]. Schmerz. 1999;13(3):183–195.
23. Tegeder I, Lotsch J, Geisslinger G. Pharmacokinetics of opioids in liver disease. Clin Pharmacokinet. 1999;37(1):17–40.
24. Dean M. Opioids in renal failure and dialysis patients. J Pain Symptom Manag. 2004;28(5):497–504.
25. Murtagh FE, Chai MO, Donohoe P, Edmonds PM, Higginson IJ. The use of opioid analgesia in end-stage renal disease patients managed without dialysis: recommendations for practice. J Pain Palliat Care Pharmacother. 2007;21(2):5–16.
26. Cherny N, Ripamonti C, Pereira J, Davis C, Fallon M, McQuay H, et al. Strategies to manage the adverse effects of oral morphine: an evidence-based report. J Clin Oncol. 2001;19(9):2542–54.
27. Miller M, Sturmer T, Azrael D, Levin R, Solomon DH. Opioid analgesics and the risk of fractures in older adults with arthritis. J Am Geriatr Soc. 2011;59(3):430–8.
28. Rolita L, Spegman A, Tang X, Cronstein BN. Greater number of narcotic analgesic prescriptions for osteoarthritis is associated with falls and fractures in elderly adults. J Am Geriatr Soc. 2013;61(3):335–40.
29. Solomon DH, Rassen JA, Glynn RJ, Garneau K, Levin R, Lee J, et al. The comparative safety of opioids for nonmalignant pain in older adults. Arch Intern Med. 2010;170(22):1979–86.

30. Morrison RS, Magaziner J, Gilbert M, Koval KJ, McLaughlin MA, Orosz G, et al. Relationship between pain and opioid analgesics on the development of delirium following hip fracture. J Gerontol A Biol Sci Med Sci. 2003;58(1):76–81.
31. Caraceni A, Hanks G, Kaasa S, Bennett MI, Brunelli C, Cherny N, et al. Use of opioid analgesics in the treatment of cancer pain: evidence-based recommendations from the EAPC. Lancet Oncol. 2012;13(2):e58–68.
32. Hanks GW, Conno F, Cherny N, Hanna M, Kalso E, McQuay HJ, et al. Morphine and alternative opioids in cancer pain: the EAPC recommendations. Br J Cancer. 2001;84(5):587–93.
33. Shoff C, Yang TC, Shaw BA. Trends in opioid use disorder among older adults: analyzing Medicare data, 2013-2018. Am J Prev Med. 2021;60(6):850–5.
34. Edlund MJ, Steffick D, Hudson T, Harris KM, Sullivan M. Risk factors for clinically recognized opioid abuse and dependence among veterans using opioids for chronic non-cancer pain. Pain. 2007;129(3):355–62.
35. Toupin April K, Bisaillon J, Welch V, Maxwell LJ, Juni P, Rutjes AW, et al. Tramadol for osteoarthritis. Cochrane Database Syst Rev. 2019;5:CD005522.
36. Veal FC, Peterson GM. Pain in the frail or elderly patient: does Tapentadol have a role? Drugs Aging. 2015;32(6):419–26.
37. Lee J, Lakha SF, Mailis A. Efficacy of low-dose oral liquid morphine for elderly patients with chronic non-cancer pain: retrospective chart review. Drugs Real World Outcomes. 2015;2(4):369–76.
38. Gianni W, Ceci M, Bustacchini S, Corsonello A, Abbatecola AM, Brancati AM, et al. Opioids for the treatment of chronic non-cancer pain in older people. Drugs Aging. 2009;26(Suppl 1):63–73.
39. Vadivelu N, Hines RL. Management of chronic pain in the elderly: focus on transdermal buprenorphine. Clin Interv Aging. 2008;3(3):421–30.
40. Lugo RA, Satterfield KL, Kern SE. Pharmacokinetics of methadone. J Pain Palliat Care Pharmacother. 2005;19(4):13–24.
41. Pickering G, Marcoux M, Chapiro S, David L, Rat P, Michel M, et al. An algorithm for neuropathic pain management in older people. Drugs Aging. 2016;33(8):575–83.
42. Haslam C, Nurmikko T. Pharmacological treatment of neuropathic pain in older persons. Clin Interv Aging. 2008;3(1):111–20.
43. Wiffen PJ, Derry S, Moore RA, Aldington D, Cole P, Rice AS, et al. Antiepileptic drugs for neuropathic pain and fibromyalgia—an overview of Cochrane reviews. Cochrane Database Syst Rev. 2013;(11):CD010567.
44. Goldstein DJ, Lu Y, Detke MJ, Lee TC, Iyengar S. Duloxetine vs. placebo in patients with painful diabetic neuropathy. Pain. 2005;116(1–2):109–18.
45. Finnerup NB, Attal N, Haroutounian S, McNicol E, Baron R, Dworkin RH, et al. Pharmacotherapy for neuropathic pain in adults: a systematic review and meta-analysis. Lancet Neurol. 2015;14(2):162–73.
46. Moore RA, Derry S, Aldington D, Cole P, Wiffen PJ. Amitriptyline for neuropathic pain in adults. Cochrane Database Syst Rev. 2015;(7):CD008242.
47. Pisani S, McGoohan K, Velayudhan L, Bhattacharyya S. Safety and tolerability of natural and synthetic cannabinoids in older adults: a systematic review and meta-analysis of open-label trials and observational studies. Drugs Aging. 2021;38:887.

Hypertension

18

Timo E. Strandberg, Mirko Petrovic, and Athanase Benetos

Hypertension is a leading cause of disability and major risk factor for cardiovascular diseases (CVD), which are common among older people, such as stroke, heart failure, and coronary heart disease. Hypertension is also an important risk factor for cognitive decline. In modern societies, systolic blood pressure generally starts to rise after 50 years of age, and consequently systolic hypertension and antihypertensive treatment are very prevalent among older people.

The most recent meta-analysis of randomized controlled trials (RCT) of pharmacotherapy clearly demonstrates that antihypertensive treatment is effective in the prevention of CVD irrespective of older age and blood pressure level at randomization [1]. However, evidence from age 85 and older is weaker, probably because of a relatively small number of oldest-old participants in trials. Besides prevention of CVD, it is noteworthy that according to systematic reviews of RCTs, medical treatment of hypertension is actually the only method proven to prevent adjudicated incident dementia—not only cognitive decline [2–4].

Results from RCTs also show that besides chronological age, strict blood pressure goals are irrelevant [1] and the benefit from treatment depends on the overall risk of the patient. Because "physiologically" normal blood pressure is as low as

T. E. Strandberg (✉)
University of Helsinki and Helsinki University Hospital, Helsinki, Finland

University of Oulu, Oulu, Finland
e-mail: timo.strandberg@oulu.fi

M. Petrovic
Section of Geriatrics, Department of Internal Medicine and Paediatrics, Ghent University, Ghent, Belgium
e-mail: mirko.petrovic@ugent.be

A. Benetos
Department of Geriatrics, University Hospital of Nancy, FHU-CARTAGE Profiles and INSERM DCAC, Université de Lorraine, Vandeoeuvre-les-Nancy, France
e-mail: a.benetos@chru-nancy.fr

A. Cherubini et al. (eds.), *Optimizing Pharmacotherapy in Older Patients*,
Practical Issues in Geriatrics, https://doi.org/10.1007/978-3-031-28061-0_18

<115/75 mmHg—a finding dating back long before the development of antihypertensive drugs [5]—this would make practically all older people candidates for antihypertensive treatment. On the other hand, a repeating finding in unselected epidemiological cohorts is that low blood pressure is often associated with worse prognosis [6–10]. Interestingly, this negative association between SBP and morbidity/mortality was observed mainly in very frail subjects receiving antihypertensive treatment and not in subjects without blood pressure lowering drugs [11–14]. How should all this information be taken into account when assessing treatment of blood pressure in an older patient?

18.1 Hypertension Is Multifaceted in an Older Patient

Observational studies cannot confirm cause and effect and may even involve reverse causality. In other words, frailty, subclinical disease, and low cardiac output may lower blood pressure and simultaneously worsen prognosis leading to a biased relationship between high blood pressure and better prognosis. Therefore, it is urgent to include in future therapeutic trials very frail older patients, i.e., those who usually have been excluded from clinical trials in the past. Presently, we have evidence for the relatively robust older patients (i.e., those with the "HYVET or SPRINT profile") in which our strategy should be very close to that proposed for the "younger-old" subjects, i.e., 65–75 years old community-dwelling subjects. European guidelines propose targeting BP levels <140/90 in these populations though for very old frail subjects, such targets should be individualized. A treatment algorithm and goals in various situations are presented in Fig. 18.1.

More generally, when antihypertensive treatment has been started earlier in life and continuing without problems, the common sense indicates that the treatment must not be modified or stopped due to age alone. As a whole, antihypertensive treatment should be started clearly earlier, i.e., in midlife, to reach the full benefit of treatment during the life course [15]. Good adherence and sufficient control of blood pressure are essential also in an older patient, and prudent lifestyle advice about diet and physical activity are useful. If problems, such as orthostatic

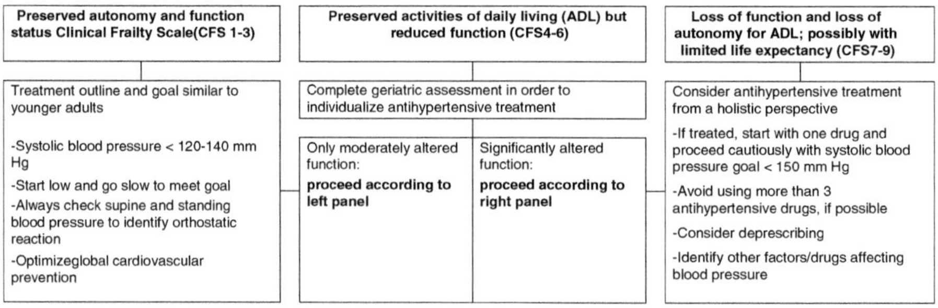

Fig. 18.1 A treatment algorithm and goals in various situations of older patients with hypertension

hypotension, electrolyte disturbances, or kidney dysfunction emerge, drug treatment must be adequately revised.

Orthostatic hypotension (OH) is common among older people and may cause problems for effective treatment of hypertension. It is defined as a reduction of blood pressure more than 20/10 mmHg (with or without symptoms) after 1–3 min of standing from 5 min in supine position. Although several drugs may increase risk of OH, the most common etiology of OH is aging-related arterial stiffness and declined intrinsic capacity to resist abrupt blood pressure drop. In fact, appropriate control of high blood pressure may paradoxically reduce OH predisposition [16, 17]. In the SPRINT trial, intensive control of blood pressure, as compared to standard treatment, was not associated with increased tendency for OH [18]. Therefore, reducing antihypertensive treatment in a patient with OH must be carefully considered, and also other medications (such as alpha-blockers) with hypotensive effects must be taken into account. Furthermore, it is important to advice a patient with OH to stand up gradually, have adequate hydration, and possible use of support stockings. Nevertheless, orthostatic test is indicated before treatment is started and when treatment changes are made, and this is emphasized in a patient with frailty.

At end of life, with development of frailty and comorbidities, it is appropriate to consider deprescribing, i.e., reducing or even stopping antihypertensive drugs [19]. However, deprescribing is not an end itself but must be based on a careful and complete geriatric assessment. It is also important to consider the drug to be deprescribed, e.g., low-dose beta-blocker may be more feasible to remove than a calcium-channel blocker [20]. Trials on this topic have been short and equivocal, and before more information from randomized trials, it is vital that discontinuation does not harm the patient [21].

Starting antihypertensive treatment in old age, >80 years of age, also requires careful consideration. The general fears of antihypertensive treatment in older patients—prevents CVD but increases total mortality due to falls and hypotension—were put to rest especially by the HYVET and SPRINT trials. They showed that total mortality was decreased when antihypertensive drug treatment was compared to placebo (HYVET, start of treatment >80 years of age [22] or when intensive blood pressure control was compared to standard treatment (SPRINT, 75+ [23–25]).

However, people aged 75 years and older are a very heterogenous group from fully functional to individuals with frailty and multimorbidity, and these are important to take into account when assessing treatment [26, 27]. Although in the HYVET [28] and SPRINT [25] cohorts benefits were seen irrespective of the frailty status, the trials did not include the frailest and most multimorbid patients [29]. While intensive treatment reduced mortality in SPRINT, it was nevertheless associated with more hypotension and electrolyte and kidney adverse effects, which are obviously accentuated in the frailest patients.

An unsettled question is effects of low diastolic pressure, i.e., <60 mmHg [30, 31]. There is no consensus of potential harms for coronary circulation if diastolic pressure is too low. Because systolic pressure is simultaneously also lowered, the burden for the heart is reduced. Too low diastolic may be harmful for brain circulation [32, 33] and vulnerable patients must be carefully monitored.

18.2 Diagnostic Procedures

It is important to exclude secondary hypertension also in the older patient, and the diagnostic procedures are similar to those in younger patients. Especially in an older patient, it is mandatory to measure blood pressure in both supine and standing position in order to detect OH predisposing to falls. It is recommended that a 3-min orthostatic test is always performed before medication changes. Isolated office ("white coat") hypertension is relatively common in an older patient, and its detection may require ambulatory measurement. On the other hand, office and its counterpart isolated masked (home) hypertension are not innocuous phenomena [34] and may indicate treatment, or at least careful follow-up. Pseudohypertension refers to a situation when brachial blood pressure measurement gives a high reading due to the pronounced arteriosclerosis. However, pseudohypertension is not so common, and one should pose this diagnosis very carefully in order to avoid underestimation of the importance of very elevated SBP levels in high-risk populations such as patients with diabetes or severe renal failure. The condition may be a reason for "resistant" hypertension and should be remembered, although confirmation may be difficult without direct arterial measurement.

18.3 Treatment Modalities

18.3.1 Lifestyle

There are surrogate data of the effects of lifestyle modification and hypertension in old age. Prudent advice on a healthy diet, especially salt intake, and exercise are recommended. Substituting ordinary salt to mineral salt is beneficial [35]. For obese, weight reduction could lower blood pressure [36], but trial evidence is nonexistent for people 75 years and older, and malnutrition and development of sarcopenia are possible hazards. Physical activity adjusted to clinical condition is always recommended to sustain general health and functional capacity, but again without specific trial evidence for the treatment of hypertension in an older patient. In general, when treatment for hypertension is indicated, lifestyle modification alone is seldom sufficient.

18.3.2 Drug Treatment

There are no specific differences in the selection of drug treatment between younger and older patients, although it is often best to start low and go slow [26]. The main drug classes of antihypertensives, i.e., diuretics, angiotensin-converting enzyme inhibitors, angiotensin II receptor blockers, and calcium channel blockers, can be used and with doses ultimately adjusted individually to reach appropriate targets. As in younger patients, beta blockers are not recommended as first-line treatment without specific indications. An interesting new possibility are the SGLT2-inhibitors, which were initially developed as antidiabetic drugs. They lower blood pressure, prevented CVD endpoints in RCTs, and are effective for heart failure (both systolic and diastolic) even in nondiabetic patients [37, 38]. Experience of SGLT2-inhibitors is accumulating also in older patients. Other drugs affecting blood pressure like nitrates, alpha-blockers, and various psychotropic drugs must be remembered, especially as they may be prescribed by other specialists than general practitioners or geriatricians. Although psychotropic drugs may not directly affect blood pressure, they can nevertheless make a frail patient more susceptible to falls.

The general principle should be to start with monotherapy when treating older patients especially frail patients over 80 years old. However, in most subjects, one single BP-lowering drug is not enough to control BP, and therefore, patients and their caregivers should be informed from the beginning about the possible adaptation after the initiation of the treatment. Combining low doses of drugs with different mode of action is usually better than increasing the dose of a single drug. Dividing doses for morning and evening may be indicated, and there is ongoing debate about the potential benefits of evening dosing [39]. Although maximum of three drugs are sometimes recommended, this cannot be absolute, and treatment must be individualized also for this.

Potential adverse effects and special considerations when using antihypertensives for older patients are listed in Table 18.1.

A special case, not uncommon in an older patient with hypertension, is the acute or subacute rise of blood pressure to very high levels ("hypertensive crisis") [40, 41]. It is defined as systolic and diastolic blood pressure of >200 mmHg and >130 mmHg, respectively, and divided to an emergency (signs of end-organ damage) or urgency state without specific symptoms except blood pressure rise. Emergency requires immediate treatment in a hospital setting and intensive care unit, whereas urgency state can usually be treated ambulatory by enhancing oral antihypertensive treatment with close follow-up. In both states, it is important to avoid exaggerated treatment and reduce blood pressure safely.

Table 18.1 Adverse effects and precautions of antihypertensives in older patients

Drug type	Potential adverse effects	Special considerations in older patients
Calcium channel blockers (CCB) Dihydropyridine CCB Non-dihydropyridine CCB	Signs related to sympathetic activation (flushing, headache, tachycardia) are less frequent than in younger subjects Lower limb edema (LLO) Bradycardia, AV block, worsening heart failure, constipation (verapamil), fatigue, dyspnea	LLO, which is relatively frequent with these drugs, can be erroneously interpreted as a clinical sign of heart failure. In addition, LLO can contribute to the decrease in social and physical activities for practical reasons (difficulties in walking with shoes) Second-line selection, diltiazem can also cause LLO With verapamil, LLO is unusual, but constipation may be a major problem in very old individuals, as it can lead to fecal impaction, with nausea, anorexia, delirium, and functional decline Never combine verapamil with β-blockers
Diuretics Thiazides, loop diuretics (not usually for hypertension)	Hyponatremia, hypokalemia, hyperuricemia and gout attacks, hypotension, dehydration	Diuretic should be titrated according to the patient's volemic status. Creatinine and electrolyte monitoring is warranted after each dose change Association with SSRI antidepressants increases the risk of severe hyponatremia Risk of aggravation of urine incontinence. Small doses (up to 25 mg of hydrochlorothiazide or equivalent) are safe and well tolerated Loop diuretics are not indicated for hypertension unless there is severe renal insufficiency (estimated creatinine clearance <30 mL/[min·1.73 m^2]), or indicated for heart failure Thiazide-like indapamide has been tested in the only RCT specific for subjects aged 80 years and older
Angiotensin-converting enzyme inhibitors	Dry cough, hyperkalemia, rash, angioedema, dizziness, fatigue, acute renal failure	Angiotensin-converting enzyme inhibitors have been tested in the only randomized placebo-controlled Specific for patients aged 80 years and over Avoid if you suspect dehydration, do not simultaneously increase diuretics to avoid a worsening in renal function Regular control of creatinine and potassium levels
Angiotensin II receptor blockers	Hyperkalemia, rash, dizziness, fatigue, acute renal failure	The same as for angiotensin-converting enzyme inhibitors: Do not combine angiotensin receptor blockers with angiotensin-converting enzyme inhibitors or renin inhibitor. Be cautious with aldosterone antagonist because of increased risk of hyperkalemia

Table 18.1 (continued)

Drug type	Potential adverse effects	Special considerations in older patients
Beta-blockers	Bradycardia, cardiac decompensation, peripheral vasoconstriction, bronchospasm, fatigue, depression, dizziness, confusion, hypoglycemia	Fatigue can be accentuated. Sleep disturbances, depression, and confusion may be present especially for the beta-blockers crossing the blood brain barrier Cardiac conduction problems can also be aggravated Caution when used in combination with acetylcholinesterase inhibitors (for memory disorders): risk of major bradycardia
Aldosterone antagonists	Hyperkalemia, hyponatremia, and gastrointestinal disturbances, including cramps and diarrhea, gynecomastia	Aldosterone antagonist should not be given in instances of severe renal insufficiency, estimated creatinine clearance <30 mL/(min·1.73 m^2) or hyperkalemia. Creatinine and electrolyte monitoring is warranted after each dose change
α-adrenoreceptor antagonists (α-blockers)	Dizziness, fatigue, nausea, urinary incontinence, orthostatic hypotension, syncope	Usually not indicated Risk of hypotension (orthostatic, postprandial) and syncope
Central α-adrenoreceptor agonists	Drowsiness, dry mouth, dizziness, constipation, depression, anxiety, fatigue, urinary problems, orthostatic hypotension, confusion, and delirium	High risk of delirium Depression can be aggravated

CCB calcium channel blockers, *LLO* lower limb edema

References

1. The Blood Pressure Lowering Treatment Trialists' Collaboration. Age-stratified and blood pressure-stratified effects of blood pressure-lowering pharmacotherapy for the prevention of cardiovascular disease and death: an individual participant-level data meta-analysis. Lancet. 2021;398:1053–64.
2. Hughes D, Judge C, Murphy R, et al. Association of blood pressure lowering with incident dementia or cognitive impairment: a systematic review and meta-analysis. JAMA. 2020;323:1934–44.
3. SPRINT MIND Investigators for the SPRINT Research Group, Williamson JD, Pajewski NM, Auchus AP, et al. Effect of intensive vs standard blood pressure control on probable dementia: a randomized clinical trial. JAMA. 2019;321:553–61.
4. Strandberg TE, Benetos A, Petrovic M. Editorial: incident dementia in trials of antihypertensive treatments. J Nutr Health Aging. 2019;23:914–5.
5. Strandberg TE. Blood pressure in a 100-year perspective. Circulation. 2019;140:101–2.
6. Boshuizen HC, Izaks GJ, van Buuren S, et al. Blood pressure and mortality in elderly people aged 85 and older: community-based study. BMJ. 1998;316:1780–4.
7. Hakala SM, Tilvis RS, Strandberg TE. Blood pressure and mortality in an older population. A 5-year follow-up of the Helsinki Ageing Study. Eur Heart J. 1997;18:1019–23.

8. Rastas S, Pirttilä T, Viramo P, et al. Association between blood pressure and survival over 9 years in a general population aged 85 and older. J Am Geriatr Soc. 2006;54:912–8.
9. van Bemmel T, Gussekloo J, Westendorp RG, et al. In a population-based prospective study, no association between high blood pressure and mortality after age 85 years. J Hypertens. 2006;24:287–92.
10. van Bemmel T, Holman ER, Gussekloo J, et al. Low blood pressure in the very old, a consequence of imminent heart failure: the Leiden 85-plus study. J Hum Hypertens. 2009;23:27–32.
11. Aparicio LS, Thijs L, Boggia J et al, International Database on Home Blood Pressure in Relation to Cardiovascular Outcome (IDHOCO) Investigators. Defining thresholds for home blood pressure monitoring in octogenarians. Hypertension. 2015;66:865–873.
12. Benetos A, Labat C, Rossignol P, et al. Treatment with multiple blood pressure medications, achieved blood pressure, and mortality in older nursing home residents: the PARTAGE study. JAMA Intern Med. 2015;175:989–95.
13. Mossello E, Pieraccioli M, Nesti N, et al. Effects of low blood pressure in cognitively impaired elderly patients treated with antihypertensive drugs. JAMA Intern Med. 2015;175:578–85.
14. Streit S, Poortvliet RKE, Gussekloo J. Lower blood pressure during antihypertensive treatment is associated with higher all-cause mortality and accelerated cognitive decline in the oldest-old-data from the Leiden 85-plus study. Age Ageing. 2018;47(4):545–50. https://doi.org/10.1093/ageing/afy072.
15. Suvila K, Niiranen TJ. Age of hypertension onset: potential for improving risk estimation and hypertension management? Hypertension. 2021;78:1475–7.
16. Lipsitz LA. A 91-year-old woman with difficult-to-control hypertension a clinical review. JAMA. 2013;310:1274–80.
17. Masuo K, Mikami H, Ogihara T, et al. Changes in frequency of orthostatic hypotension in elderly hypertensive patients under medications. Am J Hypertens. 1996;9:263–8.
18. Juraschek SP, Taylor AA, Wright JT Jr. Orthostatic hypotension, cardiovascular outcomes, and adverse events: results from SPRINT. Hypertension. 2020;75:660–7.
19. Sheppard JP, Burt J, Lown M et al.; OPTIMISE Investigators. Effect of antihypertensive medication reduction vs usual care on short-term blood pressure control in patients with hypertension aged 80 years and older: the OPTIMISE randomized clinical trial. JAMA. 2020;323:2039–2051.
20. Sheppard JP, Lown M, Burt J, et al. Blood pressure changes following antihypertensive medication reduction, by drug class and dose chosen for withdrawal: exploratory analysis of data from the OPTIMISE trial. Front Pharmacol. 2021;12:619088.
21. Applegate WB, Williamson JD, Berlowitz D. Deprescribing antihypertensive medication in elderly adults. JAMA. 2020;324:1682.
22. Beckett NS, Peters R, Fletcher AE, et al. Treatment of hypertension in patients 80 years of age or older. N Engl J Med. 2008;358:1887–98.
23. SPRINT Research Group, Wright JT Jr, Williamson JD, et al. A randomized trial of intensive versus standard blood-pressure control. N Engl J Med. 2015;373:2103–16.
24. SPRINT Research Group, Lewis CE, Fine LJ, Beddhu S, et al. Final report of a trial of intensive versus standard blood-pressure control. N Engl J Med. 2021;384:1921–30.
25. Williamson JD, Supiano MA, Applegate WB et al.; SPRINT Research Group. Intensive vs standard blood pressure control and cardiovascular disease outcomes in adults aged ≥75 years: a randomized clinical trial. JAMA. 2016;315:2673–2682.
26. Benetos A, Rossignol P, Cherubini A, Joly L, Grodzicki T, Rajkumar C, Strandberg TE, Petrovic M. Polypharmacy in the aging patient: management of hypertension in octogenarians. JAMA. 2015;314:170–80.
27. Benetos A, Petrovic M, Strandberg T. Hypertension management in older and frail older patients. Circ Res. 2019;124:1045–60.
28. Warwick J, Falaschetti E, Rockwood K, et al. No evidence that frailty modifies the positive impact of antihypertensive treatment in very elderly people: an investigation of the impact of frailty upon treatment effect in the HYpertension in the Very Elderly Trial (HYVET) study, a

double-blind, placebo-controlled study of antihypertensives in people with hypertension aged 80 and over. BMC Med. 2015;13:78.
29. Sheppard JP, Lown M, Burt J, et al. Generalizability of blood pressure lowering trials to older patients: cross-sectional analysis. J Am Geriatr Soc. 2020;68:2508–15.
30. Somes GW, Pahor M, Shorr RI, et al. The role of diastolic blood pressure when treating isolated systolic hypertension. Arch Intern Med. 1999;159:2004–9.
31. Wang JG, Staessen JA, Franklin SS, et al. Systolic and diastolic blood pressure lowering as determinants of cardiovascular outcome. Hypertension. 2005;45:907–13.
32. Blanco PJ, Müller LO, Spence JD. Blood pressure gradients in cerebral arteries: a clue to pathogenesis of cerebral small vessel disease. Stroke Vasc Neurol. 2017;2:108–17.
33. Qiu C, Winblad B, Fratiglioni L. The age-dependent relation of blood pressure to cognitive function and dementia. Lancet Neurol. 2005;4:487–99.
34. Sivén SS, Niiranen TJ, Kantola IM, et al. White-coat and masked hypertension as risk factors for progression to sustained hypertension: the Finn-Home Study. J Hypertens. 2016;34:54–60.
35. Jafarnejad S, Mirzaei H, Clark CCT, Taghizadeh M, Ebrahimzadeh A. The hypotensive effect of salt substitutes in stage 2 hypertension: a systematic review and meta-analysis. BMC Cardiovasc Disord. 2020;20(1):98. https://doi.org/10.1186/s12872-020-01347-x.
36. Horvath K, Jeitler K, Siering U, et al. Long-term effects of weight-reducing interventions in hypertensive patients: systematic review and meta-analysis. Arch Intern Med. 2008;168:571–80.
37. Brown E, Heerspink HJL, Cuthbertson DJ, Wilding JPH. SGLT2 inhibitors and GLP-1 receptor agonists: established and emerging indications. Lancet. 2021;398:262–76.
38. Drazner MH. SGLT2 inhibition in heart failure with a preserved ejection fraction—a win against a formidable foe. N Engl J Med. 2021;385:1522–4.
39. Ho CLB, Chowdhury EK, Doust J, Nelson MR, Reid CM. The effect of taking blood pressure lowering medication at night on cardiovascular disease risk. A systematic review. J Hum Hypertens. 2021;35:308–14.
40. Perez MI, Musini VM. Pharmacological interventions for hypertensive emergencies. Cochrane Database Syst Rev. 2008;2008:CD003653.
41. Varon J. Treatment of acute severe hypertension: current and newer agents. Drugs. 2008;68:283–97.

Heart Failure 19

T. L. De Backer and A. A. Mangoni

19.1 Introduction

Older people represent an ever-growing population with a variety of health states ranging from healthy to multimorbid and frail, and in whom biological as well as chronological age should be considered. This heterogeneity makes a careful individualised management plan necessary.

In general, increased age comes with increased morbidity and mortality. Heart failure (HF) is a typical example of an increasingly prevalent disease in the older population.

Many older patients with heart failure show multimorbidity often leading to polypharmacy with overprescribing as well as underprescribing, frailty, sarcopenia, and cognitive decline. All these factors have to be considered when initiating a treatment plan [1, 2]. These patients are excluded in most randomised clinical trials. One has to ask if the treatment goal is improving prognosis and/or improving symptoms and so quality of life. This should be discussed within a multidisciplinary team

T. L. De Backer (✉)
Cardiovascular Department, Ghent University Hospital, Ghent, Belgium

Clinical Pharmacology, Ghent University, Ghent, Belgium
e-mail: tine.debacker@ugent.be

A. A. Mangoni
Discipline of Clinical Pharmacology, Flinders University and Flinders Medical Centre, Adelaide, South Australia
e-mail: arduino.mangoni@flinders.edu.au

A. Cherubini et al. (eds.), *Optimizing Pharmacotherapy in Older Patients*, Practical Issues in Geriatrics, https://doi.org/10.1007/978-3-031-28061-0_19

including primary and secondary healthcare staff as well as with the patient and/or her/his caregivers (Figs. 19.1 and 19.2).

Optimising pharmacotherapy in older patients with heart failure is discussed. Device-based treatments (cardiac resynchronisation therapy, implantable cardioverter defibrillator, assist devices) and heart transplantation considered for selected advanced heart failure patients do not fall within this scope.

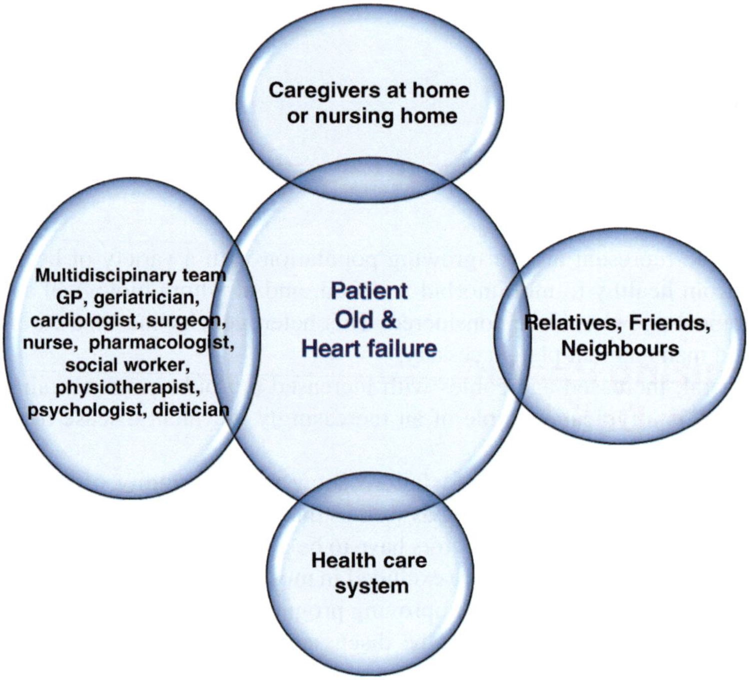

Fig. 19.1 Parties involved in the care of the old heart failure patient

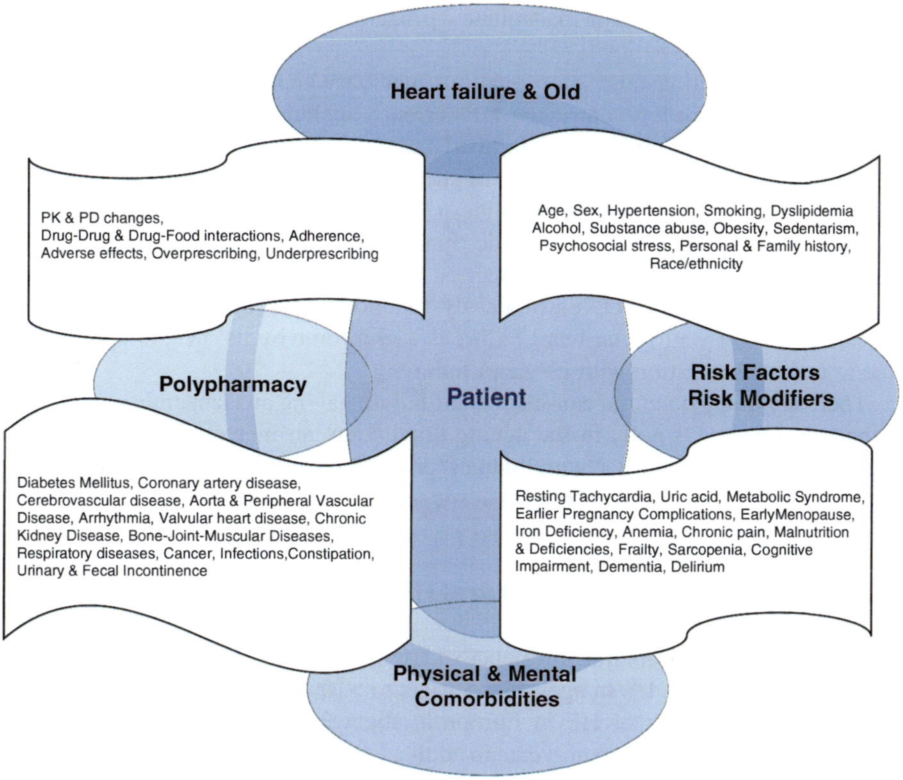

Fig. 19.2 Holistic approach of the old heart failure patient

19.2 Definition of Heart Failure

Heart failure is defined as a clinical syndrome consisting of cardinal symptoms (e.g. breathlessness, ankle swelling, fatigue) that may be accompanied by signs (e.g. elevated jugular venous pressure, pulmonary crackles, peripheral oedema). Underlying structural and/or functional abnormalities of the heart result in elevated intracardiac pressures and/or inadequate cardiac output at rest and/or during exercise [3].

Although definitions and interpretations may vary and may be somewhat artificial, the definition of left ventricular HF currently includes three phenotypes based on left ventricular ejection fraction: heart failure with preserved ejection fraction (HFpEF, LVEF ≥50%, with evidence of structural and/or functional cardiac abnormalities and/or raised natriuretic peptides (NPs)), mildly reduced (HFmrEF, LVEF 41–49%, mildly reduced LV systolic function), and reduced ejection fraction (HFrEF, LVEF <40%, significant reduction in LV systolic function) [3]. Heart failure can also be due to right ventricular dysfunction assessed by RV function measurements. Right ventricular heart failure is a syndrome by its own, however often due to and in association with LV heart failure.

There are many potential causes of heart failure having an ischaemic and/or non-ischaemic origin. Of note, in the ageing population, an increased prevalence and incidence of senile cardiac amyloidosis or wild-type transthyretin amyloidosis (ATTRwt) often in combination with aortic valve stenosis are noted.

19.3 Epidemiology and Natural History of Heart Failure

In the general population, the prevalence of HF in adults is around 1–2%, increasing with age from around 1% in ages 45–55 years to >10% in ages 70 years and older. In 2022, the incidence of HF in Europe is about 3/1000 person-years (all age-groups) or about 5/1000 person-years in adults, and over 50% of the HF patients are women. Although the age-adjusted incidence of HF may be falling, presumably related to better CVD management, the overall incidence of HF is increasing due to increasing age. In a general primary care practice, 1 out of 6 patients >65 years presenting with exertional dyspnoea are diagnosed with heart failure [3, 4]. Of the population affected by heart failure, the majority, up to 75% are 75 years or older [5].

Mainly based on studies in hospitalised patients, it is assumed that of all cases with HF, about 50% have HFrEF and about 50% have FpEF/HFmrEF [6–9].

In an ambulatory setting, the ESC Long-Term (ESC-HF-LT) Registry found 60% having HFrEF, 24% having HFmrEF, and only 16% having HFpEF. This latter relatively low number might be due to the inclusion of a younger, predominantly male population and the strict inclusion of patients from cardiology departments or specialised HF units caring mostly for HFrEF patients, while HFpEF patients rather present with worsening non-cardiac comorbidities and, therefore, are more likely to be admitted and followed in internal medicine or geriatric wards. One of the conclusions from this ESC-HF-LT Registry is that chronic HF patients stratified by categories of EF (i.e., <40%, 40–49%, ≥50%) represent different phenotypes in terms of demography, clinical presentation, aetiology, mechanical and electrical remodelling, and pharmacotherapies. Outcomes at 1 year showed that HFrEF patients had a significantly higher mortality rate than HFpEF patients, all-cause mortality in HFmrEF did not differ significantly from mortality in HFrEF or in HFpEF, while non-cardiovascular mortality was higher in patients with HFmrEF and HFpEF compared to HFrEF [10].

Although prognosis of patients with HF, mainly HFrEF, has improved since the publication and emergence on the market of successful HF treatment trials, prognosis remains poor, and quality of life (QOL) markedly reduced.

Mortality rates are higher in observational studies than in clinical trials [11]. In the Olmsted County cohort, 1-year and 5-year mortality rates after diagnosis, for all types of HF patients, were 20% and 53% [12]. In a report combining results of the Framingham Heart Study (FHS) and Cardiovascular Health Study (CHS) cohorts, mortality rate within 5 years following diagnosis was 67% [13].

A better overall survival in HFmrEF and HfpEF compared to HfrEF was considered. The MAGGIC meta-analysis concluded that the adjusted mortality risk in patients with HfpEF was lower than in patients with HfrEF. However, most observational studies show that this difference is negligible [12, 13]. In the Olmsted county cohort of hospitalised patients, it was shown that the prevalence of HFpEF over 15 years increased together with an increase in hypertension, atrial fibrillation, and diabetes and that the death rate remained unchanged (29% at 1 years and 65% at 5 years) which was minimally lower than the death rate for HFrEF (32% and 68%, respectively) [14].

The various and evolving definitions and categorisations of the heart failure syndrome over time together with heterogeneity in patient characteristics and the evolution in prevention and treatment also may contribute to the varying numbers in epidemiological data. Data from GWTG-HF (Get With The Guidelines–Heart Failure) linked to Medicare data looking at 5-year outcomes and median survival in patients hospitalised for heart failure showed a median survival of 2.1 years and a similar high 5-year mortality, 75%, in HFrEF, HFbEF(borderline, =mrEF), and HFpEF. Also, the composite of mortality and rehospitalisation was similar for all subgroups, with cardiovascular and HF readmission rates being higher in HFrEF and HFbEF compared to HFpEF. Conclusion was that patients with HF across all ages and EF groups had a markedly lower median survival compared to the overall population [15, 16].

Age by itself is an independent risk factor for mortality. Patients >75 years have significantly higher in-hospital mortality rates than patients <75 years (11.2% vs 4.4%) (www.nicor.org.uk). Two nationwide cohorts of patients hospitalised for new-onset heart failure based on linkage of the Dutch Hospital Discharge Registry and the National Cause of Death registry assessed overall and cause-specific mortality rates over time stratified by age and sex. Mortality rates at 1 year were high and increased considerably with age similarly in men and women, from 10.5% in women aged 25–54 years to 46.1% in women aged >85 years and from 9.8% in men aged 25–54 years to 53.4% in men >85 years, although the overall 1-year absolute risk of death across all ages declined by 4.0% in men and 3.2% in women [17]. The Cardiovascular Health Study, a longitudinal cohort study of community-dwelling older adults >65 years in the USA, reported 1-, 5-, and 10-year mortality rates of 19%, 56%, and 83%, respectively, following the onset of HF [13]. The Canadian Chronic Disease Surveillance System data confirmed that once HF develops, mortality increases exponentially with age [18]. Hospital admissions and readmissions are frequent in heart failure patients for cardiac as well as non-cardiac reasons and negatively impact prognosis. The proportion of hospitalisations related to decompensated HF sharply increases after the age of 65 years, with 1 in 7 HF hospitalisations occurring in patients ≥80 years of age [19].

19.4 Pharmacological Management of HF

The aim of treatment of heart failure is to improve survival, to prevent (repeated) hospitalisations due to heart failure, to reduce symptoms, and to improve functional capacity and quality of life. Together with non-pharmacological measures, pharmacotherapy is the cornerstone of treatment of heart failure.

Optimising drug therapy in older patients is a complex process because of the presence of physical and mental comorbidities, age-related changes in pharmacokinetics and pharmacodynamics, polypharmacy, under- and overprescribing, and issues with adherence [2, 20]. Management of HF patients should be planned in a multidisciplinary setting with a cardiogeriatrics team involving primary and secondary-tertiary care, and the patients and their caregivers should be educated about the HF syndrome and self-management [21] (Figs. 19.1, 19.2, and 19.3).

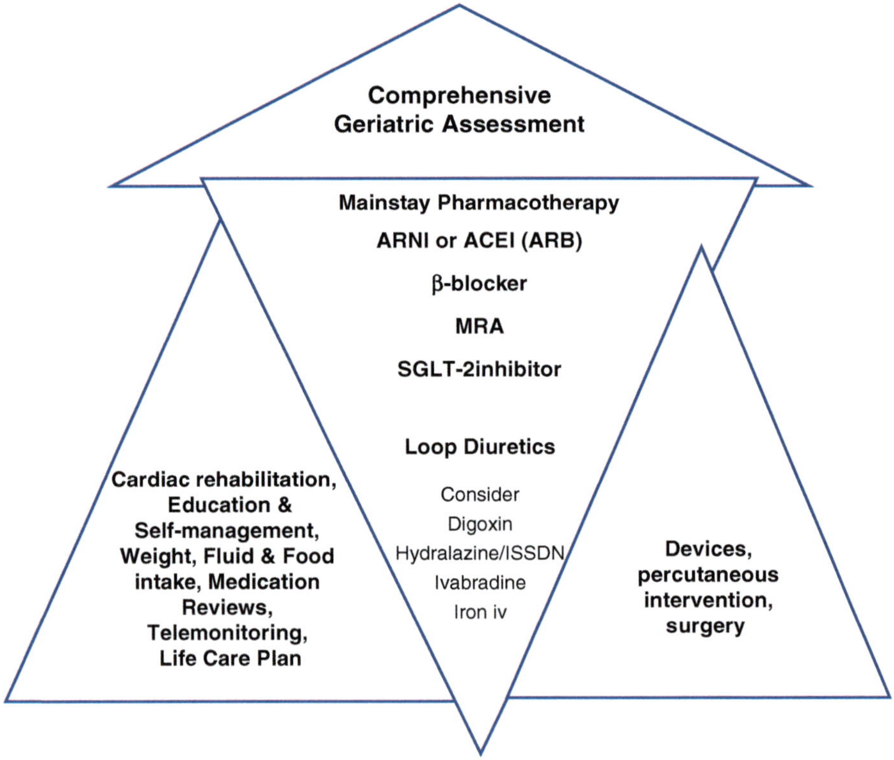

Fig. 19.3 Management of the old patient with heart failure

19.5 Pharmacological Treatment of Heart Failure in Older Persons (Fig. 19.3)

The ageing population is growing, heart failure increases with age, and age is an independent predictor of morbidity and mortality. With a few exceptions, hard evidence on the best treatment for heart failure specifically in older persons is lacking since they were largely excluded from major HF trials [22]. In the earlier studies over the past 40 years, the upper limit of age was often put at patients of 65 up to 70–75 years old and with little or no comorbidities. The more recent trials also allowed patients >75 years old, being appropriate and logical given the growing older population. However, evidence in the very old and/or multimorbid and/or frail older person is virtually non-existent.

Most drug trials until now provided evidence for a positive benefit-risk effect on morbidity and mortality mainly in HFrEF, while almost none could prove significant benefit on hard outcomes as mortality in HFpEF. Few trials demonstrated symptomatic benefit and reduced hospitalisations in HFpEF.

The recent EMPEROR-preserved and DELIVER trials showed a significant reduction by empagliflozin and dapagliflozin in the combined endpoint of CV death and HF hospitalisations, driven by a reduction in hospitalisation [23]. Treatment of HFpEF is quite individualised and mainly involves treatment of risk factors (such as hypertension) and comorbidities (such as atrial fibrillation, coronary artery disease, diabetes, renal insufficiency, pulmonary hypertension, thyroid disorder, etc.) and control of symptoms (fluid balance).

To deal with age, most trials specified subgroup analyses looking at different age ranges or at older versus younger participants, often defined as <65 years and >65 years old. This was done for most trials with ACE inhibitors (ACE-I), beta-blockers (BB), angiotensin receptor blockers (ARB), digoxin, hydralazine/ISDN, aldosterone antagonists/mineralocorticoid receptor antagonist (MRA), ivabradine, angiotensin receptor-neprilysin inhibitors (ARNI), and sodium-glucose cotransporter 2 inhibitors (SGLT2i).

An increasing number of post hoc analyses of the effectiveness of HF treatment in a broader range of older patients are performed.

A BIOSTAT-CHF analysis assessing the association between up-titration of angiotensin-converting enzyme inhibitors (ACEI), angiotensin receptor blockers (ARB), and beta-blockers and outcome across the age spectrum in HFrEF patients showed that achieving higher doses of ACEI/ARB was associated with improved outcome regardless of age, while achieving higher doses of beta-blockers was associated with improved outcome only in younger but not in older patients. The inconsistent association between beta-blocker dosage and heart rate in older patients is hypothesised to be due to a decreased cardiovascular responsiveness to beta-adrenergic stimulation, already acting as an intrinsic beta-blockade, as reflected by the lower resting heart rate in older patients [24]. Heart rate reduction might be more important than the achieved beta-blocker dose in HFrEF. For example, in CIBIS-ELD, the achieved heart rate target rather than beta-blocker dose (carvedilol or bisoprolol) was significantly associated with outcome (see further, [25, 26]).

Also, the higher prevalence of atrial fibrillation in older patients might lower the beneficial effects of beta-blockers.

One systematic review and meta-analysis of the efficacy (mortality and hospitalisations for cardiovascular causes) and safety of MRA treatment in older HF patients ≥65 years reported overall benefit from MRA therapy with no significant treatment interaction for age in patients with HFrEF, while no significant effect on any efficacy outcome in patients with HFpEF. In a subanalysis in patients ≥75 years with HErEF, the effect of MRA treatment on overall mortality seemed uncertain, mainly due to heterogeneity [25].

In an IPD meta-analysis of RALES, EMPHASIS-HF, and TOPCAT in patients ≥75 years versus <75 years of age, the primary outcome (composite of death from cardiovascular causes or hospitalisation for HF), cardiovascular death, and all-cause death were reduced by MRAs without significant between-trial or age (younger vs. older) heterogeneity. Worsening renal function (without more hyperkalaemia) was found more frequently in older patients. The reduction in morbidity and mortality was more marked in patients with HFrEF however overall homogenous across HFrEF and HFpEF (in HFpEF lower events, but not statistically significant). The authors pleaded for measures to increase MRA treatment in the older population [26].

A cohort study using US Medicare fee-for-service claims data (2014–2017) in patients >65 years with HFrEF evaluating the effectiveness of angiotensin receptor-neprilysin inhibitor (ARNI) versus renin-angiotensin system inhibition (RAS) found that ARNI treatment was associated with lower risk of the composite effectiveness endpoint (worsening HF or all-cause mortality) compared with RAS blockade alone [27].

In the PARADIGM-HF trial (LCZ696 vs. enalapril), efficacy (CV death or heart failure hospitalisation) and safety according to age (<55 years (n = 1624), 55–64 years (n = 2655), 65–74 years (n = 2557), and ≥75 years (n = 1563)) were consistent across all age categories with LCZ696 having a favourable benefit–risk profile in all age groups [28].

A meta-analysis of the effects of the SGLT2 inhibitors dapagliflozin (DAPA-HF) and empagliflozin (EMPEROR-reduced) on cardiovascular outcomes in patients with HFrEF with or without diabetes showed a significant reduction in all-cause death (−13%), cardiovascular death (−14%), combined endpoint of cardiovascular death or first hospitalisation for heart failure (−24%), composite endpoint of recurrent hospitalisations for heart failure or cardiovascular death (−25%), and composite endpoint of renal events (−38%). Analysis based on age groups, < and >65 years, showed a persistent 25% reduction in the composite endpoint of cardiovascular death or hospitalisation for heart failure [29].

Empagliflozin in patients with HFpEF (in the EMPEROR-Preserved trial defined as EF >40%) and with or without diabetes lowered the composite of cardiovascular death or hospitalisation for heart failure by 21%, mainly due to lower risk of hospitalisation for heart failure (29% reduction). Based on age, the endpoint reduction in patients <70 years was −12% (0.88, 0.70–1.11), while it was −25% (0.75, 0.64–0.87) in patients >70 years. If confirmed in other trials (confirmed for dapagliflozin in

DELIVER trial) and in real-world data, SGLT2 inhibitors are the first class showing significant beneficial effect in HFpEF (subgroup analysis showed significance in EF >40 to <50% and >50% to <60%, in EF >60% NS) [23].

Pooled data on the safety (12 studies) and efficacy (9 studies; outcome: HbA1c reduction) of the SGLT2 inhibitor dapagliflozin 10 mg/day monotherapy or combined with oral antidiabetic drugs or with insulin in older patients >65 years (20% of the studied populations) with type 2 diabetes showed HbA1c reductions across age subgroups (<65 years and >65 years) with greater reductions in HbA1c in patients aged <65 years than in patients aged >65 years. Hypoglycaemia, volume depletion, and renal AEs (predefined serum creatinine thresholds) occurred more often in patients aged >65 years, reflecting the lower eGFR in the older persons. Orthostatic hypotension occurred in <0.1% in both age groups. Urinary tract and genital infections were similar for both DAPA-treated age groups. It was concluded that DAPA's efficacy and safety observations indicate a practical, new approach to the treatment of T2DM patients aged >65 years [30].

Very few trials investigated the efficacy and safety of drug therapy specifically in an older population.

The PEP-CHF trial in patients >70 years of age and with evidence of diastolic dysfunction, comparing placebo with perindopril 4 mg/day, showed a clear trend towards reduction in the primary endpoint of combined all-cause mortality and heart failure hospitalisation (HR 0.692: 95% CI 0.474–1.010; $P = 0.055$), however not reaching statistical significance due to insufficient power. A significant reduction in hospitalisation for heart failure and a significant improvement in functional class and 6-min walking distance at 1 year were observed in patients receiving perindopril [31].

The SENIORS trial assessed the effect of nebivolol, a beta-blocker with vasodilating properties, on mortality and cardiovascular hospital admission in older patients >70 years with heart failure, regardless of ejection fraction, compared to placebo. The primary outcome, a composite of all-cause mortality or cardiovascular hospital admission, was reduced by 34%(HR, 0.86; 95% CI, 0.74–0.99; $P = 0.039$), with no significant influence of age, gender, or ejection fraction on the effect of nebivolol on the primary outcome. For all-cause mortality HR was 0.88 (95% CI, 0.71–1.08; $P = 0.21$). Nebivolol was considered an effective and well-tolerated treatment for heart failure in the older population [32].

As part of the larger CIBIS trial, the CIBIS–ELD trial was a tolerability superiority study of bisoprolol versus carvedilol comparing the tolerability and clinical effects of the two beta-blockers in older patients with heart failure with reduced or preserved left ventricular ejection fraction. The primary endpoint tolerability, defined as reaching and maintaining guideline-recommended target doses after 12 weeks treatment, was comparable, 24% versus 25%. Bisoprolol treatment resulted in greater reduction of heart rate (adjusted mean difference, 2.1 bpm; 95% CI, 0.5–3.6; $P = 0.008$) and more, dose-limiting, bradycardic adverse events (16 vs. 11%; $P = 0.02$), while carvedilol intake resulted in a reduction of forced expiratory volume (adjusted mean difference, 50 mL; 95% CI, 4–95; $P = 0.03$) and more, non-dose-limiting, pulmonary adverse events (10 vs. 4%; $P = 0.001$). It was concluded that overall tolerability to target doses was comparable, while the pattern of intolerance was different with bradycardia occurring more often in the bisoprolol group, whereas pulmonary adverse events occurring more often in the carvedilol group [33].

A 4-year follow-up study of the CIBIS-ELD trial investigated the prognostic value of achieved heart rate after beta-blocker optimisation on long-term mortality. Heart rate increases by 10 bpm following beta-blocker up-titration which was associated with a subsequent mortality hazard ratio of 1.19 (95% CI, 1.02–1.38; $P = 0.023$). The heart rate range with the lowest mortality and the fewest treatment-related adverse events was 55–64 bpm. The achieved beta-blocker dose was not associated with mortality risk. It was concluded that the achieved heart rate after up-titration, but not the beta-blocker dose, predicted all-cause mortality risk in older patients with chronic

heart failure and that titration should aim for resting heart rates between 55 and 64 bpm [34].

Several smaller, mainly Japanese, studies looked at real-world data on the effectiveness and safety of SGLT2 inhibition in older persons.

The STELLA-ELDER study was a post-marketing surveillance (PMS) study investigating real-world evidence on the safety of ipragliflozin in older (>65 years) Japanese patients with type 2 diabetes mellitus. Of all patients, 16.91% experienced 1880 adverse drug reactions (ADR), of which 165 ADRs were considered serious in 1.49% of the patients. The most common ADRs were skin and subcutaneous tissue disorders (3.25%), renal and urinary disorders (2.74%), and infections (2.23%). Of special interest were skin complications, volume depletion, polyuria/pollakisuria, genital and urinary tract infection, renal disorders, hypoglycaemia, cerebrovascular disease, cardiovascular disease, malignant tumour, fracture, and ketone body-related events. Risk factors identified for hypoglycaemia were BMI (<18.5 kg/m^2 vs. ≥22.0 to <25.0 kg/m^2; OR, 9.356) and concomitant insulin use (vs. no; OR, 4.946), and risk factors identified for volume depletion were age (≥75 years vs. <75 years; OR, 1.737) and concomitant loop diuretic use (vs. no; OR, 2.105). Overall, there were no safety concerns that were not previously observed in pre-marketing trials. The conclusion was that this PMS revealed probable ADRs in older Japanese patients with T2DM taking ipragliflozin with no new safety concerns and that PMS should help physicians to identify possible treatment-emergent ADRs in ipragliflozin-treated patients in real-world settings [35].

Another Japanese study assessing the use of sodium-glucose cotransporter 2 inhibitors in older patients (mean age 73.7 ± 10 years) with type 2 diabetes mellitus did not report events associated with oral administration of SGLT-2 inhibitors after a mean follow-up period of 289.3 days. Fasting blood glucose and glycosylated haemoglobin levels at 6 months were significantly lowered without signs of intravascular collapse or changes in creatinine, blood urea nitrogen/creatinine ratio, or estimated glomerular filtration rate. Treatment with SGLT-2 inhibitors did significantly increase haemoglobin and haematocrit levels. In a small subgroup with a brain natriuretic peptide level exceeding the normal upper limit before treatment with SGLT-2 inhibitors, the brain natriuretic peptide levels significantly decreased after 6 months of treatment. SGLT-2 inhibitors at 6 months exerted a favourable hypoglycaemic effect and no signs of dehydration were observed [36].

A small Spanish study of real-world safety and efficacy of SGLT-2 inhibitors in older patients with DM also concluded that these drugs are safe and effective in not well-controlled elderly (>65 years, however mean age being (only) 67 years) DM2 patients and that effect on systolic BP should be considered and so the antihypertensive treatment be reviewed [37].

Because of concerns on muscle wasting with the use of SGLT-2 inhibitors mainly in the older population, a highly represented population in Japan, Japanese investigators launched the EMPA-ELDERLY trial (ClinicalTrials.gov NCT04531462), a randomised, double-blind, placebo-controlled trial to assess the efficacy and safety of the sodium-glucose cotransporter-2 inhibitor empagliflozin 10 mg in patients >65 years of age with type 2 diabetes (with BMI > 22). The primary endpoint is the change in HbA1c level from baseline to week 52. Secondary endpoints include changes from baseline to week 52 in body composition, including muscle mass and body fat, skeletal muscle index, grip strength, and time in the five-time chair stand test. Other endpoints include changes in patient-reported outcomes (including quality of life), cognitive function, and safety (hypoglycaemia, hepatic injury, diabetic ketoacidosis, decreased renal function and lower-limb amputation) (ClinicalTrials.gov Identifier: NCT04531462; Recruitment Status: Active, not recruiting) [38].

Finally, a systematic review and meta-analysis (11 studies; 93,502 patients) of GLP-1 receptor agonists and SGLT2 inhibitors for older people with type 2 diabetes assessed the cardiovascular effects of glucagon-like peptide-1 receptor agonists (GLP-1 RAs) and sodium-glucose co-transporter-2 (SGLT2) inhibitors in older people (>65 years) with type 2 diabetes. Comparable to the overall population, GLP-1 RAs significantly reduced major adverse cardiovascular events (MACE) and all its subcomponents (hazard ratio [HR], 0.86; 95% CI, 0.80–0.92) in the patients ≥65 years. SGLT2 inhibitors reduced MACE (HR, 0.90; 95% CI, 0.83–0.98) (however, neutral effect on its subcomponents), reduced heart failure hospitalisation (HR, 0.62; 95% CI, 0.51–0.76), and the composite renal endpoint (HR, 0.57; 95% CI, 0.43–0.77). Similar results were obtained in patients ≥75 years. From this systematic review and meta-analysis, it was concluded that in older adults with diabetes, GLP-1 RAs reduced MACE and its components and that SGLT2 inhibitors reduced MACE, heart failure, and renal outcomes [39].

Summarising the results, overall, in heart failure, ACE-I reduced all-cause mortality around 20%, while ARBs did not significantly reduce all-cause mortality; however, around 18% reduction in CV death or HF hospitalisation was shown, an outcome more and more used as primary endpoint in heart failure RCTs. Beta-blockers showed an all-cause mortality reduction around 20–30%. MRA showed a 15% (eplerenone) to 30% (spironolactone) all-cause mortality reduction, with eplerenone also showing reduction of CV death or HF hospitalisation by 37%. Digoxin did not significantly reduce all-cause mortality but did reduce HF hospitalisations by 28%. Ivabradine did not show effect on all-cause mortality, however reduced CV deaths or HF hospitalisation by 18%. Sacubitril-Valsartan reduced CV deaths or HF hospitalisation by 20%. The SGLT2 inhibitors (empagliflozin and dapagliflozin) gave a 13% reduction in all-cause death, 14% reduction in cardiovascular death, 26% reduction in the combined risk of cardiovascular death or first hospitalisation for heart failure, and 25% reduction in the composite of cardiovascular death or recurrent hospitalisations for heart failure. For patients with HFpEF with or without diabetes, empagliflozin reduced the composite of cardiovascular death or hospitalisation for heart failure by 21% in the overall population and 25% in patients >70 years. If confirmed in other trials and in real-world data, SGLT 2 inhibitors are the first class showing beneficial effect in HFpEF. As a comparison, in earlier trials, the ARB candesartan, MRA spironolactone, and Sacubitril-Valsartan also showed some modest effect on CV death and HF hospitalisation (up to 15% risk reduction) in HfpEF patients, however mainly in the groups with an EF 40–49% considered as mildly reduced EF [23].

Overall, it can be assumed that older patients also benefit from these evidence-based pharmacological treatments and that guideline recommended HF treatment aiming at improving the quality of patient care should also be applied in older people. A guideline gives an advice, not an order, and a benefit-risk balance should be made for each individual patient.

Current mainstay drug therapy recommended for all heart failure patients are ARNI or ACE-I if ARNI not tolerated (ARB only if ARNI and ACE-I not tolerated), beta-blockers, MRA, and SGLT2i as they improve prognosis by reduction of morbidity and mortality. Dosage should be started low and slow and then progressively increased based on tolerance. Symptomatic treatment with loop diuretics and acetazolamide in certain cases (ADVOR trial) is given in case of congestion to improve symptoms, exercise tolerance, and reduce HF hospitalisations.

The following drugs should or might be considered in specific conditions. Ivabradine, an If channel blocker, should be considered in case of EF <35%, sinus rhythm with a heart rate >70 bpm in patients on mainstay HF therapy (with or without a beta-blocker). Digoxin might be considered for symptomatic patients on baseline HF therapy. Hydralazine/isosorbide dinitrate might be considered in symptomatic patients not tolerating any of the baseline therapies.

Some other drug classes for use in HF are being investigated; however, current evidence is limited. The soluble guanylate cyclase stimulator vericiguat might be considered in patients with HFrEF, on top of standard therapy to further reduce the risk of CV mortality and hospitalisations for HF (VICTORIA study) [40]. The cardiac myosin activator omecamtiv mecarbil might be considered for HFrEF patients on top of standard therapy to reduce the risk of CV mortality and HF hospitalisation (GALACTIC-HF study) [41–44].

Besides optimal HF drug therapy, other cardiovascular and non-CV therapies, including non-pharmacological strategies, should be applied in the setting of cardiovascular and non-cardiovascular risk factors and comorbidities, which may play a role in initiating and worsening of heart failure directly and/or indirectly (Fig. 19.3).

19.6 Risk Factors and Comorbidities

In older patients, heart failure seldom comes alone. Several factors may play a role in the initiation and/or worsening of heart failure, may compromise or hamper optimal therapy, and may as such influence prognosis. The list of risk factors and comorbidities is inexhaustive. Some risk factors and comorbidities, important in the setting of ageing and heart failure, are shortly discussed. Guideline-based therapies proven to prevent or stabilise cardiovascular diseases have to be weighed by an overall benefit-risk balance. Many conditions to be taken into account and to be taken care of in clinical practice (impact of ageing on PK, polypharmacy, drug-drug-food interactions, adverse drug reactions, inappropriate prescribing, geriatric syndromes & chronic conditions, multimorbidity & frailty, COPD, Diabetes, chronic kidney disease, sarcopenia, falls, pain, sleep disorders, dementia, delirium, constipation, incontinence) are discussed in detail in the other book chapters.

19.6.1 Risk Factors

Prevention of cardiovascular disease and early recognition and treatment of disease might increase survival and/or improve quality of life [3, 45].

Smoking is a strong and independent risk factor for cardiovascular and respiratory diseases and cancer. Patients should be encouraged to stop smoking to prevent cardiovascular, respiratory and cancer diseases or the worsening of it. After 1 year of smoking cessation, the risk for a myocardial infarction is reduced by 50%, and the risk for stroke becomes similar as for a non-smoker. After 5 years of smoking cessation, the risk of lung cancer is reduced by 50%.

Sedentary lifestyle should be avoided and physical activity increased to reduce morbidity and all-cause and CV mortality. Exercise-based cardiac rehabilitation is recommended in HF patients to improve functional capacity and quality of life and to reduce hospitalisations. Especially in the older people, this should also prevent further muscle wasting, frailty, and osteoporosis. For all adults of all ages at least 150–300 min a week of moderate intensity and/or 75–150 min a week of vigorous intensity aerobic physical activity are recommended. People who cannot perform 150 min of moderate-intensity physical activity a week should stay as active as their abilities and health condition allow. Anyhow at least some light activity throughout the day is recommended. Along with this, obesity prevention and weight control can be supported through a balanced food intake and energy expenditure.

Alcohol intake should not exceed 100 g a week, and binge drinking should be avoided. In alcoholic cardiomyopathy, alcohol should be forbidden. Also, other substance abuse should be checked and handled appropriately. While for some older patients an occasional drink might be part of social contact, excessive alcohol might harm physical and mental health. In patients taking (multiple) medications, drug-alcohol interactions as well as alcohol by itself might cause adverse reactions and influence adherence [46].

Fluid and *salt* intake. In HF patients, excessive fluid and salt intake should be avoided and are often restricted to a maximum of 1.5–2 l a day and to <5 g a day, respectively. Intake of fluid and salt should be modified following the hydration status. For example, in case of vomiting, diarrhoea, and prolonged heath, dehydration and electrolyte disturbances must be avoided by temporarily increasing fluid intake. A healthy varied diet should help risk factor control and prevent malnutrition. Nutrition should be more flexible in the old patient than in the young patient.

Especially older patients with HF have increased risk for malnutrition and deficiencies, which should be checked for and treated accordingly [47]. In the OPTIMIZE-HF study, low sodium serum levels was a predictor of in-hospital mortality [48].

Psychosocial stress (mental, financial, familial, loneliness, anxiety, etc.) increases cardiovascular risk and should be assessed (e.g., via Patient Health Questionnaire), and psychosocial support should be given when necessary. Increased attention and support in patients with mental disorders and cardiovascular disease is recommended to help improve adherence to lifestyle changes and medication.

Blood pressure should be regularly measured, and hypertension, an important risk factor in heart failure, should be prevented and/or efficiently treated with lifestyle interventions (no smoking, salt intake <5 g/day, physical exercise, weight control, stress reduction) and antihypertensive drugs (main classes: RAS inhibitors, diuretics, calcium channel blockers, beta-blockers). Blood pressure should also be measured in the standing position and/or after a meal to detect orthostatic and/or postprandial hypotension, especially in older persons. A blood pressure target of <140/90 mmHg with ranges of SBP <140 to 130 and DBP <80 to 70 mmHg are recommended, if tolerated. In older persons >80 years with good functionality, an antihypertensive treatment as given to younger adults should be considered. In the older persons with a moderate functional limitation and preserved autonomy for the activities of daily living, a geriatric risk assessment might be performed to decide on the individual treatment approach. Patients with few comorbidities and only very limited loss of autonomy can be considered to receive the same antihypertensive regimen as the older persons with good functionality. In older persons with severe functional limitations and loss of autonomy and/or very reduced life expectancy, quality of life and symptom control is the main aim, and treatment should be regularly reviewed and discussed in a multidisciplinary context. Because of safety reasons, treatment might be reduced or stopped [49–52].

Hypercholesterolemia should be treated with lifestyle measures (physical activity, healthy diet) and lipid-lowering drugs (mainly statins). The targets depend on the overall cardiovascular risk and tolerance. In calculating cardiovascular risk in older persons, often important non-CVD risk has to be taken into account, and therefore the Older Person SCORE and LIFE-CVD scores are more appropriate. Guidelines recommend statins in older people (>65 years) with atherosclerotic cardiovascular disease in the same way as in younger people. In primary prevention, according to level of risk, statins are recommended in older people <75 years. In people >75 years, initiation of statins may be considered if at high risk. In older patients, one should be alert for myopathy. Although there is less direct evidence of benefits in the primary prevention setting among patients older than 75 years, results from RCTs support the use of statins in older patients at high or very high risk of ASCVD. The results from the STAREE (Statin Therapy for Reducing Events in the Elderly; NCT02099123), from the SITE/SAGA (Statins In The Elderly; NCT02547883), and PREVENTABLE (Pragmatic Evaluation of Events and Benefits of Lipid-Lowering in Older Adults; NCT04262206) trials will be of help to elucidate some of the questions that remain unanswered. Shared decision-making on statin therapy in 75+-year-old people in primary prevention should be based on good clinical judgment, comorbidities, frailty, patient preferences, and life expectancy [53].

Diabetes mellitus, considered more as a comorbidity, should be as much as possible prevented by lifestyle measures (weight control, physical activity). Once DM is established, pharmacological treatment should be installed taking into account age, risk factors, and comorbidities. SGLT2 inhibitors are the preferred choice in the setting of CV disease and heart failure. Overall, in diabetes patients, an HbA1c target of <7% is recommended. Based on personal physical and mental health status, less rigorous HbA1c and glucose targets should be considered in older patients, ranging from <7.5% in healthy older persons up to <8.5–9% in very complex older patients with a poor overall health status [54, 55].

19.6.2 Cardiovascular Comorbidities

19.6.2.1 Atrial Fibrillation and Conduction Abnormalities

Atrial Fibrillation

The incidence and prevalence of atrial fibrillation (AF), the most frequent cardiac arrhythmia worldwide, typically increases with age and with HF severity [56].

AF and HF frequently coexist and can cause or exacerbate each other through several mechanisms such as structural cardiac remodelling, activation of neurohormonal systems, and heart rate-related LV impairment [57–60]. However, if AF is the cause of HF (called tachycardiomyopathy), the clinical course may be more favourable than with other causes of HF [61]. On the contrary, if AF develops in patients with chronic HF, prognosis seems worse, with increased stroke and increased mortality [62, 63].

The management of patients with concomitant HF and AF includes identification and treatment of potential causes and/or triggers of AF, management of HF, prevention of thromboembolic events, rate control, and/or rhythm control.

Potential causes or precipitating factors, such as thyroid disorders, electrolyte disturbances, infections, uncontrolled hypertension, and valve disease, should be checked and corrected. Heart failure should be optimally managed with the mainstay therapy, and increased congestion due to AF should be managed with diuretics.

Oral anticoagulants (OACs) are the cornerstone of treatment of AF to reduce the risk for stroke/systemic thromboembolism, and—unless contraindicated—long-term oral anticoagulant therapy is recommended in all patients with HF and paroxysmal, persistent, or permanent AF and CHA2DS2-VASc score >2 in men and >3 in women. Four large randomised controlled trials (RCTs) have shown that non-vitamin K antagonist oral anticoagulants (NOACs) also called direct oral anticoagulants (DOACs) are non-inferior to vitamin K antagonists (VKAs) in preventing stroke and systemic embolism, as well as regarding their risk for major bleeding. Direct-acting oral anticoagulants (DOACs) are preferred for the prevention of thromboembolic events in patients with AF—except in patients with moderate or severe mitral valve stenosis and mechanical prosthetic heart valves—as they have similar efficacy to vitamin K antagonists (VKAs) and a lower risk of intracranial haemorrhage [64]. Vulnerable geriatric patients with AF were underrepresented in trials, making the choice of the right anticoagulant in real-life patients particularly challenging. In these vulnerable patients, NOACs tend to be underused and/or underdosed due to concerns of fall-related intracranial bleeding, cognitive impairment, drug-drug interactions, low body weight, or impaired renal function. The SAFIR trial was the first large-scale prospective study assessing bleeding risk in geriatric patients aged ≥80 years with AF newly treated with rivaroxaban compared to patients treated with VKA. While ischemic stroke and all-cause mortality rates were similar, major bleeding rates were significantly lower with rivaroxaban than with VKAs (hazard ratio of 0.67 (95% CI, 0.45–0.99)) and with a lower intracranial bleeding rate (HR = 0.52; 0.21–1.28) [65]. An individual benefit-risk assessment and shared decision-making are key elements in the decision on whether to anticoagulate in the vulnerable geriatric patient with AF at high thromboembolic as well as high bleeding risk. A comprehensive geriatric assessment (CGA) in hospitalised older patients with AF may help guide clinicians in this individual benefit-risk assessment [66].

In patients with HF and AF who have a contraindication to oral anticoagulation left atrial appendage closure can be considered, although trials did not include patients with contraindications to oral anticoagulants [67, 68].

The debate and research on rate control versus rhythm control is ongoing, and no clear benefit of one strategy over the other has been shown in patients with AF and HF (except for symptomatic improvement with catheter ablation). Overall, higher heart rates are associated with worse outcomes in observational studies [69, 70].

The ESC Atrial Fibrillation Guidelines [56] advice beta-blockers for rate control in patients with HFrEF, HFmrEF, and HFpEF because of their proven safety in these patients. Digoxin can be considered when the ventricular rate remains high, despite beta-blockers, or when beta-blockers are contraindicated or not tolerated.

AV node ablation can be considered in patients with poor ventricular rate control despite medical treatment not eligible for rhythm control by catheter ablation or in patients with biventricular pacing.

Urgent electrical cardioversion is recommended in the setting of acute worsening HF in patients presenting with rapid ventricular rates and haemodynamic instability, after consideration of the thromboembolic risk. Electrical cardioversion may also be considered to improve symptoms in patients with persistent and symptomatic AF, despite optimal pharmacological management. In case of pharmacological cardioversion, amiodarone is the preferred drug as other antiarrhythmic drugs (flecainide, propafenone, dronedarone) are associated with worse outcomes in HFrEF. Amiodarone also can help maintain sinus rhythm after cardioversion.

Catheter ablation should be considered for the prevention or treatment of AF if there is a clear association between paroxysmal or persistent AF and worsening of HF symptoms, which persist despite medical therapy [56].

Symptomatic Conduction Abnormalities

Due to the ageing process degeneration of the conduction system can occur involving the sinus node, atria, AV node, His bundle, and the Purkinje system. The use of pacemakers is growing worldwide as people live longer. In older people, although the periprocedural risk is mildly increased, the implantation of a pacemaker is relatively safe. In patients with HF, the indications for pacemaker therapy do not differ from patients with other CV diseases.

Long-term RV pacing is associated with potential adverse effect on LV systolic function leading to HF (pacemaker-induced cardiomyopathy) [71]. In older patients with sinus node disease, DDD pacing programmed to minimal ventricular pacing is advised, while in the very old patients with intermittent atrioventricular block, VVI pacing may be preferred. In patients with HF and in need of frequent ventricular pacing, implantation of a CRT pacemaker should be considered (BLOCK-HF trial) [72]. More physiological pacing methods are developed and increasingly implanted. His bundle pacing, compared to RV pacing, showed less HF hospitalisation and a trend in reduced mortality [73]. In patients with a higher pacing burden (>40%), His bundle pacing showed a lower risk of new-onset atrial fibrillation compared to RV pacing [74].

Leadless pacemakers avoiding complications of access site and at the pulse generator are increasingly used instead of the classic VVIR pacemakers.

When deciding about device implantation in an older patient, general physical and mental status, risk factors and comorbidities, and physiological age rather than chronological age should be decisive for device implantation selection for survival and quality of life [75].

Valve Disease

The prevalence of valve disease is increasing with age, with more than 10% of people aged 75 years and older having moderate or severe valve disease.

Improved surgical techniques and percutaneous valve interventions increase the treatment options for older patients with or without comorbidities.

Aortic valve stenosis and mitral valve and tricuspid valve regurgitation are common in older people. Aortic valve stenosis and mitral valve regurgitation are the two most prevalent left-sided valve pathologies observed in older people.

Aortic Valve Stenosis (AS)

Degenerative or calcific aortic valve disease is common in older patients with varying numbers of prevalence reported with a prevalence of severe aortic stenosis going from 1 to 2% in people aged 75 years to 6–18% in people aged 85 years and further increasing in people over 90 years old. A systematic review and meta-analysis of population-based studies found a prevalence of 12.4% for AS and 3.4% for severe AS among the elderly [76–78].

Isolated aortic valve regurgitation is uncommon in older adults; however, aortic valve stenosis might be accompanied by aortic valve regurgitation.

Risk factors associated with the development of AS in older adults may be similar to those for atherosclerosis. In the Cardiovascular Health Study evaluating 5201 persons aged ≥65 years old, the overall incidence of aortic sclerosis and AS was 26% and 2% increasing up to 37% and 2.6% in the 75 years old. Major independent clinical risk factors for degenerative aortic valve disease were age with a twofold increased risk for each 10-year increase in age, male sex with a twofold excess risk, current cigarette smoking with a 35% increased risk, and hypertension with a 20% increased risk. High serum concentrations of lipoprotein(a) and low-density lipoprotein cholesterol were also significant risk factors [77]. Aortic valve stenosis may cause or worsen HF by increasing LV afterload with consequent LV hypertrophy and remodelling [79].

Once heart failure symptoms (angina, dyspnoea, syncope) occur in patients with severe aortic valve stenosis, the prognosis is very poor. There are no pharmacological therapies specifically for improving outcomes of AS. However, HF patients with symptomatic aortic valve stenosis should receive standard HF therapy, paying extra attention to the risk of hypotension.

Aortic valve intervention is recommended in patients with HF symptoms and severe, high-gradient aortic valve stenosis (valve area <1 cm^2, mean gradient >40 mmHg), regardless of LVEF and with a life expectancy of >1 year.

In low-gradient aortic valve stenosis, haemodynamic assessment (with dobutamine) might be necessary to determine further management [80].

Older patients have higher in-hospital mortality than younger patients, due to a poorer preoperative general status, more extensive age-related valve calcifications, and fragile connective tissues, and if CABG, aneurysm repair, and mitral valve surgery are concomitantly performed. Death after 30 days is more likely (up to 70%) due to non-cardiac causes as pneumonia, stroke, and malignancy. However, older patients who do survive the perioperative period, mostly do well with a functional and quality of life improvement. In older patients referred for cardiac surgery, a global assessment integrating frailty, disability, and risk scores should characterise elderly patients better and identify those at increased risk [81].

Transcatheter aortic valve implantation (TAVI) is non-inferior to surgical aortic valve replacement (SAVR) in reducing clinical events and mortality and disabling stroke in patients at high and intermediate risk for surgery [82–84]. In low-risk patients, SAVR is recommended in patients <75 years and at low surgical risk (STS-PROM score or EurCORE II <4%), whereas TAVI is recommended in patients >75 years or at high surgical risk (STS-PROM score or EuroSCORE II >8%). In specific cases, balloon aortic valvuloplasty may be considered as in highly symptomatic patients with acute heart failure and shock as a bridge to TAVI or SAVR [80].

A multidisciplinary team (cardiologists, cardiac surgeons, geriatricians, nurses) should make the benefit risk balance of TAVI and SAVR according to the patients age, medical history, clinical features, anatomical aspects, life expectancy, and patient preference.

Mitral Regurgitation

Mitral regurgitation is a common valve abnormality in older adults with an estimated odds ratio of 1.3 per 10-year increase in age.

Mitral regurgitation can be caused by organic or primary mitral regurgitation and functional or secondary ischemic or non-ischaemic mitral regurgitation.

Organic or primary mitral regurgitation is due to intrinsic disease of the mitral leaflets or subvalvular apparatus such as calcific degeneration, mitral valve prolapse, flail mitral leaflet, and ruptured chordae tendineae. Surgery, preferably repair, is recommended in patients with severe primary MR and HF symptoms.

Functional or secondary mitral regurgitation is mainly a disease of the left ventricle. Functional or secondary ischemic mitral regurgitation is due to ischaemia or papillary muscle infarction, with or without rupture, associated with an acute myocardial infarction. Functional secondary non-ischaemic mitral regurgitation is due to apical displacement of the papillary muscles associated with annular dilatation and left atrial dilatation caused by left ventricular dilatation of any origin. Secondary mitral regurgitation is a dynamic condition, and echocardiographic quantification during exercise may be helpful in patients with moderate regurgitation at rest and developing symptoms during physical activity [80, 85].

In older patients, the most common causes of mitral regurgitation referred for mitral valve surgery are prolapse due to myxomatous degeneration and ischaemic heart disease. Moderate or severe mitral regurgitation is associated with a poor prognosis in patients with HF [86, 87]. Follow-up by a multidisciplinary heart team is recommended. Optimal medical therapy, including cardiac resynchronisation therapy, should be considered. In patients with severe mitral regurgitation and HFrEF requiring revascularisation, mitral valve surgery and CABG should be considered. Isolated mitral valve surgery may be considered in symptomatic patients with severe mitral regurgitation despite optimal therapy and at low surgical risk [80].

Chronic mitral regurgitation is the second most common reason for valve surgery in older adults, after aortic valve surgery. While in younger asymptomatic patients with early evidence of left ventricular dysfunction, surgery is recommended, in patients over 80 years old, surgery might be considered only when symptoms are present since postoperative outcomes are less favourable in this group. The risk associated with the intervention, repair as well as with replacement, increases with the presence of ischaemic heart disease, extent of calcification, and concomitant interventions. Outcome after surgery in older patients varies with age and disease severity and is better after mitral valve repair than replacement. However, late surgery might contribute more than age to worse outcome in mitral valve surgery in older adults <80 years.

Mitral valve repair, if feasible, is the surgical treatment of choice for mitral regurgitation and HF symptoms, also in older patients, as well as in primary MR and secondary MR. If surgery is contraindicated or considered at high risk, then percutaneous repair may be considered [80, 88–90].

Various percutaneous edge-to-edge mitral valve repair techniques are currently being evaluated and showed very different results (Mitra-FR and COAPT). The procedure may be considered to improve symptoms in patients with severe heart failure, severe mitral regurgitation, and severe symptoms and not eligible for surgery [91].

Other percutaneous mitral valve repair systems, such as transcatheter indirect annuloplasty, are available for treatment of secondary mitral regurgitation. IPD meta-analysis showed trends towards improvement in mean 6MWT distance and symptoms and reduction in HF hospitalisations [92–95]. Transcatheter mitral valve replacement is a possible alternative option [96, 97].

Mitral valve interventions are not recommended in patients with a life expectancy of <1 year due to extracardiac conditions. A personal care plan including palliative care should be discussed with the patient [80].

19.6.3 Non-cardiovascular Comorbidities

19.6.3.1 Cancer

As heart failure increases with age, so does cancer. The incidence rates for cancer overall go from fewer than 25 cases per 100,000 people in age groups under 20 years, to about 350 per 100,000 people in ages 45–49 years, to more than 1000 per 100,000 people in ages 60 years and older.

On the one hand, the risk of heart failure is increased in cancer patients determined by the cancer itself, cancer treatments, age, and underlying existing cardiovascular risk factors and comorbidities. Older people compared to younger people seem more susceptible to cardiotoxicity related to cancer therapies. The cardiotoxic effects of cancer therapies may be directly through cardiomyocyte damage or indirectly through ischaemia, myocarditis, systemic arterial hypertension, pulmonary hypertension, valvular heart disease, and arrhythmia.

On the other hand, the risk of worse cancer outcome in HF patients is increased due to not starting or withdrawing anticancer therapies [98].

Management of HF in cancer patients should be done in a multidisciplinary approach by preference in a cardio-oncology service and according to the standard guidelines of heart failure. Baseline cv risk assessment and a HFA-ICOS risk assessment to define the risk for cardiotoxicity are advised [99]. Close clinical and echocardiographic follow-up from the start, during, and after cancer treatment is advised. An absolute drop of >10% in LVEF to <50% indicates cardiac dysfunction. Global longitudinal strain is more sensitive to detect cardiac dysfunction at earlier stages. Monitoring of biomarkers such as (pro-NT)BNPs and troponin is also advised, especially in patients on immunotherapy with immune checkpoint inhibitors being at increased risk of myocarditis [100]. People who survived cancer should remain monitored in the long term as HF may develop several years after cancer treatment.

Fear for increased cardiotoxicity often leads to undertreatment of cancer in older people, and in clinical oncology trials, older people are underrepresented. A careful benefit risk assessment where quality of life might be more important than prolonged survival should be performed within a multidisciplinary team (family physician, cardiologist, oncologist, geriatrician) and in a shared decision with the patient.

19.6.3.2 Iron Deficiency and Anaemia

Iron deficiency and anaemia are prevalent in patients with heart failure (up to 55% in chronic HF and up to 80% in acute HF) and are independently associated with reduced exercise capacity, recurrent HF hospitalisations, and high CV and all-cause mortality. Anaemia in older people is highly prevalent due to chronic kidney disease, chronic inflammatory diseases, and iron deficiency.

In older HF patients with anaemia, the rate of death is doubled over 3 years with patients with low haematocrit being more likely to die from worsening heart failure [101].

Prevalence of iron deficiency in heart failure patients aged 75 years or older was found to be very high in very old patients with heart failure (73.8%; 95% CI: 65.7–80.8%), irrespective of type of heart failure, however more in those with HF with mid-range EF (78.4% (95% CI: 61.8–90.2%)) or HF with preserved EF(86.5% (95% CI: 74.2%–94.4%)) compared to HF with reduced EF 57.7% (95% CI: 43.2–71.3%) [102].

In patients with HF, iron deficiency is defined as either a serum ferritin concentration of <100 ng/mL or 100–299 ng/mL with transferrin saturation (TSAT) of <20%. The cause of iron deficiency in heart failure may be increased loss, reduced intake or absorption, and/or impaired iron metabolism related to the chronic inflammatory activation of HF, although the exact cause of iron deficiency in HF is not fully clear [103].

Iron deficiency by itself may impair functional capacity and skeletal muscle function and precipitate circulatory decompensation. It is associated with frailty, irrespective of anaemia [104]. It is recommended that all patients with HF are regularly screened for anaemia and iron deficiency with full blood count, serum ferritin concentration, and TSAT. In case of anaemia and/or iron deficiency, appropriate investigations should define their cause.

Based on RCTs and meta-analyses, iron supplementation with iv ferric carboxymaltose should be considered for the improvement of symptoms, exercise capacity, and QOL in patients with HF and LVEF <45% and should also be considered for the reduction of HF rehospitalisations in patients with LVEF <50% recently hospitalised for worsening HF (Ferric HF, FAIR HF, AFFIRM AHF). Similar benefits were seen in older and younger ages [105].

Oral iron therapy is not effective in iron repletion and in improvement of exercise capacity in patients with HFrEF and iron deficiency; therefore, it is not recommended for the treatment of iron deficiency in patients with HF. Erythropoietin-stimulating agents are not indicated for the treatment of anaemia in HF due to negative benefit-risk.

19.6.3.3 Infections

Infections, viral or bacterial, may trigger acute heart failure and may worsen chronic HF. Due to diminished activity of the immune system and underlying chronic disorders such as COPD, older persons are more susceptible for infections. On top of that, in the older patient, infection may lead to severe physical and mental dysregulation and rapid global deterioration. Sepsis can cause myocardial damage and depression leading to severe heart failure, with higher risk in people with pre-existing heart failure.

Older people and people with cardiovascular morbidity have a higher risk for all types of pneumonia (community acquired, healthcare related, and aspiration pneumonia) with increased risk for a severe course leading to respiratory and cardiac failure. An observational retrospective study identified clinical characteristics and risk factors of pulmonary infection in older patients with heart failure and found that age ≥70 years, diabetes, NYHA III, LVEF <55%, and CRP ≥10 mg/L are higher risks of pulmonary infections. Preventive measures targeting these risk factors might reduce pulmonary infections [106]. Influenza and coronavirus disease 2019 (COVID-19 (SARS-COV-2)) are major causes of morbidity and mortality, including heart failure. Course of the disease and case fatality rates are highest at older ages [107–109]. The multicentre, multinational PCHF-COVICAV registry assessed the outcome of hospitalised COVID-19 patients with heart failure (HF) compared with patients with other cardiovascular disease and/or risk factors (arterial hypertension, diabetes, or dyslipidaemia). Hospitalised COVID-19 patients with HF were at 1.5-fold increased risk for in-hospital death. In-hospital worsening of HF or acute HF de novo was common and associated with a further increase in in-hospital mortality(threefold increased likelihood) [110]. In observational studies and retrospective analyses, influenza vaccination is associated with a reduced risk of all-cause death in patients with HF [111]. Influenza, COVID-19 vaccination, and pneumococcal vaccination should be considered in patients with HF.

19.7 Considerations

As life expectancy continues to rise worldwide, the number of geriatric patients substantially increases.

Given the complexity of the older patient as well as of heart failure, the management requires a multidisciplinary team involving general practitioners, geriatricians, cardiologists, liaison nurses, pharmacists, physiotherapists, dieticians, psychologists, social workers, surgeons, and other healthcare workers.

Regular patient follow-up with global assessment of general status, mental and physical functional status, nutritional status, and full clinical exam should be performed, accompanied each time by a medication review, checking appropriate and inappropriate drugs and medication adherence. Educational support to the patient and family/caregivers should be given. Optimal care should translate in reduced hospital admissions.

If feasible, remote monitoring and/or teleconsultations might be provided.

An increase in resource utilisation and economic costs are expected in the growing older population with multiple comorbidities and with broad discrepancies in outcomes. Implementation of prospective databases, quality checks, and cost-efficiency of treatment plans is essential [112].

The ESC 2021 cardiovascular disease prevention guidelines are a major step forward by considering age more appropriately in the risk estimation scores (SCORE2-OP) and in risk factor management (lifetime benefit estimation of treatment), taking into account comorbidities and patient preferences.

Future guidelines should focus more on the ageing population, an ever-growing yet highly heterogeneous population which makes a tailored holistic personal approach more than necessary.

References

1. Unlu O, Levitan EB, Reshetnyak E, Kneifati-Hayek J, Diaz I, Archambault A, et al. Polypharmacy in older adults hospitalized for heart failure. Circ Hear Fail. 2020;13(11):e006977.
2. Cherubini A, Laroche ML, Petrovic M. Mastering the complexity: drug therapy optimization in geriatric patients. Eur Geriatr Med [Internet]. 2021;12(3):431–4. https://doi.org/10.1007/s41999-021-00493-5.
3. McDonagh TA, Metra M, Adamo M, Gardner RS, Baumbach A, Böhm M, et al. 2021 ESC guidelines for the diagnosis and treatment of acute and chronic heart failure. Eur Heart J [Internet]. 2021;42(36):3599–726. https://academic.oup.com/eurheartj/article/42/36/3599/6358045.
4. Jankowska EA, Vitale C, Uchmanowicz I, Tkaczyszyn M, Drozd M, Ponikowski P. Drug therapy in elderly heart failure patients. Eur Hear J Suppl. 2019;21:L8–L11.
5. Damy T, Chouihed T, Delarche N, Berrut G, Cacoub P, Henry P, et al. Diagnosis and management of heart failure in elderly patients from hospital admission to discharge: Position paper. 2021.
6. Ceia F, Fonseca C, Mota T, Morais H, Matias F, De Sousa A, et al. Prevalence of chronic heart failure in Southwestern Europe: the EPICA study. Eur J Heart Fail. 2002;4(4):531.
7. Van Riet EES, Hoes AW, Limburg A, Landman MAJ, Van Der Hoeven H, Rutten FH. Prevalence of unrecognized heart failure in older persons with shortness of breath on exertion. Eur J Heart Fail. 2014;16(7):772.
8. Bleumink GS, Knetsch AM, Sturkenboom MCJM, Straus SMJM, Hofman A, Deckers JW, et al. Quantifying the heart failure epidemic: prevalence, incidence rate, lifetime risk and prognosis of heart failure—the Rotterdam study. Eur Heart J. 2004;25(18):1614.
9. Koh AS, Tay WT, Teng THK, Vedin O, Benson L, Dahlstrom U, et al. A comprehensive population-based characterization of heart failure with mid-range ejection fraction. Eur J Heart Fail. 2017;19(12):1624.
10. Chioncel O, Lainscak M, Seferovic PM, Anker SD, Crespo-Leiro MG, Harjola VP, et al. Epidemiology and one-year outcomes in patients with chronic heart failure and preserved, mid-range and reduced ejection fraction: an analysis of the ESC heart failure long-term registry. Eur J Heart Fail. 2017;19(12):1574.
11. Heiat A, Gross CP, Krumholz HM. Representation of the elderly, women, and minorities in heart failure clinical trials. Arch Intern Med. 2002;162:1682–8.
12. Gerber Y, Weston SA, Redfield MM, Chamberlain AM, Manemann SM, Jiang R, et al. A contemporary appraisal of the heart failure epidemic in Olmsted County, Minnesota, 2000 to 2010. JAMA Intern Med. 2015;175(6):996–1004.

13. Tsao CW, Lyass A, Enserro D, Larson MG, Ho JE, Kizer JR, et al. Temporal trends in the incidence of and mortality associated with heart failure with preserved and reduced ejection fraction. JACC Heart Fail. 2018;6(8):678.
14. Owan TE, Hodge DO, Herges RM, Jacobsen SJ, Roger VL, Redfield MM. Trends in prevalence and outcome of heart failure with preserved ejection fraction. N Engl J Med. 2006;355(3):251.
15. Groenewegen A, Rutten FH, Mosterd A, Hoes AW. Epidemiology of heart failure. Eur J Heart Fail. 2020;22:1342–56.
16. Shah KS, Xu H, Matsouaka RA, Bhatt DL, Heidenreich PA, Hernandez AF, et al. Heart failure with preserved, borderline, and reduced ejection fraction: 5-year outcomes. J Am Coll Cardiol. 2017;70(20):2476.
17. Buddeke J, Valstar GB, Van Dis I, Visseren FLJ, Rutten FH, Den Ruijter HM, et al. Mortality after hospital admission for heart failure: improvement over time, equally strong in women as in men. BMC Public Health. 2020;20(1):36.
18. Blais C, Dai S, Waters C, Robitaille C, Smith M, Svenson LW, et al. Assessing the burden of hospitalized and community-care heart failure in Canada. Can J Cardiol. 2014;30(3):352.
19. Dai S, Walsh P, Wielgosz A, Gurevich Y, Bancej C, Morrison H. Comorbidities and mortality associated with hospitalized heart failure in Canada. Can J Cardiol. 2012;28(1):74.
20. Guerra F, Brambatti M, Matassini MV, Capucci A. Current therapeutic options for heart failure in elderly patients. Biomed Res Int. 2017;2017:1483873. (Table 1).
21. Hill E, Taylor J. Chronic heart failure care planning: considerations in older patients. Card Fail Rev. 2017;3(1):46.
22. Journal TP, Beezer BJ, Beezer J. Heart failure, older people and frailty diagnosis of heart failure and frailty can often be masked by other long-term conditions, making the delivery. 2021;(July 2019):1–16.
23. Anker SD, Butler J, Filippatos G, Ferreira JP, Bocchi E, Böhm M, et al. Empagliflozin in heart failure with a preserved ejection fraction. N Engl J Med. 2021;385(16):1451–61.
24. Mordi IR, Ouwerkerk W, Anker SD, Cleland JG, Dickstein K, Metra M, et al. Heart failure treatment up-titration and outcome and age: an analysis of BIOSTAT-CHF. Eur J Heart Fail. 2021;23(3):436.
25. Japp D, Shah A, Fisken S, Denvir M, Shenkin S, Japp A. Mineralocorticoid receptor antagonists in elderly patients with heart failure: a systematic review and meta-analysis. Age Ageing. 2017;46:18–25.
26. Ferreira JP, Rossello X, Eschalier R, McMurray JJV, Pocock S, Girerd N, et al. MRAs in elderly HF patients: individual patient-data meta-analysis of RALES, EMPAHSIS-HF, and TOPCAT. JACC Heart Fail. 2019;7(12):1012–21.
27. Desai RJ, Patorno E, Vaduganathan M, Mahesri M, Chin K, Levin R, et al. Effectiveness of angiotensin-neprilysin inhibitor treatment versus renin-angiotensin system blockade in older adults with heart failure in clinical care. Heart. 2021;107(17):1407.
28. Jhund PS, Fu M, Bayram E, Chen CH, Negrusz-Kawecka M, Rosenthal A, et al. Efficacy and safety of LCZ696 (sacubitril-valsartan) according to age: insights from PARADIGM-HF. Eur Heart J. 2015;36(38):2576.
29. Zannad F, Ferreira JP, Pocock SJ, Anker SD, Butler J, Filippatos G, et al. SGLT2 inhibitors in patients with heart failure with reduced ejection fraction: a meta-analysis of the EMPEROR-reduced and DAPA-HF trials. Lancet. 2020;396(10254):819.
30. Fioretto P, Bruin T, Johnsson E, Ptaszynska A, Parikh S, List JF. Safety and efficacy of the SGLT2 inhibitor dapagliflozin in older patients with type 2 diabetes. Diabetologia. 2013;56.
31. Cleland JGF, Tendera M, Adamus J, Freemantle N, Polonski L, Taylor J. The perindopril in elderly people with chronic heart failure (PEP-CHF) study. Eur Heart J. 2006;27(19):2338–45.
32. Flather MD, Shibata MC, Coats AJS, Van Veldhuisen DJ, Parkhomenko A, Borbola J, et al. FASTTRACK randomized trial to determine the effect of nebivolol on mortality and cardiovascular hospital admission in elderly patients with heart failure (SENIORS). Eur Heart J. 2005;26(3):215.

33. Düngen HD, Apostolović S, Inkrot S, Tahirović E, Töpper A, Mehrhof F, et al. Titration to target dose of bisoprolol vs. carvedilol in elderly patients with heart failure: the CIBIS-ELD trial. Eur J Heart Fail. 2011;13(6):670.
34. Düngen HD, Musial-Bright L, Inkrot S, Apostolović S, Edelmann F, Lainščak M, et al. Heart rate following short-term beta-blocker titration predicts all-cause mortality in elderly chronic heart failure patients: insights from the CIBIS-ELD trial. Eur J Heart Fail. 2014;16(8):907.
35. Yokote K, Terauchi Y, Nakamura I, Sugamori H. Real-world evidence for the safety of ipragliflozin in elderly Japanese patients with type 2 diabetes mellitus (STELLA-ELDER): final results of a post-marketing surveillance study. Expert Opin Pharmacother. 2016;17(15):1995.
36. Kambara T, Shibata R, Osanai H, Nakashima Y, Asano H, Sakai K, et al. Use of sodium–glucose cotransporter 2 inhibitors in older patients with type 2 diabetes mellitus. Geriatr Gerontol Int. 2018;18(1):108.
37. Trescoli Serrano C, Fajardo CJ, Arazo J, Tarazona-Santabalbina FJ. Real world safety and efficacy of SGLT-2 inhibitors in elderly type 2 diabetic patients. Innov Aging. 2017;1(Suppl 1):148.
38. Yabe D, Shiki K, Suzaki K, Meinicke T, Kotobuki Y, Nishida K, et al. Rationale and design of the EMPA-ELDERLY trial: a randomised, double-blind, placebo-controlled, 52-week clinical trial of the efficacy and safety of the sodium-glucose cotransporter-2 inhibitor empagliflozin in elderly Japanese patients with type 2 diabetes. BMJ Open. 2021;11(4):e045844.
39. Karagiannis T, Tsapas A, Athanasiadou E, Avgerinos I, Liakos A, Matthews DR, et al. GLP-1 receptor agonists and SGLT2 inhibitors for older people with type 2 diabetes: a systematic review and meta-analysis. Diabetes Res Clin Pract. 2021;174:108737.
40. Armstrong PW, Roessig L, Patel MJ, Anstrom KJ, Butler J, Voors AA, et al. A multicenter, randomized, double-blind, placebo-controlled trial of the efficacy and safety of the oral soluble guanylate cyclase stimulator: the VICTORIA trial. JACC Heart Fail. 2018;6(2):96–104.
41. Screever EM, Meijers WC, van Veldhuisen DJ, de Boer RA. New developments in the pharmacotherapeutic management of heart failure in elderly patients: concerns and considerations. Expert Opin Pharmacother. 2017;18:645.
42. Patel PH, Nguyen M, Rodriguez R, Surani S, Udeani G. Omecamtiv mecarbil: a novel mechanistic and therapeutic approach to chronic heart failure management. Cureus. 2021;13(1):e12419.
43. Teerlink JR, Diaz R, Felker GM, McMurray JJV, Metra M, Solomon SD, et al. Omecamtiv mecarbil in chronic heart failure with reduced ejection fraction: rationale and design of GALACTIC-HF. JACC Heart Fail. 2020;8:329.
44. Swedberg K. Stimulation of contractility in systolic heart failure. N Engl J Med. 2021;384(2):178.
45. Visseren FLJ, Mach F, Smulders YM, Carballo D, Koskinas KC, Bäck M, et al. 2021 ESC guidelines on cardiovascular disease prevention in clinical practice. Eur Heart J [Internet]. 2021;42(34):3227–3337. https://academic.oup.com/eurheartj/article/42/34/3227/6358713.
46. Burnier M, Egan BM. Adherence in hypertension: a review of prevalence, risk factors, impact, and management. Circ Res. 2019;124(7):1124.
47. OH, JFA, AB, GB, JPE, PF, et al. Guidelines for the management and diagnosis of congestive heart failure in the elderly adult. Rev Geriatr. 2004;29(8).
48. Abraham WT, Fonarow GC, Albert NM, Stough WG, Gheorghiade M, Greenberg BH, et al. Predictors of in-hospital mortality in patients hospitalized for heart failure. Insights from the Organized Program to Initiate Lifesaving Treatment in Hospitalized Patients with Heart Failure (OPTIMIZE-HF). J Am Coll Cardiol. 2008;52(5):347–56.
49. Detremerie C, De Backer T, Petrovic M. Polypharmacy and management of hypertension in frail elderly. Tijdschr Geneeskd. 2017;73(3).
50. Benetos A, Rossignol P, Cherubini A, Joly L, Grodzicki T, Rajkumar C, et al. Polypharmacy in the aging patient: management of hypertension in octogenarians. JAMA J Am Med Assoc. 2015;314(2):170.
51. Williams B, Mancia G, Spiering W, Rosei EA, Azizi M, Burnier M, et al. 2018 ESC/ESH guidelines for the management of arterial hypertension. J Hypertens. 2018;36:1956–2041.

52. Hanon O, Belmin J, Benetos A, Chassagne P, De Decker L, Jeandel C, et al. Consensus of experts from the French Society of Geriatrics and Gerontology on the management of heart failure in very old subjects. Arch Cardiovasc Dis. 2021;114(3):246.
53. Mach F, Baigent C, Catapano AL, Koskinas KC, Casula M, Badimon L, et al. 2019 ESC/EAS guidelines for the management of dyslipidaemias: lipid modification to reduce cardiovascular risk. Russ J Cardiol. 2020;25(5):3826.
54. Leung E, Wongrakpanich S, Munshi MN. Diabetes management in the elderly. Diabetes Spectrum. 2018;31:245.
55. Cosentino F, Grant PJ, Aboyans V, Bailey CJ, Ceriello A, Delgado V, et al. 2019 ESC guidelines on diabetes, pre-diabetes, and cardiovascular diseases developed in collaboration with the EASD. Eur Heart J. 2020;41(2):255–323.
56. Hindricks G, Potpara T, Dagres N, Bax JJ, Boriani G, Dan GA, et al. 2020 ESC guidelines for the diagnosis and management of atrial fibrillation developed in collaboration with the European Association for Cardio-Thoracic Surgery (EACTS). Eur Heart J. 2021;42:373–498.
57. Carlisle MA, Fudim M, DeVore AD, Piccini JP. Heart failure and atrial fibrillation, like fire and fury. JACC Heart Fail. 2019;7:447–56.
58. Gorenek B, Halvorsen S, Kudaiberdieva G, Bueno H, Van Gelder IC, Lettino M, et al. Atrial fibrillation in acute heart failure: a position statement from the Acute Cardiovascular Care Association and European Heart Rhythm Association of the European Society of Cardiology. Eur Heart J Acute Cardiovasc Care. 2020;9(4):348–57.
59. Slawik J, Adrian L, Hohl M, Lothschütz S, Laufs U, Böhm M. Irregular pacing of ventricular cardiomyocytes induces pro-fibrotic signalling involving paracrine effects of transforming growth factor beta and connective tissue growth factor. Eur J Heart Fail. 2019;21(4):482.
60. Kotecha D, Lam CSP, Van Veldhuisen DJ, Van Gelder IC, Voors AA, Rienstra M. Heart failure with preserved ejection fraction and atrial fibrillation: vicious twins. J Am Coll Cardiol. 2016;68:2217.
61. Smit MD, Moes ML, Maass AH, Achekar ID, Van Geel PP, Hillege HL, et al. The importance of whether atrial fibrillation or heart failure develops first. Eur J Heart Fail. 2012;14(9):1030.
62. Swedberg K, Olsson LG, Charlesworth A, Cleland J, Hanrath P, Komajda M, et al. Prognostic relevance of atrial fibrillation in patients with chronic heart failure on long-term treatment with beta-blockers: results from COMET. Eur Heart J. 2005;26(13):1303.
63. Mogensen UM, Jhund PS, Abraham WT, Desai AS, Dickstein K, Packer M, et al. Type of atrial fibrillation and outcomes in patients with heart failure and reduced ejection fraction. J Am Coll Cardiol. 2017;70(20):2490.
64. Lip GYH, Banerjee A, Boriani G, Chiang CE, Fargo R, Freedman B, et al. Antithrombotic therapy for atrial fibrillation: CHEST guideline and expert panel report. Chest. 2018;154(5):1121.
65. Hanon O, Chaussade E, David JP, Boulloche N, Vinsonneau U, Fauchier L, et al. SAFIR cohort: one-year prospective follow-up of very old and frail patients treated with direct oral anticoagulant, rivaroxaban. Arch Cardiovasc Dis Suppl. 2020;12(1):115.
66. Grymonprez M, Steurbaut S, De Backer TL, Petrovic M, Lahousse L. Effectiveness and safety of oral anticoagulants in older patients with atrial fibrillation: a systematic review and meta-analysis. Front Pharmacol. 2020;11:583311.
67. Reddy VY, Holmes D, Doshi SK, Neuzil P, Kar S. Safety of percutaneous left atrial appendage closure: results from the watchman left atrial appendage system for embolic protection in patients with AF (PROTECT AF) clinical trial and the continued access registry. Circulation. 2011;123(4):417.
68. Holmes DR, Kar S, Price MJ, Whisenant B, Sievert H, Doshi SK, et al. Prospective randomized evaluation of the watchman left atrial appendage closure device in patients with atrial fibrillation versus long-term warfarin therapy: the PREVAIL trial. J Am Coll Cardiol. 2014;64(1):1.
69. Hess PL, Sheng S, Matsouaka R, DeVore AD, Heidenreich PA, Yancy CW, et al. Strict versus lenient versus poor rate control among patients with atrial fibrillation and heart failure (from the get with the guidelines—Heart Failure Program). Am J Cardiol. 2020;125(6):894.

70. Sartipy U, Savarese G, Dahlström U, Fu M, Lund LH. Association of heart rate with mortality in sinus rhythm and atrial fibrillation in heart failure with preserved ejection fraction. Eur J Heart Fail. 2019;21(4):471.
71. Cho SW, Bin GH, Hwang JK, Chun KJ, Park KM, On YK, et al. Clinical features, predictors, and long-term prognosis of pacing-induced cardiomyopathy. Eur J Heart Fail. 2019;21(5):643.
72. St. John Sutton M, Plappert T, Adamson PB, Li P, Christman SA, Chung ES, et al. Left ventricular reverse remodeling with biventricular versus right ventricular pacing in patients with atrioventricular block and heart failure in the BLOCK HF trial. Circ Heart Fail. 2015;8(3):510–8.
73. Abdelrahman M, Subzposh FA, Beer D, Durr B, Naperkowski A, Sun H, et al. Clinical outcomes of his bundle pacing compared to right ventricular pacing. J Am Coll Cardiol. 2018;71(20):2319.
74. Ravi V, Beer D, Pietrasik GM, Hanifin JL, Ooms S, Ayub MT, et al. Development of new-onset or progressive atrial fibrillation in patients with permanent his bundle pacing versus right ventricular pacing: results from the RUSH HBP registry. J Am Heart Assoc. 2020;9(22):e018478.
75. Fauchier L, Alonso C, Anselme F, Blangy H, Bordachar P, Boveda S, et al. Position paper for management of elderly patients with pacemakers and implantable cardiac defibrillators Groupe de rythmologie et stimulation cardiaque de la Société française de cardiologie et Société française de gériatrie et gérontologie. Gériatrie Psychol Neuropsychiatr du Viellissement. 2019;14(3):239.
76. Vaes B, Rezzoug N, Pasquet A, Wallemacq P, Van Pottelbergh G, Matheï C, et al. The prevalence of cardiac dysfunction and the correlation with poor functioning among the very elderly. Int J Cardiol. 2012;155(1):134.
77. Stewart BF, Siscovick D, Lind BK, Gardin JM, Gottdiener JS, Smith VE, et al. Clinical factors associated with calcific aortic valve disease. J Am Coll Cardiol. 1997;29(3):630.
78. Osnabrugge RLJ, Mylotte D, Head SJ, Van Mieghem NM, Nkomo VT, Lereun CM, et al. Aortic stenosis in the elderly: disease prevalence and number of candidates for transcatheter aortic valve replacement: a meta-analysis and modeling study. J Am Coll Cardiol. 2013;62(11):1002.
79. Généreux P, Stone GW, O'Gara PT, Marquis-Gravel G, Redfors B, Giustino G, et al. Natural history, diagnostic approaches, and therapeutic strategies for patients with asymptomatic severe aortic stenosis. J Am Coll Cardiol. 2016;67:2263.
80. Vahanian A, Beyersdorf F, Praz F, Milojevic M, Baldus S, Bauersachs J, et al. 2021 ESC/EACTS guidelines for the management of valvular heart disease. Eur Heart J. 2022;43(7):561–632.
81. Afilalo J, Mottillo S, Eisenberg MJ, Alexander KP, Noiseux N, Perrault LP, et al. Addition of frailty and disability to cardiac surgery risk scores identifies elderly patients at high risk of mortality or major morbidity. Circ Cardiovasc Qual Outcomes. 2012;5(2):222–8.
82. Leon MB, Smith CR, Mack M, Miller DC, Moses JW, Svensson LG, et al. Transcatheter aortic-valve implantation for aortic stenosis in patients who cannot undergo surgery. N Engl J Med. 2010;363(17):1597.
83. Smith CR, Leon MB, Mack MJ, Miller DC, Moses JW, Svensson LG, et al. Transcatheter versus surgical aortic-valve replacement in high-risk patients. Surv Anesthesiol. 2012;56(1):4.
84. Makkar RR, Fontana GP, Jilaihawi H, Kapadia S, Pichard AD, Douglas PS, et al. Transcatheter aortic-valve replacement for inoperable severe aortic stenosis. N Engl J Med. 2012;366(18):1696.
85. Bertrand PB, Schwammenthal E, Levine RA, Vandervoort PM. Exercise dynamics in secondary mitral regurgitation: pathophysiology and therapeutic implications. Circulation. 2017;135:297.
86. Dziadzko V, Clavel MA, Dziadzko M, Medina-Inojosa JR, Michelena H, Maalouf J, et al. Outcome and undertreatment of mitral regurgitation: a community cohort study. Lancet. 2018;391(10124):960.

87. Goliasch G, Bartko PE, Pavo N, Neuhold S, Wurm R, Mascherbauer J, et al. Refining the prognostic impact of functional mitral regurgitation in chronic heart failure. Eur Heart J. 2018;39(1):39.
88. Ghoreishi M, Dawood MY, Gammie JS. Mitral valve surgery in elderly patients with mitral regurgitation: repair or replacement with tissue valve? Curr Opin Cardiol. 2013;28:164.
89. Farid S, Ladwiniec A, Hernández-Sánchez J, Povey H, Caruana E, Ali A, et al. Early outcomes after mitral valve repair versus replacement in the elderly: a propensity matched analysis. Heart Lung Circ. 2019;28(2):314–9.
90. Feldman T, Foster E, Glower DD, Kar S, Rinaldi MJ, Fail PS, et al. Percutaneous repair or surgery for mitral regurgitation. N Engl J Med. 2011;364(15):1395.
91. Coats AJS, Anker SD, Baumbach A, Alfieri O, von Bardeleben RS, Bauersachs J, et al. The management of secondary mitral regurgitation in patients with heart failure: a joint position statement from the Heart Failure Association (HFA), European Association of Cardiovascular Imaging (EACVI), European Heart Rhythm Association (EHRA), and European Association of Percutaneous Cardiovascular Interventions (EAPCI) of the ESC. Eur Heart J. 2021;42(13):1254–69.
92. Ruf TF, Kreidel F, Tamm AR, Geyer M, Hahad O, Zirbs JC, et al. Transcatheter indirect mitral annuloplasty induces annular and left atrial remodelling in secondary mitral regurgitation. ESC Heart Fail. 2020;7(4):1400.
93. Geyer M, Keller K, Sotiriou E, Tamm AR, Ruf TF, Kreidel F, et al. Association of transcatheter direct mitral annuloplasty with acute anatomic, haemodynamic, and clinical outcomes in severe mitral valve regurgitation. ESC Heart Fail. 2020;7(6):3336.
94. Giallauria F, Di Lorenzo A, Parlato A, Testa C, Bobbio E, Vigorito C, et al. Individual patient data meta-analysis of the effects of the CARILLON® mitral contour system. ESC Heart Fail. 2020;7(6):3383.
95. Malik AH, Zaid S, Yandrapalli S, Shetty S, Aronow WS, Ahmad H, et al. Trends and outcomes with Transcatheter versus surgical mitral valve repair in patients ≥80 years of age. Am J Cardiol. 2020;125(7):1083.
96. Del Val D, Ferreira-Neto AN, Wintzer-Wehekind J, Dagenais F, Paradis JM, Bernier M, et al. Early experience with transcatheter mitral valve replacement: a systematic review. J Am Heart Assoc. 2019;8(17):e013332.
97. Fiorilli PN, Herrmann HC, Szeto WY. Transcatheter mitral valve replacement: latest advances and future directions. Ann Cardiothorac Surg. 2021;10(1):85.
98. Reddy P, Shenoy C, Blaes AH. Cardio-oncology in the older adult. J Geriatr Oncol. 2017;8:308.
99. Lyon AR, Dent S, Stanway S, Earl H, Brezden-Masley C, Cohen-Solal A, et al. Baseline cardiovascular risk assessment in cancer patients scheduled to receive cardiotoxic cancer therapies: a position statement and new risk assessment tools from the Cardio-Oncology Study Group of the Heart Failure Association of the European Society of Cardiology in collaboration with the International Cardio-Oncology Society. Eur J Heart Fail. 2020;22(11):1945–60.
100. Anker MS, Von Haehling S, Anker SD. Novel biomarkers in heart failure and cardio-oncology. Kardiol Pol. 2019;77:329.
101. McDonagh T, Damy T, Doehner W, Lam CSP, Sindone A, van der Meer P, et al. Screening, diagnosis and treatment of iron deficiency in chronic heart failure: putting the 2016 European Society of Cardiology heart failure guidelines into clinical practice. Eur J Heart Fail. 2018;20:1664.
102. Mini P, Marc B, Fabien S, Chuzeville M. Prevalence of iron deficiency in patients aged 75 years or older with heart failure. J Geriatr Cardiol. 2018;15(11):682–6.
103. von Haehling S, Ebner N, Evertz R, Ponikowski P, Anker SD. Iron deficiency in heart failure: an overview. JACC Heart Fail. 2019;7:36–46.
104. Stugiewicz M, Tkaczyszyn M, Kasztura M, Banasiak W, Ponikowski P, Jankowska EA. The influence of iron deficiency on the functioning of skeletal muscles: experimental evidence and clinical implications. Eur J Heart Fail. 2016;18:762.

105. Ponikowski P, Macdougall IC, Bohm M, Comin Colet J, Filippatos G, Roubert B, et al. An individual patient data meta-analysis of outcomes in 4 randomized double-blind trials of iron-deficient patients with HFrEF and renal dysfunction treated with IV ferric carboxymaltose. Eur J Heart Fail. 2017;19.
106. Peng Q, Yang Q. Risk factors and management of pulmonary infection in elderly patients with heart failure. Medicine (Baltimore). 2021;100(38):e27238.
107. Tomasoni D, Italia L, Adamo M, Inciardi RM, Lombardi CM, Solomon SD, et al. COVID-19 and heart failure: from infection to inflammation and angiotensin II stimulation. Searching for evidence from a new disease. Eur J Heart Fail. 2020;22:957.
108. Rey JR, Caro-Codón J, Rosillo SO, Iniesta AM, Castrejón-Castrejón S, Marco-Clement I, et al. Heart failure in COVID-19 patients: prevalence, incidence and prognostic implications. Eur J Heart Fail. 2020;22(12):2205.
109. Vardeny O, Solomon SD. Influenza and heart failure: a catchy comorbid combination. JACC Heart Fail. 2019;7:118–20.
110. Sokolski M, Trenson S, Sokolska JM, D'Amario D, Meyer P, Poku NK, et al. Heart failure in COVID-19: the multicentre, multinational PCHF-COVICAV registry, vol. 8. ESC Heart Fail; 2021. p. 4955.
111. Modin D, Jørgensen ME, Gislason G, Jensen JS, Køber L, Claggett B, et al. Influenza vaccine in heart failure. Circulation. 2019;139(5):575–86.
112. Iyngkaran P, Liew D, Neil C, Driscoll A, Marwick TH, Hare DL. Moving from heart failure guidelines to clinical practice: gaps contributing to readmissions in patients with multiple comorbidities and older age. Clin Med Insights Cardiol. 2018;12:1179546818809358.

Pharmacological Treatment of Cognitive and Behavioral Disorders in Dementia

20

F. Trotta, L. Biscetti, and A. Cherubini

20.1 Introduction

Dementia (now called major neurocognitive disorder according to the DSM-5) is a syndrome, characterized by a decline in one or more cognitive domains (learning and memory, language, executive function, complex attention, perceptual-motor, social cognition) that interferes with independence in everyday activities. These cognitive deficits do not occur exclusively in the context of delirium, and they are not better explained by another mental disorder (e.g., major depressive disorder, schizophrenia). The major neurocognitive disorder differs from mild cognitive impairment (MCI) due to the presence of functional impairment that is related to the cognitive deficits [1, 2].

The incidence of dementia increases exponentially with increasing age [3]. Dementia and cognitive impairment are the leading chronic disease contributors to disability and dependence among older people worldwide. The need for support from a caregiver often starts early in the dementia course, intensifies as the illness progresses over time, and continues until death. Furthermore, behavioral disturbances are common in people with major neurocognitive disorder and cause significant impairment in quality of life and healthcare outcomes. Therefore, care and assistance to people with dementia requires a significant practical, psychological, and economic burden for families and society. Based on the etiology, there are several subtypes of dementia.

F. Trotta · A. Cherubini (✉)
Geriatria, Accettazione geriatrica e Centro di ricerca per l'invecchiamento, IRCCS INRCA, Ancona, Italy
e-mail: f.trotta@inrca.it; a.cherubini@inrca.it

L. Biscetti
Neurologia, IRCCS INRCA, Ancona, Italy
e-mail: l.biscetti@inrca.it

A. Cherubini et al. (eds.), *Optimizing Pharmacotherapy in Older Patients*, Practical Issues in Geriatrics, https://doi.org/10.1007/978-3-031-28061-0_20

20.1.1 Alzheimer's Disease (AD)

The most common (60–80% of all dementia cases) is Alzheimer's disease (AD). AD has a complex etiology, and our understanding of the relationships between the numerous pathways involved in the development of AD and subsequent neurodegeneration is still incomplete. AD is characterized by extracellular amyloid plaques, intracellular neurofibrillary tangles, and nerve cell death [4–6]. The typical form of Alzheimer's disease is characterized by a progressive episodic memory loss, subsequently accompanied by cognitive deficits involving non-amnestic domains, e.g., language and executive functions.

20.1.2 Vascular Dementia (VaD)

Vascular dementia (VaD) is considered the second most common cause of dementia in the elderly. VaD is defined as any form of dementia caused by cerebrovascular disease or impaired blood flow. VaD can develop after stroke and can have a stepwise progression; otherwise, it can develop in individuals without clinical strokes and can have a gradual progression [7].

20.1.3 Dementia with Lewy Bodies (DLB)

Dementia with Lewy bodies (DLB) is a neurodegenerative dementia with distinctive clinical features including fluctuations of cognitive ability, early and persistent visual hallucinations, parkinsonism, and sleep disorders. Lewy bodies are spherical, eosinophilic neuronal cytoplasmic inclusions composed of aggregates of alpha-synuclein, a synaptic protein. Between 3 and 7% of patients with dementia were found to meet the criteria for DLB [8].

20.1.4 Frontotemporal Dementia (FTD)

Frontotemporal dementia (FTD) is a disorder characterized by focal degeneration of the frontal and/or temporal lobes [9]. Age of onset is typically in the late 50s or early 60s. About half of frontotemporal dementias are genetically inherited: most of the mutations involve chromosome 17q21–22 and cause abnormalities in the microtubule-associated protein tau. The primary initial clinical manifestations include changes in personality and social behavior or language, while there is less memory impairment than in Alzheimer's disease; then, the disease progresses over time to a more global dementia affecting other cognitive domains. Symptoms of extrapyramidal or motor neuron involvement, including generalized muscle wasting, weakness, fasciculations, bulbar symptoms (e.g., dysphagia, dysphonia), and increased risk of aspiration pneumonia and premature death, may also occur in a subset of patients. FTD accounts for 2.5% of the dementias across all age groups and 10.2% in those aged <65 [10–12]. There are different types of frontotemporal dementia, depending on which part of the brain is affected: behavioral variant (frontal) and primary progressive aphasia.

20.1.5 Other Neurocognitive Disorders

Other subtypes are neurocognitive disorder due to Parkinson's disease, Huntington's disease, traumatic brain injury, HIV infection, and prion disease [2]. In very old patients, mixed dementia is quite common.

20.2 Pharmacologic Management of Cognitive Impairment

Currently, in the management of dementia, the main goals are to treat symptoms related to cognitive decline and to reduce the burden of the disease on caregivers. The recommended treatment strategy includes symptomatic pharmacological therapy of cognitive deficits, cognitive rehabilitation, environmental adaptations to reduce the impact of cognitive deficits and behavioral symptoms, nonpharmacological and pharmacological treatment of behavioral symptoms, and prevention and treatment of complications (e.g., falls, malnutrition, incontinence, bed rest; planning of care and family support; education and support of caregivers).

First of all, it is necessary to evaluate the medical history: The presence of drugs with anticholinergic effect can induce a worsening of cognitive functions. An increased risk for dementia was seen in people with higher use of anticholinergics (e.g., antihistamines, gastrointestinal tract antispasmodics, antivertigo agents/antiemetic, antidepressants, bladder antimuscarinics, skeletal muscle relaxant, antipsychotics, antiarrhythmic, antiparkinsonians). Therefore, prescribers should be aware of this potential association, and alternative drugs should be considered when possible. If no therapeutic alternative exists, prescribers should use the lowest effective dose and discontinue therapy if ineffective [13]. Some tools have been developed to quantify the cumulative anticholinergic effect of the drugs and their impact on cognitive functions and activities of life: Anticholinergic Drug Scale (ADS), the Anticholinergic Burden Scale (ACS), the Anticholinergic Risk Scale (ARS), and the Drug Burden Index (DBI) [14–17]. In the advanced stages of dementia, the worsening of the impairment of cognitive functions makes it impossible to carry out the activities of daily living. This leads to an increased risk of malnutrition, pneumonia, and pressure sores. As the disease progresses, treatment should be aimed to preserve the patient's well-being, rather than trying to prolong life. Provision of palliative care was empirically recognized as a care step in the management of dementia. However, as several studies have shown, the palliative care pathway for patients with dementia is still far from being accepted, shared, and applied [18–20]. Holmes criteria have been developed for the appropriateness of prescribing drugs in advanced dementia [21].

Dementia severity can be categorized by different instruments. Mini Mental State Examination (MMSE) and Montreal Cognitive Assessment (MoCA) are screening tools only evaluating the global cognitive functioning. Clinical Dementia Rating (CDR) and FAST Scale evaluate both the patient's cognitive and functional performance. Both nonpharmacological [22] and pharmacological approaches are used for dementia management, but in this chapter, only the latter will be presented [12]. There are no disease-modifying therapies approved for dementia; therefore, management is currently based on the treatment of neurological and neuropsychiatric symptoms in order to improve the quality of life of patients and their caregivers. Treatment for major cognitive impairment differs according to the etiologic subtype.

Until now, the only pharmacological treatments approved for dementia can be used on label in AD field. The use of the same drugs in other forms of dementia is off-label.

20.2.1 Acetylcholinesterase Inhibitors

The acetylcholinesterase inhibitors inhibit the brain acetylcholinesterase enzyme, responsible for the breakdown of the neurotransmitter acetylcholine, enhancing cholinergic neurotransmission in the brain by relative increase in acetylcholine at the synaptic cleft. They are considered symptomatic therapies and are not believed to be neuroprotective or to alter the underlying disease progression.

Cochrane reviews found that all three acetylcholinesterase inhibitors improve global and cognitive symptoms in people with mild to moderate AD. They all demonstrated efficacy compared with placebo, and a limited number of direct comparisons do not suggest major differences in efficacy or tolerability among the three drugs [23–27]. In a metanalysis review of 13 randomized, double-blinded, placebo-controlled trials, they were associated with slower decline [28]; however, the magnitude of the clinically relevant benefits is uncertain. Modest improvements were observed in activities of daily living and behaviors. Real-life studies found that treatment with these drugs reduced the rate of cognitive decline and increased survival during a follow-up lasting up to 8 years [29, 30].

Therefore, for patients with newly diagnosed mild to moderate AD dementia, a cholinesterase inhibitor therapy should be introduced. For patients with severe dementia, the efficacy of anticholinesterase inhibitors may be less clinically important, and fewer studies have been performed. Not all patients have a clinical benefit from these drugs. Studies have tried to investigate whether gene alterations can affect the clinical response to AChEI: the most relevant genes influencing AChEI efficacy and safety are APOE and CYPs [31].

Most of the studies of cholinesterase inhibitors have been performed in patients with a clinical diagnosis of AD, and data are more limited and less consistent for other forms of dementia. Evidence of mixed pathology at the time of autopsy is common, especially the combination of Alzheimer's disease and vascular pathology. Therefore, many experts find it reasonable to offer a trial of a cholinesterase inhibitor in patients with a clinical diagnosis of other types of dementia, including vascular dementia and Parkinson's disease dementia [32, 33].

Cholinesterase inhibitors are also suggested in most patients with DLB and may have comparatively greater symptomatic benefits (cognition, fluctuations, psychotic symptoms, activities of daily living, and reduced caregiver burden) than those observed in patients with AD. In some instances, the response is dramatic but temporary. A meta-analysis [34] concludes that donepezil and rivastigmine improved cognitive function and visual hallucinations in patients with DLB, but rivastigmine appears to induce more side effects than placebo. Evidence for galantamine in DLB remains sparse, limited to only open-label trials.

Conversely, the available data do not support the use of cholinesterase inhibitors in FTD except when there is uncertainty about whether the patient has FTD or AD [35–39].

Each drug is available for use orally, tablet or other formulations useful in dysphagia patients (donepezil as disintegrating sublingual tablet or transdermal patch, galantamine as oral solution, rivastigmine as transdermal patch or oral solution). A slow titration dosing regimen over 4–8 weeks is recommended to reach the target dose and minimize adverse effects. Selection of an agent is based largely upon ease of use, individual patient tolerability, cost, and clinician and patient preference. In a pragmatic, open-label trial, patients were randomly assigned to donepezil, galantamine, or rivastigmine using dosing and formulations at the discretion of the treating clinician. At 18 weeks, rates of discontinuation for any reason were similar for the three drugs; side-effect rates and profiles were largely similar among groups [26].

Cholinesterase inhibitors should be avoided in patients with baseline bradycardia or known cardiac conduction system disease (e.g., sick sinus syndrome, incomplete heart block) related to cholinergic toxicity and consequently risk of syncope, falls, and fractures. They should be used with caution in combination with drugs that induce bradycardia or alter nodal conduction [40, 41]. Other relative contraindications are asthma and peptic ulcer disease. The main features of cholinesterase inhibitors are summarized in Tables 20.1 and 20.2 [26, 42–46].

20.2.1.1 Treatment Monitoring

Dementia patients taking AChEI should be periodically reevaluated concerning cognition, function, neuropsychiatric and behavioral symptoms, and medication reconciliation [47–50].

After the introduction of anticholinesterase inhibitor, patients should be seen for follow-up at 3 and 6 months to assess drug tolerance and response. Patients on a stable dose of drug are then seen every 6–12 months thereafter. During treatment with anticholinesterase inhibitor, cardiac rate should be monitored and a drug discontinuation should be considered in the presence of bradycardia. Caregiver impression of change, behavioral symptoms, sleep, and other neuropsychiatric symptoms should also be assessed at each visit.

Table 20.1 Acetylcholinesterase inhibitors

AChE inhibitors	Formulation	Dose	Dose adjustments
Donepezil	– Once-daily tablet – Once-daily disintegrating sublingual tablet – Once-weekly patch formulation (not in Europe)	Starting dose: – 5 mg once daily Increasing to 10 mg per day after 4–6 weeks[a]	None
Galantamine	– Once-daily extended-release capsule – Twice-daily tablet – Twice-daily solution[b]	Starting dose: – 8 mg daily Increasing to 16 mg daily after 4 weeks Target maintenance dose: 24 mg daily after four more weeks[c]	Moderate renal (creatinine clearance 9–59 mL/min) or hepatic impairment: maximum dose 16 mg daily End-stage kidney disease (eGFR <9 mL/min) or severe hepatic impairment (Child-Pugh >9): **contraindicated**
Rivastigmine	– Oral capsule – Oral solution – Daily transdermal patch[d]	Transdermal patch starting dose: – 4.6 mg/24 htitrated upwards every 4 weeks until 13.3 mg/24 h Oral capsule or solution starting dose: – 1.5 mg twice daily Increasing to 1.5 mg twice-daily in 2- to 4-week intervals[e]	Body weight <50 kg and mild to moderate hepatic impairment: 4.6 mg/24 h Severe hepatic impairment: the patch has not been studied

[a] Withdrawal and adverse events were higher the higher the dose [42]

[b] Given with meals to decrease the risk of nausea

[c] Galantamine improves global and cognitive symptoms at doses of 16 mg/day or greater, in people with mild to moderate AD, for at least 6 months [43]

[d] The patch is preferred due to superior pharmacokinetics and tolerability (less nausea, vomiting, weight loss, dizziness) with similar efficacy [44]

[e] One trial found that side effects of oral rivastigmine may be ameliorated and higher daily doses achieved when it is given three times a day, rather than twice daily [44]

There is not a universal consensus on how long to continue cholinesterase inhibitors in patients who are tolerating therapy. Therapy should not be continued in patients who do not appear to be benefiting or who have significant side effects: in the absence of subjective or objective improvement after a 6-month trial, some clinicians, patients, and families may choose to stop treatment. An alternative cholinesterase inhibitor is not typically used in this setting, while another drug approved in AD field, memantine, can be added or substituted in patients with moderate to severe dementia, or it can be used as a single agent among patients who do not tolerate cholinesterase inhibitors.

Table 20.2 Cholinesterase inhibitors: Side effects

Side effects	Drugs	Actions
Gastrointestinal upset [26, 45, 46] (upset stomach, nausea, diarrhea, anorexia)	Donepezil seems to be less likely to cause gastrointestinal upset than the other two drugs	• Switching to donepezil may be reasonable in patients who do not tolerate galantamine or rivastigmine even if they are taken with meals
Weight loss, anorexia		• Nutritional counseling • If comorbid depression exist, mirtazapine is a good choice of antidepressant because it can augment appetite
Bradycardia, Hypotension		• If no other modifiable cause is identified, cholinergic therapy should be discontinued in patients who develop symptomatic bradycardia and/or hypotension
Sleep disturbances (insomnia, vivid dreams, nightmares, and other sleep disturbances)	More common with donepezil	• Recognize and treat, as they are a major contributor to caregiver distress and are associated with an increased likelihood of institutionalization
Others	Donepezil → rare cases of rhabdomyolysis and/or neuroleptic malignant syndrome in post-marketing surveillance Rivastigmine transdermal patch → skin irritation: application sites should be rotated	

20.2.2 Memantine

Memantine is a moderate affinity uncompetitive N-methyl-D-aspartate (NMDA) receptor antagonist licensed for use in moderate and severe AD. Glutamate is the principal excitatory amino acid neurotransmitter in cortical and hippocampal neurons. One of the receptors activated by glutamate is the NMDA receptor, which is involved in learning and memory. Excessive NMDA stimulation can be induced by ischemia and lead to excitotoxicity.

A Cochrane review found a small clinical benefit for cognitive function and for behavior and mood of memantine in people with moderate to severe AD regardless the concomitant acetylcholinesterase inhibitor assumption, but no benefit in people with mild AD [51]. Memantine does not appear to have significant side effects: dizziness, headache, and constipation are the most common ones, while confusion and hallucinations are infrequent, but increased agitation and delusional behaviors may occur in some patients with AD. The dosage of memantine is 10–20 mg, which should be slowly titrated (an increase of 5 mg each week, starting from a dosage of 5 mg). The standard dosage is 20 mg, with the exception of patients with moderate-severe renal failure (glomerular filtration rate 5–29 mL/min), for which the maximum dosage is 10 mg per day. A fixed-dose combination with donepezil and memantine was approved for moderate to severe AD who are on stable donepezil therapy [52].

In DLB, whether memantine should be used as monotherapy or together with cholinesterase inhibitors remains unclear and requires further study.

20.2.3 Aducanumab

Aducanumab is a recombinant monoclonal antibody directed against amyloid beta. The US Food and Drug Administration (FDA) has approved aducanumab for the treatment of mild AD using the accelerated approval pathway, based on the positive results of one of the two pivotal phase III trials (the results in the other were negative) and aducanumab's effect on a surrogate endpoint of reducing amyloid beta plaques in the brain [53].

The approval of aducanumab has caused on ongoing controversy in the scientific community as it is not still clear whether the reduction of beta amyloid plaques induced by the drug leads to clinical benefits. In fact, faced to a robust effect of aducanumab with respect to reduction in brain amyloid levels, observed benefits on clinical endpoints have been small and inconsistent and therefore uncertain [54].

To date, aducanumab has been administered primarily in research settings in the USA limited to the following patients [55]:

- Mild cognitive impairment or mild AD (MMSE ≥21, MoCA ≥17, or CDR 0.5–1)
- Documented amyloid pathology: Clinicians should limit use of aducanumab to those patients proven to be amyloid positive (by amyloid positron emission tomography [PET] scan or lumbar puncture)

Contraindications Cases where aducanumab therapy should not be offered:

- Cognitive decline attributed to non-AD pathologies
- AD in the setting of Down syndrome
- High risk of hemorrhagic side effects (hemorrhagic findings on brain MRI including >4 microhemorrhages, any areas of superficial siderosis, prior macro-hemorrhage, and underlying brain lesion or vascular malformation; anticoagulant or antiplatelet use other than aspirin 81 mg daily, bleeding disorders, or any other condition leading to increased risk of central nervous system hemorrhage)
- Unstable medical/ psychiatric conditions
- Pregnancy or breastfeeding

Furthermore, patients with an apolipoprotein E epsilon allele have a greater risk of side effects.

Adverse effects Adverse effects observed with aducanumab include the following [56]:

- Amyloid-related imaging abnormalities (ARIA), especially in APOE ε4 carriers
- Hypersensitivity, including angioedema and urticaria
- Headache, falls, diarrhea, and confusion (except for diarrhea, these may reflect symptoms of ARIA)

In addition, up to 0.6% of patients in the clinical trials developed aducanumab antibodies, and no determination was made as to whether such antibodies are neutralizing.

In Europe, Biogen withdrew its application for a marketing authorization of Aducanumab for the treatment of Alzheimer's disease on April 20, 2022.

Other monoclonal antibodies against beta-amyloid, such as gantenerumab, crenezumab, and lecanemab, are being tested in clinical trials enrolling patients with mild AD and individuals with early cognitive impairment. Furthermore, gantenerumab and solanezumab are also being studied in preclinical patients with autosomal dominant AD mutations, but without cognitive symptoms. So far, none of these drugs has been approved by regulatory agencies in the USA and Europe for clinical use.

20.2.4 Vascular Risk Modifications

Patients with cognitive impairment and clinical or radiological evidence of cerebrovascular disease must undergo screening and treatment for vascular risk factors: this intervention is essential in the prevention of dementia since stroke is associated with a greater risk of cognitive intervention and post-stroke dementia is associated with higher mortality [57–59].

Treatment of cardiovascular risk factors is based on antihypertensive therapy [60, 61], diabetes management, statins [62–64], and antithrombotic therapy [64].

20.2.5 Other Therapies

Other agents have been studied for VaD, but the trials have mostly been small and without conclusive results [65]: nimodipine, ergot alkaloids (hydergine, nicergoline), cerebrolysin, vitamin E, ginkgo biloba, xanthine derivatives (propentofylline, pentoxifylline, and denbufylline), cytidinediphosphocholine, and piracetam. None of these therapies are recommended at this time.

20.2.6 Other Considerations

There is no specific therapy for frontotemporal dementias. Treatment is generally supportive: The environment should be bright, cheerful, and familiar and should be designed to reinforce orientation (e.g., placing large clocks and calendars in the room). Symptoms are treated as needed: behavioral disturbances and parkinsonism (patients with FTD who have parkinsonism typically do not respond to dopaminergic medications).

In DLB also, there are currently no treatments with evidence of disease-modifying effects, and treatment is primarily symptomatic and targeted toward specific disease manifestations: cognition and neuropsychiatric symptoms, parkinsonian symptoms, REM sleep behavior disorder, orthostatic hypotension, and urinary symptoms.

20.3 Behavioral and Psychological Symptoms

In 1996, a definition of behavioral and psychological symptoms in dementia (BPSD) was proposed as a heterogeneous group of clinical manifestations observed in patients with dementia and characterized by alterations in perception, thought content, mood, and behavior, including agitation, aggression, delusions, hallucinations, paranoia, wandering, depression, apathy, disinhibition, and sleep disturbances (IPA Consensus conference; 1996).

Most patients with dementia develop one or more BPSD [66]. BPSD can have serious consequences: they are associated with worsening cognition and progression to more severe stages of dementia and lead to individual suffering and impact the caregiver burden; they increase the risk for secondary complications such as falls and fractures leading to emergency room admissions, and ultimately institutionalization and result in higher costs of therapy and caregiving.

The pathophysiology of BPSD is complex and multifactorial [67]. Considering that BPSD tend to occur in clusters, often co-present, a multiple neurotransmitter dysregulation maybe involved (monoamine 5-hydroxytryptamine, serotonin, dopaminergic system, and histamine) [68, 69].

In order to measure treatment effects, frequency and severity of BPSD should be quantified at baseline, possibly using a validity scale, such as the Neuropsychiatric Inventory (NPI) and Behavioral Pathology in Alzheimer's Disease Rating Scale (BEHAVE-AD) [69].

First, Garre-Olmo identified four clusters of symptoms [70]:

1. "psychotic" cluster ("delusions" and/or "hallucinations" items)
2. "emotional" cluster ("agitation/aggression" and/or "depression/dysphoria" and/or "anxiety" and/or "irritability" items)
3. "behavioral" cluster ("euphoria/elation" and/or "apathy" and/or "disinhibition" and/or "aberrant motor behavior" items)
4. "sleep and night-time behavior disorders" and "appetite and eating disorders"

Apathy, depression, anxiety, and agitation were found to be the most frequent forms of BPSD. However, a recent systematic review revealed substantial variation in the reported prevalence, incidence, and longitudinal course among different studies. In an individual patient, the type and severity of BPSD tend to change over time, but some forms such as wandering seem to be more persistent. Overall, the "natural course" of BPSD over time is still largely unknown [70].

The treatment of BPSD is often highly challenging. BPSD management requires both a patient-centered and caregiver-centered focus. Treating concomitant somatic diseases can reduce BPSD. Effective pain management is part of successful BPSD treatment. It is important to always consider medication toxicity, such as anticholinergic side effects, or abrupt discontinuation of chronic therapies. Pharmacotherapy for BPSD is frequently provided, but it carries the risk of serious side effects. Therefore, nonpharmacological therapies are the first choice, and they should be continued also when pharmacotherapy is necessary.

The topic of depression is treated in a separate chapter, so below we will only deal with the management of hyperactivity/agitation.

20.3.1 Treatment of Hyperactivity-Impulsivity-Irritiability-Disinhibition-Aggression-Agitation (HIDA) Domain

The hyperactivity-impulsivity-irritability-disinhibition-aggression-agitation (HIDA) domain represents one of the most difficult sets of symptoms to manage and accounts for much of the burden for caregivers and hospital staff. These symptoms can arise from a variety of underlying causes in patients with dementia, and identifying the genesis of the abnormal behavior is critical to effective management (e.g., delirium, depression, sleep disorders, misperception). Many studies suggest non-pharmacological treatments for HIDA domain symptoms as first line, for instance, music therapy, sensory interventions, and person-centered communication skill for caregivers [71].

When non-pharmacological intervention fails and neuropsychiatric symptoms produced severe distress or safety issues, acute pharmacologic therapy with an antipsychotic drug is often necessary [72]. NICE Guidelines recommend (1) to use the lowest effective dose for the shortest possible time, (2) to reassess the patients at least every 6 weeks, (3) to check whether they still need medication, and (4) to stop treatment with antipsychotics if the person with dementia is not getting a clear ongoing benefit from taking these drugs (after discussion with the person taking them and their family members or careers when appropriate). To this regard, it should be acknowledged that many of these drugs may increase mortality, and most of them are not approved for treatment of behavioral disorders in patients with dementia by FDA. Despite the warnings issued by the FDA, the EMA and the UK Medicines and Healthcare Products Regulatory Agency mainly related to increased risk of death, cerebrovascular adverse events (CVAEs), parkinsonism, sedation, gait disturbance, cognitive decline, and pneumonia, antipsychotics are often used in individuals with dementia for sustained periods (≥6 months). It is noteworthy that the drug-related mortality risk remains elevated for at least 2 years, with a risk of death that is greater than the longer duration of use [69].

Benzodiazepines are not recommended for the management of neuropsychiatric symptoms in elderly patients with dementia because they can induce worsening of gait and balance, potential paradoxical agitation, and physical dependence [73].

20.3.1.1 Antipsychotic Drugs

Antipsychotic drugs, also known as **neuroleptics**, are a class of psychotropic medication primarily used to manage psychosis (including delusions, hallucinations, paranoia, or disordered thought), principally in schizophrenia but also in a range of other psychotic disorders. They have a complex mechanism of action, interacting with several different class of receptors, mainly dopaminergic and serotoninergic. Specifically, all antipsychotic drugs block dopaminergic D2 receptors with different grade of affinity, and some of them show also a significant interaction with serotoninergic 5HT2A receptors. Based on their potency as dopamine D2 receptor antagonists and their actions on serotonin 5-HT2A receptors, antipsychotics are commonly classed as either typical or atypical, with the latter showing a more effective modulation of 5HT2A receptors.

Typical (or First-Generation) Antipsychotics

Typical antipsychotics have significant potential to cause extrapyramidal side effects (i.e., drug-related parkinsonism) and tardive dyskinesia due to their strong block of D2 receptors. This propensity to cause movement disorders is the primary difference between typical and atypical antipsychotics. The main mechanism of action of all typical antipsychotics indeed appears to be postsynaptic blockade of brain dopamine D2 receptors [74]. Evidence supporting this mechanism includes strong antagonism of D2 receptors in both cortical and striatal areas, a high correlation between D2 receptor binding and clinical potency, and a consistent requirement of about 65% D2 receptor occupancy for antipsychotic efficacy in functional imaging studies. Aside from their common activity as D2 antagonists, each typical antipsychotic drug has distinct effects on neuronal 5-HT2a, alpha-1, histaminic, and muscarinic receptors, which generally correspond to their individual side effect profiles.

Based on their chemical structures, they are grouped into several classes: (1) phenothiazines (e.g., chlorpromazine and fluphenazine), (2) butyrophenones (e.g., haloperidol), (3) benzamides (e.g., sulpiride and tiapride).

The pharmacologic differences are the basis for the classification of typical antipsychotics as either high- or low-potency drugs. The high-potency typical antipsychotics (fluphenazine, haloperidol, loxapine, perphenazine, pimozide, thiothixene, and trifluoperazine) have low activity on histaminic and muscarinic receptors. They are associated with relatively small risk of sedation and weight gain but a high risk for extrapyramidal side effects.

The low-potency typical antipsychotics (chlorpromazine and thioridazine), instead, have high histaminic and muscarinic activity with a corresponding increased prevalence of sedation and anticholinergic effects but lower risk of extrapyramidal side effects compared to high-potency antipsychotics.

All these drugs can be administered in oral and/or i.m. and/or i.v. formulation, and all of these can cause QTc prolongation (in particular, haloperidol, for which QTc prolongation is an absolute contraindication).

Nowadays, a long-acting injectable formulation of some antipsychotic medications, for instance, haloperidol, is also available. However, the American Psychiatric Association (APA) recommends that in individuals with dementia complicated by agitation or psychosis, a long-acting injectable antipsychotic medication should not be utilized unless it is otherwise indicated for a co-occurring chronic psychotic illness [72] (Recommendation 1B). From a general point of view, the use of all typical antipsychotic medications is off-label in dementia context, due to a non-clear evidence of a favorable risk/benefit profile.

Atypical (or Second-Generation) Antipsychotics

Atypical antipsychotic drugs (AAPs), also known as nonconventional, are more active on serotoninergic receptors (mainly on 5HT2A) and less active on dopaminergic receptors than typical antipsychotics. Based on this pharmacodynamic profile, unconventional antipsychotics, compared to conventional antipsychotics, may cause less cognitive impairment, induce significantly fewer extrapyramidal symptoms and a lower risk of tardive dyskinesia, and have few or no effects on prolactin production (with exception of risperidone, which increases prolactin as conventional antipsychotics). On the other hand, most of these drugs can generate a metabolic syndrome, with insulin resistance, weight gain, and hypertension. Very relevant are also the risk of falls and fractures and of QTc prolongation.

In general, adverse events with the use of these drugs in patients with dementia are dose related.

The atypical antipsychotics are very similar to each other in efficacy but differ in adverse effects, so the selection of a specific drugs should be based on consideration of side effects and individual patient characteristics: For instance, olanzapine, which has a relatively high rate of sedation, may be prescribed for patients with agitation or insomnia; furthermore, it could be useful in patients with loss of appetite because weight gain is a frequent side effect of this drug.

Among AAPs, only risperidone is indicated for the short-term management of persisting and severe aggression in individuals with AD, even if, in clinical practice, also other antipsychotic therapies are used off-label.

Typical Vs Atypical Antipsychotics

Many clinical studies have systematically compared atypical with typical antipsychotics in terms of efficacy, quality of life, tolerability, dropout, and side effects, and most of them demonstrated a better outcome with atypical ones in several aspects. From a general point of view, even if not all atypical antipsychotics drugs have achieved the same results, AAPs have been shown to have an improved pharmacological profile in the treatment of positive and negative symptoms compared to the prototypical typical haloperidol, with clozapine being probably the most effective [75]. To this regard, it is noteworthy the uniqueness of clozapine's clinical effect based on its ideal activity on dopamine and serotonin receptors, strongly in favor of the second, and also on other targets, i.e., muscarinic and noradrenergic receptors, glycine transporter, and BDNF. Conversely, risperidone's activity is mostly based on a similar antagonism at dopamine and serotonin receptors, making it the least atypical in the family of atypical antipsychotics. For these reasons, some authors proposed a continuum spectrum of atypia that ranges from risperidone, the least atypical, to clozapine, the most atypical. On the continuum spectrum of atypia, there are three levels of atypicality, based on the molecular profiles, wherein risperidone is the least atypical (level I) and clozapine is the most atypical (level III), while all others (*aripiprazole, amisulpride, luraseride, ziprasidone, asenapine, quetiapine, olanzapine*) fall within these two extremes of the spectrum (level II) [76].

Anyway, it is important to underline that although clozapine has a good efficacy and a low risk of extrapyramidal side effects, its use requires regular blood monitoring due to a risk of agranulocytosis. Therefore, clozapine should be used with caution, and generally, it should be introduced only if other drugs are ineffective (however, in some cases, for instance, for the treatment of Parkinson's disease patients with psychosis, clozapine represents the first-choice drug).

Risperidone

Risperidone, at low dosages (1–2 mg per day), shows higher affinity for 5-HT 2A than for D2, while at high dosages (3–6 mg per day), the affinity for D2 overcomes that for 5-HT2A. Risperidone has shown good efficacy in treating positive symptoms. However, the strong binding to 5-HT 2C, α1, and H1 is responsible for the side effects, such as weight gain, sedation, orthostatic hypotension, and parkinsonism.

Aripiprazole

Together with amisulpride, aripiprazole represents an exception among AAPs, given the relatively low affinity to 5HT2A receptor. It is associated to a low risk of extrapyramidal side effects, and it is efficacious against both positive and negative symptoms. Aripiprazole causes minimal weight gain and sedation and does not produce elevation in serum prolactin levels; most importantly, unlike other neuroleptics, it does not significantly lengthen QTc interval. However, based on randomized controlled trial performed to test efficacy and safety of aripiprazole in the context of Alzheimer's dementia [77], faced to a small but statistically significant efficacy in controlling BPSD in AD patients, aripiprazole resulted to be associated to higher mortality and higher risk of stroke compared to placebo. Although a real causal role of the drug in inducing these severe side effects is still controversial, the prevalent expert opinion suggests that aripiprazole should be used with caution in AD patients [78].

Olanzapine

Olanzapine can be started at a dose of 2.5 mg daily and titrated up to a maximum of 5 mg twice a day (the incidence of extrapyramidal symptoms is quite low at doses of 5 mg per day). It appears to be quite effective for treating neuropsychiatric symptoms in Alzheimer's disease or vascular dementia [79]. Metabolic side effects (weight gain, diabetes, and hypercholesterolemia) are more common compared to other antipsychotic drugs.

Quetiapine

Quetiapine generally is used at a dose of 25 mg at bedtime and titrating up a maximum of 75 mg twice a day. It has different effects based on the dose administrated: antipsychotic effect with 600 mg per day, antidepressant with 300 mg per day, hypnotic effect with 50 mg per day. Because of its effects on the cardiac repolarization, it is necessary to check the QTc before the prescription.

In conclusion, it must be highlighted that only three drugs are licensed for BPSD treatment in dementia: *pimavanserin* (only in the USA) and *clozapine* for hallucinations and delusions associated with Parkinson's disease (PD) psychosis and *risperidone* for short-term treatment of persistent aggression in moderate-to-severe Alzheimer's disease (AD). In the remaining cases, the use of antipsychotics is off-label and guided by the physician's judgment.

Risperidone, aripiprazole, and olanzapine have been evaluated in multiple studies and show improvement in symptoms like severe agitation, aggression, and psychosis (such as delusions and hallucinations) in patients with dementia.

Maximal duration of antipsychotic treatment should be limited according to 3Ts (target symptom, titration, time) whereby the duration of the treatment should not exceed 3 months due to an increased risk of mortality, and regular reassessment is necessary.

Antipsychotics are generally to be avoided when diagnosing dementia with Lewy bodies due to particular sensitivity of these patients to extrapyramidal side effects. A use with caution of quetiapine and clozapine is possible [80, 81].

References

1. American Psychiatric Association. Diagnostic and statistical manual of mental disorders, fifth edition (DSM-5). American Psychiatric Publishing; 2013.
2. Hugo J, Ganguli M. Dementia and cognitive impairment: epidemiology, diagnosis, and treatment. Clin Geriatr Med. 2014;30(3):421–42.
3. Prince M, Wimo A, Guerchet M, Ali GC, Wu YT, Prina M. World Alzheimer report 2015, the global impact of dementia: an analysis of prevalence, incidence, cost and trends. Alzheimer's Disease International; 2015.
4. Selkoe DJ, Hardy J. The amyloid hypothesis of Alzheimer's disease at 25 years. EMBO Mol Med. 2016;8(6):595–608.
5. Iqbal K, del C Alonso A, Chen S, Chohan MO, El-Akkad E, Gong CX, Khatoon S, Li B, Liu F, Rahman A, Tanimukai H, Grundke-Iqbal I. Tau pathology in Alzheimer disease and other tauopathies. Biochim Biophys Acta. 2005;1739(2–3):198–210.
6. Mufson EJ, Counts SE, Perez SE, Ginsberg SD. Cholinergic system during the progression of Alzheimer's disease: therapeutic implications. Expert Rev Neurother. 2008;8(11):1703–18.
7. Wolters FJ, Ikram MA. Epidemiology of vascular dementia. Arterioscler Thromb Vasc Biol. 2019;39(8):1542–9.
8. Erkkinen MG, Kim MO, Geschwind MD. Clinical neurology and epidemiology of the major neurodegenerative diseases. Cold Spring Harb Perspect Biol. 2018;10(4):a033118.
9. The Lund and Manchester Groups. Clinical and neuropathological criteria for frontotemporal dementia. J Neurol Neurosurg Psychiatry. 1994;57(4):416.
10. Lopez OL, Kuller LH. Epidemiology of aging and associated cognitive disorders: prevalence and incidence of Alzheimer's disease and other dementias. Handb Clin Neurol. 2019;167:139–48.
11. Oh ES, Rabins PV. Dementia. Ann Intern Med. 2019;171(5):ITC33–48.
12. Arvanitakis Z, Shah RC, Bennett DA. Diagnosis and management of dementia: review. JAMA. 2019;322(16):1589–99.
13. Gray SL, Anderson ML, Dublin S, Hanlon TJ, Hubbard R, Walker R, Yu O, Crane PK, Larson EB. Cumulative use of strong anticholinergics and incident dementia: a prospective cohort study. JAMA Intern Med. 2015;175(3):401–7.

14. Rudolph JL, Salow MJ, Angelini MC, McGlinchey RE. The anticholinergic risk scale and anticholinergic adverse effects in older persons. Arch Intern Med. 2008;168(5):508–13.
15. O'Connell J, Burke É, Mulryan N, O'Dwyer C, Donegan C, McCallion P, McCarron M, Henman MC, O'Dwyer M. Drug burden index to define the burden of medicines in older adults with intellectual disabilities: an observational cross-sectional study. Br J Clin Pharmacol. 2018;84(3):553–67.
16. Salahudeen MS, Duffull SB, Nishtala PS. Anticholinergic burden quantified by anticholinergic risk scales and adverse outcomes in older people: a systematic review. BMC Geriatrics. 2015;15:31.
17. Sargent L, Nalls M, Amella EJ, Mueller M, Lageman SK, Bandinelli S, Colpo M, Slattum PW, Singleton A, Ferrucci L. Anticholinergic drug induced cognitive and physical impairment: results from the InCHIANTI Study. J Gerontol A Biol Sci Med Sci. 2020;75(5):995–1002.
18. Mataqi M, Aslanpour Z. Factors influencing palliative care in advanced dementia: a systematic review. BMJ Support Palliat Care. 2020;10(2):145–56.
19. Mitchell SL, Teno JM, Kiely DK, Shaffer ML, Jones RN, Prigerson HG, Volicer L, Givens JL, Hamel MB. The clinical course of advanced dementia. N Engl J Med. 2009;361(16):1529–38.
20. Sampson EL, Candy B, Davis S, Gola AB, Harrington J, King M, Kupeli N, Leavey G, Moore K, Nazareth I, Omar RZ, Vickerstaff V, Jones L. Living and dying with advanced dementia: a prospective cohort study of symptoms, service use and care at the end of life. Palliat Med. 2018;32(3):668–81.
21. Holmes HM, Sachs GA, Shega JW, Hougham GW, Cox HD, Dale W. Integrating palliative medicine into the care of persons with advanced dementia: identifying appropriate medication use. J Am Geriatr Soc. 2008;56:1306–11.
22. Abraha I, Rimland JM, Trotta FM, Dell'Aquila G, Cruz-Jentoft A, Petrovic M, Gudmundsson A, Soiza R, O'Mahony D, Guaita A, Cherubini A. Systematic review of systematic reviews of non-pharmacological interventions to treat behavioural disturbances in older patients with dementia. The SENATOR-OnTop series. BMJ Open. 2017;7(3):e012759.
23. Wilcock G, Howe I, Coles H, Lilienfeld S, Truyen L, Zhu Y, Bullock R, Kershaw P, GAL-GBR-2 Study Group. A long-term comparison of galantamine and donepezil in the treatment of Alzheimer's disease. Drugs Aging. 2003;20(10):777.
24. Ancoli-Israel S, Amatniek J, Ascher S, Sadik K, Ramaswamy K. Effects of galantamine versus donepezil on sleep in patients with mild to moderate Alzheimer disease and their caregivers: a double-blind, head-to-head, randomized pilot study. Alzheimer Dis Assoc Disord. 2005;19(4):240.
25. Bullock R, Touchon J, Bergman H, Gambina G, He Y, Rapatz G, Nagel J, Lane R. Rivastigmine and donepezil treatment in moderate to moderately-severe Alzheimer's disease over a 2-year period. Curr Med Res Opin. 2005;21(8):1317.
26. Campbell NL, Perkins AJ, Gao S, Skaar TC, Li L, Hendrie HC, Fowler N, Callahan CM, Boustani MA. Adherence and tolerability of Alzheimer's disease medications: a pragmatic randomized trial. J Am Geriatr Soc. 2017;65(7):1497.
27. Chodosh J, Colaiaco BA, Connor KI, et al. Dementia care management in an underserved community: the comparative effectiveness of two different approaches. J Aging Health. 2015;27(5):864–93.
28. Birks J. Cholinesterase inhibitors for Alzheimer's disease. Cochrane Database Syst Rev. 2006;2006(1):CD005593.
29. Xu H, Garcia-Ptacek S, Jönsson L, Wimo A, Nordström P, Eriksdotter M. Long-term effects of cholinesterase inhibitors on cognitive decline and mortality. Neurology. 2021;96(17):e2220–30.
30. Zuin M, Cherubini A, Volpato S, Ferrucci L, Zuliani G. Acetyl-cholinesterase-inhibitors slow cognitive decline and decrease overall mortality in older patients with dementia. Sci Rep. 2022;12(1):12214.
31. Cacabelos R. Pharmacogenetic considerations when prescribing cholinesterase inhibitors for the treatment of Alzheimer's disease. Expert Opin Drug Metab Toxicol. 2020;16(8):673–701.
32. Gorelick PB, Scuteri A, Black SE, Decarli C, Greenberg SM, Iadecola C, Launer LJ, Laurent S, Lopez OL, Nyenhuis D, Petersen RC, Schneider JA, Tzourio C, Arnett DK, Bennett DA, Chui

HC, Higashida RT, Lindquist R, Nilsson PM, Roman GC, Sellke FW, Seshadri S, American Heart Association Stroke Council, Council on Epidemiology and Prevention, Council on Cardiovascular Nursing, Council on Cardiovascular Radiology and Intervention, and Council on Cardiovascular Surgery and Anesthesia. Vascular contributions to cognitive impairment and dementia: a statement for healthcare professionals from the American Heart Association/ American Stroke Association. Stroke. 2011;42(9):2672–713.
33. Kalaria RN, Ballard C. Overlap between pathology of Alzheimer disease and vascular dementia. Alzheimer Dis Assoc Disord. 1999;13(Suppl 3):S115.
34. Meng YH, Wang PP, Song YX, Wang JH. Cholinesterase inhibitors and memantine for Parkinson's disease dementia and Lewy body dementia: a meta-analysis. Exp Ther Med. 2019;17(3):1611–24.
35. Mendez MF, Shapira JS, McMurtray A, Licht E. Preliminary findings: behavioral worsening on donepezil in patients with frontotemporal dementia. Am J Geriatr Psychiatry. 2007;15(1):84.
36. Kimura T, Takamatsu J. Pilot study of pharmacological treatment for frontotemporal dementia: risk of donepezil treatment for behavioral and psychological symptoms. Geriatr Gerontol Int. 2013;13(2):506.
37. Arciniegas DB, Anderson CA. Donepezil-induced confusional state in a patient with autopsy-proven behavioral-variant frontotemporal dementia. J Neuropsychiatry Clin Neurosci. 2013;25(3):E25.
38. Kertesz A, Morlog D, Light M, Blair M, Davidson W, Jesso S, Brashear R. Galantamine in frontotemporal dementia and primary progressive aphasia. Dement Geriatr Cogn Disord. 2008;25(2):178.
39. Moretti R, Torre P, Antonello RM, Cattaruzza T, Cazzato G, Bava A. Rivastigmine in frontotemporal dementia: an open-label study. Drugs Aging. 2004;21(14):931.
40. Hernandez RK, Farwell W, Cantor MD, Lawler EV. Cholinesterase inhibitors and incidence of bradycardia in patients with dementia in the veterans affairs new England healthcare system. J Am Geriatr Soc. 2009;57(11):1997.
41. Gill SS, Anderson GM, Fischer HD, Bell CM, Li P, Normand SL, Rochon PA. Syncope and its consequences in patients with dementia receiving cholinesterase inhibitors: a population-based cohort study. Arch Intern Med. 2009;169(9):867.
42. Birks JS, Harvey RJ. Donepezil for dementia due to Alzheimer's disease (Review). Cochrane Database Syst Rev. 2018;6(6):CD001190.
43. Loy C, Schneider L. Galantamine for Alzheimer's disease and mild cognitive impairment. Cochrane Database Syst Rev. 2006;2006(1):CD001747.
44. Winblad B, Cummings J, Andreasen N, Grossberg G, Onofrj M, Sadowsky C, Zechner S, Nagel J, Lane R. A six-month double-blind, randomized, placebo-controlled study of a transdermal patch in Alzheimer's disease—rivastigmine patch versus capsule. Int J Geriatr Psychiatry. 2007;22(5):456–67.
45. Doody RS, Geldmacher DS, Gordon B, Perdomo CA, Pratt RD, Donepezil Study Group. Open-label, multicenter, phase 3 extension study of the safety and efficacy of donepezil in patients with Alzheimer disease. Arch Neurol. 2001;58(3):427–33.
46. Winblad B, Engedal K, Soininen H, Verhey F, Waldemar G, Wimo A, Wetterholm AL, Zhang R, Haglund A, Subbiah P, Donepezil Nordic Study Group. A 1-year, randomized, placebo-controlled study of donepezil in patients with mild to moderate AD. Neurology. 2001;57(3):489–95.
47. Lin JS, O'Connor E, Rossom RC, Perdue LA, Eckstrom E. Screening for cognitive impairment in older adults: a systematic review for the U.S. Preventive Services Task Force. Ann Intern Med. 2013;159(9):601–12. Review.
48. US Department of Health and Human Services, Assistant Secretary for Planning and Evaluation, Office of Disability, Aging and Long-Term Care Policy. Examining models of dementia care: final report. 9 2016.
49. Epperly T, Dunay MA, Boice JL. Alzheimer disease: pharmacologic and nonpharmacologic therapies for cognitive and functional symptoms. Am Fam Physician. 2017;95(12):771–8.

50. Molony SL, Kolanowski A, Van Haitsma K, Rooney KE. Person-centered assessment and care planning. Gerontologist. 2018;58(suppl_1):S32–47.
51. McShane R, Westby MJ, Roberts E, Minakaran N, Schneider L, Farrimond LE, Maayan N, Ware J, Debarros J. Memantine for dementia. Cochrane Database Syst Rev. 2019;3(3):CD003154.
52. Irvine, C.A. Namzaric (memantine and donepezil hydrochlorides). Full prescribing information, Allergan USA, Inc. 2016.
53. FDA Grants Accelerated Approval for Alzheimer's Drug. US Food and Drug Administration. https://www.fda.gov/news-events/press-announcements/fda-grants-accelerated-approval-alzheimers-drug. Accessed 7 June 2021.
54. McCleery J, Quinn TJ. Aducanumab and the certainty of evidence. Age Ageing. 2021;50(6):1899–900.
55. Cummings J, Salloway S. Aducanumab: appropriate use recommendations. Alzheimers Dement. 2021;18(3):531–3.
56. Aduhelm (Aducanumab-AVWA injection). US FDA approved product information. Cambridge: Biogen Inc; 2021.
57. Droś J, Klimkowicz-Mrowiec A. Current view on post-stroke dementia. Psychogeriatrics. 2021;21(3):407–17.
58. Mijajlović MD, Pavlović A, Brainin M, Heiss WD, Quinn TJ, Ihle-Hansen HB, Hermann DM, Assayag EB, Richard E, Thiel A, Kliper E, Shin YI, Kim YH, Choi S, Jung S, Lee YB, Sinanović O, Levine DA, Schlesinger I, Mead G, Milošević V, Leys D, Hagberg G, Ursin MH, Teuschl Y, Prokopenko S, Mozheyko E, Bezdenezhnykh A, Matz K, Aleksić V, Muresanu D, Korczyn AD, Bornstein NM. Post-stroke dementia—a comprehensive review. BMC Med. 2017;15(1):11.
59. Leys D, Hénon H, Mackowiak-Cordoliani MA, Pasquier F. Poststroke dementia. Lancet Neurol. 2005;4(11):752–9.
60. Williamson JD, Supiano MA, Applegate WB, Berlowitz DR, Campbell RC, Chertow GM, Fine LJ, Haley WE, Hawfield AT, Ix JH, Kitzman DW, Kostis JB, Krousel-Wood MA, Launer LJ, Oparil S, Rodriguez CJ, Roumie CL, Shorr RI, Sink KM, Wadley VG, Whelton PK, Whittle J, Woolard NF, Wright JT Jr, Pajewski NM, SPRINT Research Group. Intensive vs standard blood pressure control and cardiovascular disease outcomes in adults aged ≥75 years: a randomized clinical trial. JAMA. 2016;315(24):2673.
61. Bavishi C, Bangalore S, Messerli FH. Outcomes of intensive blood pressure lowering in older hypertensive patients. J Am Coll Cardiol. 2017;69(5):486.
62. Corvol JC, Bouzamondo A, Sirol M, Hulot JS, Sanchez P, Lechat P. Differential effects of lipid-lowering therapies on stroke prevention: a meta-analysis of randomized trials. Arch Intern Med. 2003;163(6):669.
63. Oesterle A, Laufs U, Liao JK. Pleiotropic effects of statins on the cardiovascular system. Circ Res. 2017;120(1):229.
64. Kernan WN, Ovbiagele B, Black HR, Bravata DM, Chimowitz MI, Ezekowitz MD, Fang MC, Fisher M, Furie KL, Heck DV, Johnston SC, Kasner SE, Kittner SJ, Mitchell PH, Rich MW, Richardson D, Schwamm LH, Wilson JA, American Heart Association Stroke Council, Council on Cardiovascular and Stroke Nursing, Council on Clinical Cardiology, and Council on Peripheral Vascular Disease. Guidelines for the prevention of stroke in patients with stroke and transient ischemic attack: a guideline for healthcare professionals from the American Heart Association/American Stroke Association. Stroke. 2014;45(7):2160.
65. Smith EE, Cieslak A, Barber P, Chen J, Chen YW, Donnini I, Edwards JD, Frayne R, Field TS, Hegedus J, Hanganu V, Ismail Z, Kanji J, Nakajima M, Noor R, Peca S, Sahlas D, Sharma M, Sposato LA, Swartz RH, Zerna C, Black SE, Hachinski V. Therapeutic strategies and drug development for vascular cognitive impairment. J Am Heart Assoc. 2017;6(5):e005568.
66. Cummings J, Ritter A, Rothemberg K. Advances in management of neuropsychiatric syndromes in neurodegenerative diseases. Curr Psychiatry Rep. 2019;21:79.
67. Tible OP, Riese F, Savaskan E, von Gunten A. Best practice in the management of behavioural and psychological symptoms of dementia. Ther Adv Neurol Disord. 2017;10(8):297–309.

68. Eissa N, Sadeq A, Sasse A, Sadek B. Role of neuroinflammation in autism spectrum disorder and the emergence of brain histaminergic system. Lessons also for BPSD? Front Pharmacol. 2020;11:886.
69. Calsolaro V, Femminella GD, Rogani S, Esposito S, Franchi R, Okoye C, Rengo G, Monzani F. Behavioral and psychological symptoms in dementia (BPSD) and the use of antipsychotics. Pharmaceuticals. 2021;14(3):246.
70. Garre-Olmo J, López-Pousa S, Vilalta-Franch J, de Gracia Blanco M, Vilarrasa AB. Grouping and trajectories of the neuropsychiatric symptoms in patients with Alzheimer's disease, part I: symptom clusters. J Alzheimers Dis. 2010;22(4):1157–67.
71. Livingston G, Kelly L, Lewis-Holmes E, Baio G, Morris S, Patel N, Omar RZ, Katona C, Cooper C. Non-pharmacological interventions for agitation in dementia: systematic review of randomised controlled trials. Br J Psychiatry. 2014;205(6):436–42.
72. Reus VI, Fochtmann LJ, Eyler AE, Hilty DM, Horvitz-Lennon M, Jibson MD, Lopez OL, Mahoney J, Pasic J, Tan ZS, Wills CD, Rhoads R, Yageret J. The American Psychiatric Association practice guideline on the use of antipsychotics to treat agitation or psychosis in patients with dementia. Am J Psychiatry. 2016;173(5):543–6.
73. Markota M, Rummans TA, Bostwick JM, Lapid MI. Benzodiazepine use in older adults: dangers, management, and alternative therapies. Mayo Clin Proc. 2016;91(11):1632–9.
74. Brücke T, Roth J, Podreka I, Strobl R, Wenger S, Asenbaum S. Striatal dopamine D2-receptor blockade by typical and atypical neuroleptics. Lancet. 1992;339(8791):497.
75. Faay MDM, Czobor P, Sommer IEC. Efficacy of typical and atypical antipsychotic medication on hostility in patients with psychosis-spectrum disorders: a review and meta-analysis. Neuropsychopharmacology. 2018;43(12):2340–9.
76. Aringhieri S, Carli M, Kolachalam S, Verdesca V, Cini E, Rossi M, McCormick PJ, Corsini GU, Maggio R, Scarselli M. Molecular targets of atypical antipsychotics: from mechanism of action to clinical differences. Pharmacol Ther. 2018;192:20–41.
77. Mintzer JE, Tune LE, Breder CD, Swanink R, Marcus RN, McQuade RD, Forbes A. Aripiprazole for the treatment of psychoses in institutionalized patients with Alzheimer dementia: a multicenter, randomized, double-blind, placebo-controlled assessment of three fixed doses. Am J Geriatr Psychiatry. 2007;15(11):918–31.
78. De Deyn PP, Drenth AF, Kremer BP, Oude Voshaar RC, Van Dam D. Aripiprazole in the treatment of Alzheimer's disease. Expert Opin Pharmacother. 2013;14(4):459–74.
79. Schneider LS, Tariot PN, Dagerman KS, Davis SM, Hsiao JK, Ismail MS, Lebowitz BD, Lyketsos CG, Ryan JM, Stroup TS, Sultzer DL, Weintraub D, Lieberman JA, CATIE-AD Study Group. Effectiveness of atypical antipsychotic drugs in patients with Alzheimer's disease. N Engl J Med. 2006;355(15):1525–38.
80. Kales HC, Gitlin LN, Lyketsos CG. Assessment and management of behavioral and psychological symptoms of dementia. BMJ. 2015;350:h369.
81. Tampi RR, Tampi DJ, Balachandran S, Srinivasan S. Antipsychotic use in dementia: a systematic review of benefits and risks from meta-analyses. Ther Adv Chronic Dis. 2016;7:229–45.

Pharmacological Treatment of Osteoporosis in Older Patients

21

Marian Dejaeger, Jolan Dupont, Michaël R. Laurent, and Evelien Gielen

21.1 Epidemiology of Osteoporosis and Osteoporotic Fractures in Old Age

Osteoporosis is a systemic bone disease, characterized by low bone mass and disruptions in the micro-architectural structure of bone tissue, resulting in an increase in bone fragility and fracture risk [1]. The incidence of osteoporotic fractures increases with age, and osteoporosis at advanced age is a challenge because of coexisting comorbidities and the major post-fracture implications in terms of morbidity, loss of mobility, and mortality. Currently, the cumulative incidence of hip and vertebral fractures in women at the age of 80 years is close to 30% and more than 40%, respectively. Women over the age of 80 represent more than 30% of all osteoporotic fractures and even more than 60% of all non-vertebral fractures [2–4]. Age is also one of the main determinants of the type of osteoporotic fracture. Between the ages of 55 and 75, the risk of vertebral fractures peaks in women, whereas beyond the age of 75, women become increasingly at risk of non-vertebral fractures, e.g., hip fractures [5]. The burden of osteoporosis will only increase further because of the aging society.

M. Dejaeger · J. Dupont · E. Gielen (✉)
Geriatrics & Gerontology, Department of Public Health and Primary Care, KU Leuven, Leuven, Belgium

Department of Geriatric Medicine, University Hospitals Leuven, Leuven, Belgium

Centre for Metabolic Bone Diseases, University Hospitals Leuven, Leuven, Belgium
e-mail: marian.dejaeger@uzleuven.be; jolan.dupont@uzleuven.be; evelien.gielen@uzleuven.be

M. R. Laurent
Centre for Metabolic Bone Diseases, University Hospitals Leuven, Leuven, Belgium

Geriatrics Department, Imelda Hospital, Bonheiden, Belgium
e-mail: Michael.Laurent@imelda.be

A. Cherubini et al. (eds.), *Optimizing Pharmacotherapy in Older Patients*, Practical Issues in Geriatrics, https://doi.org/10.1007/978-3-031-28061-0_21

21.2 Older Persons with Osteoporotic Fractures Are Frail

Osteoporosis and osteoporotic fractures tend to occur in a part of the older population already suffering from frailty [6]. Indeed, older persons with osteoporotic fractures are not “average” older persons but frail individuals with a high prevalence of underlying comorbidities and at risk of disabilities [7]. This frailty is reflected in the poor post-fracture outcomes of these patients. For example, 1 year post-fracture, 40% of the patients are still unable to walk independently, 33% are institutionalized or totally dependent, and 20% are deceased [8, 9]. These poor outcomes are not restricted to hip fractures alone, as similar observations have been made in older persons with other types of non-vertebral fractures and even vertebral fractures [10]. Moreover, the excess mortality is not only observed within the first year after the fracture but persists in the years thereafter due to the underlying comorbidities of these frail older persons [11, 12].

21.3 Diagnosis of Osteoporosis and Intervention Thresholds in Old Age

Despite the high prevalence and significant burden of osteoporosis, this condition remains to be underdiagnosed and undertreated. This is most prominent in women aged ≥80 years [13]. To illustrate, according to a study in more than 700,000 persons aged ≥75 years in Sweden, 16.1% of women and 3.4% of men used osteoporosis medication, lower than the estimated prevalence of osteoporosis in that country. In particular in persons ≥90 years, osteoporosis was largely undertreated [14].

Yet, the operational definition of osteoporosis also applies to older persons. The World Health Organization (WHO) defines osteoporosis as a bone mineral density (BMD) value at the lumbar spine or the proximal femur of at least −2.5 standard deviations (SD) below the peak bone mass of a young healthy individual [15]. However, sensitivity of dual-energy X-ray absorptiometry (DXA) for fracture is low, as the majority of fractures occurs in persons with a T-score above −2.5. This implies that factors other than BMD contribute to fracture risk [16]. More specifically, an existing osteoporotic fracture is the most significant predictor of future fracture risk, resulting in a doubling of fracture risk compared to persons without previous fractures. Also, increasing age itself is an important risk factor for fractures as over a 4 SD interval of BMD (+1 to −3 SD), a 14-fold increase in hip fracture risk is seen at the age of 50, but a 145-fold increase at the age of 80 [17, 18]. Therefore, fracture risk assessment tools based on age and other clinical risk factors are increasingly being used to target osteoporosis therapy. Among these is the FRAX algorithm, which includes the weight of various clinical risk factors for fractures, with or without femoral neck BMD, to estimate the 10-year probability of hip fracture and major osteoporotic fractures (clinical spine, forearm, hip, or shoulder fractures) [19]. The main goal of FRAX is to identify individuals at higher fracture risk who qualify for osteoporosis treatment. Three approaches can be distinguished, which, especially in older persons, differ in the threshold above which treatment is recommended: fixed, age-dependent, and hybrid thresholds.

First, according to the fixed model of the USA National Osteoporosis Foundation (NOF), treatment should be initiated when the 10-year fracture risk of a person exceeds the 10-year fracture probability at which treatment becomes cost-effective [20, 21]. Second, the age-dependent model of the UK National Osteoporosis Guideline Group (NOGG) indicates that treatment should be considered when the fracture probability of an individual exceeds the FRAX intervention threshold, defined as the age-specific fracture probability of a man or woman with a previous fragility fracture, no other risk factors, an average BMI (24 kg/m^2), and without knowledge of BMD [22, 23]. The rationale is that in general, a person with a previous fragility fracture is considered to qualify for treatment. Third, as the previous model induces inequalities in access to therapy especially at older age, an alternative threshold using a hybrid model has been proposed by the NOGG. According to this model, the intervention threshold rises with age but remains constant from the age of 70, being at 20% for a major osteoporotic fracture and 5.4% for a hip fracture [23, 24].

21.4 Treatment of Osteoporosis in Older Persons

In this section, we will discuss the efficacy and safety of the pharmacological treatment options for osteoporosis in older persons. Osteoporosis treatment for older persons should be proven to be effective in this cohort, not only against vertebral fractures but even more so against non-vertebral fractures, as these account for the majority of negative outcomes (e.g., morbidity, mortality). Treatment should also be safe in frail older adults, with underlying comorbidities and at increased risk of adverse events.

21.4.1 Calcium and Vitamin D Supplementation in Old Age

One of the main determinants of bone loss and fracture risk in old age is calcium and vitamin D deficiency. Therefore, combined supplementation of calcium and vitamin D has become one of the main treatment strategies for reducing bone loss and fracture risk in old age. Low vitamin D status and insufficient dietary calcium intake can lead to secretion of parathyroid hormone (age-related hyperparathyroidism), stimulating bone resorption and increasing the fracture risk.

Despite a high degree of consensus on the essential role of vitamin D for bone health and other extra-skeletal effects, there remains some lack of consensus regarding the optimal concentration of total 25-hydroxyvitamin D (25(OH)D). Yet, it is clear that vitamin D insufficiency occurs in all age groups. In fact, a gradual decline in 25(OH)D levels from healthy adults over independent older adults to institutionalized individuals and hip fracture patients can be observed [25]. Severe vitamin D deficiency (<10 μg/L) is seen in almost 4 out of 5 institutionalized people [25]. The intestinal absorption of vitamin D is adequate, even at very advanced ages [25]. However, the vitamin D status deteriorates with aging above 70 years due to a very low dietary intake, decreased sun exposure, and a reduced capacity to produce vitamin D in the skin with aging [25, 26].

There has been some debate whether calcium and vitamin D supplementation has an influence on fracture prevention. A meta-analysis of Bolland et al., for example, found that vitamin D co-administered with calcium reduced hip fracture risk in institutionalized but not in community-dwelling older persons [27]. This and other meta-analyses and individual RCTs may have failed to demonstrate a reduction in fracture risk with calcium and vitamin D because of an insufficient dose, therapeutic incompliance, or lack of targeting of supplementation to persons at risk of vitamin D deficiency or a negative calcium balance [28–31]. Calcium and vitamin D supplementation indeed need to be directed to persons with documented or at risk of calcium and/or vitamin D deficiency, which is, as mentioned before, highly prevalent in osteoporosis patients, home-bound frail persons, and institutionalized persons [25]. A recent systematic review and meta-analysis of the effectiveness of calcium and vitamin D showed a significant reduction in the risk of total fractures and hip fractures and concluded that the minimum effective dose of calcium is 1200 mg while vitamin D should not be below 800 IU [32].

In addition to the effect on bone loss, a daily intake of 800 IU to 1000 IU vitamin D lowers the risk of falling by 20% in older adults, independent of calcium intake [33]. Efficacy of doses higher than 1000 IU/day has not been observed in RCTs. On the contrary, intermittent supplementation with very high doses, such as a single oral dose of 500,000 IU, even increases the risk of falls, especially in the first months after intake when serum 25(OH)D levels are >45 ng/mL [34]. Also, an increased risk of falls was seen at a monthly intake of 60,000 IU vitamin D compared to 24,000 IU [35]. Therefore, an intake of >1000 IU of vitamin D per day is not recommended to prevent falls in all older adults [31]. Both the International Osteoporosis Foundation as the American Geriatrics Society recommend 800–1000 IU of vitamin D per day in community-dwelling and institutionalized older adults [33, 36].

To conclude, the combination of calcium and vitamin D has become an essential part in fracture risk prevention in the aged population. A daily intake of 1200 mg calcium per day (but not more than 2000 mg/day) is recommended in older adults at risk of fracture. As some cardiovascular safety issues have been raised about the use of calcium supplements (that, however, were not confirmed in other studies), the preferable source of calcium is by food intake of dairy products [27]. When the daily recommended intake cannot be achieved by food intake, oral supplements should be considered.

21.4.2 Pharmacological Osteoporosis Treatment in Old Age

Besides optimizing calcium and vitamin D intake, osteoporosis treatment should be in added in older persons with osteoporosis and osteoporotic fractures. Currently available osteoporosis medications are classified as antiresorptive (bisphosphonates, denosumab, and selective estrogen receptor modulators) and anabolic (teriparatide, abaloparatide, romosozumab) drugs.

When considering drug therapy for osteoporosis in older persons, one should bear in mind that these older adults often have a reduced intestinal absorption, metabolism, and excretion of drugs as well as polypharmacy, therapeutic incompliance, and concomitant disorders [37]. Aging is, for example, associated with a reduced kidney function. Since about 50% of the bisphosphonates are excreted by the kidneys, reduced kidney function may result in an accumulation of these drugs, which potentially affects efficacy and safety [38]. In the following paragraphs, evidence in older persons about the efficacy (Table 21.1) and safety of the available osteoporosis medications will be elucidated. The evidence is mostly based on subgroup analyses of the landmark osteoporosis trials in postmenopausal women.

21.4.2.1 Antiresorptive Treatment for Osteoporosis

Alendronate

The efficacy of alendronate in postmenopausal women was demonstrated by the Fracture Intervention Trial (FIT). The FIT Vertebral Fracture Arm (FIT I) included women who suffered from vertebral fracture(s), while the FIT Clinical Fracture Arm (FIT II) included women with a *T*-score of ≤ -1.6 at the femoral neck (mean age 70.8 years and 67.7 years, respectively) [39, 40].

Two sub-analyses of the FIT trials have been undertaken to determine the anti-fracture efficacy and safety of alendronate in older persons. A post hoc analysis of FIT I has focused on the efficacy of alendronate in postmenopausal women with the highest fracture risk, including a subgroup of women aged ≥75 years (range 75–82 years) [41]. In order to prevent one new vertebral fracture, eight women aged ≥75 years (RR = 0.62; 95% CI, 0.41–0.94) needed to be treated for 3 years with alendronate compared with nine women aged <75 years (RR = 0.49; 95% CI, 0.35–0.68). Another analysis, based on pooled data from both FIT arms, aimed to calculate age-specific fracture rates by treatment group (55 to <65 years, 65 to <70 years, 70 to <75 years, and 75–85 years) [42]. Relative risk reductions were comparable among age groups for hip (RR = 0.47; 95% CI, 0.27–0.81; $p < 0.01$) and vertebral (RR = 0.55; 95% CI, 0.37–0.83; $p < 0.01$) fractures, revealing an even greater absolute risk reduction as age increases, which can be explained by the age-related increase in fracture risk in the placebo group [42]. A study on older patients (range 71–92 years) with a previous fracture showed also a significant reduction in hip fracture risk (hazard ratio (HR) = 0.72; 95% CI, 0.61–0.85, $p < 0.001$), which was maintained across all age quartiles [43]. Finally, using a national database of men and women undergoing a fall risk assessment at a Swedish healthcare facility, the efficacy of alendronate treatment was investigated in patients aged ≥80 years (mean age of 85.7+/− 3.9 years) and history of fracture [43]. Alendronate was associated with a lower hip fracture risk (HR = 0.66; 95% CI, 0.51–0.86; $P < 0.01$).

The post hoc analysis of FIT I and the pooled analysis from both FIT arms did not report safety data in older persons [41, 42]. The Swedish study reported a reduced mortality risk in patients treated with alendronate (HR = 0.88; 95% CI,

Table 21.1 Relative risk (95% CI) of new vertebral, hip and non-vertebral fractures compared with placebo in older women receiving currently available osteoporosis treatments

	RCT	Included participants	N	Mean age (years)	Vertebral fractures	Hip fractures	Non-vertebral fractures
Alendronate	Post hoc analysis FIT I (3 years) (Ensrud 1997)	Women aged 75–82 y	539	Not specified	**RR = 0.62; 95% CI 0.41–0.94. $p < 0.05$** $p_{interact < 75 \& \geq 75 y}$ NS	–	–
	Pooled analysis FIT I and FIT II (3–4 years) (Hochberg 2005)	Women aged 55–80 y 55–<65 y 65–<70 y 70–<75 y 75–85 y	3658		**RR = 0.55; 95% CI 0.37–0.83** (constant RR)	**RR = 0.47; 95% CI 0.27–0.81** (constant RR)	–
	Axelsson et al. (5 years) (Axelsson 2016)	Women aged 71.1–92.3 y with a prior fracture	110.190	82.4 y	–	**HR = 0.72; 95% CI: 0.61–0.85; $p < 0.001$**	–
Risedronate	HIP - arm 2 (3 years) (McClung 2001)	Women aged ≥80 y with at least one non-skeletal risk factor for hip fracture or *T*-score at FN < −4 or <−3 + hip axis length of ≥11.1 cm	3886	83 y	–	RR = 0.8; 95% CI 0.6–1.2; $p = 0.35$	10.8% (Risedronate) *vs* 11.9% (placebo); $p = 0.43$
	Post hoc pooled analysis VERT-NA, VERT-MN and HIP (3 years) (Boonen 2004b)	Women aged ≥80 y with *T*-score <−2.5 at FN or at least one prevalent vertebral fracture	1392	83 y	**HR = 0.56; 95% CI 0.39–0.81; $p = 0.003$** $p_{interact < 80 \& \geq 85 y}$ NS	–	14.0% (Risedronate) *vs* 16.2% (placebo); $p = 0.66$

Zoledronic acid	Post hoc analysis HORIZON-PFT and RFT (3 years) (Boonen 2010)	Women aged ≥75 y with T-score ≤−2.5 at FN or ≥1 vertebral or hip fracture	3888	79.4 y	**HR = 0.34; 95% CI 0.21–0.55; $p < 0.001$** $p_{interact < 75 \& \geq 75 y}$ NS	HR = 0.82; 95% CI 0.56–1.2; $p = 0.297$ $\boldsymbol{p_{interact < 70 \& \geq 75 y}}$ **SS**	**HR = 0.73; 95% CI 0.60–0.90; $p = 0.002$** $p_{interact < 70 \& \geq 75 y}$ NS
Denosumab	Post hoc analysis FREEDOM (3 years) (Boonen 2011)	Women aged ≥75 y	2471	78.2 y	–	**0.9% (Denosumab) *vs* 2.3% (placebo); $p < 0.01$; ARR 1.4%** $p_{interact < 75 \& \geq 75 y}$ NS	–
	Preplanned analysis FREEDOM (3 years) (McClung 2012)	Women aged ≥75 y	2471	78.2 y	**3.1% (Denosumab) *vs* 8.6% (placebo); RR = 0.36; 95% CI 0.25–0.53** $p_{interact < 75 \& \geq 75 y}$ NS	–	7.9% (Denosumab) *vs* 9.0% (placebo); RR = 0.84; 95% CI 0.63–1.12 $p_{interact < 75 \& \geq 75 y}$ NS
	FREEEDOM Extension (6 years) (Papapoulos 2012)	Women aged ≥75 y	662	78 y	3.6% (Denosumab) (no placebo group)	1.0% (Denosumab) (no placebo group)	5.4% (Denosumab) (no placebo group)
Teriparatide	Prespecified subgroup analysis FPT (19 months) (Boonen 2006a)	Women aged ≥75 y	244	78.3 y	**RR = 0.35, $p < 0.05$** $p_{interact < 75 \& \geq 75 y}$ NS	–	RR = 0.75; $p = 0.661$ (not powered) $p_{interact < 75 \& \geq 75 y}$ NS
Abalopratide	Posthoc analysis ACTIVE (18 months) McClung 2018	Women aged ≥80 y	94	81.7	0 fractures (Aboloparatide) *vs* 2 fractures (placebo)		1 fracture (Abaloparatide) *vs* 2 fractures (placebo)
	Posthoc analysis ACTIVE (18 months) Cosman 2017	Women aged ≥75 y	303	NA	<65 y, 65–75 y, ≥75 y: consistent fracture risk reduction		<65 y, 65–75 y, ≥75 y: consistent fracture risk reduction

(continued)

Table 21.1 (continued)

	RCT	Included participants	N	Mean age (years)	Vertebral fractures	Hip fractures	Non-vertebral fractures
Romosozumab	FRAME (2 years) Cosman 2016	Women 55–90 y	7180	70.9 y	12 months (Romo *vs* placebo): **RR = 0.27; 95% CI 0.16–0.47** 24 months (Romo/ Dmab *vs* placebo/ Dmab): **RR = 0.25; 95% CI 0.16–0.40**	12 months (Romo *vs* placebo): HR = 0.54; 95% CI 0.22–1.35 24 months (Romo/ Dmab *vs* placebo/ Dmab): HR = 0.50; 95% CI 0.24–1.04	12 months (Romo *vs* placebo): HR = 0.75; 95% CI 0.53–1.05 24 months (Romo/ Dmab *vs* placebo/ Dmab): HR = 0.75; 95% CI 0.57–0.97
	ARCH (2 years) Saag 2017	Women 55–90 y	4093	74.3 y	12 months (Romo *vs* ALN): **RR = 0.63; 95% CI 0.47–0.85** 24 months (Romo/ ALN *vs* ALN/ALN): **RR = 0.52; 95% CI 0.40–0.66**	12 months (Romo *vs* ALN): HR = 0.64; 95% 0.33–1.26 Primary analysis (Romo/ALN *vs* ALN/ ALN): **HR = 0.62; 95% CI 0.42–0.92**	12 months (Romo *vs* ALN): HR = 0.74; 95% CI 0.54–1.01 Primary analysis (Romo/ALN *vs* ALN/ ALN): HR = **0.81; 95% CI 0.66–0.99**

FN Femoral neck, *LS* Lumbar spine, *y* Years, *ITT* Intention to treat, *NS* Not significant, *RR* Risk ratio, *HR* Hazard ratio, *Romo* Romosozumab, *Dmab* Denosumab, *ALN* Alendronate. **Results in bold indicate significant results**

Table adapted from: Vandenbroucke A et al. Pharmacological treatment of osteoporosis in the oldest old. Clinical Interventions in Aging 2017:12; 1065–1077. Dove Medical Press Limited

0.82–0.95) as well as an increased risk of mild upper gastrointestinal symptoms (UGI) (HR = 1.58; 95% CI, 1.12–2.24). The association between alendronate and mild UGI, however, did not change with age. Furthermore, the Number Needed to Harm (NNH) was 91, as compared to the Number Needed to Treat (NNT) of 26 for hip fracture, which is considered as a favorable risk-benefit ratio [43]. Together, these data illustrate that alendronate is safe in older persons, with reduced vertebral and hip fracture risk, and suggest that older persons, who intrinsically have a higher baseline fracture risk, benefit more from osteoporosis treatment than younger persons.

Risedronate

The Vertebral Efficacy with Risedronate Therapy North America (VERT-NA) and Multinational (VERT-MN) studies showed both that risedronate can efficiently reduce vertebral and non-vertebral fractures rates [44, 45] in postmenopausal women with one or more vertebral fractures (mean age +/− 70 years) [44, 45]. In addition, the HIP trial has studied the effect of risedronate on hip fracture risk in two different arms, of which the first arm included postmenopausal women with a mean age of 74 years [46]. To determine the efficacy of risedronate in older persons, the second arm of the HIP trial included 3886 women, aged ≥80 years (mean age 83 years). These older women were included based on having a low BMD at the femoral neck or at least one nonskeletal risk factor for hip fracture (e.g., poor gait or a propensity to fall) [46]. After 3 years of risedronate use, no significant reduction in the risk of hip fractures was observed (RR = 0.8; 95% CI, 0.6–1.2; $p = 0.35$). Only in the subgroup of women (16%) included based on low BMD, a significant reduction in hip fracture rate was seen. However, most of the participants (58%) were included on the basis of a nonskeletal risk factor. A second analysis on pooled data from these three studies (VERT-NA, VERT-MN, and HIP trials) focused on older individuals [47]. This analysis included 1392 women aged ≥80 years (mean age 83 years) with osteoporosis (T-score <−2.5 or at least one vertebral fracture). After 1 year, the vertebral fracture risk decreased by 81% (HR = 0.19; 95% CI, 0.09–0.40; $P < 0.001$) and after 3 years by 44% (HR = 0.56; 95% CI, 0.39–0.81; $p = 0.003$). Regarding non-vertebral fractures, the incidence did not differ significantly between the treatment group and the placebo group ($p = 0.66$).

This gap in benefit for vertebral vs non-vertebral fractures in both analyses in older persons might be explained by the knowledge that bisphosphonates impact on BMD, demonstrated by the significant reduction of vertebral fractures [46, 47]. In spite of this, bisphosphonates do not intervene with the nonskeletal risk factors of fractures such as gait disturbances, impaired balance, and fall risk. These nonskeletal factors play a major role in the occurrence of non-vertebral fractures, such as hip fractures, in older persons, who are more at risk of falling [48]. On the contrary, vertebral fractures are often spontaneous or atraumatic, thus less influenced by these nonskeletal risk factors. Furthermore, the discrepancy *between the older* and younger population in preventing non-vertebral fractures might be explained, at least partly, due to insufficient statistical power in the older age group [47].

Older women (aged ≥80 years) in the HIP trial had a marginally higher incidence of death, other serious adverse events, and discontinuation due to adverse events than younger women [46]. However, the overall occurrence and types of adverse events, including those involving the upper gastrointestinal tract, were comparable in the risedronate and placebo group, aside from age. Additionally, in women aged ≥80 years in the pooled analysis of the VERT-NA, VERT-MN, and HIP trials, adverse events were similar in the risedronate and placebo group [47]. Even in older persons with active gastrointestinal tract disease at baseline or on aspirin, nonsteroidal anti-inflammatory drugs (NSAIDs), or proton pump inhibitors (PPIs), the incidence of adverse events was similar in both treatment groups.

Thus, safety data of oral bisphosphonates confirm that they are well tolerated in older persons and not associated with an increased risk of adverse events as compared to placebo. Nonetheless, in clinical practice, treatment with oral bisphosphonates may be challenging, as the rather demanding intake instructions (e.g., to stay upright for at least 30 min after the intake) may be difficult for physically or cognitively impaired persons. Inappropriate administration, however, increases the risk of adverse events and potentially further decreases the already low oral bioavailability (around 1%–2%) [38, 49, 50]. Furthermore, oral osteoporosis medication rises the pill burden in older persons, which contributes to low compliance. Indeed, almost 50% of those who have been prescribed an oral bisphosphonate have discontinued treatment after 1 year [51].

Zoledronic Acid

Usage of an intravenous bisphosphonate, such as zoledronic acid, might provide an alternative in older persons that cannot tolerate or adhere to oral bisphosphonates [52]. The Health Outcomes and Reduced Incidence with Zoledronic Acid Once Yearly Pivotal Fracture Trial (HORIZON-PFT) demonstrated that once-yearly infusion of zoledronic acid significantly reduces the risk of vertebral, hip, and non-vertebral fractures in postmenopausal women with osteoporosis (mean age 73 years) [53]. In a second analysis in participants with surgical repair of a low-trauma hip fracture (mean age 74.4 years), the HORIZON-Recurrent Fracture Trial (HORIZON-RFT), zoledronic acid significantly lowers the risk of new vertebral and new non-vertebral fractures [54].

Additional post hoc pooled analysis of the HORIZON-PFT and HORIZON-RFT was performed, focusing on older persons, by including postmenopausal women aged ≥75 years (mean age 79.4 years) with osteoporosis (*T*-score ≤−2.5 at the femoral neck or ≥1 prevalent vertebral or hip fracture) [52]. After 3 years of treatment, incidence of any clinical vertebral (1.1% vs 3.7%) and non-vertebral fracture (9.9% vs 13.7%) was significantly lower in the zoledronic acid group compared to the placebo group (HR = 0.34; 95% CI 0.21–0.55; $p < 0.001$ and HR = 0.73; 95% CI 0.6–0.9; $p = 0.002$ respectively). This benefit was similar to the relative risk reduction in subjects younger than 75 years in the HORIZON-PFT and HORIZON-RFT. Hence, zoledronic acid is an efficient treatment option for the prevention of vertebral and non-vertebral fractures in older persons. However, in patients aged ≥75 years, the incidence of hip fractures decreased with zoledronic acid, but this did not reach statistical significance (HR = 0.82; 95% CI 0.56–1.2; $P = 0.297$). Presumably, the sample size was not statistically powered to observe a reduction of hip fracture risk in this older age group. An alternative explanation is the large influence of nonskeletal risk factors for hip fractures with ageing [47, 52].

In the post hoc analysis of the HORIZON-PFT and RFT trial in women aged ≥75 years, incidence of adverse events and post-administration symptoms occurring within 3 days of the infusion (pyrexia, myalgia, and influenza-like illness) was higher with zoledronic acid than with placebo [52]. The incidence of renal events, serious adverse events, and death was similar in the two treatment arms. An increased risk of atrial fibrillation, suggested in the HORIZON-PFT, which could be a concern in older persons, was not observed in the post hoc analysis evaluating older persons on zoledronic acid [52].

Denosumab

Denosumab is a human monoclonal antibody that acts on RANKL, a mediator of bone resorption. In the Fracture Reduction Evaluation of Denosumab in Osteoporosis Every 6 months (FREEDOM) trial, 7800 women between 60 and 90 years (mean age 72.3 years) with a BMD T-score of <−2.5 but not <−4.0 at the lumbar spine or total hip received denosumab or placebo for 3 years. Denosumab was linked with a significant reduction in the risk of vertebral, hip, and non-vertebral fractures [55].

An additional post hoc analysis of the FREEDOM trial focused on the effect of denosumab in populations at high risk of fractures, among which women aged ≥75 years [56]. In this age group (mean age 78.2 years), denosumab lowered the risk of hip fractures by 62% (2.3% placebo vs 0.9% denosumab; $p < 0.01$). This risk reduction in older patients is similar with the risk reduction in the overall study population of the FREEDOM trial. One more analysis of the FREEDOM trial confirmed that denosumab lowers the risk of vertebral fractures to the same extent in subjects aged ≥75 years (RR = 0.36; 95% CI, 0.25–0.53) as in subjects <75 years (RR = 0.30; 95% CI, 0.22–0.41; interaction *p*-value, 0.482) [57]. Moreover, the effect on non-vertebral fractures in persons older than 75 years (RR = 0.84; 95% CI, 0.63–1.12) was comparable to younger persons (RR = 0.78; 95% CI, 0.63–0.96; interaction *p*-value, 0.642). Also, the FREEDOM Extension trial demonstrated that also in women aged ≥75 years, denosumab for up to 6 years was associated with a persistently low incidence of new vertebral, hip, and non-vertebral fractures, with a fracture incidence similar to that observed after 3 years [58].

Hence, denosumab is effective in preventing vertebral *and* hip fractures in older persons [56, 57]. In contrast, as indicated, no significant reduction in hip fracture risk was shown for the bisphosphonates risedronate and zoledronic acid in older persons, although, as mentioned, this might be explained by lack of statistical power [41, 42, 52]. However, it is tempting to speculate that this observation of hip fracture reduction with denosumab is due to the mechanism of action of denosumab, different from that of bisphosphonates, with distinct effects on cortical bone [59]. Cortical porosity is indeed one of the main determinants of non-vertebral fracture risk, including hip fracture risk.

Denosumab was well tolerated in postmenopausal women in the FREEDOM trial [55]. In the post hoc analysis of women aged ≥75 years, no significant differences were noted regarding safety between placebo- and denosumab-treated subjects, and the incidence of adverse events was similar to those in the overall FREEDOM population [56]. Importantly, the efficacy of denosumab is not influenced by kidney function, so older persons with renal impairment will profit the same anti-fracture efficacy as patients with normal kidney function [60]. However, since the use of denosumab is associated with a high rate of severe hypocalcemia in patients with advanced chronic kidney disease, close monitoring and replacement of calcium and vitamin D is required to avoid hypocalcemia in these patients.

Finally, denosumab, like the bisphosphonates, may be associated with very rare but severe adverse events, such as atypical femoral fractures and osteonecrosis of the jaw. In particular for denosumab, treatment interval should be respected, and discontinuation without alternative treatment should be avoided, in order to avoid rebound phenomena. Denosumab has a washout period of 6 months, following the 6-month dosing interval, and there is no persistent effect on BMD and BTM (bone turnover makers) after discontinuation, in contrast to long-acting bisphosphonates [61]. In case of discontinuation, BTM rise to levels above the pre-treatment baseline levels [62]. Subsequently, several case reports and a post hoc analysis of the FREEDOM trial confirmed that vertebral fracture rate increased after denosumab discontinuation to a level comparable with untreated patients [63–66]. These rebound phenomena might be counteracted by using a potent bisphosphonate (e.g., zoledronic acid or alendronate) as alternative treatment upon discontinuation [67]. However, clinical studies have not yet determined the optimal approach for preventing the effects of denosumab discontinuation [68]. These findings highlight the importance of respecting dosage intervals and avoiding noncompliance in persons treated with denosumab, even in older adults. To our knowledge, there is no evidence that these events are independently associated with age [69]. Since there are no guidelines about the optimal duration of denosumab and no definitive answers yet about the sequential treatment with a bisphosphonate after stopping denosumab, a lifelong treatment with denosumab may be the preferred approach, especially in older patients [70].

Selective Estrogen Receptor Modulators (SERM)
Raloxifene and bazedoxifene are approved for osteoporosis treatment, but like the bisphosphonate ibandronate, SERMS have only a proven preventive effect on vertebral fractures. As such, these drugs are reserved for young postmenopausal women that are at low risk of hip fractures.

21.4.2.2 Anabolic Treatment for Osteoporosis

Currently available anabolic drugs for osteoporosis are teriparatide, abaloparatide, and romosozumab. Teriparatide and abaloparatide are parathyroid hormone analogues administered in a once-daily injection inducing an anabolic effect on bone formation. Romosozumab is a human monoclonal antibody, administered once-monthly, that binds to and inhibits sclerostin. Romosozumab has a dual mode of action, by increasing bone formation and decreasing bone resorption. In patients that have received a course with anabolic treatment (which lasts 1 to 2 years), it is recommended to continue with antiresorptive therapy to maintain the gain in bone mass (sequential therapy).

Teriparatide

In the Fracture Prevention Trial (FPT), teriparatide lowered the risk of vertebral fractures by 65% (HR = 0.35; 95% CI, 0.22–0.55; $P < 0.001$) and the risk of non-vertebral fractures by 53% (HR = 0.47; 95% CI, 0.25–0.88; $P = 0.04$) in postmenopausal women with a prior vertebral fracture (mean age 69.5 years) [71]. In a subgroup analysis on the FPT study, Boonen et al. investigated the effect of teriparatide in persons aged ≥75 years after 19 months of treatment (mean age 78.3 years) [72]. About 5.2% of the older persons in the teriparatide group and 15.1% in the placebo group suffered a new vertebral fracture (RR = 0.35, $P < 0.05$). Hip fracture incidence was not a primary endpoint in this trial. Treatment-by-age interaction was not significant ($p = 0.99$), indicating that there was no significant difference in the effect of teriparatide in younger vs older patients. Also in the older subgroup, 3.2% of the women in the teriparatide group and 4.2% in the placebo group had a new non-vertebral fracture (RR = 0.75; $p = 0.661$). Again, the treatment-by-age interaction was not significant ($p = 0.42$). The nonsignificant effect on non-vertebral fracture risk in older persons can be justified by the small number of non-vertebral fractures in the older subgroup, resulting in a lack of power for this aspect [72]. In conclusion, teriparatide has a significant effect on vertebral and non-vertebral fracture risk in young as well as in older fracture patients.

In the post hoc analysis of the FPT trial in women aged ≥75 years, there was no rise in adverse events in women treated with teriparatide compared to placebo [72]. On the contrary, back pain, cataract, and pruritus were significantly less present in those treated with teriparatide. Treatment-by-age interaction (≥75 vs <75 years) was not significant for the major adverse events. Cataract, deafness, pruritus, and weight loss were reported to be less frequent in the older compared to the younger age group, whereas only diarrhea was reported to be more frequent. Thus, in older persons, the safety profile of teriparatide is comparable to placebo. In clinical practice, the major disadvantages of teriparatide are the cost and the daily subcutaneous administration which may be a hamper for older patients.

Abaloparatide

The pivotal phase 3 trial ACTIVE (Abaloparatide Comparator Trial In Vertebral Endpoints) and its extension (ACTIVExtend) showed that 18 months of abaloparatide, a 34-amino acid PTH-related peptide (PTHrP), followed by sequential treatment with alendronate for an additional 24 months, significantly reduced the risk of vertebral, non-vertebral, clinical, and major osteoporotic fractures in postmenopausal women with osteoporosis (mean age of 68.8 years) [73].

Two post hoc analyses, by McClung et al. and Cosman et al., investigated the efficacy and safety of abaloparatide in women aged ≥80 years [74] and ≥75 years [75], respectively. In the analysis of McClung et al., abaloparatide was associated with numerical, but not statistically significant reductions in the risk of vertebral and non-vertebral fractures (two vertebral and two non-vertebral fractures in the placebo group vs. zero and one fracture, respectively, in the abaloparatide group) [74]. These numerical reductions in fracture risk are consistent with the effectiveness of abaloparatide in the overall ACTIVE population, but the difference is not statistically significant, which may be explained by the very small number of fractures in the older age group [74]. In the analysis by Cosman et al., the effect of abaloparatide on vertebral and non-vertebral fracture risk reduction was consistent across different age groups (<65 vs. 65 to <75 vs. ≥75 years) [75]. In these separate age groups, vertebral and non-vertebral fracture risk reduction was not significant, which may be explained by the small number of participants and events in these subgroups.

Regarding tolerability and safety, the proportion of women reporting adverse events was similar in the older age group (≥80 years) and the overall ACTIVE population [74]. However, the older patients reported more serious adverse events than the overall ACTIVE population. This may not be unexpected for an older population but, more importantly, did not differ between abaloparatide and placebo [74].

Romosozumab

In the FRAME (Fracture Study in Postmenopausal Women with Osteoporosis) study in postmenopausal women aged 55–90 years with osteoporosis, romosozumab was associated with a lower risk of vertebral fractures than placebo at 12 months and, after the transition to denosumab, at 24 and 36 months [76, 77]. At 12 months, the risk of clinical fracture was also significantly lower with romosozumab than with placebo. The ARCH study (Active-Controlled Fracture Study in Postmenopausal Women with Osteoporosis at High Risk) showed that in postmenopausal women aged 55 to 90 years at high risk of fracture, 12 months of romosozumab followed by alendronate resulted in a significantly lower risk of clinical, vertebral, non-vertebral, and hip fractures compared to alendronate alone [78].

No post hoc analyses have been performed regarding the efficacy of romosozumab in older persons, but the mean age in FRAME and ARCH was 71 years and 74.3 years, respectively, with 31.2% and 52% of included women being ≥75 years.

21.4.2.3 Osteoporosis Treatment in Men

There is little evidence from studies in men, but it is recommended that 1000 mg of calcium and 800 IU of vitamin D should be taken, similar as in women [79]. Medical agencies such as the US Food and Drug Administration (FDA) and European Medicines Agency (EMA) state that it is not necessary to demonstrate antifracture efficacy in men for drugs that already have shown antifracture efficacy in postmenopausal osteoporosis. Hence, majority of clinical trials in men only have effects on BMD and BTM as outcome parameters.

In a meta-analysis, bisphosphonates (alendronate and risedronate) significantly reduced vertebral fracture risk and possibly also non-vertebral fracture risk in men [80]. There is only one study in men evaluating zoledronic acid that has been sufficiently powered for vertebral fracture. This study showed that men treated with zoledronic acid had fewer vertebral fractures than those on placebo [81]. The effect of denosumab was investigated in the ADAMO trial in 242 men, showing a significant increase of BMD at the spine and hip after 12 months of treatment vs placebo [82]. The study was not powered for fractures. Teriparatide significantly increases BMD in men with osteoporosis and is licensed by the FDA and EMA as treatment for osteoporosis in men [83]. Romosozumab for 12 months increased BMD at the spine and hip in men in the BRIDGE study, yet fracture endpoints were not included. According to the authors, based on the observed BMD gains and similar fracture risk, the fracture reduction observed in the FRAME study in postmenopausal women can be extrapolated to men [84]. While in some countries (Japan, Australia, etc.) romosozumab is approved for men at high risk of fractures, this is not the case in Europe. Finally, testosterone replacement results in a small increase in BMD but not as large as osteoporosis treatments and no data are available on fracture risk. Thus, testosterone (taking also the potential side effects into account) is not considered as an adequate treatment option for osteoporosis in men.

Hence, we conclude that men seem to respond to the available osteoporosis treatments in the same way as women, and therefore, the treatment approach, for the most part, is similar in both genders.

21.4.2.4 Effectiveness of Osteoporosis Treatment in Older Persons in the Clinical Setting

Older persons in clinical practice may differ from the persons included in trials, both in terms of patient characteristics and comorbidities. Patients in clinical practice may also be less compliant or take the medication for a longer or shorter time period than recommended. These aspects may impact the effectiveness of medication. Therefore, the real-word effectiveness of osteoporosis treatments was compared between persons aged ≥80 years and younger women (60–79 years) using the Swedish health register data [85]. The results showed that osteoporosis medication is effective in women older than 80 years, with an effect size similar to that in younger women and to that reported in RCTs [85].

21.4.2.5 Lag Time to Benefit from Osteoporosis Treatment

In clinical practice, physicians may have doubts about starting osteoporosis treatment in very old patients with a rather short life expectancy. However, in the landmark osteoporosis trials, most pharmacological therapies for osteoporosis obtained a significant reduction in fracture risk within 12 months of treatment, at least for vertebral fractures. A recent meta-analysis about the time to benefit of bisphosphonate therapy found that 12.4 months were needed to avoid one non-vertebral fracture per 100 postmenopausal women receiving bisphosphonate therapy. In addition, 200 postmenopausal women would need to be treated with a bisphosphonate for 12.1 months and 20.3 months to avoid one clinical vertebral fracture and one hip fracture, respectively [86]. These results suggest that starting osteoporosis treatment is appropriate for persons with a life expectancy greater than 1 year [70, 87]. In 2015, the average life expectancy at 80 years in the EU was 9.2 years [88].

21.5 Conclusion

Osteoporosis is one of the most common age-associated conditions causing increased bone fragility and risk of fractures. In old age, osteoporosis and osteoporotic fractures tend to occur in a subset of frail people. Treatment of osteoporosis is of particular concern in older persons because of the substantial impact of osteoporotic fractures on morbidity, mortality, and economic cost. Moreover, as the risk of a subsequent fracture is the highest in the year following a fragility fracture, international guidelines and scientific bodies highly recommend focus on secondary fracture prevention.

The treatment window for osteoporosis is never closed, not even in older patients with the most severe degree of osteoporosis and not even in those who have already suffered an osteoporotic fracture. Calcium and vitamin D supplementation is a crucial component but not sufficient in the management of osteoporosis in old age. Adding osteoporosis treatment significantly lowers the risk of fractures, at least for vertebral fractures and possibly also for hip fractures. In frail older persons with documented osteoporosis, osteoporosis treatment may even be more effective than in younger patients, with more fractures avoided and decreased numbers needed to treat.

Data in older persons clearly indicate that the existing osteoporosis therapies are relatively safe, with no significant differences in the incidence of most adverse events in the treated group compared to that in the placebo group. Also, the incidence of adverse events in older persons is not higher than reported in the general population. In the clinical setting, specific issues such as comorbidity and polypharmacy should be taken into account in older persons and may influence the choice of therapy. However, real-word data confirmed that osteoporosis medication is safe and effective in older persons. All together, these data in older persons indicate that age in itself is no reason to withhold osteoporosis treatment in old persons with osteoporosis or at high fracture risk.

References

1. Cosman F, de Beur SJ, LeBoff MS, Lewiecki EM, Tanner B, Randall S, et al. Clinician's guide to prevention and treatment of osteoporosis. Osteoporos Int. 2014;25(10):2359–81.
2. Cooper C, Campion G, Melton LJ 3rd. Hip fractures in the elderly: a world-wide projection. Osteoporos Int. 1992;2(6):285–9.
3. Grados F, Marcelli C, Dargent-Molina P, Roux C, Vergnol JF, Meunier PJ, et al. Prevalence of vertebral fractures in French women older than 75 years from the EPIDOS study. Bone. 2004;34(2):362–7.
4. Seeman E, Boonen S, Borgstrom F, Vellas B, Aquino JP, Semler J, et al. Five years treatment with strontium ranelate reduces vertebral and nonvertebral fractures and increases the number and quality of remaining life-years in women over 80 years of age. Bone. 2010;46(4):1038–42.
5. Sambrook P, Cooper C. Osteoporosis. Lancet. 2006;367(9527):2010–8.
6. Boonen S, Autier P, Barette M, Vanderschueren D, Lips P, Haentjens P. Functional outcome and quality of life following hip fracture in elderly women: a prospective controlled study. Osteoporos Int. 2004;15(2):87–94.

7. Gielen E, Verschueren S, O'Neill TW, Pye SR, O'Connell MD, Lee DM, et al. Musculoskeletal frailty: a geriatric syndrome at the core of fracture occurrence in older age. Calcif Tissue Int. 2012;91(3):161–77.
8. Leibson CL, Tosteson AN, Gabriel SE, Ransom JE, Melton LJ. Mortality, disability, and nursing home use for persons with and without hip fracture: a population-based study. J Am Geriatr Soc. 2002;50(10):1644–50.
9. Schnell S, Friedman SM, Mendelson DA, Bingham KW, Kates SL. The 1-year mortality of patients treated in a hip fracture program for elders. Geriatr Orthop Surg Rehabil. 2010;1(1):6–14.
10. Gielen E, Vanderschueren D, Callewaert F, Boonen S. Osteoporosis in men. Best Pract Res Clin Endocrinol Metab. 2011;25(2):321–35.
11. Haentjens P, Magaziner J, Colon-Emeric CS, Vanderschueren D, Milisen K, Velkeniers B, et al. Meta-analysis: excess mortality after hip fracture among older women and men. Ann Intern Med. 2010;152(6):380–90.
12. Tran T, Bliuc D, Hansen L, Abrahamsen B, van den Bergh J, Eisman JA, et al. Persistence of excess mortality following individual nonhip fractures: a relative survival analysis. J Clin Endocrinol Metab. 2018;103(9):3205–14.
13. Feldstein A, Elmer PJ, Orwoll E, Herson M, Hillier T. Bone mineral density measurement and treatment for osteoporosis in older individuals with fractures: a gap in evidence-based practice guideline implementation. Arch Intern Med. 2003;163(18):2165–72.
14. Johnell K, Fastbom J. Undertreatment of osteoporosis in the oldest old? A nationwide study of over 700,000 older people. Arch Osteoporos. 2009;4(1–2):17–23.
15. Kanis JA, Melton LJ 3rd, Christiansen C, Johnston CC, Khaltaev N. The diagnosis of osteoporosis. J Bone Miner Res. 1994;9(8):1137–41.
16. Thomas-John M, Codd MB, Manne S, Watts NB, Mongey AB. Risk factors for the development of osteoporosis and osteoporotic fractures among older men. J Rheumatol. 2009;36(9):1947–52.
17. Melton LJ 3rd, Atkinson EJ, Cooper C, O'Fallon WM, Riggs BL. Vertebral fractures predict subsequent fractures. Osteoporos Int. 1999;10(3):214–21.
18. Kanis JA, Johnell O, Oden A, Dawson A, De Laet C, Jonsson B. Ten year probabilities of osteoporotic fractures according to BMD and diagnostic thresholds. Osteoporos Int. 2001;12(12):989–95.
19. FRAX®. Fracture Risk Assessment Tool. http://www.shef.ac.uk/FRAX/.
20. Kanis JA, McCloskey EV, Johansson H, Cooper C, Rizzoli R, Reginster JY, et al. European guidance for the diagnosis and management of osteoporosis in postmenopausal women. Osteoporos Int. 2013;24(1):23–57.
21. Tosteson AN, Melton LJ 3rd, Dawson-Hughes B, Baim S, Favus MJ, Khosla S, et al. Cost-effective osteoporosis treatment thresholds: the United States perspective. Osteoporos Int. 2008;19(4):437–47.
22. Compston J, Bowring C, Cooper A, Cooper C, Davies C, Francis R, et al. Diagnosis and management of osteoporosis in postmenopausal women and older men in the UK: National Osteoporosis Guideline Group (NOGG) update 2013. Maturitas. 2013;75(4):392–6.
23. McCloskey E, Kanis JA, Johansson H, Harvey N, Oden A, Cooper A, et al. FRAX-based assessment and intervention thresholds—an exploration of thresholds in women aged 50 years and older in the UK. Osteoporos Int. 2015;26(8):2091–9.
24. Kanis JA, Harvey NC, Cooper C, Johansson H, Oden A, McCloskey EV, et al. A systematic review of intervention thresholds based on FRAX : a report prepared for the National Osteoporosis Guideline Group and the international osteoporosis foundation. Arch Osteoporos. 2016;11(1):25.
25. Lips P. Vitamin D deficiency and secondary hyperparathyroidism in the elderly: consequences for bone loss and fractures and therapeutic implications. Endocr Rev. 2001;22(4):477–501.
26. MacLaughlin J, Holick MF. Aging decreases the capacity of human skin to produce vitamin D3. J Clin Invest. 1985;76(4):1536–8.

27. Bolland MJ, Grey A, Gamble GD, Reid IR. The effect of vitamin D supplementation on skeletal, vascular, or cancer outcomes: a trial sequential meta-analysis. Lancet Diabetes Endocrinol. 2014;2(4):307–20.
28. Jackson RD, LaCroix AZ, Gass M, Wallace RB, Robbins J, Lewis CE, et al. Calcium plus vitamin D supplementation and the risk of fractures. N Engl J Med. 2006;354(7):669–83.
29. Grant AM, Avenell A, Campbell MK, McDonald AM, MacLennan GS, McPherson GC, et al. Oral vitamin D3 and calcium for secondary prevention of low-trauma fractures in elderly people (Randomised Evaluation of Calcium Or vitamin D, RECORD): a randomised placebo-controlled trial. Lancet. 2005;365(9471):1621–8.
30. Boonen S, Vanderschueren D, Haentjens P, Lips P. Calcium and vitamin D in the prevention and treatment of osteoporosis - a clinical update. J Intern Med. 2006;259(6):539–52.
31. Bouillon R, Van Schoor NM, Gielen E, Boonen S, Mathieu C, Vanderschueren D, et al. Optimal vitamin D status: a critical analysis on the basis of evidence-based medicine. J Clin Endocrinol Metab. 2013;98(8):E1283–304.
32. Eleni A, Panagiotis P. A systematic review and meta-analysis of vitamin D and calcium in preventing osteoporotic fractures. Clin Rheumatol. 2020;39(12):3571–9.
33. Dawson-Hughes B, Mithal A, Bonjour JP, Boonen S, Burckhardt P, Fuleihan GE, et al. IOF position statement: vitamin D recommendations for older adults. Osteoporos Int. 2010;21(7):1151–4.
34. Sanders K. ACP journal Club: a single, annual, high dose of oral vitamin D increased falls and fractures in older women. Ann Intern Med. 2010;153(6):JC3.
35. Bischoff-Ferrari HA, Dawson-Hughes B, Orav EJ, Staehelin HB, Meyer OW, Theiler R, et al. Monthly high-dose vitamin D treatment for the prevention of functional decline: a randomized clinical trial. JAMA Intern Med. 2016;176(2):175–83.
36. American Geriatrics Society Workgroup on Vitamin DSfOA. Recommendations abstracted from the American Geriatrics Society consensus statement on vitamin D for prevention of falls and their consequences. J Am Geriatr Soc. 2014;62(1):147–52.
37. Rizzoli R, Branco J, Brandi ML, Boonen S, Bruyere O, Cacoub P, et al. Management of osteoporosis of the oldest old. Osteoporos Int. 2014;25(11):2507–29.
38. Vondracek SF, Linnebur SA. Diagnosis and management of osteoporosis in the older senior. Clin Interv Aging. 2009;4:121–36.
39. Black DM, Cummings SR, Karpf DB, Cauley JA, Thompson DE, Nevitt MC, et al. Randomised trial of effect of alendronate on risk of fracture in women with existing vertebral fractures. Fracture Intervention Trial Research Group. Lancet. 1996;348(9041):1535–41.
40. Cummings SR, Black DM, Thompson DE, Applegate WB, Barrett-Connor E, Musliner TA, et al. Effect of alendronate on risk of fracture in women with low bone density but without vertebral fractures: results from the Fracture Intervention Trial. JAMA. 1998;280(24):2077–82.
41. Ensrud KE, Black DM, Palermo L, Bauer DC, Barrett-Connor E, Quandt SA, et al. Treatment with alendronate prevents fractures in women at highest risk: results from the fracture intervention trial. Arch Intern Med. 1997;157(22):2617–24.
42. Hochberg MC, Thompson DE, Black DM, Quandt SA, Cauley J, Geusens P, et al. Effect of alendronate on the age-specific incidence of symptomatic osteoporotic fractures. J Bone Miner Res. 2005;20(6):971–6.
43. Axelsson KF, Wallander M, Johansson H, Lundh D, Lorentzon M. Hip fracture risk and safety with alendronate treatment in the oldest-old. J Intern Med. 2017;282(6):546–59.
44. Harris ST, Watts NB, Genant HK, McKeever CD, Hangartner T, Keller M, et al. Effects of risedronate treatment on vertebral and nonvertebral fractures in women with postmenopausal osteoporosis: a randomized controlled trial. Vertebral Efficacy with Risedronate Therapy (VERT) Study Group. JAMA. 1999;282(14):1344–52.
45. Reginster J, Minne HW, Sorensen OH, Hooper M, Roux C, Brandi ML, et al. Randomized trial of the effects of risedronate on vertebral fractures in women with established postmenopausal osteoporosis. Vertebral Efficacy with Risedronate Therapy (VERT) Study Group. Osteoporos Int. 2000;11(1):83–91.

46. McClung MR, Geusens P, Miller PD, Zippel H, Bensen WG, Roux C, et al. Effect of risedronate on the risk of hip fracture in elderly women. Hip Intervention Program Study Group. N Engl J Med. 2001;344(5):333–40.
47. Boonen S, McClung MR, Eastell R, El-Hajj Fuleihan G, Barton IP, Delmas P. Safety and efficacy of risedronate in reducing fracture risk in osteoporotic women aged 80 and older: implications for the use of antiresorptive agents in the old and oldest old. J Am Geriatr Soc. 2004;52(11):1832–9.
48. Tom SE, Adachi JD, Anderson FA Jr, Boonen S, Chapurlat RD, Compston JE, et al. Frailty and fracture, disability, and falls: a multiple country study from the global longitudinal study of osteoporosis in women. J Am Geriatr Soc. 2013;61(3):327–34.
49. Cryer B, Bauer DC. Oral bisphosphonates and upper gastrointestinal tract problems: what is the evidence? Mayo Clin Proc. 2002;77(10):1031–43.
50. Porras AG, Holland SD, Gertz BJ. Pharmacokinetics of alendronate. Clin Pharmacokinet. 1999;36(5):315–28.
51. Lo JC, Pressman AR, Omar MA, Ettinger B. Persistence with weekly alendronate therapy among postmenopausal women. Osteoporos Int. 2006;17(6):922–8.
52. Boonen S, Black DM, Colon-Emeric CS, Eastell R, Magaziner JS, Eriksen EF, et al. Efficacy and safety of a once-yearly intravenous zoledronic acid 5 mg for fracture prevention in elderly postmenopausal women with osteoporosis aged 75 and older. J Am Geriatr Soc. 2010;58(2):292–9.
53. Black DM, Delmas PD, Eastell R, Reid IR, Boonen S, Cauley JA, et al. Once-yearly zoledronic acid for treatment of postmenopausal osteoporosis. N Engl J Med. 2007;356(18):1809–22.
54. Lyles KW, Colon-Emeric CS, Magaziner JS, Adachi JD, Pieper CF, Mautalen C, et al. Zoledronic acid in reducing clinical fracture and mortality after hip fracture. N Engl J Med. 2007;357:nihpa40967.
55. Cummings SR, San Martin J, McClung MR, Siris ES, Eastell R, Reid IR, et al. Denosumab for prevention of fractures in postmenopausal women with osteoporosis. N Engl J Med. 2009;361(8):756–65.
56. Boonen S, Adachi JD, Man Z, Cummings SR, Lippuner K, Torring O, et al. Treatment with denosumab reduces the incidence of new vertebral and hip fractures in postmenopausal women at high risk. J Clin Endocrinol Metab. 2011;96(6):1727–36.
57. McClung MR, Boonen S, Torring O, Roux C, Rizzoli R, Bone HG, et al. Effect of denosumab treatment on the risk of fractures in subgroups of women with postmenopausal osteoporosis. J Bone Miner Res. 2012;27(1):211–8.
58. Papapoulos S, McClung M, Franchimont N, Adachi J, Bone H, Benhamou C, et al. Low fracture incidence is maintained in postmenopausal women ≥75 years with osteoporosis with long-term denosumab treatment. J Bone Miner Res. 2012;27(Suppl 1)
59. Genant HK, Libanati C, Engelke K, Zanchetta JR, Hoiseth A, Yuen CK, et al. Improvements in hip trabecular, subcortical, and cortical density and mass in postmenopausal women with osteoporosis treated with denosumab. Bone. 2013;56(2):482–8.
60. Jamal SA, Ljunggren O, Stehman-Breen C, Cummings SR, McClung MR, Goemaere S, et al. Effects of denosumab on fracture and bone mineral density by level of kidney function. J Bone Miner Res. 2011;26(8):1829–35.
61. Tsourdi E, Zillikens MC. Certainties and uncertainties about denosumab discontinuation. Calcif Tissue Int. 2018;103(1):1–4.
62. Bone HG, Bolognese MA, Yuen CK, Kendler DL, Miller PD, Yang YC, et al. Effects of denosumab treatment and discontinuation on bone mineral density and bone turnover markers in postmenopausal women with low bone mass. J Clin Endocrinol Metab. 2011;96(4):972–80.
63. Cummings SR, Ferrari S, Eastell R, Gilchrist N, Jensen JB, McClung M, et al. Vertebral fractures after discontinuation of denosumab: a post hoc analysis of the randomized placebo-controlled FREEDOM trial and its extension. J Bone Miner Res. 2018;33(2):190–8.
64. Anastasilakis AD, Polyzos SA, Makras P, Aubry-Rozier B, Kaouri S, Lamy O. Clinical features of 24 patients with rebound-associated vertebral fractures after denosumab discontinuation: systematic review and additional cases. J Bone Miner Res. 2017;32(6):1291–6.

65. Dupont J, Laurent MR, Dedeyne L, Luyten FP, Gielen E, Dejaeger M. Rebound-associated vertebral fractures after stopping denosumab: report of four cases. Joint Bone Spine. 2020;87(2):171–3.
66. Dupont J, Laurent MR, Dedeyne L, Luyten FP, Gielen E, Dejaeger M. Vertebral fractures after denosumab cessation. Cleve Clin J Med. 2020;87(6):337–8.
67. Grassi G, Chiodini I, Palmieri S, Cairoli E, Arosio M, Eller-Vainicher C. Bisphosphonates after denosumab withdrawal reduce the vertebral fractures incidence. Eur J Endocrinol. 2021;185(3):387–96.
68. Solling AS, Harslof T, Langdahl B. Treatment with zoledronate subsequent to denosumab in osteoporosis: a 2-year randomized study. J Bone Miner Res. 2021;36(7):1245–54.
69. Low A. Should all elderly women receive bisphosphonates to prevent osteoporotic fractures? Can J Hosp Pharm. 2012;65(1):45–8.
70. Sanchez-Rodriguez D, Bergmann P, Body JJ, Cavalier E, Gielen E, Goemaere S, et al. The Belgian Bone Club 2020 guidelines for the management of osteoporosis in postmenopausal women. Maturitas. 2020;139:69–89.
71. Neer RM, Arnaud CD, Zanchetta JR, Prince R, Gaich GA, Reginster JY, et al. Effect of parathyroid hormone (1-34) on fractures and bone mineral density in postmenopausal women with osteoporosis. N Engl J Med. 2001;344(19):1434–41.
72. Boonen S, Marin F, Mellstrom D, Xie L, Desaiah D, Krege JH, et al. Safety and efficacy of teriparatide in elderly women with established osteoporosis: bone anabolic therapy from a geriatric perspective. J Am Geriatr Soc. 2006;54(5):782–9.
73. Miller PD, Hattersley G, Riis BJ, Williams GC, Lau E, Russo LA, et al. Effect of abaloparatide vs placebo on new vertebral fractures in postmenopausal women with osteoporosis: a randomized clinical trial. JAMA. 2016;316(7):722–33.
74. McClung MR, Harvey NC, Fitzpatrick LA, Miller PD, Hattersley G, Wang Y, et al. Effects of abaloparatide on bone mineral density and risk of fracture in postmenopausal women aged 80 years or older with osteoporosis. Menopause. 2018;25(7):767–71.
75. Cosman F, Hattersley G, Hu MY, Williams GC, Fitzpatrick LA, Black DM. Effects of Abaloparatide-SC on fractures and bone mineral density in subgroups of postmenopausal women with osteoporosis and varying baseline risk factors. J Bone Miner Res. 2017;32(1):17–23.
76. Cosman F, Crittenden DB, Adachi JD, Binkley N, Czerwinski E, Ferrari S, et al. Romosozumab treatment in postmenopausal women with osteoporosis. N Engl J Med. 2016;375(16):1532–43.
77. Lewiecki EM, Dinavahi RV, Lazaretti-Castro M, Ebeling PR, Adachi JD, Miyauchi A, et al. One year of romosozumab followed by two years of denosumab maintains fracture risk reductions: results of the FRAME extension study. J Bone Miner Res. 2019;34(3):419–28.
78. Saag KG, Petersen J, Brandi ML, Karaplis AC, Lorentzon M, Thomas T, et al. Romosozumab or alendronate for fracture prevention in women with osteoporosis. N Engl J Med. 2017;377(15):1417–27.
79. Watts NB, Adler RA, Bilezikian JP, Drake MT, Eastell R, Orwoll ES, et al. Osteoporosis in men: an Endocrine Society clinical practice guideline. J Clin Endocrinol Metab. 2012;97(6):1802–22.
80. Nayak S, Greenspan SL. Osteoporosis treatment efficacy for men: a systematic review and meta-analysis. J Am Geriatr Soc. 2017;65(3):490–5.
81. Boonen S, Reginster JY, Kaufman JM, Lippuner K, Zanchetta J, Langdahl B, Rizzoli R, Lipschitz S, Dimai HP, Witvrouw R, Eriksen E, Brixen K, Russo L, Claessens F, Papanastasiou P, Antunez O, Su G, Bucci-Rechtweg C, Hruska J, Incera E, Vanderschueren D, Orwoll E. N. Fracture risk and zoledronic acid therapy in men with osteoporosis. Engl J Med. 2012;367(18):1714–23.
82. Orwoll E, Teglbjaerg CS, Langdahl BL, Chapurlat R, Czerwinski E, Kendler DL, et al. A randomized, placebo-controlled study of the effects of denosumab for the treatment of men with low bone mineral density. J Clin Endocrinol Metab. 2012;97(9):3161–9.

83. Orwoll ES, Scheele WH, Paul S, Adami S, Syversen U, Diez-Perez A, et al. The effect of teriparatide [human parathyroid hormone (1-34)] therapy on bone density in men with osteoporosis. J Bone Miner Res. 2003;18(1):9–17.
84. Lewiecki EM, Blicharski T, Goemaere S, Lippuner K, Meisner PD, Miller PD, et al. A phase III randomized placebo-controlled trial to evaluate efficacy and safety of romosozumab in men with osteoporosis. J Clin Endocrinol Metab. 2018;103(9):3183–93.
85. Strom O, Lauppe R, Ljunggren O, Spangeus A, Ortsater G, O'Kelly J, et al. Real-world effectiveness of osteoporosis treatment in the oldest old. Osteoporos Int. 2020;31(8):1525–33.
86. Deardorff WJ, Cenzer I, Nguyen B, Lee SJ. Time to benefit of bisphosphonate therapy for the prevention of fractures among postmenopausal women with osteoporosis: a meta-analysis of randomized clinical trials. JAMA Intern Med. 2022;182(1):33–41.
87. Gielen E, Bergmann P, Bruyere O, Cavalier E, Delanaye P, Goemaere S, et al. Osteoporosis in frail patients: a consensus paper of the Belgian Bone Club. Calcif Tissue Int. 2017;101(2):111–31.
88. Eurostat; 2017. https://ec.europa.eu/eurostat/web/products-eurostat-news/-/EDN-20170930-1?inheritRedirect=true&redirect=%2Feurostat%2F.

22 Chronic Respiratory Disease: COPD, IPF

Raffaele Antonelli Incalzi and Filippo Luca Fimognari

22.1 Introduction

Chronic obstructive pulmonary disease (COPD) may be considered an age-related condition for biological and epidemiological reasons. Indeed, pathogenetic mechanisms largely mimic aging-associated changes in bronchial tree and alveoli, and a distinctive phenotype of aging lung, the secretory one, may be considered a proxy of the bronchitic type of COPD [1]. On the other hand, age itself does not account for emphysematous changes, but the longer the exposure to pollutants, not only to smoke, the greater the possibility that emphysematous and bronchitic changes, in variable proportion, occur. This explains why COPD prevalence dramatically increases with age, though the earliest pathological expressions of the disease date back to the young adulthood. Similarly, severity of COPD increases with age so that chronic respiratory failure complicates COPD mainly in the geriatric population: the main age of people under long-term oxygen therapy, the vast majority of whom suffers from COPD, is well over 70 years [2].

Treatment of COPD has been the object of international guidelines, the Global Initiative for Lung Disease (GOLD), which are updated yearly. The last GOLD release dates 2022 (2022 GOLD Reports—Global Initiative for Chronic Obstructive Lung Disease, https://goldcopd.org). These guidelines are a framework for the approach to COPD in older adults. However, they only to some extent take into

R. A. Incalzi (✉)
Department of Internal Medicine and Geriatrics, Campus Bio-Medico University, Rome, Italy
e-mail: R.Antonelli@policlinicocampus.it; r.antonelli@unicampus.it

F. L. Fimognari
Department of Medicine and Unit of Geriatrics, Azienda Ospedaliera "Annunziata, Mariano Santo, S. Barbara", Cosenza, Italy

A. Cherubini et al. (eds.), *Optimizing Pharmacotherapy in Older Patients*, Practical Issues in Geriatrics, https://doi.org/10.1007/978-3-031-28061-0_22

consideration selected distinctive features of COPD in the elderly, especially in the oldest old. First, rating COPD severity is troublesome because coexisting morbidities co-determinate symptoms and frequently COPD is not the main disease, although it largely accounts for health status impairment. Thus, the therapeutic approach should be decided in the perspective of multimorbidity including COPD rather than of COPD and comorbid diseases. Second, spirometry, a key diagnostic exam, requires cognitive and physical function which is frequently defective in the elderly [3]. Thus, tailoring the therapy on symptoms and respiratory function may be impossible or difficult. Furthermore, polypharmacy, a typical trait of the elderly multimorbid patient, requires a judicious choice of topical anti-inflammatory and bronchodilating drugs: acting locally, they are variably absorbed, have systemic effects, and the potential for important pharmacokinetic interactions. In addition, impaired praxic abilities could limit the quality of the inhaling maneuver. Finally, measuring the effects of the therapy requires that different outcomes be pursued and measured according to individual conditions. This implies that a multidimensional geriatric assessment guides the choice and the ensuing tailoring of the therapy.

22.2 Therapy of COPD: An Overview

It is difficult to image a disease requiring such an articulate and comprehensive therapy as COPD in the elderly (Table 22.1). The pharmacological component of the therapy may be poorly effective in patients requiring mainly educational and

Table 22.1 Components of the therapy of COPD in the elderly

Intervention	Comment
Smoking cessation	Highly effective at any age
Education	Proved to decrease the frequency and to improve the management of exacerbations. It also reduces the risk of adverse drug reactions
Rehabilitation	It improves personal capabilities and health status besides decreasing the risk of exacerbations and contrasting depression
Telerehabilitation	Proposed as an alternative to traditional approaches, it has been promoted during the COVID-19 pandemic
Vaccines	Flu, pneumococcus, pertussis, zoster
Mucus clearance devices	Important in the bronchitic (secretory) form of COPD
Sleep hygiene	If sleep problems are present, exclude comorbid OSAS or night time hypoxia
Nutrition	Selected interventions tailored to the individual needs can improve nutritional status and independence
Cognitive training	Overall ineffective, should not be further recommended
Topically acting bronchodilators	Effective at any age, should be carefully chosen according to the individual conditions

Table 22.1 (continued)

Intervention	Comment
Topically acting steroids	Able to prevent the desensitization and to promote the expression of the beta receptor, are a key measure at any age
Theophylline and related compounds	Though they are no further recommended (GOLD 2020), they maintain efficacy in carefully selected patients, mainly to sustain the nocturnal respiratory drive. Due to their low cost, they may be considered as an alternative to topical drugs in low-income countries as well as in patients with major praxic problems
Roflumilast	In difficult to control bronchitic forms of severe COPD
Mucolytics (erdosteine, carbocysteine, NAC)	Likely decrease the frequency of exacerbations in the bronchitic type
Long-term oxygen therapy	For $SpO2 < 93\%$ at rest or during sleep or exercise
Noninvasive ventilation	To contrast dyspnea in end-stage COPD or to prevent muscle exhaustion in cachectic patients. Of primary importance in severe acute exacerbations
Endoscopic therapeutic procedures	Giant bullectomy, lung sealants, large airway stenting, coil, thermal vapor ablation
Lung volume reduction surgery	Upper lobe emphysema and low exercise capacity
Remote monitoring	Effective if performed according to a standardized model and tailored to the individual patient
Palliative care	It might be started before the patient enters the end stage of COPD because it can largely improve the quality of life, mainly by relieving dyspnea
Pharmacological assessment	A comprehensive revision of the pharmacological therapy for any problem allows to identify drugs having the potential for worsening the respiratory status

rehabilitation measures. Thus, therapy may be considered as a mix of integrated measures aimed at optimizing the health status. However, important caveats should be considered because coexisting diseases and social, cognitive, and functional problems have the potential for waning the effects of the therapy. Some problems potentially affecting the diagnosis of exacerbation or limiting the efficacy of the therapy of COPD in the elderly are reported in Table 22.2. Thus, a preliminary comprehensive geriatric assessment is needed to optimize the cost/effectiveness of the therapeutic approach. Interestingly, the approach to COPD changes as a function of the specialty of the caring physician [4]. Thus, efforts should be made to promote the awareness of the complex clinical picture and related needs of the older COPD patient in different specialists.

For obvious reasons, we will present individual components of the therapy, but we will do it in a relational and dynamic perspective. Missing the network of therapeutic measures, i.e., considering each of them as an isolated intervention, would negatively affect the cumulative effect of the therapy.

Table 22.2 Main problems affecting the diagnosis of exacerbation or limiting the efficacy of therapy of COPD in the elderly

Coexistent OSASs	Frequently it manifests with nocturia due to brisk changes in abdominal pressure and, then, is misinterpreted as a prostatic symptom
Cognitive impairment/linguistic barriers	Attention should be paid to tailor the therapeutic plan to the individual capabilities and to provide a follow-up
Impaired dexterity	As above
Coexisting CHF	Nt-proBNP should be measured and, if high, cardiological work-up performed
Malnutrition	MNA might be used as a screening test
Anorexia	Pharyngeal or esophageal mycosis is a frequently missed cause of anorexia with or without dysphagia
Atypical exacerbation	Delirium, gait problems, lethargy, CHF-like presentation, no or mild dyspnea, thoracic pain may confound the examiner
Arrhythmias	Atrial fibrillation, flutter, atrial chaotic tachycardia could account for hemodynamic instability and require urgent dedicated intervention besides the correction of the blood gas derangement
Concealed chronic kidney disease	An important cause of fluid retention and a risk factor for drug toxicity
Frequently defective enteroception	Mainly in patients with diabetes or hyposmia it could make the patient unaware of her/his true health status

22.3 Therapy of COPD: The Main Individual Components

22.3.1 Education

Making the patient aware of her/his disease, able to recognize significant changes and to disregard minor ones, and able to adopt pertinent behaviors are a primary therapeutic objective. Indeed, empowerment and promotion of the enteroception have been associated with decreased frequency and more timely treatment of exacerbations as well as with better disease-related health status [5]. Furthermore, education decreases the risk of adverse drug reactions and the use, mainly the improper use, of healthcare services. To pursue this objective, either individual education or group programs proved effective. Furthermore, a well-informed patient is able to appreciate the individual and cumulative values of each therapeutic measure, which promotes the adherence to maintenance rehabilitation, periodical control visits, and so on. Finally, an important objective of education is a periodical check of adherence to and retraining the correct use of inhaler devices. Indeed, it has been demonstrated that even mild cognitive impairment, as reflected by a MMSE < 24 or a defective performance in the copy of the two pentagons test, identifies people who will have difficulty with inhalers [6].

22.3.2 Rehabilitation

Once considered a typical post-acute therapeutic measure, rehabilitation is presently recognized as a leading therapeutic tool all over the course of COPD at any age and for any stage of COPD severity [7]. Rehabilitation is effective also during the acute exacerbations, but it plays a primary role as a continuous aid, "maintenance rehabilitation," with positive effects on both physical and affective domains [8]. Also patients with disabling COPD benefit from rehabilitation, else more than patients with mild to moderate COPD [9]. Besides the classical respiratory rehabilitation, worthy of attention are general rehabilitation; upper limb exercise, mainly for the emphysematous patient; and occupational therapy. If possible, rehabilitation should be tailored to the individual needs by taking into account the mainly hypersecretive or dyspneic trait of COPD, exercise-related fatigue, ability to retain the inherent information, and mood. Thus, a comprehensive assessment is functional to plan the best rehabilitation for the individual patient. However, if such an approach is unavailable, it is well proved that also simple exercise such as walking is effective at improving exercise tolerance and health status [10]. Finally, selected forms of rehabilitation, such as rehabilitation of swallowing [11], may be of benefit on individual bases.

22.3.3 Devices Promoting Airways Mucus Clearance

The mucus changes physical status, from more to less dense, by absorbing kinetic energy (thixotropism). Thus, exercise itself is the primary promoter of mucus clearance. However, mainly in sarcopenic or disabled hypersecretive patients, some mechanical aids may improve mucus clearance. Among these is the flutter, which, by delivering kinetic energy, loosens the mucus from the airway walls and increases airways patency. A comparable effect is obtained by the oscillating positive expiratory pressure devices. Other devices produce a negative pressure in the mouth and, thus, a favorable gradient for mucus clearance; however, their use should be limited to patient with an efficient cough reflex. Finally, high-frequency and low-frequency chest compression devices are simple and totally passive mucus clearance promoters [12]. These tools should not be regarded as an alternative to rehabilitation, but they have the potential for complementing and speeding it in the hypersecretive phenotype of COPD, mainly in patients whom early fatigability makes unable to take the full benefit from rehabilitation.

22.3.4 Vaccinations

Vaccination is a key measure of care for older COPD patients [13]. Annual influenza vaccination prevents exacerbations and is associated with decreased mortality [14]. Pneumococcal 13-valent polysaccharide vaccine (PPSV13), to be repeated every 5 years, has been proved to prevent acute exacerbations and bacteremia from pneumococcus in the elderly. Current CDC recommendations bend toward PPSV23, which has been proved to decrease pneumonia in COPD patients under 65 years or FEV1 <40% or comorbidities. Given that pertussis or whooping cough is a primary cause and a severity factor of COPD exacerbations, a dTaP/dTPa vaccination is recommended for patients who were not vaccinated in adolescence. However, immunity wanes in a few years and a booster dose should be provided after 10 years and should be repeated every 10 years. Vaccination anti-herpes zoster is also indicated in people over 65 years. COPD patients are at special risk of immunodepression to malnutrition, steroid use, and chronic inflammation. The adjuvant zoster vaccine is safe and effective also in immunocompromised patients. Finally, COVID-19 vaccine is strongly advocated for COPD patients, given that COPD qualifies as a severity factor for COVID-19 disease [15].

22.3.5 Sleep Hygiene

Sleep is essential to life, but it is frequently impaired in elderly and diseased patients. COPD is a major cause of sleep troubles [16], but unrecognized obstructive sleep apnea frequently contributes to disrupt the sleep architecture. Interestingly, nocturia, commonly considered a clue to urologic problems, may be an effect of OSAS [17]. Furthermore, defective tailoring of oxygen supplementation to changing needs at night may account for hypoxia and related sleep troubles in COPD patients under long-term oxygen therapy. Thus, any COPD patient should undergo at least one nocturnal oximetry in standard conditions, i.e., the ones characterizing her/his usual health status, to exclude or, if present, to correct nocturnal hypoxia, e.g., by increasing O_2 delivery or providing nocturnal ventilation as needed. Furthermore, a careful scrutiny of pharmacological therapy, including over-the-counter drugs and nutritional supplementations, is mandatory to identify possible pharmacological-related sleep troubles. For instance, antidepressants are associated with a variety of sleep disturbances besides carrying some risk respiratory depression [18]. Thus, a thorough pharmacological revision is needed to disentangle the potential effects of COPD, comorbidity, and drugs on the quality of sleep.

22.3.6 Nutrition

Obesity and, mainly, undernutrition are traditionally considered severity factors of COPD, and the emphysematous cachexia the hallmark of malnutrition. While these problems maintain importance, both sarcopenia, also in the presence of normal or increased body mass index (sarcopenic obesity), and more subtle nutritional deficits are gaining importance as an expression of malnutrition. Worthy of interest are deficits of folate, D vitamin, iron, and B12 vitamin [19]. Even if isolated, these deficits have important health implications; thus, they should be object of screening and, if demonstrated, correction (Table 22.3). Several definitions of sarcopenia do exist [20]; an universal consensus lacking the one by Crutz Jentoft seems the most convenient [21]; the ultrasound might help to rate sarcopenia [22]. Overall, the screening of malnutrition may rely upon the Mini Nutritional Assessment, freely available online. More sophisticated questionnaires, such as the EPIC, are used only for a point estimate of nutrient intake.

Table 22.3 Main nutritional deficits in COPD

Deficit	Screening	Clinical meaning	Correction
Overall malnutrition	Mini nutritional assessment	Worsened heath status and respiratory conditions, severity factor in the event of exacerbation	Tailored dietetic intervention
Vitamin D	Serum level <30 pg/mL	Increased risk of fracture and infection	Oral supplementation. Provide 1alpha25 dihydrotachysterol if eGFR <30 mL/1.72 m²/min
Iron	Ferritin <100 mcg/L or ferritin <300 mcg/L, but transferrin saturation <20%	Muscle weakness, anemia, worsened dyspnea, and respiratory failure	Per os or iv (Fe-carboxymaltose) correction as for clinical judgment
B12 vitamin	Serum cyanocobalamin <200 pg/mL	Anemia, postural instability, neuropathic pain	I. B12 supplementation
Folate	Serum level <3.4 ng/mL or 5 mg/dL	Depression, cognitive impairment	Per os folate supplementation (e.g., 5 mg daily)
Sarcopenia	See Ref. [19]	Fatigability, worsened dyspnea, and respiratory failure	Both exercise and nutrient supplementation are needed

Iv Intravenous, *Im* Intramuscular

Age does not decrease the nutrient needs. Thus, the elderly COPD patient should receive a balanced and complete diet, not differently from an adult one. Dietary supplementation shown to improve muscle strength is branched amino acids and PUFA, though the strength of the evidence is only moderate [23, 24]. In hypercatabolic status characterizing selected patients, a greater caloric and protein intake should be provided, but several obstacles, like digestive problems (early satiety, epigastric burn) and sarcopenia (mastication, exhaustion, etc.), make such an objective difficult to reach. Furthermore, dysphagia is highly prevalent, though unreported, in severe, mainly emphysematous, COPD, and can manifest either as malnutrition or as chronic cough and/or ab ingestis pneumonia.

22.3.7 Pharmacological Therapy

Overall, it should conform to GOLD guidelines. However, selected factors should be considered to tailor the therapy to the older patient:

1. Polypharmacy is very common in the elderly multimorbid patient. Thus, pharmacokinetic interactions should be prevented by choosing drugs having the least potential for interactions. Among LABA, salmeterol serum levels may increase for coadministration of inhibitors of the CYP3A4, like antifungal azoles and clarithromycin. While the available data are inconclusive for olodaterol,

vilanterol, and indacaterol, formoterol is known to undergo direct metabolization with only a marginal role of CYP3A4, and, thus, it is less exposed to important serum level fluctuations. Furthermore, formoterol has an early onset of action and, thus, can promptly relieve dyspnea. It is worth considering that, even if inhaled, LABA are variably absorbed, and their non-respiratory side effects, like tremor, anxiety, and arrhythmias, prove it.

2. Beta2 receptor desensitization occurs more easily in the elderly. Thus, promoting the alpha to beta receptor conversion through a steroid seems of special interest for the elderly. Accordingly, besides being first choice in the bronchitic type of COPD, the ICS-LABA may be tried every time the suspicion of defective response to LABA arises.
3. Side effects of ICS are of special interest in the elderly; while the risk of pneumonia is well recognized, attention should be paid to oral or esophageal candidiasis, which may manifest simply with dysphagia or anorexia or dysphonia or low-grade fever.
4. LAMA are usually well tolerated in the elderly, but they carry some risk of acute urinary retention. It is likely that aclidinium bromide, being metabolized be endothelial esterase and not by the kidney, is safer in patients with depressed renal function.
5. The 2023 GOLD update suggests a LAMA-LABA combination as the preferred therapy for patients not amenable or unresponsive to a single drug treatment and, in the event of poor effectiveness, a triple therapy (LAMA+LABA+ICS) rather than a trial with ICS + LABA.
6. Loss of dexterity and cognitive abilities makes the elderly patient at risk of misusing inhalers. Accordingly, a trial of use should be performed rather than merely prescribing a given drug, and the most reliable technical solution should be identified. The use of distancers enables many disabled or sarcopenic patients to benefit from topical therapy. Only in severely impaired patients aerosol therapy should be considered a therapeutic option, although it is less effective than topical long-acting drugs.
7. Theophylline: once largely prescribed, it is actually considered a second-line drug with an unfavorable cost/benefit ratio. However, it is also accredited of biologically interesting actions such as immunostimulance, which are evident for low and safe doses, and may represent a therapeutic option for elderly patients with nocturnal slowing of the respiratory drive.
8. The possibility that bronchiectases complicate the COPD lung increases with age and carries some risk of selecting Gram negative bacteria, mainly the *Pseudomonas aeruginosa*, and of hemoptysis. Thus, in the event of exacerbations, an antibiotic therapy active on Gram- bacteria may be required.
9. In patients with highly symptomatic bronchitic type of COPD, especially if bronchiectases coexist, a long-term (6–12 months) therapy with low-dose azithromycin (250 mg every other day or 500 mg three times a week) may benefit due to the immunostimulant action of macrolides. Thus, the direct antimicrobial effect is unlikely to account for clinical benefit. In the older adult, attention should be paid to the risk of pharmacokinetic interactions.

22.3.8 Oxygen Therapy

Oxygen should be prescribed like a drug, i.e., at the correct dosage, not more and not less. Indeed, excess oxygen may depress the respiratory drive, causing hypercarbia until carbonarcosis, but in the elderly, it carries an important additional risk, the one of coronary or cerebral vasoconstriction [25]. Thus, efforts should be made to obtain and maintain an arterial oxygen saturation (SaO_2) of 90–95%; higher values might be associated with adverse effects. Importantly, percutaneous oxygen saturation (SpO_2) is frequently unreliable in the elderly due to hypotension, fever, tremor, chills, atrial fibrillation, and other causes. Thus, SpO_2 >90% should not deter from performing an arterial blood gas analysis if one or more of these confounding conditions occur and/or if the inherent information may be of value to assess the metabolic status, e.g., in patients on high-dose diuretics or renal failure. Attention should be paid to modulate the inspired fraction of oxygen according to potentially changing needs with sleep and exercise.

High-flow oxygen therapy is safe and effective in elderly patients who are severely hypoxemic while on Ventimask, but moderate to severe hypercarbia carries an important risk of ineffectiveness or respiratory depression. Thus, its effects should be checked timely and, then, monitored to prevent adverse events. Finally, for people using oxygen concentrators, it is important to know that the provided fraction of oxygen varies with the respiratory rate and, for selected models, dramatically declines for increasing respiratory rate [26].

22.3.9 Noninvasive Ventilation (NIV)

Besides being a vital support in severe acute exacerbation, NIV plays an important role in the chronic care of elderly COPD patients either as a component of palliative care, to relieve dyspnea, or as an intermittent aid to patient experiencing fatigue and respiratory muscle exhaustion. Thus, it should not be considered a measure dedicated to acute care; else its use is gaining importance in the chronic patient. There are no age-related changes in the operating rules; else NIV is highly efficacious in the elderly [27, 28]. However, extra caution is needed to prevent pneumothorax or pneumomediastinum and CHF worsening due to increased intrathoracic barrage, both of which are more likely to occur in the elderly. In patients experiencing frequent lung atelectases due to either hypoexpansion or defective mucus clearance, NIV has the potential for preventing atelectases. Finally, NIV may be of value to assist the patient proved or likely to undergo nocturnal depression of the respiratory drive which cannot be compensated by changing the inspired fraction of oxygen. However, the individual needs should be carefully scrutinized; in the event of coexisting OSAS, C-PAP should be preferred.

22.3.10 Remote Monitoring

It has been proved to prevent exacerbations and improve the quality of life, but only few studies reach high-quality standards. Nevertheless, there is evidence that a well-organized telemonitoring system is highly cost-effective and has positive indirect effects by improving empowerment and confidence in the caregivers [29].

22.3.11 Palliative Care

Dyspnea and, to a lesser extent, pain are the two symptoms which characterize end stage COPD. Being deeply generated and phylogenetically ancient sensations, they are perceived also in end-stage COPD. Thirst and hunger also are "hard" sensation. Thus, the end-stage COPD patients should be the object of a comprehensive care aimed at relieving these untoward sensations through a properly tailored strategy. However, the principles and practice of palliative care should not be the patrimony of preterminal care. It has been proved that even in patients with severe COPD, mainly of the emphysematous type, but not in preterminal stage, using these principles and practice can significantly improve the health status. For instance, low-dose morphine has the potential for relieving dyspnea without causing major respiratory depression. Furthermore, it can improve the amount and quality of sleep.

22.4 Therapy of Acute COPD Exacerbations

GOLD recommendations apply to patients of any age. However, selected points are worthy of comment for elderly COPD patients:

1. Concurrent conditions like acutely decompensated heart failure or pulmonary embolism frequently underlie the sudden worsening of the health status in these patients. Thus, exacerbation of COPD should not be invariably considered as the cause of acute respiratory distress.
2. Older age does not affect the response to NIV. Thus, NIV should be provided at any age if indicated on clinical and pathophysiological ground.
3. In frequent exacerbators, sputum cultures are desirable to redirect the antibiotic therapy, if needed. Fungi could also sustain the exacerbation.
4. Delirium is a common presentation of acute exacerbation in the elderly.
5. Dyspnea may play a marginal role in the clinical picture of an exacerbation of the elderly.
6. Arrhythmias, mainly atrial fibrillation or atrial chaotic rhythm, frequently complicate the exacerbation. They may subside after reverting the acute respiratory failure and decreasing the adrenergic drive but frequently must be timely reversed because of severe hemodynamic effects.
7. Anorexia, besides being common in advanced COPD, is highly prevalent during the acute exacerbation. The nutrient intake should be monitored and integrated, if needed.
8. Fluid retention is frequently due to hypoxia and hypercarbia related renal function impairment and, thus, revert with blood gases normalization. However, diuretic therapy is frequently needed and should be adopted on an individual basis.

9. Hypoxia, malnutrition, and immobility make the older patient at special risk of developing pressure ulcers. Thus, preventative measures are highly recommended.
10. A severely hypoxic and normo- or hypocarbic exacerbation should raise the suspicion of pulmonary embolism or heart failure.
11. Once a worsening of the lung problem and a cardiac complication has been excluded, a sudden increase or worsening of hypercarbia likely reflects muscle exhaustion.
12. In older COPD patients hospitalized for severe exacerbations, any effort should be made to guarantee family and social contacts and to provide a supportive environment as a strategy preventing delirium.

22.5 Idiopathic Pulmonary Fibrosis and Other Interstitial Lung Diseases in the Elderly

22.5.1 An Overview

The interstitial lung diseases (ILDs) constitute a group of parenchymal lung diseases that affect the interstitial space with different grades of inflammation and fibrosis (Table 22.4). Some ILDs are secondary to known etiologies, including drug

Table 22.4 Classification of interstitial lung diseases

Idiopathic interstitial pneumonias
Chronic fibrosing idiopathic interstitial pneumonias
• Idiopathic pulmonary fibrosis
• Idiopathic nonspecific interstitial pneumonia
Smoking-related idiopathic interstitial pneumonias
• Respiratory bronchiolitis-interstitial lung disease
• Desquamative interstitial pneumonia
Acute/subacute idiopathic interstitial pneumonias
• Cryptogenic organizing pneumonia
• Acute interstitial pneumonia
Rare idiopathic interstitial pneumonias
• Lymphocytic interstitial pneumonia
• Idiopathic pleuroparenchymal fibroelastosis
Unclassifiable idiopathic interstitial pneumonias
ILD of known association
• Connective tissues diseases
• Drugs (amiodarone, nitrofurantoin, methotrexate)
• Occupational or environmental exposure (asbestosis and silicosis)
Sarcoidosis (granulomatous interstitial lung disease)
Hypersensitivity pneumonitis
Miscellaneous interstitial lung diseases
• Lymphangioleiomyomatosis
• Pulmonary Langerhans' cell histiocytosis/histiocytosis X
• Eosinophilic pneumonia

From references [30–32], and, with changes

toxicity, exposure to occupational or environmental factors (e.g., asbestosis and silicosis), allergens like mold, animal dander, and others (hypersensitivity pneumonitis), or represent the lung manifestation of sarcoidosis and connective tissue diseases (CTDs) such as systemic sclerosis (SSc) and rheumatoid arthritis (RA) [30].

The "idiopathic" ILDs encompass a composite family of ILDs without any recognizable origin [31, 32]. *Idiopathic pulmonary fibrosis (IPF)*, the most common (about 50% of all idiopathic ILDs), is characterized by histopathologic and high-resolution computed tomography (HRTC) pattern of usual interstitial pneumonia (UIP). IPF is a highly severe illness and is usually diagnosed in men older than 60 years, although it may rarely occur in younger adults. Smoking is a risk factor. Thus, IPF is typical of older patients and may also initially manifest with an "acute exacerbation," that is featured by acute respiratory failure, dyspnea, and ground-glass infiltrates. Later on, acute exacerbations will punctuate the natural history of IPF, along with progressive lung deterioration [31, 32]. HRTC hallmarks of typical UIP pattern include basilar and subpleural predominant reticulation and honeycombing, with frequently present traction bronchiectasis and traction bronchiolectasis [33]. This HRTC phenotype, but without honeycombing, qualifies the "probable" UIP pattern. The typical UIP pattern in a typical patient, together with the exclusion of other known causes of ILD, may authorize the diagnosis of IPF without resorting to cellular analysis of bronchoalveolar lavage (BAL) or to surgical lung biopsy (SLB). When clinical suspicion is associated with "probable," "indeterminate," or "alternative diagnosis" HRTC patterns, BAL or even SLB may be recommended to obtain a diagnosis [33]. Transbronchial lung cryobiopsy (TLC) is a less invasive alternative to SLB but is burdened by not negligible complications [33]. Many frail older patients, however, present with advanced disease and multiple comorbidities and are not suitable to SLB or TLC, owing to the unfavorable risk/benefit ratio.

Nonspecific interstitial pneumonia (NSIP) is the second idiopathic ILD for frequency (25% of all idiopathic ILDs; median age of onset 40–50 years; no association with smoking). NSIP has a more favorable prognosis compared to IPF and exhibits some response to corticosteroids, but evolution to end-stage fibrosis and death may occur, causing death 5 years after diagnosis in 20% of patients [34]. HRTC pattern includes extensive, prevalently basal, ground-glass opacities, reticular lines, traction bronchiectasis, and subpleural preservation [34]. Smoking-related idiopathic ILDs encompass *respiratory bronchiolitis-interstitial lung disease (RB-ILD)* and *desquamative interstitial pneumonia (DIP)*. The first is more frequent and can be diagnosed in middle-aged current smokers showing at HRTC patchy ground-glass opacities and centrilobular nodules mainly in the upper field. The outcome of RB-ILD is good, and the majority of patients improve after smoking cessation and/or treatment with corticosteroids. DIP is considered to represent the end of the spectrum of RB-ILD and may progress to respiratory failure, but the overall survival is about 70% after 10 years [31, 32]. The acute/subacute idiopathic ILDs are *cryptogenic organizing pneumonia (COP)* and *acute interstitial pneumonia (AIP)* [31, 32]. Organizing pneumonia (OP) is a nonspecific response to lung injuries secondary to infections, drugs, aspiration, CTDs, acute exacerbation of IPF, and other conditions. When OP occurs without a specific cause, COP is diagnosed. There is no association with smoking, and patients have a mean age of 55 years. The HRTC pattern is represented by peripheral bilateral (but also unilateral) and diffuse ground-glass opacities or alveolar consolidations with air bronchograms, which are often migratory, spare the subpleural space, more frequently involve the lower lobes, and can spontaneously disappear. COP is known for its excellent response to corticosteroids, although relapse is common with corticosteroid tapering or discontinuation [35]. AIP is similar to the acute respiratory distress syndrome (ARDS), but while ARDS is provoked by identifiable associated conditions, AIP is idiopathic. Mean age of patients is 50 years, and there is no relation with smoking. AIP develops as a severe form of diffuse alveolar damage (DAD), and mortality is around 50%. Management relies on supportive care, even though steroid therapy is often tried, without any demonstrated benefit. HRTC pattern is characterized by bilateral, basal, ground-glass attenuation or consolidation in the dependent areas, in the late phase followed by architectural distortion, traction bronchiectasis, and honeycombing in the nondependent areas [31, 32]. Very rare idiopathic ILDs are *lymphoid interstitial pneumonia* (*LIP*: ground-glass opacities at HRTC and polyclonal lymphocytes in BAL, good response to corticosteroids) and *idiopathic pleuroparenchymal fibroelastosis* (PPFE, death in 40% of patients). A category of *unclassifiable idiopathic interstitial pneumonias* [31, 32] completes the idiopathic ILDs classification (Table 22.4).

Idiopathic ILDs are rare, but their histopathologic and HRTC patterns (UIP, NSIP, OP, LIP, DAD, and others) represent "prototypes" recurring in more frequent ILDs, including those associated with CTDs, drugs, vasculitis, and in the hypersensitivity pneumonitis (HP). NSIP is common in most CTDs, particularly SSc, but in RA and vasculitis, the UIP pattern predominates [36]. HP is an immune-mediated inflammatory and fibrotic pulmonary response to the inhalation of several antigens (mainly organic, including avian and microbial agents). HP has been recently categorized as non-fibrotic HP (ground-glass opacities and mosaic attenuation, associated with centrilobular nodules on inspiratory images or air trapping in expiratory images) and fibrotic HP. The fibrotic phenotype is clinically more severe, and patients are often older [37].

22.5.2 Therapeutic Approach

22.5.2.1 Antifibrotic Therapy in IPF: Implications in Elderly Patients

In 2012, the PANTHER-IPF trial (prednisone, azathioprine, and n-acetyl cysteine for pulmonary fibrosis) conclusively showed that immunosuppression, previously the "gold standard" of IPF therapy, is ineffective and associated with increased risk of hospitalization and death compared to placebo [38].

Two antifibrotic agents, nintedanib and pirfenidone, have been recently approved for the treatment of IPF, ushering in a new era. Nintedanib, an oral tyrosine kinase inhibitor, at a dosage of 150 mg twice daily reduced the rate of decline of forced vital capacity (FVC) in IPF patients by about 50%, without affecting the time to the first IPF acute exacerbation [39–41]. The mean age of patients enrolled in the INPULSIS 1 and INPULSIS 2 trials was around 67 years, and eligibility criteria included age ≥40 years, FVC ≥50%, and diffusing capacity of the lung for carbon monoxide (DL_{CO}) ≥30% [39]. An analysis of prespecified subgroups from the INPULSIS trials demonstrated a similar benefit of nintedanib in older (≥65 years) compared to younger (<65 years) patients [42]. Diarrhea was the most common adverse effect but caused drug discontinuation in less than 5% of study patients [39]. Nintedanib is a substrate of P-glycoprotein (P-gp) and CYP3A4, and concurrent use of P-gp and CYP3A4 inhibitors (e.g., ketoconazole) or inducers (e.g., carbamazepine) may, respectively, reduce or increase nintedanib exposure [43].

Pirfenidone, an orally administered pyridine, regulates the expression of TGF-β and inhibits collagen synthesis, exerting anti-inflammatory, antioxidant, and anti-fibrotic actions. The recommended dosage of 801 mg 3 times per day is reached after a 2-week dose titration starting from 267 mg 3 times daily on the first day [43]. In the ASCEND trial, pirfenidone treatment was associated—compared to placebo—with a reduced rate of FVC decline (by about 45%), a lower proportion of patients who reported a decreased distance at the 6-min walk test, and with an increased progression-free survival (neither disease progression nor death) [44]. Pooled data from ASCEND and CAPACITY [45] trials demonstrated lower overall and IPF-related mortality in the pirfenidone group [44]. The two trial-enrolled patients aged between 40 and 80 years (mean age was about 67 years), who had baseline FVC ≥50%, together with DL_{CO} ≥30% in ASCEND and ≥35% in CAPACITY. However, a recent post hoc analysis from ASCEND and CAPACITY trials that included a small sample of patients who had more impaired respiratory function (FVC <50% and/or DL_{CO} <35%) and a mean age of 70 years confirmed pirfenidone-related clinical benefits, including lower FVC decline and decreased all-cause mortality [46]. Possible adverse effects are gastrointestinal symptoms (nausea, dyspepsia), photosensitivity rash, and elevation in aminotransferase level; these side effects led to discontinuation of study drug in less than 3% of patients enrolled in the ASCEND trial. Pirfenidone is metabolized by CYP1A2, and the concurrent use of CYP1A2 inhibitors (e.g., fluvoxamine, ciprofloxacin) should warrant dosage reduction [43].

Nintedanib and pirfenidone provide similar benefits in terms of reduction of FVC decline: the choice of administering one agent or the other should be individualized according to patient's preference, age, and possible side effects. Since the eligibility criteria of clinical trials (FVC >50%; DL_{CO} >30–35%; age less than 80 years for pirfenidone) were translated into clinical practice as clinical conditions required for authorizing treatment, these agents are prescribed only to patients with mild to moderate IPF, and very elderly patients with advanced disease, comorbidities, and respiratory failure are always excluded from such treatments. In addition, possible drug-drug interactions are an obvious concern in frail patients affected by several illnesses and treated with multiple drugs [30].

22.5.2.2 Corticosteroids and Immunosuppressive Cytotoxic Therapy in Non-IPF ILDs

Therapy may not be indicated when ILD is mild and asymptomatic. In symptomatic ILDs, however, corticosteroids and/or cytotoxic immunosuppressive drugs are usually prescribed, even though this therapeutic approach is not supported by randomized controlled trials, except for SSc-ILD. NSIP, the most frequent idiopathic ILD after IPF, is currently treated with corticosteroids (starting from 0.5–1 mg/kg/day or 40–60 mg of prednisone, followed by gradual tapering until maintenance dose). One cytotoxic drug, mainly cyclophosphamide (CYC), but also azathioprine (AZA) or mycophenolate mofetil (MMF), can be added to implement or replace corticosteroid treatment in more severe NSIP cases. There is no agreement about the length of treatment that should be individualized [34]. The dramatic response to corticosteroids (in general beginning with prednisone 0.75 mg/kg/day) is a clinical distinctive characteristic of COP [35].

The efficacy of CYC in SSc-ILD was proven by two randomized controlled trials versus placebo [47, 48]. In another randomized trial, oral MMF was as effective as oral CYC in improving FVC in SSc-ILD and caused fewer adverse effects [49]. These three trials included elderly patients, but the mean age of enrolled patients did not exceed 55 years. MMF (first line) or CYC (second line) are thus recommended as induction therapy in SSc-ILD. Based on uncontrolled studies, MMF and CYC are also recommended in RA-ILD, together with corticosteroids [50].

Corticosteroids (prednisone 0.5 mg/kg/day followed by gradual tapering to reach maintenance dose of 10 mg/day) are used to treat HP, together with MMF or AZA as steroid-sparing agents in patients with disease progression or in whom it is impossible to avoid exposure to the inciting antigen [37].

Sarcoidosis, the most common ILD (28–38% of all ILDs), can remit spontaneously, and the first challenge is to identify patients deserving treatment due to progressive organ involvement and quality of life impairment. The first line of treatment relies on corticosteroids (prednisone 0.5 mg/kg/day for 4–8 weeks, followed by gradual tapering to maintenance dose). Second-line and steroid-sparing agents include methotrexate or, less commonly, AZA. Antitumor necrosis factor (TNF) α agents (especially infliximab) represent the third line, and the three lines of therapy can be administered concomitantly [51].

22.5.2.3 Antifibrotic Treatment in Progressive Fibrosing Non-IPF ILDs

Some non-IPF ILDs—including idiopathic NSIP, CTDs-ILD, fibrotic-HP, unclassifiable ILDs, exposure-related IPF (asbestosis and silicosis), and sarcoidosis—at a certain time of their natural history may develop progressive fibrosis, worsening clinical course, and more accelerated FVC decline, despite standard therapy with corticosteroids and immunosuppressive agents. The umbrella terminology of "non-IPF progressive fibrosing ILDs" (non-IPF PF-ILDs) is used to indicate this phenotype of non-IPF ILDs with progressive fibrosis [52]. Because IPF, the prototype of fibrotic ILD, responds to antifibrotic agents, it is hypothesized that such drugs could exert a similar benefit also in non-IPF PF-ILDs. There is no agreement on a precise clinical definition of PF-ILD, but rapid FVC decline (e.g., ≥10% in 24 months), worsening of respiratory symptoms directly attributable to the ILD, and growing extent of fibrosis and honeycombing on HRTC are all useful signals to establish fibrotic disease progression [52]. Recent randomized controlled trials proved the efficacy of nintedanib versus placebo in decreasing the rate of FVC decline in a mixed group of patients with PF-ILDs (26% with HP, 26% CTDs-ILDs, and 19% NSIP) [53] and in SSc-ILD [54]. Similar results were obtained for pirfenidone in patients with unclassifiable ILDs [55] and in a mixed PF-ILDs group [56]. Since the conventional therapeutic approach to non-IPF ILDs of corticosteroids and immunosuppressive agents offers uncertain benefits and could be harmful, particularly among older frail patients, the possibility to treat non-IPF-ILDs with antifibrotic agents may have promising implications. The proportion of older patients enrolled in non-IPF PF-ILDs trials, however, was low.

22.5.2.4 Practical Considerations on the Therapeutic Management of IPF and Other ILDs in the Elderly

The diagnostic and therapeutic management of IPF and other ILDs in older patients poses relevant challenges (Table 22.5) [30]. The restrictive spirometric pattern of ILD can be observed in about 15% of older subjects without ILDs [57]. Indeed, restriction is the ventilator epiphenomenon of frequent age-related chronic non-respiratory disorders, such as diabetes, metabolic syndrome, congestive heart failure, obesity, sarcopenia, or rib cage deformity, and is associated with increased mortality [58]. Thus, while taking decisions on ILD treatment in elderly patients, the accelerated FVC decline should be carefully interpreted in the context of other

Table 22.5 Practical considerations on therapeutic management of ILDs older patients

• Differential diagnosis should be accurate: the treatment of IPF (nintedanib or pirfenidone) is different from that of non-IPF ILDs (corticosteroids and/or immunosuppressive agents)
• In older patients, a typical HRTC pattern of UIP may be sufficient to diagnose IPF
• Before starting treatment, overall patient's prognosis should be estimated by the comprehensive geriatric assessment
• The efficacy of corticosteroids and/or immunosuppressive agents in non-IPF ILDs is not proved by controlled trials, and expected benefits should be weighed against possible harmful effects
• Management of comorbid conditions should be optimized.
• If IPF is diagnosed, therapy with nintedanib or pirfenidone should be initiated in eligible older patients with mild-to-moderate IPF
• Older IPF patients treated with nintedanib or pirfenidone should undergo careful monitoring of adverse drug effects and drug-drug interactions
• Consideration of treatment with antiacid therapy is recommended in all IPF older patients
• Pulmonary rehabilitation improves the capacity of exercise and should be offered to all suitable older IPF patients
• High-flow nasal cannula oxygen therapy is useful as end-of-life treatment in patients requiring high flows of oxygen and can facilitate the transition from hospital to home

Abbreviations: ILDs Interstitial lung diseases, *IPF* Idiopathic pulmonary fibrosis, *HRTC* High-resolution computed tomography, *UIP* Usual interstitial pneumonia comorbidities and not hastily attributed to progressive lung fibrosis. IPF is prevalent in the elderly, but also CTD-ILDs and occupational or environmental ILDs tend to manifest clinically with advancing age. Differential diagnosis should be accurate, because the standard treatment of IPF (nintedanib or pirfenidone) is different from that of non-IPF ILDs (immunosuppression). HRTC is a crucial diagnostic tool, but the current gold standard for ILD diagnosis is a multidisciplinary discussion [33]. Once a diagnosis of non-IPF ILD is obtained in elderly patients, the expected benefits of corticosteroids and/or immunosuppressive agents should be weighed against possible drug-related complications, comorbidities, overall prognosis estimated by the comprehensive geriatric assessment, and patient's expectations. If a confident diagnosis of IPF is ascertained, nintedanib or pirfenidone should not be denied to eligible older patients with mild to moderate IPF, accompanied by a strict monitoring of possible drug-related side effects and drug-drug interactions. The gastroesophageal reflux disease is highly prevalent in IPF, and episodes of reflux with microaspiration are believed to contribute to IPF pathogenesis and to the onset of acute exacerbations. Since a survival benefit was suggested in patients treated with antiacid agents [59], this treatment should be considered in all IPF patients. Pulmonary rehabilitation is a crucial intervention in the symptom-centered management of IPF and improves the capacity of exercise [60]. High-flow nasal cannula oxygen therapy is gaining a role as end-of-life palliative treatment of patients requiring very high flow of oxygen that cannot be guaranteed by conventional oxygen therapy [61] and may facilitate the transition from hospital to home in frail end-stage ILD patients.

References

1. Kumar M, et al. Senescence-associated secretory phenotype and its possible role in chronic obstructive pulmonary disease. Am J Respir Cell Mol Biol. 2014;51:323–33.
2. Melloni B, Mounier L, Laaban JP, Chambellan A, Foret D. Muir JF home-based care evolution in chronic respiratory failure between 2001 and 2015 (Antadir federation observatory). Respiration. 2018;96:446–54.
3. Bellia V, et al. Quality control of spirometry in the elderly. The SA.R.A. study. Salute Respiration nell'Anziano = Respiratory Health in the Elderly. Am J Respir Crit Care Med. 2000;161:1094–100.
4. Paladini L, et al. Procalcitonin vs clinical and chest film findings to diagnose community-acquired pneumonia in patients with acute asthma or acute exacerbations of chronic bronchitis. Chest. 2011;140:1667–8.
5. Effing T, et al. 2007 Self-management education for patients with chronic obstructive pulmonary disease. Cochrane Rev. 2007:CD002990.
6. Board M, et al. A simple drawing test to identify patients who are unlikely to be able to learn to use an inhaler. Int J Clin Pract. 2006;60:510.
7. Corhay JL, et al. Should we exclude elderly patients with chronic obstructive pulmonary disease from a long-time ambulatory pulmonary rehabilitation programme? J Rehabil Med. 2012;44:466–72.
8. Alexopoulos GS, et al. Outcomes of depressed patients undergoing inpatient pulmonary rehabilitation. Am J Geriatr Psych. 2006;5:466–75.
9. Di Meo F, et al. Age does not hamper the response to pulmonary rehabilitation of COPD patients. Age Ageing. 2008;37:530–5.

10. Maltals F, et al. Effects of home-based pulmonary rehabilitation in patients with chronic obstructive pulmonary disease: a randomized trial. Ann Intern Med. 2008;149:869–78.
11. Diez Gross R, et al. The coordination of breathing and swallowing in chronic obstructive pulmonary disease. Am J Respir Crit Care Med. 2009;179:559.
12. O'Clock G, et al. High-frequency and low-frequency chest compression: effects on lung water secretion, mucus transport, heart rate, and blood pressure using a trapezoidal source pressure waveform. IEEE Trans Biomed Eng. 2012;59:106–14.
13. Antonelli Incalzi R, et al. Manifesto on the value of adult immunization: "we know, we intend, we advocate". Vaccines (Basel). 2021;9(11):1232.
14. Ontario Health Technology Assessment Series; Vol. 12(3), pp. 1–64; 2012.
15. Higham A, Mathioudakis A, Vestbo J, Singh D. COVID-19 and COPD: a narrative review of the basic science and clinical outcomes. Eur Respir Rev. 2020;29(158):200199.
16. Bellia V, Catalano F, Scichilone N, Incalzi RA, Spatafora M, Vergani C, Rengo F. Sleep disorders in the elderly with and without chronic airflow obstruction: the SARA study. Sleep. 2003;26:318–23.
17. Endeshaw YW, et al. Sleep-disordered breathing and nocturia in older adults. JAGS. 2004;52:957–60.
18. Wichniak A, Wierzbicka A, Walęcka M, Jernajczyk W. Effects of antidepressants on sleep. Curr Psychiatry Rep. 2017;19:63.
19. Antonelli Incalzi R et al. Nutritional status in aging and lung disease. In Molecular basis of nutrition and aging: a volume in the molecular nutrition series; 2016, pp. 411–421.
20. Bhasin S, et al. Sarcopenia definition: the position statements of the sarcopenia definition and outcomes consortium. JAGS. 2020;68:1410–8.
21. Cruz-Jentoft AJ, Sayer AA. Sarcopenia. Lancet. 2019;393:2636–46.
22. Perkisas S, et al. Application of ultrasound for muscle assessment in sarcopenia: 2020 SARCUS update. Eur Geriatr Med. 2021;12:45–59.
23. Engelen MP, Rutten EP, De Castro CL, Wouters EF, Schols AM, Deutz NE. Supplementation of soy protein with branched-chain amino acids alters protein metabolism in healthy elderly and even more in patients with chronic obstructive pulmonary disease. Am J Clin Nutr. 2007;85:431–9.
24. Broekhuizen R, Wouters EF, Creutzberg EC, Weling-Scheepers CA, Schols AM. Polyunsaturated fatty acids improve exercise capacity in chronic obstructive pulmonary disease. Thorax. 2005;60:376–82.
25. Moradkhan R, et al. Revisiting the role of oxygen therapy in cardiac patients. JACC. 2010;56:1013–6.
26. Dunne PJ. The clinical impact of new long-term oxygen therapy technology. Respir Care. 2009;54:1100–11.
27. Comer DM, et al. Domiciliary non-invasive ventilation in the elderly. Effective, tolerated and justified. Ulster Med J. 2015;84:22–5.
28. Laudisio A, et al. Noninvasive ventilation in older adults admitted to a pneumogeriatric unit. JAGS. 2014;62:1195.
29. Pedone C, et al. Efficacy of multiparametric telemonitoring on respiratory outcomes in elderly people with COPD: a randomized controlled trial. BMC: Health Services Res. 2013;13:82.
30. Jo HE, Randhawa S, Corte TJ, Moodley Y. Idiopathic pulmonary fibrosis and the elderly: diagnosis and management considerations. Drugs Aging. 2016;33:321–34.
31. American Thoracic Society; European Respiratory Society. American Thoracic Society/European Respiratory Society international multidisciplinary consensus classification of the idiopathic interstitial pneumonias. Am J Respir Crit Care Med. 2002;165:277–304.
32. Travis WD, Costabel U, Hansell DM, King TE Jr, Lynch DA, Nicholson AG, et al. ATS/ERS Committee on idiopathic interstitial pneumonias. An official American Thoracic Society/European Respiratory Society statement: update of the international multidisciplinary classification of the idiopathic interstitial pneumonias. Am J Respir Crit Care Med. 2013;188:733–48.
33. Raghu G, Remy-Jardin M, Myers JL, Richeldi L, Ryerson CJ, Lederer DJ, et al. American Thoracic Society, European Respiratory Society, Japanese Respiratory Society, and Latin

American Thoracic Society. Diagnosis of idiopathic pulmonary fibrosis. An official ATS/ERS/JRS/ALAT clinical practice guideline. Am J Respir Crit Care Med. 2018;198:e44–68.
34. Belloli EA, Beckford R, Hadley R, Flaherty KR. Idiopathic non-specific interstitial pneumonia. Respirology. 2016;21:259–68.
35. Raghu G, Meyer KC. Cryptogenic organising pneumonia: current understanding of an enigmatic lung disease. Eur Respir Rev. 2021;30:210094.
36. Doyle TJ, Dellaripa PF. Lung manifestations in the rheumatic diseases. Chest. 2017;152:1283–95.
37. Alberti ML, Rincon-Alvarez E, Buendia-Roldan I, Selman M. Hypersensitivity pneumonitis: diagnostic and therapeutic challenges. Front Med (Lausanne). 2021;8:718299.
38. Idiopathic Pulmonary Fibrosis Clinical Research Network, Raghu G, Anstrom KJ, King TE Jr, Lasky JA, Martinez FJ. Prednisone, azathioprine, and N-acetylcysteine for pulmonary fibrosis. N Engl J Med. 2012;366:1968–77.
39. Richeldi L, du Bois RM, Raghu G, Azuma A, Brown KK, Costabel U, et al. INPULSIS trial investigators. Efficacy and safety of nintedanib in idiopathic pulmonary fibrosis. N Engl J Med. 2014;370:2071–82.
40. Richeldi L, Costabel U, Selman M, Kim DS, Hansell DM, Nicholson AG, et al. Efficacy of a tyrosine kinase inhibitor in idiopathic pulmonary fibrosis. N Engl J Med. 2011;365:1079–87.
41. Crestani B, Huggins JT, Kaye M, Costabel U, Glaspole I, Ogura T, et al. Long-term safety and tolerability of nintedanib in patients with idiopathic pulmonary fibrosis: results from the open-label extension study, INPULSIS-ON. Lancet Respir Med. 2019;7:60–8.
42. Costabel U, Inoue Y, Richeldi L, Collard HR, Tschoepe I, Stowasser S, et al. Efficacy of Nintedanib in idiopathic pulmonary fibrosis across prespecified subgroups in INPULSIS. Am J Respir Crit Care Med. 2016;193:178–85.
43. Morrow LE, Hilleman D, Malesker MA. Management of patients with fibrosing interstitial lung diseases. Am J Health Syst Pharm. 2022;79:129–39.
44. King TE Jr, Bradford WZ, Castro-Bernardini S, Fagan EA, Glaspole I, Glassberg MK, et al. ASCEND study group. A phase 3 trial of pirfenidone in patients with idiopathic pulmonary fibrosis. N Engl J Med. 2014;370:2083–92.
45. Noble PW, Albera C, Bradford WZ, Costabel U, Glassberg MK, Kardatzke D, et al. CAPACITY study group. Pirfenidone in patients with idiopathic pulmonary fibrosis (CAPACITY): two randomised trials. Lancet. 2011;377:1760–9.
46. Nathan SD, Costabel U, Albera C, Behr J, Wuyts WA, Kirchgaessler KU, et al. Pirfenidone in patients with idiopathic pulmonary fibrosis and more advanced lung function impairment. Respir Med. 2019;153:44–51.
47. Tashkin DP, Elashoff R, Clements PJ, Goldin J, Roth MD, Furst DE, et al. Scleroderma Lung Study Research Group. Cyclophosphamide versus placebo in scleroderma lung disease. N Engl J Med. 2006;354:2655–66.
48. Hoyles RK, Ellis RW, Wellsbury J, Lees B, Newlands P, Goh NS, et al. A multicenter, prospective, randomized, double-blind, placebo-controlled trial of corticosteroids and intravenous cyclophosphamide followed by oral azathioprine for the treatment of pulmonary fibrosis in scleroderma. Arthritis Rheum. 2006;54:3962–70.
49. Tashkin DP, Roth MD, Clements PJ, Furst DE, Khanna D, Kleerup EC, et al. Sclerodema lung study II investigators. Mycophenolate mofetil versus oral cyclophosphamide in scleroderma-related interstitial lung disease (SLS II): a randomised controlled, double-blind, parallel group trial. Lancet. Respir Med. 2016;4:708–19.
50. Kadura S, Raghu G. Rheumatoid arthritis-interstitial lung disease: manifestations and current concepts in pathogenesis and management. Eur Respir Rev. 2021;30:210011.
51. Melani AS, Bigliazzi C, Cimmino FA, Bergantini L, Bargagli E. A comprehensive review of sarcoidosis treatment for pulmonologists. Pulm Ther. 2021; in press
52. Cottin V. Treatment of progressive fibrosing interstitial lung diseases: a milestone in the management of interstitial lung diseases. Eur Respir Rev. 2019;28:190109.

53. Flaherty KR, Wells AU, Cottin V, Devaraj A, Walsh SLF, Inoue Y, et al. INBUILD trial investigators. Nintedanib in progressive fibrosing interstitial lung diseases. N Engl J Med. 2019;381:1718–27.
54. Distler O, Highland KB, Gahlemann M, Azuma A, Fischer A, Mayes MD, et al. SENSCIS trial investigators. Nintedanib for systemic sclerosis-associated interstitial lung disease. N Engl J Med. 2019;380:2518–28.
55. Maher TM, Corte TJ, Fischer A, Kreuter M, Lederer DJ, Molina-Molina M, et al. Pirfenidone in patients with unclassifiable progressive fibrosing interstitial lung disease: a double-blind, randomised, placebo-controlled, phase 2 trial. Lancet Respir Med. 2020;8:147–57.
56. Behr J, Prasse A, Kreuter M, Johow J, Rabe KF, Bonella F, et al. RELIEF investigators. Pirfenidone in patients with progressive fibrotic interstitial lung diseases other than idiopathic pulmonary fibrosis (RELIEF): a double-blind, randomised, placebo-controlled, phase 2b trial. Lancet. Respir Med. 2021;9:476–86.
57. Fimognari FL, Pasqualetti P, Moro L, Franco A, Piccirillo G, Pastorelli R, et al. The association between metabolic syndrome and restrictive ventilatory dysfunction in older persons. J Gerontol A Biol Sci Med Sci. 2007;62:760–5.
58. Pedone C, Scarlata S, Chiurco D, Conte ME, Forastiere F, Antonelli-Incalzi R. Association of reduced total lung capacity with mortality and use of health services. Chest. 2012;141:1025–30.
59. Fidler L, Sitzer N, Shapera S, Shah PS. Treatment of gastroesophageal reflux in patients with idiopathic pulmonary fibrosis: a systematic review and meta-analysis. Chest. 2018;153:1405–15.
60. Ferreira A, Garvey C, Connors GL, Hilling L, Rigler J, Farrell S, et al. Pulmonary rehabilitation in interstitial lung disease: benefits and predictors of response. Chest. 2009;135:442–7.
61. Fimognari FL, Rizzo M, Cuccurullo O, Cristiano G, Ricchio R, Ricci C, et al. High-flow nasal cannula oxygen therapy for acute respiratory failure in a non-intensive geriatric setting. Geriatr Gerontol Int. 2018;18:1652–3.

Diabetes Mellitus

23

Edoardo Mannucci and Daniele Scoccimarro

Diabetes mellitus is a heterogeneous metabolic disorder characterized by the presence of hyperglycemia. In the most frequent form of diabetes, i.e., type 2 diabetes, hyperglycemia is due to the impairment of insulin secretion, associated with different degrees of defective insulin action. Chronic hyperglycemia is associated with relatively specific long-term microvascular complications affecting eyes, kidneys, and nerves, as well as with an increased risk of cardiovascular disease (CVD).

An increasing number of newly diagnosed older adults with diabetes, together with increasing life expectancy, have led to an increase in the prevalence of diabetes in the geriatric age group [1]: it is estimated that 19.3% of people aged 65–99 years have diabetes. It is projected that the worldwide number of people older than 65 years with diabetes will reach 195.2 million by 2030 and 276.2 million by 2045 [2].

Although type 2 diabetes is the most common form of diabetes in advanced age, there are also more older adults than ever with long-standing type 1 diabetes. Older patients have unique and different needs and challenges, which should be considered when developing a treatment plan. The approach to the management of diabetes in older adults must be individualized and adapted over time, considering comorbidities, risk of hypoglycemia, social support, and patient's preferences.

E. Mannucci (✉)
University of Florence, Florence, Italy

Diabetology and Metabolic Diseases, Careggi Hospital, Florence, Italy
e-mail: edoardo.mannucci@unifi.it

D. Scoccimarro
Diabetology and Metabolic Diseases, Careggi Hospital, Florence, Italy

A. Cherubini et al. (eds.), *Optimizing Pharmacotherapy in Older Patients*, Practical Issues in Geriatrics, https://doi.org/10.1007/978-3-031-28061-0_23

23.1 Therapeutic Targets in the Elderly

The aims of treatment of diabetes are the elimination of symptoms (polyuria, polydipsia, dehydration) and the prevention of long-term diabetic complications. The elimination of symptoms can be achieved even with glucose levels well above the normal range, whereas the prevention of chronic complications requires a stricter glycemic control [3, 4]. Since the risk of developing chronic complications depends on the length of exposure to hyperglycemia, and not only on the degree of hyperglycemia, the potential benefits of accurate glucose control are inversely related to life expectancy. Thus, older patients have smaller advantages from strict glycemic control in the long term than younger individuals. In addition, the risk of some adverse events associated with pharmacological treatment (e.g., severe hypoglycemia) is increased in older patients, particularly with comorbidities. Hospital admissions for hypoglycemia are more frequent than those for hyperglycemia, and the older population is at particularly high risk: the age-related impairment of renal function and adrenergic counter-regulatory mechanisms lead to an increased risk of hypoglycemia [5, 6]. In patients with long duration of diabetes, recurrent hypoglycemic episodes and autonomic neuropathy can determine hypoglycemia unawareness, further increasing the risk of severe hypoglycemia [6]. On the other hand, hypoglycemia in older patients could be associated with a higher risk of cognitive impairment [7] and cardiovascular morbidity [8, 9]. In addition, hypoglycemia in advanced age is a major risk factor for falls and fractures [10].

The identification of appropriate glycemic targets is based on the assessment of the ratio between clinical benefits and potential risks, such as hypoglycemia and other drug-related adverse events. Most guidelines provide recommendations for desired HbA1c levels, indicating either 53 or 48 mmol/mol as a target [11–14]. Some guidelines suggest different HbA1c targets depending on current pharmacological treatments [12, 14], discriminating between patients treated or not treated with hypoglycemia-inducing drugs [12, 14]. In fact, in subjects receiving treatment with insulin or sulfonylureas, the incidence of severe hypoglycemia is markedly increased when glucose and HbA1c levels are close to the normal range [15]. As a consequence, higher HbA1c targets are recommended when patients receive hypoglycemia-inducing treatments [12, 14], sometimes indicating minimum HbA1c thresholds below which the risk-benefit ratio is no longer favorable [14].

Unfortunately, trials exploring the longer-term effects of the improvement of glycemic control in diabetes usually do not include patients aged more than 75 years [14, 16]. Results obtained in younger age groups cannot be automatically extended to older patients, since both beneficial and detrimental effects of diabetes treatment are moderated by age.

Furthermore, the complexity of treatment, in terms of need of subcutaneous injections, multiple administrations, and frequent glucose monitoring, can influence the adherence to therapy, as patients develop medical conditions that may impair their ability to follow prescribed therapies. Psychological factors, with an increased inertia, and a reduced willingness to change habits and try new medications, should also be considered. In addition, the close availability of family members or caregivers is often crucial to support self-management of T2DM in older persons.

In summary, a reasonable target for patients aged over 75 years could be that of maintaining HbA1c below 58 mmol/mol in individual treated with drugs that do not induce hypoglycemia, and between 53 and 64 mmol/mol in those treated with insulin. Higher HbA1c levels can be acceptable only in frail patients with very limited life expectancy.

23.2 Insulin Therapy in the Elderly

Basal-bolus insulin therapy is the only adequate treatment of type 1 diabetes, irrespective of age. The management of such treatment in older adults is more problematic: cognitive impairment, visual loss, and reduced ability to perform complex manual tasks can all increase the risk of inappropriate insulin administration; renal impairment, hypoglycemia unawareness, and irregularities in food intake increase the risk of severe hypoglycemia, and frailty further increases the risk of hypoglycemia-induced falls. Ability to self-manage cannot be readily passed onto family members, and older adults with type 1 diabetes are increasingly reliant on care from the community and outpatient structures.

When basal insulin is needed, long-acting analogs (glargine, detemir, and degludec insulin) are preferable to NPH human insulin, since they guarantee lower glucose variability and less hypoglycemia [17], thus allowing a more accurate dose titration [18]. Insulin glargine U-300 and degludec are ultra-long-acting analogs with a higher half-life and a lower risk for nocturnal hypoglycemia than glargine U-100, even in people aged ≥75 years [19, 20]. In addition, their longer duration of action warrants a greater flexibility in the timing of administration, which can be advantageous for patients needing third-party assistance for drug administration [21].

For the management of postprandial glycemia, short-acting analogs (lispro, aspart, glulisine) should be preferred to human regular insulin, since they allow a better control of early postprandial hyperglycemia with lower risk for late postprandial hypoglycemia [22, 23]. In addition, short-acting analogs can also be administered immediately before or even after, meals, instead of 20–30 min in advance. In older patients with irregular food intake, the administration of insulin at the end of the meal allows for the regulation of insulin dose on the basis of the amount of food actually eaten.

In patients with type 2 diabetes, insulin should be considered when glycemic control cannot be achieved otherwise. Insulin therapy schemes should be individualized, based on the patient's actual needs, as determined by the results of glucose monitoring. Thus, basal insulin should be prescribed when needed for the control of fasting glucose and prandial insulin for the management of postprandial glucose excursions. Once-daily basal insulin facilitates compliance to therapy, particularly in patients requiring caregiver assistance, and it is therefore often considered the strategy of choice. On the other hand, the age-related reduction in insulin secretion

[24] often requires the use of rapid insulin for postprandial glucose control [25, 26], which cannot be achieved otherwise. The attempt at reducing the postprandial increase of blood glucose with of basal insulin would be scarcely effective, and it would imply a high risk of inter-prandial hypoglycemia.

An adequate education of patients and/or caregivers is an integral part of insulin therapy, particularly in older adults. Such education should include the technique of insulin injection, the recognition and treatment of hypoglycemia, and the management of insulin therapy in relation to food intake and concurrent acute conditions. All those skills should be periodically verified [27]. In addition, capillary blood glucose monitoring—which could be problematic in some elderly patients with reduction in visual acuity, cognitive dysfunction, or limited motor skills—is needed in all individuals on insulin therapy.

In older patients, the complexity of the insulin treatment induces to consider insulin only when an acceptable glucose control cannot be achieved otherwise. Although insulin is still a precious therapeutic option for many elderly patients, it is associated with a relevant risk for hypoglycemia, falls, and fractures.

23.3 Non-insulin Therapy in Older Patients

Many drugs other than insulin are currently available for the treatment of type 2 diabetes. Some of those agents provide health benefits (e.g., reduction of cardiovascular risk, nephroprotection, etc.) which outreach the favorable effects of improved glucose control. However, most of available data on the effects of drugs for type 2 diabetes have been collected in adult non-geriatric populations; the risks and benefits associated with some classes of drugs could be partly different in the elderly.

23.3.1 Biguanides

The biguanide metformin exerts its glucose-lowering effect primarily by decreasing hepatic glucose production and increasing peripheral insulin sensitivity [28]. Additionally, metformin may improve glucose homeostasis by interacting with the incretin axis through the action of glucagon-like peptide 1 (GLP-1) [29]. Metformin is effective, inexpensive, and well tolerated; it does not induce hypoglycemia or weight gain; and it may reduce cardiovascular events and mortality [30–32], although specific data on cardiovascular and overall mortality in the older population from randomized controlled trials are lacking. For these reasons, most guidelines recommend metformin as first-line therapy in all people with type 2 diabetes, including older adults, if tolerated and not contraindicated [14, 33, 34].

The principal side effect of metformin is diarrhea, which can be mitigated by a gradual dose titration and by the use of extended-release formulations [35]. Severe renal failure, 3rd/4thNYHA class heart failure, liver insufficiency, and hypoxemic respiratory failure contraindicate metformin therapy because of the increased risk for lactic acidosis. In particular, the Food and Drug Administration (FDA) recommends against the use of metformin with serum creatinine above 1.5 mg/dL (114.4 mmol/L) in men and above 1.4 mg/dL (106.8 mmol/L) in women, respectively, whereas according to the European Society of Cardiology (ESC) and the European Association for the Study of Diabetes (EASD), metformin is contraindicated in patient with estimated glomerular filtration ratio (eGFR) below 30 mL/min, recommending caution and dosage reduction when eGFR is between 30 and 60 mL/min [27, 36]. Notably, creatinine levels do not always adequately reflect renal function in older patients due to sarcopenia. Moreover, older individuals are at higher risk for dehydration and acute kidney failure. For these reasons, it is advisable not to exceed a daily metformin dose of 1500 mg in patients aged more than 75 years. In addition, patients and caregivers should be instructed to suspend metformin in case of prolonged fever, vomiting, and diarrhea.

An additional concern is the development of vitamin B12 deficiency in chronic metformin users [37, 38], which could contribute to anemia, cognitive dysfunction [37], and symptomatic peripheral neuropathy [39]. Although there are no available randomized trials on the topic, some guidelines suggest that vitamin B12 levels should be monitored yearly in older patients in therapy with metformin [34].

23.3.2 Glucagon-Like Peptide 1 Receptor Agonists

Glucagon-like peptide-1 (GLP-1) released from enteroendocrine cells controls meal-related glycemic excursions through a glucose-dependent stimulation of insulin release and inhibition of glucagon secretion. Thus, GLP-1 receptor agonists (GLP-1Ras) reduce hyperglycemia in type 2 diabetes without inducing hypoglycemia. GLP-1 also inhibits food intake, determining weight loss [40].

GLP-1 RAs can be classified according to their half-life as short-acting (exenatide, lixisenatide), with a duration of action of 2–3 h, and long-acting (exenatide q.w., liraglutide, dulaglutide, semaglutide), which, administered once daily or once weekly, warrant drug circulating levels within the therapeutic range for the whole day [41]. Short-acting GLP-1 RAs are more effective than longer-acting agents on postprandial glucose increments, whereas long-acting compounds have a wider effect on fasting glucose and HbA1c [42].

In head-to-head trials, GLP1-RAs reduce HbA1c to a greater extent than other glucose-lowering agents, including aggressively titrated basal insulin [43, 44]. Although all drugs of the class induce weight loss, the weight-reducing action is different across molecules, mainly depending on their ability to cross the blood-brain barrier [45]. In addition, long-acting GLP-1Ras prevent cardiovascular disease in high-risk patients [46, 47], including those aged ≥65 years [46]. However, specific data on cardiovascular outcomes in patients older than 75 years are not available.

Results from clinical and preclinical studies suggest a protective effect of GLP-1RAs on cognitive decline [10]. An analysis of the REWIND study shows that long-term therapy with dulaglutide could prevent cognitive impairment in people with type 2 diabetes, including those aged ≥70 years [48], but further purposely designed studies are needed to confirm these data.

GLP-1RAs, with the only exception of oral semaglutide, are administered with subcutaneous injections, requiring adequate visual, motor, and cognitive skills. On the other hand, the possibility of once-weekly administration facilitates drug management by patients and caregivers.

The most frequent side effects of GLP-1RAs are gastrointestinal symptoms, such as nausea and, less frequently, vomiting, and diarrhea [36]. These effects usually appear in the first weeks of treatment and decrease over the time with the prosecution of therapy; an initial dose titration is needed with some molecules of the class in order to minimize side effects. Data from randomized clinical trials seem to show similar efficacy and safety across ages, with no significant differences across age classes, even if there was a trend toward higher rates of discontinuation for adverse events with increasing age [49, 50].

Since weight loss and reduced appetite are usually associated with GLP1-RAs, these drugs should not be used in malnourished or cachexic elderly patients [33]. In addition, even if obesity is associated with frailty [51], weight loss is not always desirable in the elderly because of an increased risk of sarcopenia, falls, and fractures. For this reason, although GLP1-RAs are a very interesting option for the treatment of type 2 diabetes, their use in older patients is limited by weight loss; caution is recommended in nonobese elderly patients.

23.3.3 Sodium-Glucose Transporter 2 Inhibitors

The primary action of sodium-glucose transporter 2 inhibitors (SGLT-2i) is the inhibition of glucose reabsorption in the kidney, thus inducing glycosuria and reducing both postprandial and fasting hyperglycemia. This primary renal effect of SGLT2is is independent of insulin, limiting the risk of hypoglycemia [52].

SGLT2i-induced glycosuria is associated with transient sodium excretion and osmotic diuresis, resulting in a reduction of blood pressure [53]. The risk of sustained reductions in plasma volume with SGLT2is is controversial [54, 55]. In addition, SGLT-2i induce a moderate weight loss due to the calorie loss determined by glycosuria [56].

In large-scale trials, SGLT2i reduce the incidence of cardiovascular events, hospitalization for heart failure, and progression of kidney disease in high-risk patients with type 2 diabetes [57–61]. Protection from hospitalization for heart failure and renal failure has also been shown in nondiabetic patients with heart failure and chronic kidney disease, respectively [60, 62]; however, data on patients older than 75 years are not available [58, 61].

A post hoc pooled analysis of patient-level data from clinical trials showed that the efficacy of SGLT2i on HbA1c, body weight, and blood pressure in patients aged over 60 years is not different from that observed in younger individuals [63]. However, specific RCTs assessing the efficacy and safety of SGLT2i in the patients aged >75 years are still lacking, and only very limited data have been published from observational studies. The theoretical risk of volume depletion suggests caution in prescribing SGLT2is in very old patients. SGLT2is can be an interesting option in selected healthy elderly patients with T2DM, particularly if overweight or with uncontrolled hypertension; on the other hand, these medications are not the treatment of choice in frail patients, especially when treated with loop diuretics (due to the increased risk of dehydration and orthostatic hypotension) [52]. Dose adjustments for diuretics and insulin are generally required at the initiation of SGLT2i treatment [36].

Mycotic genital infection is the most frequent adverse event with SGLT2i. Treatment with SGLT2 inhibitors has also been associated with a modest increase in the risk of urinary tract infections [64]. Genitourinary infections are more frequent in women, particularly those with a history of recurrent genital infections [65], and in current or former smokers [66]. In clinical trials, events were generally mild to moderate in intensity and rarely lead to discontinuation of treatment [67].

23.3.4 Dipeptidyl Peptidase 4-Inhibitors

The inhibition of dipeptidyl peptidase 4 (DPP-4), which is the principal enzyme responsible for the inactivation of endogenous GLP-1, increases the concentration of both active incretin hormones GLP-1 and glucose-dependent insulinotropic polypeptide (GIP) [68]. Since these hormones are mostly released by the enteroendocrine L and K cells in response to meals, DPP-4 inhibitors (DPP-4i) exert their glucose-lowering effects mainly acting on postprandial glycemia.

DPP4-I are effective and well tolerated in patients aged ≥65 years, with minimal risk of hypoglycemia [69]. Pooled analysis from phase 2 and 3 studies showed no differences across age groups in terms of safety and efficacy [70], and this was confirmed in clinical trials specifically performed in elderly patients [71, 72]. However, it should be considered that β-cells function declines with the duration of diabetes [73], and a preserved pancreatic function is required for the therapeutic action of DPP4i: in fact, the glucose-lowering effect of this class can be blunted or absent in patients with very low residual insulin secretion.

Despite increases in active GLP-1 concentrations, there are no effects of these compounds on directly measured gastric emptying and satiation [74]. For these reasons, DPP-4 inhibitors are not usually associated with typical GLP-1RAs gastrointestinal side effects, and they are neutral on body weight [75].

In cardiovascular outcome trials, DPP4 inhibitors were generally safe, without increasing, nor reducing, the risk of major cardiovascular events [76]. An increase of hospitalizations for heart failure was shown in patients treated with saxagliptin [77], but not with other molecules of the class; a possible detrimental effect on heart failure has also been suggested for alogliptin [78] and vildagliptin [79], but not with sitagliptin [80] and linagliptin [81, 82].

Experimental data suggest that DPP-4i could have neuroprotective effects, delaying cognitive decline in a glucose-independent way in animal models of Alzheimer's and Parkinson's disease [83], but to date, there is no available clinical evidence in humans supporting this hypothesis.

Efficacy, tolerability, and safety of DPP-4i in older patients with impaired kidney function have been confirmed by randomized controlled trials [71, 72], so that this class can represent a useful option in patients with declined eGFR.

Side effects are uncommon with DPP-4 inhibitors, which are a very considerable advantage in the elderly. The possibility of an increased risk of pancreatitis associated with DPP-4i is controversial [84], but it is advisable not to use these drugs in patients with a history of pancreatitis. Data from observational and randomized controlled trials also show an increased risk for bullous pemphigoid, in particular for linagliptin and vildagliptin, but the absolute risk is low [85].

DPP4 inhibitors are probably the most extensively studied class of glucose-lowering drugs in elderly patients. Available evidences show that they are safe in older individuals, with low risk of hypoglycemia and neutral effect on body weight. In addition, they are administered orally once daily, facilitating adherence and management of therapy. Therefore, despite their limited efficacy on glucose control and the lack of specific cardiovascular actions, they are an interesting treatment option in elderly, particularly in non-overweight patients with mainly postprandial hyperglycemia, as add-on to metformin, or when metformin is not tolerated or contraindicated.

23.3.5 Thiazolidinediones

Thiazolidinediones, or glitazones, enhance insulin sensitivity through the activation of nuclear PPARγ receptors, which modulate the expression of several genes, promoting differentiation of adipocytes and lipogenesis in peripheral adipocytes, increasing glucose uptake in skeletal muscle, and suppressing hepatic gluconeogenesis [86]. In patients with type 2 diabetes, glitazones reduce fasting glycemia and HbA1c, without inducing hypoglycemia. Pioglitazone is the only thiazolidinedione (TZD) available at present in Europe, while rosiglitazone is available in the USA with limited indications.

Pioglitazone is effective and potentially well tolerated in the elderly, with no risk of hypoglycemia, unless it is associated with insulin. The most frequent adverse event is fluid retention, with peripheral edema, which contributes to pioglitazone-associated weight gain. In patients with left ventricular dysfunction, fluid retention can precipitate symptoms of heart failure; for this reason, glitazones are associated with an increased risk of hospitalization for heart failure despite the lack of detrimental effects on myocardial contractility. Fluid retention, which develops predominantly within the first months of treatment, seems to be more frequent in the elderly [87, 88], particularly when glitazones are associated with insulin [88]. This suggests caution in using these drugs in advanced age, unless an undetected impairment of cardiac function can be reasonably excluded.

In addition, TZDs stimulate the differentiation of bone marrow mesenchymal stem cells into adipocytes, reducing the differentiation of osteoblasts and therefore inducing a reduction of bone mass [89]. In postmenopausal women, the use of glitazones is associated with accelerated osteoporosis [90] and increased risk of fractures [91]. This phenomenon is not observed in men, since androgens antagonize the inhibitory effect of TZDs on osteoblastogenesis [89]. As a consequence, glitazones are not among the drugs of choice in postmenopausal women. Finally, pioglitazone has been associated with an increased risk of bladder cancer [92], prompting a relative contraindication in patients with a familiar or personal history of bladder cancer.

Pioglitazone should be considered as a second-/third-line therapy in elderly patients due to its effect on bone and heart failure. It could be an effective option in selected patients, in particular male patients, provided that ventricular function is preserved.

23.3.6 Alpha-Glucosidase Inhibitors

α-Glucosidase inhibitors are competitive inhibitors of the intestinal enzymes responsible for terminal carbohydrate digestion, thereby delaying carbohydrate absorption. They need to be administered 10 min before meals, and they reduce the postprandial increment of glycemia, with a moderate efficacy on HbA1c and no relevant action on body weight. Specific trials on cardiovascular outcomes are not available.

The most common side effects are gastrointestinal adverse events, such as flatulence and diarrhea, with a relatively high rate of nonadherence and/or withdrawal [8].

α-Glucosidase inhibitors are not associated with hypoglycemia, unless they are combined with insulin or sulfonylureas. In this latter case, the drug-induced delay in digestion and absorption of disaccharides (i.e., sugar) commonly used for the self-treatment of hypoglycemia interferes with the efficacy of treatment of non-severe hypoglycemia. Insulin-treated patients who receive a prescription of α-glucosidase inhibitors should be instructed to use glucose, instead of sucrose, for the correction of hypoglycemia.

The only drug of this class widely available in Europe is acarbose (miglitol is authorized in very few countries), which can be considered a therapeutic option in elderly non-insulin-treated patients with type 2 diabetes with moderate postprandial hyperglycemia.

23.3.7 Sulfonylureas and Glinides

Sulfonylureas and glinides promote insulin release by blocking β-cell K-ATP channels, thus inducing membrane hyperpolarization, which triggers insulin secretion. Sulfonylureas stimulate insulin secretion irrespective of glucose levels [92], potentially leading to hypoglycemia. In epidemiological studies, the incidence of severe hypoglycemia with sulfonylureas is not dissimilar from that observed with insulin in type 2 diabetes [93]. This risk is even greater in elderly patients, in whom the impairment of renal function can alter the pharmacokinetic of many drugs of the class, and the recognition and early treatment of mild hypoglycemia are often compromised. Furthermore, in both randomized clinical trials and observational studies, sulfonylureas are associated with an increased risk of overall and cardiovascular mortality [94, 95]. The explanation of this phenomenon is still controversial; it is possible that the blockade of myocardial and cerebral K-ATP channels similar to those expressed in β-cells reduces the ability of adapting to ischemia [96, 97]. For all these reasons, sulfonylureas are excluded by some guidelines [14] and considered third-line treatment by many others [11–13]. An even greater caution should be taken in elderly patients, considering the greater risk of hypoglycemia and consequent falls and fractures.

23.4 Conclusion

Individuals aged more than 75 years represent a growing fraction of patients with type 2 diabetes. Despite the epidemiological relevance of this population, most intervention studies enroll only younger individuals, thus limiting available specific evidence. Clinical reasoning suggests that less ambitious glycemic goals should be chosen for older patients, in the attempt of limiting undesired side effects of pharmacological therapy. In addition, the choice of drugs requires caution, considering existing comorbidities and other factors (such as social support) possibly affecting the incidence of drug-related adverse events (Table 23.1). Most guidelines [11, 12, 14]

Table 23.1 Strengths and weaknesses of different drug classes

	Strength	General side effects	Warnings in elderly
Biguanides	Effective on HbA1c No hypoglycemia Weight loss (modest) Overall/cardiovascular mortality reduction	Diarrhea Lactic acidosis[a]	Accumulation due to higher risk of acute renal insufficiency Vitamin B12 deficiency
GLP-1 receptor agonists	Very effective on HbA1c No hypoglycemia Weight loss Protection from cognitive impairment Protection from major cardiovascular events[b] Once weekly administration[c]	Nausea/vomiting/ diarrhea	Visual and motor skills required for administration Risk of excessive weight loss
SGLT2 inhibitors	Effective on HbA1c No hypoglycemia Weight loss Nephroprotection Protection from hospitalization for heart failure and major cardiovascular events[b]	Genital infections Plasma volume depletion	Interaction with diuretics and dehydration

Table 23.1 (continued)

	Strength	General side effects	Warnings in elderly
DPP4 inhibitors	No hypoglycemia Safe and very well tolerated	Bullous pemphigoid (uncommon)	Low effectiveness on HbA1c when reduced β-cells function
Thiazolidinediones	No hypoglycemia	Fluid retention and heart failure Weight gain Bone loss and fractures (women)	Increased risk of heart failure Increased risk of pathologic bone fracture (women)
α-Glucosidase inhibitors	No hypoglycemia	Flatulence and diarrhea	Gastrointestinal tolerability
Sulfonylureas and glinides		Hypoglycemia Weight gain Mild increase of overall/ cardiovascular mortality	Higher risk for falls and fractures Frequent self-monitoring of blood glucose required
Insulin	Effective on HbA1c Adjustable dosage	Hypoglycemia Weight gain	Higher risk for falls and fractures Cognitive, visual, and motor skills required for administration Frequent self-monitoring of blood glucose required

[a]In predisposing conditions
[b]In high risk patients
[c]For dulaglutide, semaglutide, exenatide LAR

recommend metformin as the first-line pharmacological treatment irrespective of age; this position is reasonable, provided that contraindications are observed, and higher doses are avoided. The choice of the second drug, when needed, is more problematic. The majority of current guidelines supports a wide use of SGLT2 inhibitors and/or GLP1 receptor agonists, at least in patients at high cardiovascular and/or renal risk [11, 13, 14]; however, the safety of those classes could be less satisfactory in very old patients. On the other hand, other classes, such as DPP4 inhibitors, do not show relevant safety issues in the elderly, but they do not provide additional health advantages beyond the reduction of hyperglycemia. The choice of treatment should therefore be individualized, considering specific goals and concurrent conditions.

References

1. Sun H, Saeedi P, Karuranga S, Pinkepank M, Ogurtsova K, Duncan BB, Stein C, Basit A, Chan JCN, Mbanya JC, Pavkov ME, Ramachandaran A, Wild SH, James S, Herman WH, Zhang P, Bommer C, Kuo S, Boyko EJ, Magliano DJ. IDF diabetes atlas: global, regional and country-level diabetes prevalence estimates for 2021 and projections for 2045. Diabetes Res Clin Pract. 2022;183:109119.

2. Sinclair A, Saeedi P, Kaundal A, Karuranga S, Malanda B, Williams R. Diabetes and global ageing among 65–99-year-old adults: findings from the International Diabetes Federation Diabetes Atlas, 9th edition. Diabetes Res Clin Pract. 2020;162:108078. https://doi.org/10.1016/j.diabres.2020.108078. Epub 2020 Feb 14.
3. Diabetes Control and Complications Trial (DCCT)/Epidemiology of Diabetes Interventions and Complications (EDIC) Study Research Group. Intensive diabetes treatment and cardiovascular outcomes in type 1 diabetes: the DCCT/EDIC study 30-year follow-up. Diabetes Care. 2016;39(5):686–93.
4. Intensive blood-glucose control with sulphonylureas or insulin compared with conventional treatment and risk of complications in patients with type 2 diabetes (UKPDS 33). UK Prospective Diabetes Study (UKPDS) Group. Lancet. 1998;352(9131):837–53. Erratum in: Lancet 1999;354(9178):602.
5. Monami M, Aleffi S. Hyperglycemia, hypoglycemia and glycemic variability in the elderly: a fatal triad? Monaldi Arch Chest Dis. 2016;84(1–2):726.
6. Hoeldtke RD, Boden G. Epinephrine secretion, hypoglycemia unawareness, and diabetic autonomic neuropathy. Ann Intern Med. 1994;120(6):512–7.
7. Meneilly GS, Tessier DM. Diabetes, dementia and hypoglycemia. Can J Diabetes. 2016;40(1):73–6.
8. International Hypoglycaemia Study Group. Hypoglycaemia, cardiovascular disease, and mortality in diabetes: epidemiology, pathogenesis, and management. Lancet Diabetes Endocrinol. 2019;7(5):385–96.
9. Mannucci E, Monami M, Lamanna C, Gori F, Marchionni N. Prevention of cardiovascular disease through glycemic control in type 2 diabetes: a meta-analysis of randomized clinical trials. Nutr Metab Cardiovasc Dis. 2009;19(9):604–12.
10. Freeman J. Management of hypoglycemia in older adults with type 2 diabetes. Postgrad Med. 2019;131(4):241–50.
11. Standards of Medical Care in Diabetes—2022 Abridged for Primary Care Providers
12. Guideline Type 2 diabetes in adults: management—NICE; 2022.
13. 2019 Guidelines on diabetes, pre-diabetes and cardiovascular diseases developed in collaboration with the EASD—ESC Clinical Practice Guidelines.
14. Mannucci E, Candido R, Delle Monache L, Gallo M, Giaccari A, Masini ML, Mazzone A, Medea G, Pintaudi B, Targher G, Trento M, Turchetti G, Lorenzoni V, Monami M, for Società Italiana di Diabetologia (SID) and Associazione Medici Diabetologi (AMD). Italian guidelines for the treatment of type 2 diabetes. Nutr Metab Cardiovasc Dis. 2022:S0939-4753(22)00044-8.
15. Monami M, Dicembrini I, Kundisova L, Zannoni S, Nreu B, Mannucci E. A meta-analysis of the hypoglycaemic risk in randomized controlled trials with sulphonylureas in patients with type 2 diabetes. Diabetes Obes Metab. 2014;16(9):833–40.
16. Monami M, Candido R, Pintaudi B, Targher G, Mannucci E, Of the SID-AMD joint panel for Italian Guidelines on Treatment of Type 2 Diabetes. Improvement of glycemic control in type 2 diabetes: a systematic review and meta-analysis of randomized controlled trials. Nutr Metab Cardiovasc Dis. 2021;31:2539–46.
17. Pandya N, DiGenio A, Gao L, Patel M. Efficacy and safety of insulin glargine compared to other interventions in younger and older adults: a pooled analysis of nine open-label, randomized controlled trials in patients with type 2 diabetes. Drugs Aging. 2013;30(6):429–38.
18. Lee P, Chang A, Blaum C, Vlajnic A, Gao L, Halter J. Comparison of safety and efficacy of insulin glargine and neutral protamine hagedorn insulin in older adults with type 2 diabetes mellitus: results from a pooled analysis. J Am Geriatr Soc. 2012;60(1):51–9.
19. Ritzel R, et al. A randomized controlled trial comparing efficacy and safety of insulin glargine 300 units/mL versus 100 units/mL in older people with type 2 diabetes: results from the SENIOR study. Diabetes Care. 2018;41(8):1672–80.
20. Yale J-F, et al. Glycaemic control and hypoglycaemia risk with insulin glargine 300 U/mL versus glargine 100 U/mL: a patient-level meta-analysis examining older and younger adults with type 2 diabetes. Diabetes Metab. 2020;46(2):110–8.

21. Marso SP, et al. Efficacy and safety of Degludec versus glargine in type 2 diabetes. N Engl J Med. 2017;377(8):723–32.
22. Gómez-Huelgas R, et al. Safety and efficacy of a basal-plus regimen with insulin glargine and insulin glulisine for elderly patients with high cardiovascular risk and type 2 diabetes mellitus. Rev Clin Esp. 2017;217(4):201–6.
23. Mannucci E, Monami M, Marchionni N. Short-acting insulin analogues vs. regular human insulin in type 2 diabetes: a meta-analysis. Diabetes Obes Metab. 2009;11(1):53–9.
24. Helman A, et al. Effects of aging and senescence on pancreatic β-cell function. Diabetes Obes Metab. 2016;18(Suppl 1):58–62.
25. Giugliano D, Chiodini P, Maiorino MI, Bellastella G, Esposito K. Intensification of insulin therapy with basal-bolus or premixed insulin regimens in type 2 diabetes: a systematic review and meta-analysis of randomized controlled trials. Endocrine. 2016;51(3):417–28.
26. Bowering K, et al. Faster Aspart versus insulin Aspart as part of a basal-bolus regimen in inadequately controlled type 2 diabetes: the onset 2 trial. Diabetes Care. 2017;40(7):951–7.
27. Valencia WM, Florez H. Pharmacological treatment of diabetes in older people. Diabetes Obes Metab. 2014;16(12):1192–203.
28. Natali A, Ferranini E. Effects of metformin and thiazolidinediones on suppression of hepatic glucose production and stimulation of glucose uptake in type 2 diabetes: a systematic review. Diabetologia. 2006;49:434–41.
29. Mulherin AJ, Oh AH, Kim H, Grieco A, Lauffer LM, Brubaker PL. Mechanisms underlying metformin-induced secretion of glucagon-like peptide-1 from the intestinal L cell. Endocrinology. 2011;152:4610–9.
30. Look AHEAD Research Group. Eight-year weight losses with an intensive lifestyle intervention: the look AHEAD study. Obesity (Silver Spring). 2014;22(1):5–13.
31. Schlender L, Martinez YV, Adeniji C, Reeves D, Faller B, Sommerauer C, Al Qur'an T, Woodham A, Kunnamo I, Sönnichsen A, Renom-Guiteras A. Efficacy and safety of metformin in the management of type 2 diabetes mellitus in older adults: a systematic review for the development of recommendations to reduce potentially inappropriate prescribing. BMC Geriatr. 2017;17(Suppl 1):227.
32. Monami M, Candido R, Pintaudi B, Targher G, Mannucci E. SID-AMD joint panel for Italian guidelines on treatment of type 2 diabetes. Effect of metformin on all-cause mortality and major adverse cardiovascular events: an updated meta-analysis of randomized controlled trials. Nutr Metab Cardiovasc Dis. 2021;31(3):699–704.
33. Care D, Suppl SS. 12. Older adults: standards of medical care in diabetes-2020. Diabetes Care. 2020;43(January):S152–62.
34. Leroith D, et al. Treatment of diabetes in older adults: an endocrine society. J Clin Endocrinol Metab. 2019;104(5)
35. Levy J, Cobas RA, Gomes MB. Assessment of efficacy and tolerability of once-daily extended release metformin in patients with type 2 diabetes mellitus. Diabetol Metab Syndr. 2010;2:16. https://doi.org/10.1186/1758-5996-2-16. Erratum in: Diabetol Metab Syndr 2010;2:57.
36. Sesti G, et al. Management of diabetes in older adults. Nutr Metab Cardiovasc Dis. 2018;28(3):206–18.
37. Porter KM, et al. Hyperglycemia and metformin use are associated with B vitamin deficiency and cognitive dysfunction in older adults. J Clin Endocrinol Metab. 2019;104(10):4837–47.
38. Kancherla V, et al. Long-term metformin therapy and monitoring for vitamin B12 deficiency among older veterans. J Am Geriatr Soc. 2017;65(5):1061–6.
39. Out M, Kooy A, Lehert P, Schalkwijk CA, Stehouwer CDA. Long-term treatment with metformin in type 2 diabetes and methylmalonic acid: post hoc analysis of a randomized controlled 4.3year trial. J Diabetes Complicat. 2018;32(2):171–8.
40. Drucker DJ. Mechanisms of action and therapeutic application of glucagon-like Peptide-1. Cell Metab. 2018;27(4):740–56.
41. Meier JJ. GLP-1 receptor agonists for individualized treatment of type 2 diabetes mellitus. Nat Rev Endocrinol. 2012;8:728–42.

42. Anderson J. The pharmacokinetic properties of glucagon-like Peptide-1 receptor agonists and their mode and mechanism of action in patients with type 2 diabetes. J Fam Pract. 2018;67(6 suppl):S8–S13.
43. Singh S, Wright EE Jr, Kwan AY, Thompson JC, Syed IA, Korol EE, Waser NA, Yu MB, Juneja R. Glucagon-like peptide-1 receptor agonists compared with basal insulins for the treatment of type 2 diabetes mellitus: a systematic review and meta-analysis. Diabetes Obes Metab. 2017;19(2):228–38.
44. Abd El Aziz MS, Kahle M, Meier JJ, Nauck MA. A meta-analysis comparing clinical effects of short- or long-acting GLP-1 receptor agonists versus insulin treatment from head-to-head studies in type 2 diabetic patients. Diabetes Obes Metab. 2017;19(2):216–27.
45. Katsurada K, Yada T. Neural effects of gut- and brain-derived glucagon-like peptide-1 and its receptor agonist. J Diabetes Investig. 2016;7(Suppl 1):64–9.
46. Kristensen SL, et al. Cardiovascular, mortality, and kidney outcomes with GLP-1 receptor agonists in patients with type 2 diabetes: a systematic review and meta-analysis of cardiovascular outcome trials. Lancet Diabetes Endocrinol. 2019;7(10):776–85.
47. Nreu B, Dicembrini I, Tinti F, Sesti G, Mannucci E, Monami M. Major cardiovascular events, heart failure, and atrial fibrillation in patients treated with glucagon-like peptide-1 receptor agonists: an updated meta-analysis of randomized controlled trials. Nutr Metab Cardiovasc Dis. 2020;30(7):1106–14.
48. Cukierman-Yaffe T, et al. Effect of dulaglutide on cognitive impairment in type 2 diabetes: an exploratory analysis of the REWIND trial. Lancet Neurol. 2020;19(7):582–90.
49. Frias JP, Bonora E, Nevárez Ruiz L, Hsia SH, Jung H, Raha S, Cox DA, Bethel MA, Konig M. Efficacy and safety of dulaglutide 3.0 and 4.5 mg in patients aged younger than 65 and 65 years or older: post hoc analysis of the AWARD-11 trial. Diabetes Obes Metab. 2021;23(10):2279–88.
50. Mosenzon O, Miller EM, Warren ML. Oral semaglutide in patients with type 2 diabetes and cardiovascular disease, renal impairment, or other comorbidities, and in older patients. Postgrad Med. 2020;132(suppl 2):37–47.
51. Wilson PWF, Kannel WB. Obesity, diabetes, and risk of cardiovascular disease in the elderly. Am J Geriatr Cardiol. 2002;11(2):119–23, 125.
52. Scheen AJ. Sodium-glucose cotransporter type 2 inhibitors for the treatment of type 2 diabetes mellitus. Nat Rev Endocrinol. 2020;16(10):556–77.
53. Zaccardi F, et al. Efficacy and safety of sodium-glucose cotransporter 2 inhibitors in type 2 diabetes mellitus: systematic review and network meta-analysis. Diabetes Obes Metab. 2016;18:783–94.
54. Sha S, et al. Effect of the sodium glucose co-transporter 2 inhibitor canagliflozin on plasma volume in patients with type 2 diabetes mellitus. Diabetes Obes Metab. 2014;16:1087–95.
55. Lambers Heerspink HJ, de Zeeuw D, Wie L, Leslie B, List J. Dapagliflozin a glucose-regulating drug with diuretic properties in subjects with type 2 diabetes. Diabetes Obes Metab. 2013;15:853–62.
56. Lee PC, Ganguly S, Goh SY. Weight loss associated with sodium-glucose cotransporter-2 inhibition: a review of evidence and underlying mechanisms. Obes Rev. 2018;19:1630–41.
57. Zinman B, et al. Empagliflozin, cardiovascular outcomes, and mortality in type 2 diabetes. N Engl J Med. 2015;373(22):2117–28.
58. Zelniker TA, et al. SGLT2 inhibitors for primary and secondary prevention of cardiovascular and renal outcomes in type 2 diabetes: a systematic review and meta-analysis of cardiovascular outcome trials. Lancet. 2019;393(10,166):31–9.
59. Neal B, et al. Canagliflozin and cardiovascular and renal events in type 2 diabetes. N Engl J Med. 2017;377(7):644–57.
60. McMurray JJV, et al. A trial to evaluate the effect of the sodium-glucose co-transporter 2 inhibitor dapagliflozin on morbidity and mortality in patients with heart failure and reduced left ventricular ejection fraction (DAPA-HF). Eur J Heart Fail. 2019;21(5):665–75.
61. Perkovic V, et al. Canagliflozin and renal outcomes in type 2 diabetes and nephropathy. N Engl J Med. 2019;380(24):2295–306.

62. Heerspink HJL, Jongs N, Chertow GM, Langkilde AM, McMurray JJV, Correa-Rotter R, Rossing P, Sjöström CD, Stefansson BV, Toto RD, Wheeler DC, Greene T. DAPA-CKD Trial Committees and Investigators. Effect of dapagliflozin on the rate of decline in kidney function in patients with chronic kidney disease with and without type 2 diabetes: a prespecified analysis from the DAPA-CKD trial. Lancet Diabetes Endocrinol. 2021;9(11):743–54.
63. Cintra R, et al. Inhibition of the sodium-glucose co-transporter 2 in the elderly: clinical and mechanistic insights into safety and efficacy. Rev Assoc Med Bras. 2019;65:70–86.
64. Wu JH, Foote C, Blomster J, Toyama T, Perkovic V, Sundström J, Neal B. Effects of sodium-glucose cotransporter-2 inhibitors on cardiovascular events, death, and major safety outcomes in adults with type 2 diabetes: a systematic review and meta-analysis. Lancet Diabetes Endocrinol. 2016;4(5):411–9.
65. Tentolouris A, Vlachakis P, Tzeravini E, Eleftheriadou I, Tentolouris N. SGLT2 inhibitors: a review of their antidiabetic and cardioprotective effects. Int J Environ Res Public Health. 2019;16(16):2965.
66. Scoccimarro D, Cipani G, Dicembrini I, Mannucci E. Cigarette smoking as a predictor of sodium-glucose cotransporter 2 inhibitor-associated genital infections: a retrospective cohort study. Diabetes Care. 2021;44(6):e127–8.
67. Kohler S, Zeller C, Iliev H, Kaspers S. Safety and tolerability of empagliflozin in patients with type 2 diabetes: pooled analysis of phase I-III clinical trials. Adv Ther. 2017;34(7):1707–26.
68. Vella A. Mechanism of action of DPP-4 inhibitors—new insights. J Clin Endocrinol Metab. 2012;97(8):2626–8.
69. Karyekar CS, Ravichandran S, Allen E, Fleming D, Frederich R. Tolerability and efficacy of glycemic control with saxagliptin in older patients (aged ≥ 65 years) with inadequately controlled type 2 diabetes mellitus. Clin Interv Aging. 2013;8:419–30.
70. Del Prato S, et al. Efficacy and safety of linagliptin in subjects with type 2 diabetes mellitus and poor glycemic control: pooled analysis of data from three placebo-controlled phase III trials. J Diabetes Complicat. 2013;27(3):274–9.
71. Barzilai N, et al. Efficacy and tolerability of sitagliptin monotherapy in elderly patients with type 2 diabetes: a randomized, double-blind, placebo-controlled trial. Curr Med Res Opin. 2011;27(5):1049–58.
72. Barnett AH, Huisman H, Jones R, von Eynatten M, Patel S, Woerle H-J. Linagliptin for patients aged 70 years or older with type 2 diabetes inadequately controlled with common antidiabetes treatments: a randomised, double-blind, placebo-controlled trial. Lancet (London, England). 2013;382(9902):1413–23.
73. Zangeneh F, Arora PS, Dyck PJ, Bekris L, Lernmark A, Achenbach SJ, Oberg AL, Rizza RA. Effects of duration of type 2 diabetes mellitus on insulin secretion. Endocr Pract. 2006;12(4):388–93. https://doi.org/10.4158/EP.12.4.388.
74. Vella A, Bock G, Giesler PD, Burton DB, Serra DB, Saylan ML, Deacon CF, Foley JE, Rizza RA, Camilleri M. The effect of dipeptidyl peptidase-4 inhibition on gastric volume, satiation and enteroendocrine secretion in type 2 diabetes: a double-blind, placebo-controlled crossover study. Clin Endocrinol. 2008;69(5):737–44.
75. Apovian CM, Okemah J, O'Neil PM. Body weight considerations in the management of Type 2 diabetes. Adv Ther. 2019;36(1):44–58.
76. Mannucci E, Nreu B, Montereggi C, Ragghianti B, Gallo M, Giaccari A, Monami M, SID-AMD Joint Panel for Italian Guidelines on Treatment of Type 2 Diabetes. Cardiovascular events and all-cause mortality in patients with type 2 diabetes treated with dipeptidyl peptidase-4 inhibitors: an extensive meta-analysis of randomized controlled trials. Nutr Metab Cardiovasc Dis. 2021;31(10):2745–55.
77. Scirica BM, Bhatt DL, Braunwald E, Steg PG, Davidson J, Hirshberg B, Ohman P, Frederich R, Wiviott SD, Hoffman EB, Cavender MA, Udell JA, Desai NR, Mosenzon O, McGuire DK, Ray KK, Leiter LA, Raz I, SAVOR-TIMI 53 Steering Committee and Investigators. Saxagliptin and cardiovascular outcomes in patients with type 2 diabetes mellitus. N Engl J Med. 2013;369(14):1317–26.

78. Zannad F, Cannon CP, Cushman WC, Bakris GL, Menon V, Perez AT, Fleck PR, Mehta CR, Kupfer S, Wilson C, Lam H, White WB, EXAMINE Investigators. Heart failure and mortality outcomes in patients with type 2 diabetes taking alogliptin versus placebo in EXAMINE: a multicentre, randomised, double-blind trial. Lancet. 2015;385(9982):2067–76.
79. McMurray JJV, Ponikowski P, Bolli GB, Lukashevich V, Kozlovski P, Kothny W, Lewsey JD, Krum H, VIVIDD Trial Committees and Investigators. Effects of vildagliptin on ventricular function in patients with type 2 diabetes mellitus and heart failure: a randomized placebo-controlled trial. JACC Heart Fail. 2018;6(1):8–17.
80. Green JB, Bethel MA, Armstrong PW, Buse JB, Engel SS, Garg J, Josse R, Kaufman KD, Koglin J, Korn S, Lachin JM, McGuire DK, Pencina MJ, Standl E, Stein PP, Suryawanshi S, Van de Werf F, Peterson ED, Holman RR, TECOS Study Group. Effect of sitagliptin on cardiovascular outcomes in type 2 diabetes. N Engl J Med. 2015;373(3):232–42.
81. Rosenstock J, Perkovic V, Johansen OE, Cooper ME, Kahn SE, Marx N, Alexander JH, Pencina M, Toto RD, Wanner C, Zinman B, Woerle HJ, Baanstra D, Pfarr E, Schnaidt S, Meinicke T, George JT, von Eynatten M, McGuire DK, CARMELINA Investigators. Effect of linagliptin vs placebo on major cardiovascular events in adults with type 2 diabetes and high cardiovascular and renal risk: the CARMELINA randomized clinical trial. JAMA. 2019;321(1):69–79.
82. Rosenstock J, Kahn SE, Johansen OE, Zinman B, Espeland MA, Woerle HJ, Pfarr E, Keller A, Mattheus M, Baanstra D, Meinicke T, George JT, von Eynatten M, McGuire DK, Marx N, CAROLINA Investigators. Effect of linagliptin vs glimepiride on major adverse cardiovascular outcomes in patients with type 2 diabetes: the CAROLINA randomized clinical trial. JAMA. 2019;322(12):1155–66.
83. Paolisso G, Monami M, Marfella R, Rizzo MR, Mannucci E. Dipeptidyl peptidase-4 inhibitors in the elderly: more benefits or risks? Adv Ther. 2012;29(3):218–33.
84. Dicembrini I, Montereggi C, Nreu B, Mannucci E, Monami M. Pancreatitis and pancreatic cancer in patients treated with dipeptidyl peptidase-4 inhibitors: an extensive and updated meta-analysis of randomized controlled trials. Diabetes Res Clin Pract. 2020;159:107981.
85. Silverii GA, Dicembrini I, Nreu B, Montereggi C, Mannucci E, Monami M. Bullous pemphigoid and dipeptidyl peptidase-4 inhibitors: a meta-analysis of randomized controlled trials. Endocrine. 2020;69(3):504–7.
86. Lebovitz HE. Thiazolidinediones: the forgotten diabetes medications. Curr Diab Rep. 2019;19(12):151.
87. Nesto RW, et al. Thiazolidinedione use, fluid retention, and congestive heart failure: a consensus statement from the American Heart Association and American Diabetes Association. Diabetes Care. 2004;27(1):256–63.
88. Scheen AJ. Combined thiazolidinedione-insulin therapy: should we be concerned about safety? Drug Saf. 2004;27(12):841–56.
89. Benvenuti S, et al. Rosiglitazone stimulates adipogenesis and decreases osteoblastogenesis in human mesenchymal stem cells. J Endocrinol Investig. 2007;30(9):RC26–30.
90. McDonough AK, Rosenthal RS, Cao X, Saag KG. The effect of thiazolidinediones on BMD and osteoporosis. Nat Clin Pract Endocrinol Metab. 2008;4(9):507–13.
91. Kahn SE, et al. Rosiglitazone-associated fractures in type 2 diabetes: an analysis from a diabetes outcome progression trial (ADOPT). Diabetes Care. 2008;31(5):845–51.
92. Lv W, Wang X, Xu Q, Lu W. Mechanisms and characteristics of sulfonylureas and glinides. Curr Top Med Chem. 2020;20(1):37–56.
93. Mannucci E, Naletto L, Vaccaro G, Silverii A, Dicembrini I, Pintaudi B, Monami M. Efficacy and safety of glucose-lowering agents in patients with type 2 diabetes: a network meta-analysis of randomized, active comparator-controlled trials. Nutr Metab Cardiovasc Dis. 2021;31(4):1027–34.
94. Mannucci E, Monami M, Candido R, Pintaudi B, Targher G. SID-AMD joint panel for Italian Guidelines on Treatment of Type 2 Diabetes. Effect of insulin secretagogues on major cardiovascular events and all-cause mortality: a meta-analysis of randomized controlled trials. Nutr Metab Cardiovasc Dis. 2020;30(10):1601–8.

95. Phung OJ, Schwartzman E, Allen RW, Engel SS, Rajpathak SN. Sulphonylureas and risk of cardiovascular disease: systematic review and meta-analysis. Diabet Med. 2013;30(10):1160–71.
96. Scognamiglio R, Avogaro A, Vigili de Kreutzenberg S, Negut C, Palisi M, Bagolin E, Tiengo A. Effects of treatment with sulfonylurea drugs or insulin on ischemia-induced myocardial dysfunction in type 2 diabetes. Diabetes. 2002;51(3):808–12.
97. Liu R, Wang H, Xu B, Chen W, Turlova E, Dong N, Sun CL, Lu Y, Fu H, Shi R, Barszczyk A, Yang D, Jin T, Mannucci E, Feng ZP, Sun HS. Cerebrovascular safety of sulfonylureas: the role of KATP channels in neuroprotection and the risk of stroke in patients with type 2 diabetes. Diabetes. 2016;65(9):2795–809.

Stroke Therapeutics in the Care of Older Persons

24

A. Bahk, F. A. Kirkham, Y. T. Ng, and Chakravarthi Rajkumar

24.1 Background and Epidemiology

Stroke is defined as 'rapidly developing clinical signs of focal (or global) disturbance of cerebral function, with symptoms lasting 24 h or longer or leading to death, with no apparent cause other than of vascular origin' [1]. It accounts for approximately 11% of deaths worldwide [2], and over 116 million years of healthy life lost are due to stroke-related conditions. In Europe, stroke mortality has declined in recent years due to improvements in diagnosis and treatment [3], but with changing demographics and population structure, the projected number of stroke survivors in Europe is expected to increase 27% by 2047 [4].

While 87% of strokes are ischaemic compared to only 13% that are haemorrhagic [5], the World Stroke Organisation reports that 51% of all deaths from stroke occur from haemorrhages [6], defined as intracerebral or subarachnoid haemorrhages in the absence of trauma [7]. An estimated 30% of strokes occur in those over 80 years, with this group experiencing a threefold higher 30-day case fatality rate compared to their younger counterparts [8]. Older adults often present with higher NIHSS (National Institute of Health Stroke Scale) score which translates to more severe strokes, increased levels of risk factors [9] and have delayed time to thrombolysis administration, when given [10], making this patient group a particularly important focus when it comes to stroke management.

A. Bahk · F. A. Kirkham · Y. T. Ng
University Hospitals Sussex NHS Foundation Trust, Brighton, East Sussex, UK
e-mail: annabahk@nhs.net; f.kirkham@nhs.net; yiting.ng1@nhs.net

C. Rajkumar (✉)
University Hospitals Sussex NHS Foundation Trust, Brighton, East Sussex, UK

Department of Medicine, Brighton and Sussex Medical School, University of Sussex, Brighton, UK
e-mail: C.Rajkumar@bsms.ac.uk; Raj.rajkumar@nhs.net

A. Cherubini et al. (eds.), *Optimizing Pharmacotherapy in Older Patients*, Practical Issues in Geriatrics, https://doi.org/10.1007/978-3-031-28061-0_24

Transient ischaemic attack (TIA) is an episode of neurological dysfunction caused by focal brain, spinal cord, or retinal ischaemia, without acute infarction, lasting less than 24 h [11]. It is estimated that 4.7% of TIA patients will go on to have a stroke in the subsequent 90 days [12].

24.2 Ischaemic Stroke Classification

A number of different classification systems have been proposed. The most commonly used system is the TOAST criteria (trial of ORG 10172 in acute stroke treatment), focusing on the likely causative event to divide strokes predominately into large artery atherosclerotic, cardioembolic or small vessel occlusion [13] while allowing for undetermined or other causes. Approximately 45% of ischaemic strokes are due to thrombosis [14] in a large or small vessel, while one fifth are thought to derive from cardiac emboli [15].

Alternatively, Bamford classification (Table 24.1) relies on clinical findings to determine the brain territory affected, defining strokes as lacunar (LAC), total (TAC) or partial anterior (PAC), or posterior (POC) and assigning a letter following CT imaging (I for infarct, H for haemorrhage or S for syndrome) [16]. The oldest old are more likely to have large vessel (TAC/PAC) occlusion than small vessel (POC/LAC) occlusion compared to those under 80 years [17].

Table 24.1 Bamford classification of ischaemic stroke

Stroke type	Clinical findings
Lacunar (LAC)	Any of: Pure motor Pure sensory Sensorimotor Ataxic hemiparesis Dysarthria-clumsy hand syndrome Without higher cortical dysfunction.
Total anterior circulation (TAC)	All of: Higher cortical dysfunction Homonymous visual field deficit Unilateral motor and/or sensory loss affecting 2 out of 3 regions (face, upper limb, lower limb).
Partial anterior circulation (PAC)	2 out of 3: Higher cortical dysfunction Homonymous visual field deficit Unilateral motor and/or sensory loss affecting 2 out of 3 regions (face, upper limb, lower limb).
Posterior circulation (POC)	Any of: Cerebellar syndrome Homonymous visual field deficit Ipsilateral cranial nerve impairment with contralateral motor and/or sensory loss Bilateral motor and/or sensory loss.

Additionally, there are numerous 'brainstem syndromes' describing specific groups of symptoms occurring in rarer stroke subtypes, often with eponymous names and defined by their vascular supply. Examples include Wallenberg syndrome (lateral medullary syndrome) and Millard-Gubler syndrome (ventral pontine syndrome). In general, brainstem strokes are characterised by ipsilateral cranial nerve palsy and contralateral hemiparesis and/or hemisensory loss.

24.3 Pathophysiology

Hypertension is implicated in many of the changes to cerebral blood vessels associated with both ischaemic and haemorrhagic stroke. Over time, exposure to high pressure causes arterial remodelling, changes in elastic and muscular constituents of vessels and endothelial dysfunction, as well as promoting atherosclerotic plaque formation [18]. Precursors to stroke include microaneurysms and microbleeds, white matter changes [19] and subclinical infarcts.

Inflammation plays a significant role in the pathophysiology of ischaemic stroke, with increases in reactive oxidant species and endothelial dysfunction contributing to atherosclerosis, platelet aggregation and plaque rupture [20]. Impaired microvascular function secondary to chronic hypertension and age-induced vascular stiffness interacts with a systemic inflammatory state to predispose fragile vessels to bleeding and thrombosis. Further changes with age such as reduced cerebral perfusion and deposition of β-amyloid are associated with degeneration of vascular function [21].

Embolic strokes can originate from thrombosis (formed in a blood vessel, cardiac chamber or heart valve), atherosclerotic material or non-thrombotic material such as tumour, infectious vegetations, air or fat [22].

24.4 Risk Factors

The Framingham Stroke Risk Profile (FSRP) is the most commonly used tool for evaluating stroke risk [23] and has been validated for predicting cerebrovascular events in older patient groups. It incorporates the following established risk factors:

- Sex
- Age
- Smoking
- Blood pressure (treatment for hypertension or raised SBP)
- Diabetes
- Cardiovascular disease
- Atrial fibrillation

In high-income countries, almost half of global stroke mortality could be accounted for by modifiable risk factors. Additional to those included in the

FSRP, hyperlipidaemia, alcohol use, obesity, air pollution and dietary choices have been shown to contribute to increased risk of stroke [24], while higher levels of physical activity have also been shown to be inversely related to stroke risk [25].

Additional risk factors have been investigated in recent years. There is some evidence to suggest that serum biomarkers including advanced glycation end products, CRP and total homocysteine are independently associated with increased risk of stroke [26]. The role of measurable sex hormones and adipokines has been suggested; however, thus far results are inconclusive. Genetic elements have also been proposed as tools for identifying those at higher risk of stroke, and the APOEε2 allele has been shown to be protective against ischaemic stroke in those aged 71–79 years, but not in people over 80 years [27]. Psychosocial factors shown to increase stroke risk include depressive symptoms [28], low psychological well-being and reduced cognitive function [29]. Finally, low socioeconomic status not only increases the risk of having a stroke but is also associated with reduced access to care and poorer outcomes [30].

24.5 Presentation

Stroke in older patients does not always present with typical features, and the term 'stroke chameleon' has been used to describe unusual presentations. The oldest old are more likely to present with falls or reduced mobility and less likely to have sensory symptoms [31]. Other potential presentations include neuropsychiatric symptoms (such as confusion, memory loss or reduced GCS), abnormal movements, dizziness or headache [32]. The reasons for such divergent presentations are manifold, as symptoms may still be evolving with subtly different brain regions involved, alongside practical difficulties in performing comprehensive examinations in frail older people and the possibility that dual pathologies may exist simultaneously in multimorbid adults [33]. Full assessment, however, is paramount to avoid misdiagnosis or attribution of symptoms to another coincidental illness (e.g. urinary tract infection or pre-existing mobility issues). The most common misdiagnoses are delirium, syncope, hypertensive emergencies or systemic infection [34].

24.6 Assessment

The Recognition Of Stroke In the Emergency Room (ROSIER) scale is designed for use in emergency departments to aid in the diagnosis of stroke [35]. However, as older patients may present with atypical symptoms, and 'time is brain' [36], it is generally recommended to prioritise brain imaging in the form of CT for all potential strokes. Table 24.2 outlines the recommended investigations for all stroke patients being assessed in the acute setting.

Table 24.2 Investigations for older people presenting with acute stroke

Bedside investigations	Blood tests	Imaging
History and clinical examination including NIHSS score	Full blood count	CT brain within 1 h of presentation
Functional assessment	Urea and electrolytes	Chest X-ray
Blood pressure	Clotting	Consider CT angiography or diffusion-weighted MRI
12-lead ECG	Inflammatory markers	Consider echocardiography and 24-h ambulatory ECG to identify cause
Bedside glucose	Lipid profile	Consider carotid doppler US
Swallow assessment	HbA1c	

NIHSS National Institutes of Health Stroke Scale

24.7 Functional Assessment

It has been shown that in older adults, frailty score is a better predictor of stroke outcome than other measures [37]. Equally, pre-stroke cognitive function is an important determinant of cognitive recovery [38]. Therefore, it is of particular significance to assess pre-morbid frailty and cognition in this patient group.

The most widely used tools for frailty assessment include the Rockwood Clinical Frailty Scale [39] which relies on the judgement of an experienced clinician; the Fried Frailty Index [40] which focuses on independently measurable variables such as BMI and handgrip strength; or the Barthel Index [41] which looks at self-reported ability to perform activities of daily living.

The modified Rankin Scale (mRS) has been applied within stroke research and in clinical settings as a measure of disability and dependence after stroke. The scale ranges from 0 (no symptoms) to 6 (death). It can be used to evaluate pre-stroke disability with validity in prognostication.

Although it is not possible to measure pre-morbid cognitive function on presentation, it is widely accepted that cognitive assessment should be performed prior to discharge [42]. Many tools have been validated for use in older adults; however, there is limited evidence for their use in acute stroke [43]. The Montreal Cognitive Assessment (MoCA) has been suggested as the most useful for identifying cognitive impairment after stroke [44], offering a validated evaluation that is also feasible to perform regularly in clinical practice.

24.8 Hyperacute Management of Acute Stroke

The hyperacute management of stroke is largely dependent on the stroke subtype. With loss of neurons every second, rapid treatment is crucial to reduce the sequelae of further neuronal death. Stroke patients treated in a specialist stroke unit are more likely to achieve a favourable outcome, taking into account different stroke types, severity and age [45].

24.8.1 Ischaemic Stroke

The immediate treatment of acute ischaemic strokes targets the occluded cerebral artery to enable revascularisation and re-establish cerebral blood flow. The use of thrombolytic agents and mechanical thrombectomy is now widely adopted as standard practice owing to the overall net benefit in reducing disability and mortality.

Numerous studies have shown thrombolysis treatment with intravenous recombinant tissue-plasminogen activator (rt-PA), when delivered within 4.5 h, achieved significant reduction in disability [46, 47]. This was despite symptomatic intracerebral haemorrhage (sICH) of 7.7% and fatal intracerebral haemorrhage of 3.6% within the first 7 days [48].

The exclusion of patients aged ≥80 from these initial trials has led to uncertainty of potential benefits in this cohort. A major concern was the theoretically greater bleeding risk in older patients. The Third International Stroke Trial (IST-3) provided valuable safety and efficacy data in patients aged ≥80, and subsequent trials indicate that the overall benefit of treatment is comparable to younger patients [49]. While sICH rates are similar across age groups, delay in treatment time, larger strokes, hyperglycaemia and hypertension is implicated in higher bleeding risk and considered to be contraindications for thrombolysis. The presence of leukoaraiosis on brain imaging, which is more commonly seen in older patients, is also linked to increased risk of thrombolysis-related sICH [50]. However, in general, increasing age is a predictor of adverse outcome and mortality due to non-haemorrhagic complications, often associated with the ageing process. Multi-morbidity and pre-stroke frailty are also linked to poor prognosis [51]. Treatment decisions therefore require careful consideration, balancing the overall benefit and risk on an individual basis.

Research continues in the use of magnetic resonance imaging (MRI) and computed tomography perfusion (CTP) to support thrombolysis in patients with stroke of unknown time of onset or symptoms beyond 4.5 h [52]. This could potentially widen the treatment time window.

The efficacy of endovascular therapy in the hyperacute treatment of ischaemic stroke with anterior proximal large vessel occlusion is well established. Mechanical devices are deployed to remove the clot and open up the occluded cerebral artery thereby restoring blood flow (Figs. 24.1 and 24.2). The development of newer generation mechanical devices and advances in technique has led to lower mortality rates and a substantial reduction in disability at 90 days [53]. These findings have also been observed in patients aged ≥80 when compared to those given standard care [53, 54]. Where possible, it is considered to be the treatment of choice for ischaemic strokes with a proximal large vessel occlusion for several reasons. Patients who would otherwise not be eligible for thrombolysis can be offered treatment without the bleeding risks associated. These include patients with underlying bleeding tendencies and those on anticoagulation treatment. It can also be performed in conjunction with thrombolysis to achieve higher rates of recanalisation than thrombolysis alone [53]. However, the overall recanalisation rates are lower in older patients [54] with associated higher rates of adverse outcome and mortality [55].

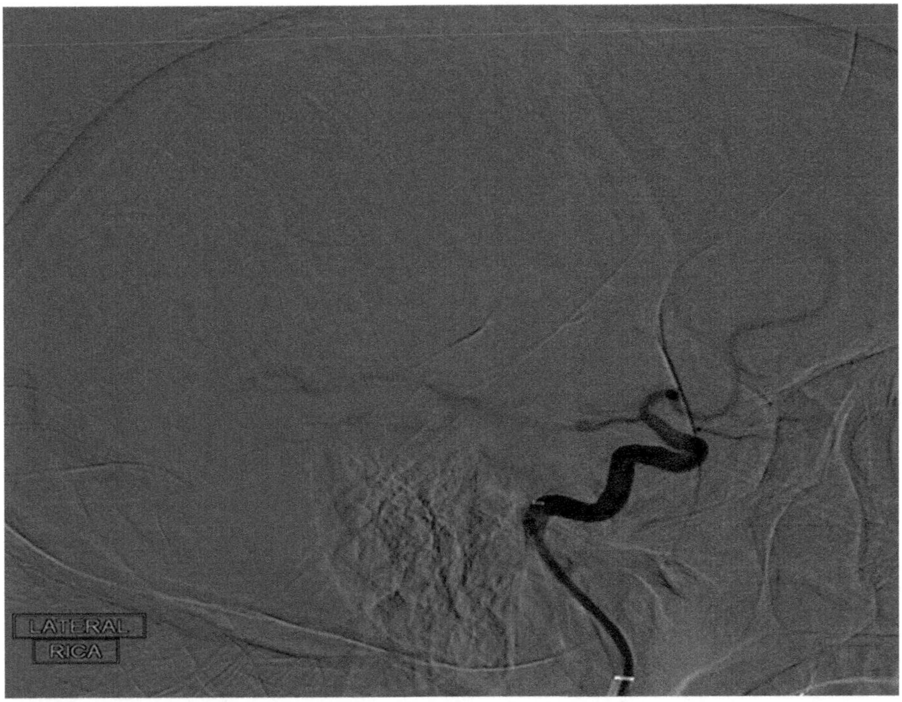

Fig. 24.1 Angiography of right middle cerebral artery occlusion

Poorer neurological reserve and higher risk of post-stroke complication are suggested to be contributing factors.

Current evidence supports the use of intravenous thrombolysis and mechanical thrombectomy in the treatment of ischaemic strokes, regardless of age. However, the utilisation of these treatments remains less in older patients [53, 56]. These decisions are likely to be based on various factors including pre-existing comorbidities and frailty, perceived risk of complications and the overall benefit. Therefore, decision to treat should be based on the individual patient to avoid potentially harmful intervention in patients who are unlikely to achieve a favourable outcome.

24.8.2 Intracerebral Haemorrhage

The management of intracerebral haemorrhage (ICH) involves measures to reduce haematoma expansion and thereby prevent further neurological deterioration. Compared to acute ischaemic strokes, patients with ICH are more likely to be commenced on end-of-life care within the first 72 h with less patients receiving higher level care, independent of premorbid mRS, age, comorbidities and level of consciousness [57]. In doing so, this could impose limitations in acute treatment and thus impact recovery and outcome [58]. Coordinated specialist stroke units and

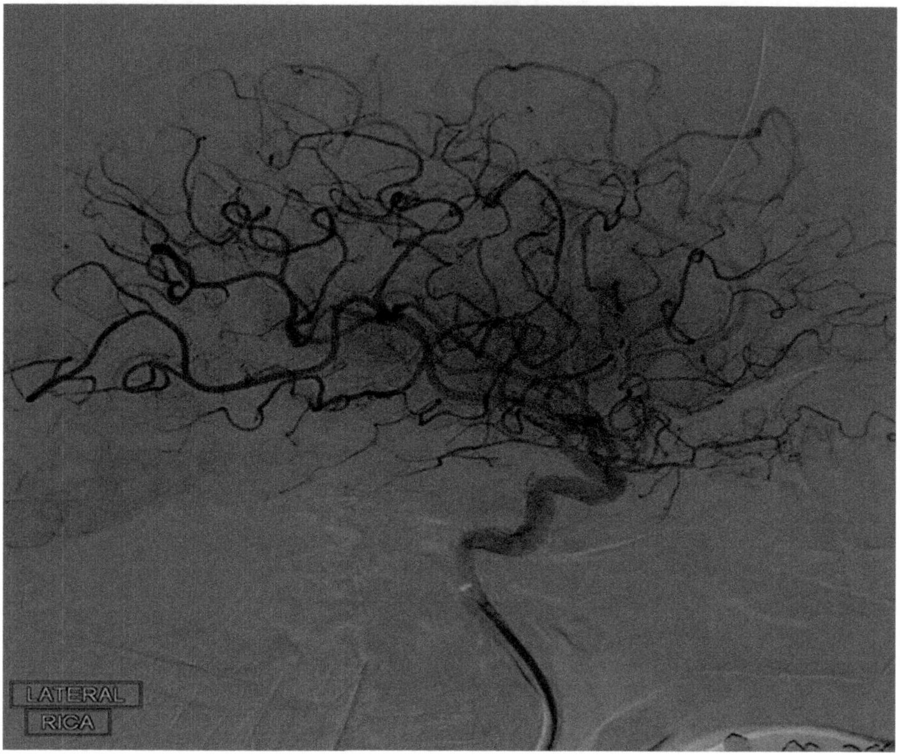

Fig. 24.2 Angiography of reperfusion in the right middle cerebral artery after mechanical thrombectomy

neurocritical care are associated with improved mortality and level of independence in patients with ICH [45].

Elevated blood pressure in the acute phase is a common physiological response in ICH. Resultant haematoma enlargement and cerebral oedema are feared complications and predictors of poor outcome [59]. Initiating intensive blood pressure lowering has shown to be safe in reducing haematoma size without added risk of neurological deterioration or recurrent stroke events. While this did not translate to significant reduction in mortality or major disability at 3 months, improved functional outcome was observed in ordinal shift analysis of mRS in the INTERACT trials with rapid lowering of blood pressure to a target systolic of 140 mmHg in the first 6 h [60]. Thus, other factors are likely to contribute to clinical outcome including time frame from symptom onset to first brain imaging, the volume of haematoma at presentation and effects of blood pressure variability in the acute phase [61, 62]. Furthermore, extrapolation of data in the oldest old population should be interpreted with caution in view of uncertainties in the blood pressure physiology of this age group.

The use of vitamin K antagonists (VKA) such as warfarin at presentation results in larger haematoma size at baseline with greater risk of haematoma expansion and mortality compared to those not on anticoagulation [63]. In comparison, haematoma size tends to be smaller with less severe stroke in patients on direct oral anticoagulant (DOAC) although with comparable case fatality rates [64]. Due to the correlation of haematoma expansion and poor outcome, rapid reversal of anticoagulants to attenuate haematoma enlargement has been widely adopted. The use of prothrombin complex concentrate (PCC) and other targeted reversal agents for DOACs has shown to be effective [65]. Currently, there is no licensed reversal agent for patients on antiplatelet therapy.

Earlier trials evaluating the clinical outcome of neurosurgery in patients with ICH concluded no overall benefit in mortality or favourable outcome [66]. There is now emerging evidence that targeted therapy using minimally invasive surgery (MIS) in select patients improves mortality and, potentially, functional outcome [67, 68]. Due to small sample size, variability in timing of surgery and haematoma size, as well as the exclusion of older patients in these studies, further research is required to appreciate the role of surgery in the treatment of ICH in older patients.

24.8.3 Transient Ischaemic Attack

Stroke prevention is central to the management of transient ischaemic attacks (TIA). Currently, guidelines for TIA management involve prompt assessment by a stroke specialist, ideally within 24 h [69]. Detailed history and clinical examination are key to confirm diagnosis and exclude mimics which can account for up to 60% of patients seen in the TIA clinic [70]. This can be particularly challenging when assessing older patients as recollection of symptoms may be vague; however, brain imaging can be helpful. Urgent investigations are performed to identify modifiable risk factors, including atrial fibrillation, carotid disease and hypertension. Immediate treatment with the combination of antithrombotic agents, blood pressure and lipid lowering strategies has been shown to reduce stroke risk by up to 80% [71]. Addressing the precipitating cause and risk factors for TIA, such as initiating anticoagulation in atrial fibrillation and surgical intervention for significant carotid stenosis, is important to secondary prevention [69]. Opportunities should be taken to promote non-pharmacological measures such as dietary adjustments, exercise and smoking cessation.

24.9 Secondary Prevention of Stroke and TIA

The success of stroke prevention with decline in stroke incidence has been offset by the rapidly ageing population. The exclusion of older patients in numerous landmark clinical trials on stroke prevention has led to a paucity of evidence in the benefits of secondary prevention measures in this cohort. However, with increasing life expectancy, even patients aged 80 of average health would benefit from secondary stroke prevention [72].

24.9.1 Antiplatelets

Antiplatelet agents are a key component in secondary prevention following a non-cardioembolic acute ischaemic stroke or TIA [73]. Thus far, aspirin is the only antiplatelet agent shown to significantly reduce recurrent ischaemic stroke risk in the acute phase [74]. Patients presenting with TIAs or minor strokes observe greater benefit with aspirin, with a risk reduction for recurrent ischaemic stroke of 60% and disabling or fatal ischaemic stroke of 70% [74]. It is therefore vital that patients suspected of a TIA or stroke (after haemorrhage has been excluded) are immediately administered aspirin. After the acute phase, clopidogrel has been shown to be a superior long-term monotherapy compared to aspirin in reducing the combined risk of ischaemic stroke, myocardial infarction or vascular death [75]. Dual antiplatelet therapy (DAPT), with aspirin and a P2Y12 inhibitor, such as clopidogrel or ticagrelor, can be used in select patients with acute minor ischaemic strokes or high-risk TIAs. By initiating early treatment and duration of up to 90 days, stroke recurrence is reduced by 24% with a small absolute increased risk of haemorrhage. Exclusion of very elderly patients in the trials with DAPT (mean age in these trials 62–68) may implicate bias in clinical practice [76].

24.9.2 Antihypertensives

Hypertension is the single most important modifiable risk factor for both ischaemic and haemorrhagic stroke, and reduction in blood pressure correlates with lower stroke risk [77].

In the hyperacute phase, blood pressure can be elevated as normal cerebral autoregulation is impaired. Lowering blood pressure may be beneficial in the management of ICH; however, in acute ischaemic stroke, elevated blood pressure is considered to have a neuroprotective effect to improve cerebral perfusion to the ischaemic areas. Optimum timing to initiate antihypertensive treatment remains uncertain, and recommendations vary from days to weeks [78]. In TIAs, antihypertensive treatment can be commenced once the diagnosis of hypertension is established [79], and there are no specific contraindications.

Comparison data between patients aged ≥65 versus <65 showed comparable risk reduction [80]. Patients aged ≥80 were underrepresented in this study; however, the Hypertension in the Very Elderly Trial (HYVET) showed that antihypertensive therapy reduced stroke risk by 30% and all-cause mortality by 21% [81]. Adverse effects of intensive blood pressure lowering in older patients include cerebral hypoperfusion and orthostatic hypotension. However, slightly higher blood pressure targets of 150/80 mmHg as seen in the HYVET trial could still achieve satisfactory outcome.

24.9.3 Lipid-Lowering Agents

Hyperlipidaemia is a common modifiable risk factor for ischaemic stroke in older patients, observed in over 50% of those aged ≥65 [82]. Reducing low-density lipoprotein (LDL) cholesterol levels to less than 70 mg/dL (1.8 mmol/L) following ischaemic stroke or TIA could lower risk of subsequent cardiovascular events [83]. Hydroxy-3-methylglutaryl-coenzyme A (HMG-CoA) reductase inhibitors, also known as statins, have proven to have protective benefits in reducing stroke risk by lowering LDL cholesterol [84]. These benefits have also been reflected in further studies examining older patients for both primary and secondary prevention and with high level of tolerability [85]. However, these findings have not been consistently replicated and only seen to be effective in patients with carotid disease [86]. Furthermore, the use of statins should be guided by the life expectancy of the patient as its benefits are observed over several years. Newer lipid-lowering agents such as PCSK9 inhibitors have been utilised in patients who are intolerant to statins. With higher rates of statin intolerance in the older patient, alternative agents may be considered, although the evidence of its role in the older population is yet to be evaluated.

24.9.4 Diabetes Treatment

Diabetes mellitus is a recognised risk factor for ischaemic stroke and is associated with a fourfold increase in stroke risk. The prevalence of type 2 diabetes increases with age, and these patients have a higher propensity for strokes and cardiovascular disease compared to those with type 1 diabetes [87]. Pre-existing diabetes is associated with recurrent ischaemic stroke and poorer prognosis [88]. However, intensive glycaemic control has not been shown to reduce cardiovascular events including stroke and can lead to adverse outcome [89]. This emphasises the need for an individualised approach to glycaemic targets and optimisation of coexisting vascular risk factors, including hypertension and hyperlipidaemia. The extent of glycaemic control should be balanced with the risk of major hypoglycaemic events. The current recommendation is to aim for a target HbA1c of 48 mmol/mol (6.5%) in type 2 diabetes [90].

24.9.4.1 Atrial Fibrillation

Atrial fibrillation (AF) accounts for up to one in three ischaemic strokes, and the incidence increases with age. It is associated with worse prognosis; however, it can be preventable [91]. The benefits of anticoagulation therapy are well established and accordingly recommended in guidelines [69, 79, 92]. The superiority of vitamin K antagonists, such as warfarin, over aspirin in stroke prevention is also widely recognised, even in older patients [93]. However, with effectiveness dependent on 'time in therapeutic range' (TTR) and the challenges of monitoring the international normalised ratio (INR), this can be particularly problematic in older patients [94]. Direct oral anticoagulants (DOAC) have been shown to be non-inferior to warfarin in stroke reduction with potentially better safety profile. Importantly, these results were also evident in those aged ≥75 years [95]. However, in clinical practice, older patients are often denied anticoagulation due to age and perceived risks of bleeding and falls [96].

While there may be valid reasons not to commence older patients on anticoagulation, individual risk assessment is vital to ensure that appropriate treatment is offered to eligible patients. A comprehensive assessment should be carried out to determine the suitability of commencing anticoagulation using risk stratification tools. The Outcome Registry for Better Informed Treatment of Atrial Fibrillation (ORBIT) score has been shown to be superior in assessing bleeding risk when compared to the HASBLED score. Stroke recurrence risk in AF can be estimated using the CHA_2DS_2VASc score. There is always a debate around avoiding anticoagulation in elderly patients due to the risk of falls. Current guidelines in the management of AF emphasise that falls alone should not be treated as a contraindication to anticoagulation [92]. The various factors which affect the patient and the benefit of anticoagulation versus not anticoagulating should be taken into account before deciding treatment. Discussions with the patient and the family on the risks and benefits of treatment are beneficial.

24.9.5 Carotid Endarterectomy

Atherosclerotic carotid stenosis is associated with 10–15% of ischaemic strokes and TIAs, with prevalence increasing with age [97]. Carotid revascularization is achieved by carotid endarterectomy (CEA) or carotid artery stenting (CAS).

The benefits of CEA are based on two landmark trials. The European Carotid Surgery Trial (ESCT) and the North American Symptomatic Carotid Endarterectomy Trial (NASCET) [98, 99]. Currently, CEA is performed for secondary stroke prevention in the context of symptomatic significant internal carotid artery stenosis in TIAs and non-disabling strokes [100]. Symptomatic carotid disease is defined as diameter reduction of ≥50% using the NASCET method [99]. The risk of recurrent stroke is highest in the first 7–14 days, and the benefits of CEA diminish beyond this period; therefore, there is emphasis on performing surgery soon after the index event (within 2 weeks). The number needed to treat (NNT) is significantly reduced when stenosis is >70%, hence the need to refer for surgical intervention early in the presence of high-grade carotid stenosis [98]. Reassuringly, advancing age was not associated with increased risk of 30-day stroke or mortality rates and conversely patients aged ≥75 years observed greater benefits following carotid surgery [101]. The short- and long-term stroke complications are not insignificant and particularly more common in patients aged ≥70 [102]. Given that the absolute risk reduction is calculated over 5 years, the decision to proceed with surgical treatment should be based on the overall prognosis.

The risks of peri-procedural stroke and mortality following CAS are higher when compared to CEA and particularly in patients aged ≥70. It is therefore currently not recommended as first-line treatment for symptomatic carotid disease. However, there is a role for CAS in patients aged ≤70 who are unable to undergo CEA in the treatment of symptomatic carotid stenosis [103].

Guidelines recommend CEA in asymptomatic carotid artery stenosis in high-risk patients despite best medical therapy. Patients aged ≥75 years with expected survival of at least 5 years may be considered following careful multidisciplinary assessment. CAS is, however, not routinely recommended in asymptomatic carotid stenosis owing to limited evidence [103].

24.9.5.1 Post-Stroke Sequelae in the Older Person

Studies estimate that up to 85% of stroke patients encounter a medical complication during hospital admission [104]. These conditions are common in older patients and can occur early or late in the stroke recovery phase, limiting the rehabilitation process. Often these conditions are preventable and treatable, emphasising the importance of organised stroke care in a hyperacute stroke unit in reducing stroke mortality and improving functional outcome [45].

Malignant middle cerebral artery (MCA) syndrome is a potentially fatal complication of middle cerebral artery ischaemic stroke. Decompressive hemicraniectomy is proven to be a life-saving treatment without increasing the risk of severe disability among patients aged 60 years or younger [105]. However, its benefits in older patients remain controversial, and further research is needed.

Seizures are common complication following a stroke and can occur early (within the first 7 days) or late (after 7 days). Seizures occurring after 7 days are diagnostic for post-stroke epilepsy and carry a risk of seizure recurrence of up to 71.5% at 10 years [106]. Anti-epileptic agents should be initiated; however, assessment is advised to determine the need for long-term treatment.

Infections are frequently seen in stroke patients, and early detection and treatment are crucial. Stroke-associated pneumonia is one of the most common forms of infection. Dysphagia, severe strokes and increasing age are independent predictors. Urinary tract infections are also seen in patients following a stroke and are often related to urinary catheterisation.

Prolonged immobility can lead to thromboembolism such as deep vein thrombosis (DVT) and pulmonary embolism (PE). The use of intermittent pneumatic compression devices has been proven to reduce rates of thromboembolic events [107]. Pressure ulcers, spasticity and contractures are also common complications related to impaired mobility. Involvement of multidisciplinary team to support early mobilisation and pressure-relieving strategies is vital for prevention. The use of botulinum toxin and neuropathic analgesia can reduce the severity of spasticity.

Post-stroke neuropsychological complications can occur in patients of all ages. Anxiety and depression can significantly limit recovery and can last for many years after stroke. Both non-pharmacological and pharmacological treatment with antidepressants can help. Post-stroke fatigue is a common problem and closely associated with mood. There is inconsistent evidence of age as a risk factor for developing post-stroke fatigue. Thus far, there is no specific treatment proven to be effective [108]. Early neuropsychological assessment and therapy are components in its management.

The incidence of dementia can be up to 50 times greater following a stroke or TIA compared to the general population. Vascular dementia is closely associated with stroke, and treatment of reversible causes will help reduce progression of the disease. Stroke burden and severity, age and premorbid dependency are risk factors for developing dementia in stroke survivors [109].

24.10 Conclusion

Stroke remains common in older patient groups, and while mortality has declined in recent years, it is a significant cause of morbidity and impaired function. In older people, presenting symptoms may be atypical, and time to treatment is often delayed, potentially resulting in poorer outcomes. With advances in imaging and novel therapeutic approaches, it is imperative for geriatricians to stay informed of up-to-date evidence and guidelines on stroke management to maximise opportunities for intervention both in the acute setting and as secondary prevention. Management within a hyperacute stroke unit by a multidisciplinary team has been shown to improve outcomes and encourage holistic care. In the future, targeted molecular therapies and nanotechnology may enable even greater reductions in mortality and enable faster detection, more effective reperfusion and prevent the complications still associated with this important condition.

References

1. Truelsen T. The global burden of cerebrovascular disease: WHO. World Health Organisation. 2006; https://www.who.int/healthinfo/statistics/bod_cerebrovasculardiseasestroke.pdf
2. WHO. The top 10 causes of death 2020. https://www.who.int/news-room/fact-sheets/detail/the-top-10-causes-of-death.
3. Shah R, Wilkins E, Nichols M, Kelly P, El-Sadi F, Wright FL, et al. Epidemiology report: trends in sex-specific cerebrovascular disease mortality in Europe based on WHO mortality data. Eur Heart J. 2019;40(9):755–64.
4. Wafa HA, Wolfe CDA, Emmett E, Roth GA, Johnson CO, Wang Y. Burden of stroke in Europe: thirty-year projections of incidence, prevalence, deaths, and disability-adjusted life years. Stroke. 2020;51(8):2418–27.
5. Virani SS, Alonso A, Aparicio HJ, Benjamin EJ, Bittencourt MS, Callaway CW, et al. Heart disease and stroke Statistics-2021 update: a report from the American Heart Association. Circulation. 2021;143(8):e254–743.
6. Lindsay MP. Global stroke factsheet 2019. WSO, World Stroke Organisation; 2019.
7. Sacco RL, Kasner SE, Broderick JP, Caplan LR, Connors JJ, Culebras A, et al. An updated definition of stroke for the 21st century: a statement for healthcare professionals from the American Heart Association/American Stroke Association. Stroke. 2013;44(7):2064–89.
8. Russo T, Felzani G, Marini C. Stroke in the very old: a systematic review of studies on incidence, outcome, and resource use. J Aging Res. 2011;2011:108785.
9. Navis A, Garcia-Santibanez R, Skliut M. Epidemiology and outcomes of ischemic stroke and transient ischemic attack in the adult and geriatric population. J Stroke Cerebrovasc Dis. 2019;28(1):84–9.
10. Birnbaum LA, Rodriguez JS, Topel CH, Behrouz R, Misra V, Palacio S, et al. Older stroke patients with high stroke scores have delayed door-to-needle times. J Stroke Cerebrovasc Dis. 2016;25(11):2668–72.
11. Easton JD, Saver JL, Albers GW, Alberts MJ, Chaturvedi S, Feldmann E, et al. Definition and evaluation of transient ischemic attack: a scientific statement for healthcare professionals from the American Heart Association/American Stroke Association Stroke Council; Council on Cardiovascular Surgery and Anesthesia; Council on Cardiovascular Radiology and Intervention; Council on Cardiovascular Nursing; and the Interdisciplinary Council on Peripheral Vascular Disease. The American Academy of Neurology affirms the value of this statement as an educational tool for neurologists. Stroke. 2009;40(6):2276–93.

12. Shahjouei S, Sadighi A, Chaudhary D, Li J, Abedi V, Holland N, et al. A 5-decade analysis of incidence trends of ischemic stroke after transient ischemic attack: a systematic review and meta-analysis. JAMA Neurol. 2021;78(1):77–87.
13. Radu RA, Terecoasă EO, Băjenaru OA, Tiu C. Etiologic classification of ischemic stroke: where do we stand? Clin Neurol Neurosurg. 2017;159:93–106.
14. Bogousslavsky J, Van Melle G, Regli F. The Lausanne stroke registry: analysis of 1,000 consecutive patients with first stroke. Stroke. 1988;19(9):1083–92.
15. Ferro JM. Cardioembolic stroke: an update. Lancet Neurol. 2003;2(3):177–88.
16. Bamford J, Sandercock P, Dennis M, Burn J, Warlow C. Classification and natural history of clinically identifiable subtypes of cerebral infarction. Lancet. 1991;337(8756):1521–6.
17. Di Carlo A, Lamassa M, Pracucci G, Basile AM, Trefoloni G, Vanni P, et al. Stroke in the very old : clinical presentation and determinants of 3-month functional outcome: a European perspective. European BIOMED Study of Stroke Care Group. Stroke. 1999;30(11):2313–9.
18. Jones WJ, Williams LS, Bruno A, Biller J. Hypertension and cerebrovascular disease. Semin Cerebrovasc Dis Stroke. 2003;3(3):144–54.
19. Pantoni L. Cerebral small vessel disease: from pathogenesis and clinical characteristics to therapeutic challenges. Lancet Neurol. 2010;9(7):689–701.
20. Allen CL, Bayraktutan U. Oxidative stress and its role in the pathogenesis of ischaemic stroke. Int J Stroke. 2009;4(6):461–70.
21. Love S, Miners S, Palmer J, Chalmers K, Kehoe P. Insights into the pathogenesis and pathogenicity of cerebral amyloid angiopathy. Front Biosci (Landmark Ed). 2009;14:4778–92.
22. Ntaios G, Hart RG. Embolic stroke. Circulation. 2017;136(25):2403–5.
23. Dufouil C, Beiser A, McLure LA, Wolf PA, Tzourio C, Howard VJ, et al. Revised Framingham stroke risk profile to reflect temporal trends. Circulation. 2017;135(12):1145–59.
24. Avan A, Digaleh H, Di Napoli M, Stranges S, Behrouz R, Shojaeianbabaei G, et al. Socioeconomic status and stroke incidence, prevalence, mortality, and worldwide burden: an ecological analysis from the Global Burden of Disease Study 2017. BMC Med. 2019;17(1):191.
25. Soares-Miranda L, Siscovick DS, Psaty BM, Longstreth WT, Mozaffarian D. Physical activity and risk of coronary heart disease and stroke in older adults: the cardiovascular health study. Circulation. 2016;133(2):147–55.
26. Singer J, Gustafson D, Cummings C, Egelko A, Mlabasati J, Conigliaro A, et al. Independent ischemic stroke risk factors in older Americans: a systematic review. Aging (Albany NY). 2019;11(10):3392–407.
27. Ferrucci L, Guralnik JM, Pahor M, Harris T, Corti MC, Hyman BT, et al. Apolipoprotein E epsilon 2 allele and risk of stroke in the older population. Stroke. 1997;28(12):2410–6.
28. Arbelaez JJ, Ariyo AA, Crum RM, Fried LP, Ford DE. Depressive symptoms, inflammation, and ischemic stroke in older adults: a prospective analysis in the cardiovascular health study. J Am Geriatr Soc. 2007;55(11):1825–30.
29. Elkins JS, O'Meara ES, Longstreth WT, Carlson MC, Manolio TA, Johnston SC. Stroke risk factors and loss of high cognitive function. Neurology. 2004;63(5):793–9.
30. Marshall IJ, Wang Y, Crichton S, McKevitt C, Rudd AG, Wolfe CD. The effects of socioeconomic status on stroke risk and outcomes. Lancet Neurol. 2015;14(12):1206–18.
31. Muangpaisan W, Hinkle JL, Westwood M, Kennedy J, Buchan AM. Stroke in the very old: clinical presentations and outcomes. Age Ageing. 2008;37(4):473–5.
32. Edlow JA, Selim MH. Atypical presentations of acute cerebrovascular syndromes. Lancet Neurol. 2011;10(6):550–60.
33. Huff JS. Stroke mimics and chameleons. Emerg Med Clin North Am. 2002;20(3):583–95.
34. Anathhanam S, Hassan A. Mimics and chameleons in stroke. Clin Med (Lond). 2017;17(2):156–60.
35. Nor AM, Davis J, Sen B, Shipsey D, Louw SJ, Dyker AG, et al. The recognition of stroke in the emergency room (ROSIER) scale: development and validation of a stroke recognition instrument. Lancet Neurol. 2005;4(11):727–34.
36. Saver JL. Time is brain—quantified. Stroke. 2006;37(1):263–6.

37. Evans NR, Wall J, To B, Wallis SJ, Romero-Ortuno R, Warburton EA. Clinical frailty independently predicts early mortality after ischaemic stroke. Age Ageing. 2020;49(4):588–91.
38. Smithard DG. Stroke in frail older people. Geriatrics (Basel). 2017;2(3)
39. Wallis SJ, Wall J, Biram RW, Romero-Ortuno R. Association of the clinical frailty scale with hospital outcomes. QJM. 2015;108(12):943–9.
40. Fried LP, Tangen CM, Walston J, Newman AB, Hirsch C, Gottdiener J, et al. Frailty in older adults: evidence for a phenotype. J Gerontol A Biol Sci Med Sci. 2001;56(3):M146–56.
41. Mahoney FI, Barthel DW. Functional evaluation: the Barthel index. Md State Med J. 1965;14:61–5.
42. Quinn TJ, Elliott E, Langhorne P. Cognitive and mood assessment tools for use in stroke. Stroke. 2018;49(2):483–90.
43. McGovern A, Pendlebury ST, Mishra NK, Fan Y, Quinn TJ. Test accuracy of informant-based cognitive screening tests for diagnosis of dementia and multidomain cognitive impairment in stroke. Stroke. 2016;47(2):329–35.
44. Burton L, Tyson SF. Screening for cognitive impairment after stroke: a systematic review of psychometric properties and clinical utility. J Rehabil Med. 2015;47(3):193–203.
45. Langhorne P, Ramachandra S. Organised inpatient (stroke unit) care for stroke: network meta-analysis. Cochrane Database Syst Rev. 2020;4(4):Cd000197.
46. Wardlaw JM, Murray V, Berge E, del Zoppo GJ. Thrombolysis for acute ischaemic stroke. Cochrane Database Syst Rev. 2014;2014(7):Cd000213.
47. Emberson J, Lees KR, Lyden P, Blackwell L, Albers G, Bluhmki E, et al. Effect of treatment delay, age, and stroke severity on the effects of intravenous thrombolysis with alteplase for acute ischaemic stroke: a meta-analysis of individual patient data from randomised trials. Lancet. 2014;384(9958):1929–35.
48. Wardlaw JM, Murray V, Berge E, del Zoppo G, Sandercock P, Lindley RL, et al. Recombinant tissue plasminogen activator for acute ischaemic stroke: an updated systematic review and meta-analysis. Lancet. 2012;379(9834):2364–72.
49. Sandercock P, Wardlaw JM, Lindley RI, Dennis M, Cohen G, Murray G, et al. The benefits and harms of intravenous thrombolysis with recombinant tissue plasminogen activator within 6 h of acute ischaemic stroke (the third international stroke trial [IST-3]): a randomised controlled trial. Lancet. 2012;379(9834):2352–63.
50. Kongbunkiat K, Wilson D, Kasemsap N, Tiamkao S, Jichi F, Palumbo V, et al. Leukoaraiosis, intracerebral hemorrhage, and functional outcome after acute stroke thrombolysis. Neurology. 2017;88(7):638–45.
51. Bhatnagar P, Sinha D, Parker RA, Guyler P, O'Brien A. Intravenous thrombolysis in acute ischaemic stroke: a systematic review and meta-analysis to aid decision making in patients over 80 years of age. J Neurol Neurosurg Psychiatry. 2011;82(7):712–7.
52. Thomalla G, Boutitie F, Ma H, Koga M, Ringleb P, Schwamm LH, et al. Intravenous alteplase for stroke with unknown time of onset guided by advanced imaging: systematic review and meta-analysis of individual patient data. Lancet. 2020;396(10,262):1574–84.
53. Goyal M, Menon BK, van Zwam WH, Dippel DW, Mitchell PJ, Demchuk AM, et al. Endovascular thrombectomy after large-vessel ischaemic stroke: a meta-analysis of individual patient data from five randomised trials. Lancet. 2016;387(10,029):1723–31.
54. Zhao W, Ma P, Zhang P, Yue X. Mechanical thrombectomy for acute ischemic stroke in octogenarians: a systematic review and meta-analysis. Front Neurol. 2019;10:1355.
55. Hilditch CA, Nicholson P, Murad MH, Rabinstein A, Schaafsma J, Pikula A, et al. Endovascular management of acute stroke in the elderly: a systematic review and meta-analysis. AJNR Am J Neuroradiol. 2018;39(5):887–91.
56. Arora R, Salamon E, Katz JM, Cox M, Saver JL, Bhatt DL, et al. Use and outcomes of intravenous thrombolysis for acute ischemic stroke in patients ≥90 years of age. Stroke. 2016;47(9):2347–54.
57. Parry-Jones AR, Paley L, Bray BD, Hoffman AM, James M, Cloud GC, et al. Care-limiting decisions in acute stroke and association with survival: analyses of UK national quality register data. Int J Stroke. 2016;11(3):321–31.

58. Morgenstern LB, Zahuranec DB, Sánchez BN, Becker KJ, Geraghty M, Hughes R, et al. Full medical support for intracerebral hemorrhage. Neurology. 2015;84(17):1739–44.
59. Rodriguez-Luna D, Piñeiro S, Rubiera M, Ribo M, Coscojuela P, Pagola J, et al. Impact of blood pressure changes and course on hematoma growth in acute intracerebral hemorrhage. Eur J Neurol. 2013;20(9):1277–83.
60. Anderson CS, Heeley E, Huang Y, Wang J, Stapf C, Delcourt C, et al. Rapid blood-pressure lowering in patients with acute intracerebral hemorrhage. N Engl J Med. 2013;368(25):2355–65.
61. Lattanzi S, Cagnetti C, Provinciali L, Silvestrini M. How should we lower blood pressure after cerebral hemorrhage? A systematic review and meta-analysis. Cerebrovasc Dis. 2017;43(5–6):207–13.
62. Al-Shahi Salman R, Frantzias J, Lee RJ, Lyden PD, Battey TWK, Ayres AM, et al. Absolute risk and predictors of the growth of acute spontaneous intracerebral haemorrhage: a systematic review and meta-analysis of individual patient data. Lancet Neurol. 2018;17(10):885–94.
63. Seiffge DJ, Goeldlin MB, Tatlisumak T, Lyrer P, Fischer U, Engelter ST, et al. Meta-analysis of haematoma volume, haematoma expansion and mortality in intracerebral haemorrhage associated with oral anticoagulant use. J Neurol. 2019;266(12):3126–35.
64. Tsivgoulis G, Wilson D, Katsanos AH, Sargento-Freitas J, Marques-Matos C, Azevedo E, et al. Neuroimaging and clinical outcomes of oral anticoagulant-associated intracerebral hemorrhage. Ann Neurol. 2018;84(5):694–704.
65. Christensen H, Cordonnier C, Kõrv J, Lal A, Ovesen C, Purrucker JC, et al. European stroke organisation guideline on reversal of oral anticoagulants in acute intracerebral haemorrhage. Eur Stroke J. 2019;4(4):294–306.
66. Mendelow AD, Gregson BA, Fernandes HM, Murray GD, Teasdale GM, Hope DT, et al. Early surgery versus initial conservative treatment in patients with spontaneous supratentorial intracerebral haematomas in the International Surgical Trial in Intracerebral Haemorrhage (STICH): a randomised trial. Lancet. 2005;365(9457):387–97.
67. Hanley DF, Thompson RE, Rosenblum M, Yenokyan G, Lane K, McBee N, et al. Efficacy and safety of minimally invasive surgery with thrombolysis in intracerebral haemorrhage evacuation (MISTIE III): a randomised, controlled, open-label, blinded endpoint phase 3 trial. Lancet. 2019;393(10175):1021–32.
68. Sondag L, Schreuder F, Boogaarts HD, Rovers MM, Vandertop WP, Dammers R, et al. Neurosurgical intervention for supratentorial intracerebral Hemorrhage. Ann Neurol. 2020;88(2):239–50.
69. Fonseca AC, Merwick Á, Dennis M, Ferrari J, Ferro JM, Kelly P, et al. European Stroke Organisation (ESO) guidelines on management of transient ischaemic attack. Eur Stroke J. 2021;6(2):V
70. Prabhakaran S, Silver AJ, Warrior L, McClenathan B, Lee VH. Misdiagnosis of transient ischemic attacks in the emergency room. Cerebrovasc Dis. 2008;26(6):630–5.
71. Rothwell PM, Giles MF, Chandratheva A, Marquardt L, Geraghty O, Redgrave JN, et al. Effect of urgent treatment of transient ischaemic attack and minor stroke on early recurrent stroke (EXPRESS study): a prospective population-based sequential comparison. Lancet. 2007;370(9596):1432–42.
72. Kaplan RC, Tirschwell DL, Longstreth WT Jr, Manolio TA, Heckbert SR, Lefkowitz D, et al. Vascular events, mortality, and preventive therapy following ischemic stroke in the elderly. Neurology. 2005;65(6):835–42.
73. Rothwell PM, Algra A, Amarenco P. Medical treatment in acute and long-term secondary prevention after transient ischaemic attack and ischaemic stroke. Lancet. 2011;377(9778):1681–92.
74. Rothwell PM, Algra A, Chen Z, Diener HC, Norrving B, Mehta Z. Effects of aspirin on risk and severity of early recurrent stroke after transient ischaemic attack and ischaemic stroke: time-course analysis of randomised trials. Lancet. 2016;388(10,042):365–75.
75. CAPRIE Steering Committee. A randomised, blinded, trial of clopidogrel versus aspirin in patients at risk of ischaemic events (CAPRIE). Lancet. 1996;348(9038):1329–39.

76. Bhatia K, Jain V, Aggarwal D, Vaduganathan M, Arora S, Hussain Z, et al. Dual antiplatelet therapy versus aspirin in patients with stroke or transient ischemic attack: meta-analysis of randomized controlled trials. Stroke. 2021;52(6):e217–e23.
77. Zhang H, Thijs L, Staessen JA. Blood pressure lowering for primary and secondary prevention of stroke. Hypertension. 2006;48(2):187–95.
78. Appleton JP, Sprigg N, Bath PM. Blood pressure management in acute stroke. Stroke Vasc Neurol. 2016;1(2):72–82.
79. National Institute for Health and Care Excellence (NICE). Stroke and transient ischaemic attack in over 16s: diagnosis and initial management. NICE guideline [NG128]; 2019.
80. Turnbull F, Neal B, Ninomiya T, Algert C, Arima H, Barzi F, et al. Effects of different regimens to lower blood pressure on major cardiovascular events in older and younger adults: meta-analysis of randomised trials. BMJ. 2008;336(7653):1121–3.
81. Beckett NS, Peters R, Fletcher AE, Staessen JA, Liu L, Dumitrascu D, et al. Treatment of hypertension in patients 80 years of age or older. N Engl J Med. 2008;358(18):1887–98.
82. Aronow WS. Managing hyperlipidaemia in the elderly: special considerations for a population at high risk. Drugs Aging. 2006;23(3):181–9.
83. Amarenco P, Kim JS, Labreuche J, Charles H, Abtan J, Béjot Y, et al. A comparison of two LDL cholesterol targets after ischemic stroke. N Engl J Med. 2020;382(1):9.
84. Amarenco P, Labreuche J, Lavallée P, Touboul PJ. Statins in stroke prevention and carotid atherosclerosis: systematic review and up-to-date meta-analysis. Stroke. 2004;35(12):2902–9.
85. Deedwania P, Stone PH, Bairey Merz CN, Cosin-Aguilar J, Koylan N, Luo D, et al. Effects of intensive versus moderate lipid-lowering therapy on myocardial ischemia in older patients with coronary heart disease: results of the Study Assessing Goals in the Elderly (SAGE). Circulation. 2007;115(6):700–7.
86. Shepherd J, Blauw GJ, Murphy MB, Bollen EL, Buckley BM, Cobbe SM, et al. Pravastatin in elderly individuals at risk of vascular disease (PROSPER): a randomised controlled trial. Lancet. 2002;360(9346):1623–30.
87. Tun NN, Arunagirinathan G, Munshi SK, Pappachan JM. Diabetes mellitus and stroke: a clinical update. (1948–9358 (Print)).
88. Shou J, Zhou L, Zhu S, Zhang X. Diabetes is an independent risk factor for stroke recurrence in stroke patients: a meta-analysis. J Stroke Cerebrovasc Dis. 2015;24(9):1961–8.
89. Turnbull FM, Abraira C, Anderson RJ, Byington RP, Chalmers JP, Duckworth WC, et al. Intensive glucose control and macrovascular outcomes in type 2 diabetes. Diabetologia. 2009;52(11):2288–98.
90. National Institute for Health and Care Excellence (NICE). Type 2 diabetes in adults: management. NICE guideline [NG28]; 2015.
91. Friberg L, Rosenqvist M, Lindgren A, Terént A, Norrving B, Asplund K. High prevalence of atrial fibrillation among patients with ischemic stroke. Stroke. 2014;45(9):2599–605.
92. National Institute for Health and Care Excellence (NICE). Atrial fibrillation: diagnosis and management. NICE guidelines [NG196]; 2021.
93. Mant J, Hobbs FD, Fletcher K, Roalfe A, Fitzmaurice D, Lip GY, et al. Warfarin versus aspirin for stroke prevention in an elderly community population with atrial fibrillation (the Birmingham Atrial Fibrillation Treatment of the Aged Study, BAFTA): a randomised controlled trial. Lancet. 2007;370(9586):493–503.
94. Björck F, Renlund H, Lip GY, Wester P, Svensson PJ, Själander A. Outcomes in a warfarin-treated population with atrial fibrillation. JAMA Cardiol. 2016;1(2):172–80.
95. Ruff CT, Giugliano RP, Braunwald E, Hoffman EB, Deenadayalu N, Ezekowitz MD, et al. Comparison of the efficacy and safety of new oral anticoagulants with warfarin in patients with atrial fibrillation: a meta-analysis of randomised trials. Lancet. 2014;383(9921):955–62.
96. Pugh D, Pugh J, Mead GE. Attitudes of physicians regarding anticoagulation for atrial fibrillation: a systematic review. Age Ageing. 2011;40(6):675–83.
97. Petty GW, Brown RD Jr, Whisnant JP, Sicks JD, O'Fallon WM, Wiebers DO. Ischemic stroke subtypes: a population-based study of incidence and risk factors. Stroke. 1999;30(12):2513–6.

98. MRC European Carotid Surgery Trial: interim results for symptomatic patients with severe (70-99%) or with mild (0-29%) carotid stenosis. European Carotid Surgery Trialists' Collaborative Group. Lancet. 1991;337(8752):1235–43.
99. Barnett HJM, Taylor DW, Haynes RB, Sackett DL, Peerless SJ, Ferguson GG, et al. Beneficial effect of carotid endarterectomy in symptomatic patients with high-grade carotid stenosis. N Engl J Med. 1991;325(7):445–53.
100. Rothwell PM, Eliasziw M, Gutnikov SA, Fox AJ, Taylor DW, Mayberg MR, et al. Analysis of pooled data from the randomised controlled trials of endarterectomy for symptomatic carotid stenosis. Lancet. 2003;361(9352):107–16.
101. Naylor AR, Sillesen H, Schroeder TV. Clinical and imaging features associated with an increased risk of early and late stroke in patients with symptomatic carotid disease. Eur J Vasc Endovasc Surg. 2015;49(5):513–23.
102. Bonati LH, Lyrer P, Ederle J, Featherstone R, Brown MM. Percutaneous transluminal balloon angioplasty and stenting for carotid artery stenosis. Cochrane Database Syst Rev. 2012;(9):Cd000515.
103. Bonati LH, Kakkos S, Berkefeld J, de Borst GJ, Bulbulia R, Halliday A, et al. European Stroke Organisation guideline on endarterectomy and stenting for carotid artery stenosis. Eur Stroke J. 2021;6(2):I.
104. Langhorne P, Stott DJ, Robertson L, MacDonald J, Jones L, McAlpine C, et al. Medical complications after stroke: a multicenter study. Stroke. 2000;31(6):1223–9.
105. Cruz-Flores S, Berge E, Whittle IR. Surgical decompression for cerebral oedema in acute ischaemic stroke. Cochrane Database Syst Rev. 2012;1:Cd003435.
106. Zelano J, Holtkamp M, Agarwal N, Lattanzi S, Trinka E, Brigo F. How to diagnose and treat post-stroke seizures and epilepsy. Epileptic Disord. 2020;22(3):252–63.
107. Dennis M, Sandercock P, Reid J, Graham C, Forbes J, Murray G. Effectiveness of intermittent pneumatic compression in reduction of risk of deep vein thrombosis in patients who have had a stroke (CLOTS 3): a multicentre randomised controlled trial. Lancet. 2013;382(9891):516–24.
108. Wu S, Kutlubaev MA, Chun HY, Cowey E, Pollock A, Macleod MR, et al. Interventions for post-stroke fatigue. Cochrane Database Syst Rev. 2015;2015(7):Cd007030.
109. Pendlebury ST, Rothwell PM. Incidence and prevalence of dementia associated with transient ischaemic attack and stroke: analysis of the population-based Oxford Vascular Study. Lancet Neurol. 2019;18(3):248–58.

Optimizing Pharmacotherapy in Older Patients with Depression or Anxiety

25

Sylvie Bonin-Guillaume

25.1 Depression

Depression occurs up to 11% in the ageing population [1] with numerous atypical presentations; only 12% of depressed older persons meet the DSM major depressive criteria [2]. This prevalence reaches 40% in long-term care and nursing homes [3].

Thus, depression in older patient is often underdiagnosed and undertreated, although it is associated with a poor prognosis (suicide [4], relapse, chronicity [5]). Depression is also independently associated with frailty [6], malnutrition [7], functional decline [8] and morbidity.

25.1.1 Pharmacological Treatment of Depression

Antidepressants are the first-line treatment for depression in older adults.

25.1.1.1 Antidepressants Efficacy

In a large meta-analysis that included 51 randomized control trials comprising of old patients with depressive disorders, all classes of antidepressant (tricyclic agents (TCAs), selective serotonin reuptake inhibitors (SSRIs) and other antidepressants) were more effective than placebo in achieving response and remission. No differences were found in remission or response rates between classes of antidepressants. The numbers needed to treat (NNT) were 14.4 (95% CI 8.3–50) for one additional remission to antidepressants compared with placebo and 6.7 (95% CI 4.8–10) for response [9], which is similar to the rates observed in younger adults [10].

S. Bonin-Guillaume (✉)
Internal Medicine and Geriatric Department, Aix Marseille University, University Hospital of Marseille, Hôpital de Sainte Marguerite, Marseille, France
e-mail: sylvie.bonin@ap-hm.fr; sylvie.bonin-guillaume@univ-amu.fr

A. Cherubini et al. (eds.), *Optimizing Pharmacotherapy in Older Patients*,
Practical Issues in Geriatrics, https://doi.org/10.1007/978-3-031-28061-0_25

Lower treatment response in elderly might be due to a vascular component in late-onset depression, executive dysfunctions and longer current depressive episode [11, 12].

Tricyclics are also very effective treatments, but they should be reserved for specific types of depression (e.g. depression with pain) or for depression that is resistant to other therapeutic classes. Indeed, their anticholinergic effects (aggravation of cognitive disorders, risk of falling, confusion) are the cause of significant adverse effects in elderly subjects, especially when there are associated cognitive disorders [13].

More recently, vortioxetine has been studied in people over 65 years of age, and the results showed its efficacy versus placebo at a dose of 5 mg/d. Preliminary data suggest that vortioxetine has promising effects in improving cognition in older adults with depressive symptoms (processing speed, as well as learning and memory [14, 15]. A recent review showed that vortioxetine had no difference in response or remission comparing with SSRIs or the serotonin noradrenaline reuptake inhibitors (SNRIs) [16]. Although well tolerated, caution should be exercised when treating patients 65 years of age and older with dosages greater than 10 mg of vortioxetine once daily.

Anyhow, old patients with depression are poorly represented in randomized control trials, and those with significant medical comorbidities are commonly excluded [17]. Moreover, antidepressant response involved defined small sample sizes populations (i.e. mostly major depressive disorders according to the DSMV [18]) and is short lasting (about 8 weeks). Then, the results reported are difficult to generalize to the real world of clinically depressed elderly patients. At last, there is a lack of efficacy studies examining relapse prevention.

25.1.1.2 Antidepressant Management

Thus, to determine the best pharmacological treatment options for individual patients, careful considerations are required (see Table 25.1): (1) ascertain depression and the type of mood disorders by trained health professionals; (2) assessing concurrent medical problem and drug therapy; and (3) looking for previous response to treatment if history of depression is known.

According to current recommendations, SSRIs are the first-line choice treatment for old patients because they are effective for treating depression with fewer side effects than other classes (see Table 25.2) [13, 19, 20].

One or two doses escalation steps are required to achieve the final daily dose and avoid side effect. The final daily dose is for most cases the same as for younger [10, 22].

In a dimensional approach and according to their action on brain monoaminergic systems, antidepressants might be selected for their expected behavioural effects. For example, psychomotor retardation and loss of energy may be linked to a reduced dopaminergic activity. Anhedonia, lack of motivation and arousal and loss of concentration are linked to noradrenergic activity, while irritability, pessimism, sadness or dysphoria are mediated by serotoninergic system [21, 23].

Table 25.1 Recommendations for a better antidepressant treatment efficiency (from [13, 19–21])

1. Discuss the choice of antidepressant with the patient
   - First choice: SSRI (selective serotonin reuptake inhibitors)
   - Efficiency and tolerability of any antidepressants previously taken
2. Inform the patient about the following:
   - Gradual development of the full antidepressant effect
   - Importance of taking medication as prescribed and the need to continue beyond remission
   - Potential side effects and drug interactions
3. Monitor AD response regularly and side effects carefully
   - Do not prescribe sub-therapeutic doses of antidepressants
   - Evaluate improvement or remission (a delayed response up to 12 weeks is usual in older patients)
   - Monitor carefully for side effects
4. Check treatment duration and adherence
   - >6 months after complete remission for the first episode (optimally 1 year after complete remission), longer if past history of depression episode
   - A step-by-step withdrawal (at least 1 month, optimally 3 months)
5. Avoid psychotropic drugs co-prescription unless:
   - Congruent psychosis symptoms present (antipsychotic should be proposed)
   - Severe anxiety (benzodiazepines might be associated with 12 weeks maximum)

Table 25.2 Antidepressant drugs [22, 23]

Drug class	Contraindication	Common side effects	Comments
Selective serotoninergic reuptake inhibitors	Association with other serotoninergic drugs (i.e. tramadol)	Nausea Hyponatremia, parkinsonism, tremor, insomnia, serotonin syndrome Changes in QT interval	First choice Monitor drug-drugs interactions
Selective serotonin noradrenaline (norepinephrine) reuptake inhibitor (SNRI)	Association with other serotoninergic drugs	Hypotension Nausea, vomiting, Anticholinergic effects for some drugs	Second choice Monitor drugs-drugs interaction
Selective inhibitors of monoamine oxidase A	Hypertension, Other IMO and antidepressants	Hypertension or hypotension, tremor, dry mouth	Only occasionally Need specific diet Monitor hepatic enzymes
Conventional tricyclic agents	Glaucoma, Enlarged prostate Heart failure Association to monoamine oxidase inhibitors	Anticholinergic effects Urinary retention Visual disturbance tachycardia, Constipation, Dry mouth delusion+++ Sedative effects, etc.	Not a first choice Monitor carefully side effects avoid when cognitive impairments
Other antidepressants Mianserine, mirtazapine, tianeptine, Agomelatine	According to the drug	Different types of side effects according to the drug	Not a first choice Use with caution in old patients

The final step in the choice of antidepressant is to provide a sedative or anxiolytic action of the antidepressant. This often avoids co-prescription of anxiolytics or sedatives, the systematic use of which is no longer recommended.

Particular attention must be paid to the monitoring of adverse effects at the beginning of treatment, which are always likely to discourage a patient if they are not managed, and clear information must be given to the patient and his or her family on the usefulness of the prescription, the time required to respond to the treatment and the expected results, taking into account comorbidities and associated treatments (possible drug-drug interactions) [19]. Yet, although SSRIs appear to be safer, they also cause many adverse effects. For example, with SSRIs, there is an increased risk of gastrointestinal bleeding, especially in combination with anticoagulants and risk of developing serotonin syndrome if combining with certain opioid analgesics (e.g. tramadol). These potential adverse effects necessitate controls of ECG and lab tests including blood count, electrolytes, serum creatinine and transaminases on a regular basis [22]. Finally, many drug interactions must be taken into account because of the action of SRIs on cytochrome P450.

25.1.1.3 Duration of Treatment

Complete remission should be the goal of antidepressant treatment and should continue. The risk of recurrence or relapse is mainly due to the premature antidepressant discontinuation [24]. The current consensus is to propose a 1-year treatment for a first episode, a 2-year treatment for a second episode and a 3-year treatment or more from the third episode [10]. If the episode was particularly severe or if minimal depressive symptoms persist, it is advisable to continue antidepressant treatment for a longer period [21]. Treatment discontinuation should be prepared with a gradual decrease steps over several weeks to avoid withdrawal effects.

25.1.1.4 Antidepressant Adherence

Poor adherence to antidepressant is common in old depressed patients. In a cohort study with more than 90,000 veteran antidepressant users, 50% of the prevalent users discontinued their treatment within 6 months and 61% within 12 months [25]. In a recent population-based study conducted on 27,865 older patients, 26.9% of the incident antidepressant users were fully adherent as recommended by guidelines (i.e. duration of treatment and daily doses) [26].

Moreover, compared with non-depressed persons, depressed medical patients are three times more likely to be non-adherents with other medication regimes or medical care [27].

Factors of poor adherence to treatment are misperceptions about mental illness and its treatment, the stigma associated with depression, the lack of family support, cognitive impairment, adverse events and drug side effects, cost of treatments and poor physician-patient communication or relationship. The choice of drug is an important factor influencing compliance. Patients and family education must be given priority, and a caring enthusiastic attitude from the caring team promotes compliance [10, 13].

25.1.1.5 Antidepressant Resistance

Treatment resistance is defined as failure to respond to two different evidence-based antidepressant treatments of adequate duration and dosage. Only 50% of elderly patients respond (generally defined as a 50% decrease in scores on depression scales) to first-line treatment and less than 40% reach remission (the patient experiences few, if any, symptoms of depression as measured on a depression scale) [10].

If depressive symptoms persist after the second treatment approach, patients should be referred to a specialist (geriatric psychiatrist), and change of antidepressant or adding a second substance should be considered with a possible improvement up to 50% [22].

25.1.1.6 Antidepressant, Depression and Neurocognitive Disorders

Efficiency of antidepressants for depression in cognitively impaired adults is controversial. Antidepressants are frequently prescribed in subjects with dementia: from 39% in the general population with dementia [28] to 69% in patients followed in memory consultations [29]. Yet the use of antidepressants in cognitive impaired patients is more often related to the control of psychobehavioural symptoms of dementia than to the treatment of identified depressive disorders.

A clinical trial comparing with three groups (two antidepressants and a placebo groups) including 326 patients with an Alzheimer's disease and a depression status according to the Cornell's scale [30] showed no superiority of antidepressants over placebo after 39 weeks of treatment [31]. This has been confirmed by a recent Cochrane review showing limited efficiency of antidepressants, regardless of the class evaluated, in old subjects with documented dementia and depression [32]. Moreover antidepressants did not affect the ability to manage daily activities and probably had little or no effect on a test of cognitive function.

Main limitations of these trials are the short duration of the trials (6–12 weeks), different depression scales used and small samples included.

Neurocognitive disorders and depression often coexist, from 30 to 50% [33]. One of the difficulties in treating depression in people with dementia is the lack of reliable diagnostic criteria for depression in this population [12, 34]. Usually, the diagnosis is based on depression scales. In addition, the depressive symptomatology changes with the progression of the disease. Finally, apathetic behaviour makes differential diagnosis complex, as it can be present in both depression and Alzheimer's disease [35]. Antidepressants are not indicated for apathy [36] especially since some, in particular SSRIs, can induce apathy [37].

Thus, the existence of documented depression in a person with Alzheimer's disease justifies antidepressant treatment. However, close monitoring and reassessment are essential to limit ineffective prolonged treatments that may aggravate psychobehavioural disorders of the dementia.

25.1.1.7 Mood Stabilizer

Lithium is the gold-standard treatment for old age bipolar disorders and the most studied in geriatric samples, although there are few older adults being often excluded from clinical trials. However, it has shown to be effective both in treating manic symptoms and in reducing depressive symptoms.

Although there can be adverse effects with lithium, it is generally well tolerated in older adults. Regular monitoring of renal function and lithium levels (0.4–0.8 mmol/L) as well as drug-drug interactions (as diuretics, angiotensin-converting enzyme (ACE) inhibitors, angiotensin receptor blockers (ARBs) and non-steroidal anti-inflammatory drugs (NSAIDs) is necessary to prevent side effects [38]. Some studies have described a positive effect of continuous lithium treatment in reducing the risk of neurocognitive disorders in older adults [39].

25.1.2 Non-pharmacological Treatment of Depression

25.1.2.1 Psychological Approach

Psychotherapy is recommended for patients with mild to moderate severity of depression [10, 20]. Evidence shows that cognitive behavioural therapy (CBT) is the most widely available structured psychotherapy for depression. A large randomized control trial provided robust evidence that CBT given as an adjunct to usual care that includes antidepressant medication is effective in reducing depressive symptoms and improving quality of life. The treatment response was maintained at the 12-month follow-up after the CBT treatment had ended [40].

However, access to this treatment is scarce in old depressed patients, and there is a lack of trained therapists skilled enough to interact with vulnerable, multimorbid and/or dependent populations.

25.1.2.2 Electroconvulsive Therapy

Electroconvulsive therapy (ECT) is considered to be the most effective treatment in severe or treatment-resistant depression in older populations (up to 75% of remission). For patients who cannot tolerate or respond poorly to medications and who are at a high risk for drug-induced toxicity or toxic drug interactions, ECT is the safest treatment option [41].

The principal adverse effects associated with ECT are confusion and memory loss. Memory impairment is usually transient and undetectable 6 months later. ECT decreases the risk of relapse when associated with antidepressant.

Clinical predictors of a good response to ECT are age, depression with melancholic features, psychotic depression, a high severity of suicide behaviour and speed of response. On the other side, the longer the duration of the depressive episode, the lower the response to ECT [42].

The strong negative attitude towards ECT that still prevails among both professionals and old patients and caregivers remains the highest limitation to its use [43].

25.1.2.3 Repetitive Transcranial Magnetic Stimulation

During the past 20 years, therapeutic effects of repetitive transcranial magnetic stimulation (rTMS) have been studied in psychiatric diseases, particularly in the treatment of depressive disorders with data suggesting its efficiency in the treatment of depression in older patients. The r-TMS is a non-invasive method of brain stimulation for the treatment of patients with no need of analgesia or induction seizure.

Literature data globally confirm that rTMS is safe and does not produce cognitive deficits, even among highly vulnerable patients. Poorer responsiveness to rTMS may be related to several patient factors, including older age and smaller frontal grey matter volumes [44].

A review comparing ECT and r-TMS concluded that ECT was superior to high-frequency rTMS in terms of response (64.4% vs. 48.7%, RR = 1.41, $p = 0.03$) and remission (52.9% vs. 33.6%, RR = 1.38, $p = 0.006$), particularly for psychotic depression [45]. However, ECI is less tolerated, whereas unilateral right prefrontal -rTMS is better, and bilateral-rTMS appears to have the most favourable balance between efficacy and acceptability [46].

25.2 Anxiety

The prevalence of anxiety disorders (generalized anxiety disorders, phobic disorders, panic attacks, and obsessive compulsive disorders) decreases with ageing and is estimated to be 13.5%. However, anxiety is frequently associated with other psychiatric disorders (coexisting with 30% of depressive disorders) or chronic conditions (heart failure, Parkinson's disease, stroke, diabetes, hyperthyroidism), or drugs side effect (corticoids, calcium channel blockers) and cognitive impairment [47].

25.2.1 Pharmacological Treatment of Anxiety

Benzodiazepines are the first-line treatment for anxiety attacks episodes but are overused in older populations. Recent studies showed that 60% of older persons on benzodiazepines are chronic users (over 5 consecutive months) [28], especially those living in nursing homes [48] or having neurocognitive disorders [29]. Guidelines recommend that benzodiazepines should not be prescribed for more than 12 weeks for acute anxiety that impacts on daily life, and no more than 4 weeks for sleep disorders [49]. Principles of benzodiazepines prescription are summarized in Table 25.3.

Table 25.3 Optimizing benzodiazepines prescription in anxiety disorders (from [21, 50])

1.	Check the indication (anxiety/insomnia)
2.	Inform patients of the treatment effect and treatment duration
3.	Inform patient of the drug side effects
4.	Prescribe for a maximum of 12 weeks for anxiety including the withdrawal
5.	Ensure patient understanding and compliance to the treatment
6.	Start with a low dose and keep the lowest dose
7.	Choose a short-lasting effect product
8.	In case of a long users, propose a step-by-step withdrawal in a specific consultation

It is well known that benzodiazepine has numerous side effects, injurious falls, fractures, drowsiness, delirium and agitation [50]. Recently, several pharmacological studies demonstrated an association between BZD users and the risk of developing neurocognitive disorders, particularly for chronic users (over 6 months) and for long-acting BZD users [51]. This risk decreases, but several months after, benzodiazepines withdrawal [52].

To avoid benzodiazepine prescription, some non-benzodiazepine drugs may be used to treat anxiety. They are considered to have fewer side effects because of different pharmacological action. However, no clinical trials have been conducted in old populations. Buspirone and etifoxine are not commonly used in this population. Hydroxyzine is more often prescribed for agitation and/or anxiety in older patients. However, because of a high anticholinergic score and the risk of a QT lengthening [53], the use of this drug is no more recommended for patients aged 75 years and over.

Benzodiazepine reduction in older patients is effective even in general practice with low risk of withdrawal symptoms [54]. This should be attempted in chronic users during a dedicated consultation with a progressive reduction regimen [49].

25.2.2 Non-pharmacological Treatment of Anxiety

Non-pharmacological treatment should be the first line for anxiety disorders management.

However, there are very few studies showing psychological approach efficiency in anxiety disorders in older adults. Most studies have tested cognitive behavioural therapies showing that CBT has more helpful than having no treatment for GAD in later life. Nevertheless, whether CBT shows long-term durability, or is superior to other commonly available treatments (such as supportive psychotherapy), remains to be tested [55]. Psychological interventions cognitive behavioural therapy and mindfulness showed better benefit in the presence of co-occurring anxiety and mood disorders in older adults, but with moderate effect sizes and few information about follow-up [56].

References

1. Castro Costa E, Dewey M, Stewart R, Barnerjee S, Huppert F, Mendoca-Lima C, et al. Prevalence of depressive symptoms and syndromes in later life in ten European countries. Br J Psychiatry. 2007;191:393–401. https://doi.org/10.1192/bjp.bp.107.036772.
2. Judd LL, Akiskal HS. The clinical and public health relevance of current research on subthreshold depressive symptoms to elderly patients. Am J Geriatr Psychiatry. 2002;10:233–8.
3. Blazer DG. Epidemiology of depression: prevalence and incidence. In: Copeland JRM, Abou-Saleh MT, Blazer DG, editors. Principles and practice of geriatric psychiatry. 2nd ed. London: John Wiley & Sons Ltd; 2002. p. 389–92.
4. Jalenques I, Gallarda T, Vaille-Perret E. Suicide. In: Clément JP, editor. Psychiatrie de la Personne âgée. Paris: Edition Flammarion; 2010. p. 262–75.
5. Beekman AT, Geerlings SW, Deeg DJ, Smit JH, Schoevers RS, de Beurs E, et al. The natural history of late-life depression : a 6-year prospective study in the community. Arch Gen Psychiatry. 2002;59:605–11. https://doi.org/10.1001/archpsyc.59.7.60.

6. Vaughan L, Corbin AL, Goveas JS. Depression and frailty in later life: a systematic review. Clin Interv Aging. 2015;10:1947–58. https://doi.org/10.2147/CIA.S69632.
7. Cabrera MA, Mesas AE, Garcia AR, de Andrade SM. Malnutrition and depression among community-dwelling elderly people. J Am Med Dir Assoc. 2007;8:582–4. https://doi.org/10.1016/j.jamda.2007.07.008.
8. Da Silva SA, Scazufca M, Menezes PR. Population impact of depression on functional disability inelderly: results from "São Paulo Ageing & Health Study" (SPAH). Eur Arch Psychiatry Clin Neurosci. 2013;263:153–8. https://doi.org/10.1007/s00406-012-0345-4.
9. Kok RM, Nolen WA, Heeren TJ. Efficacy of treatment in older depressed patients: a systematic review and meta-analysis of double-blind randomized controlled trials with antidepressants. J Affect Disord. 2012;141:103–15. https://doi.org/10.1016/j.jad.2012.02.036.
10. Kok RB, Reynolds CF III. Management of depression in older adults: a review. JAMA. 2017;317:2114–22. https://doi.org/10.1001/jama.2017.5706.
11. Calati R, Salvina Signorelli M, Balestri M, Marsano A, De Ronchi D, Aguglia E, Serretti A. Antidepressants in elderly: metaregression of double-blind, randomized clinical trials. J Affect Disord. 2013;147:1–8.
12. Pimontel MA, Rindskopf D, Rutherford BR, Brown PJ, Roose SP, Sneed JR. A meta-analysis of executive dysfunction and antidepressant treatment response in late-life depression. Am J Geriatr Psychiatry. 2016;24:31–41.
13. Alamo C, Lopez-Munoz F, Garcia-Garcia P, Garcia-Ramoz S. Risk–benefit analysis of antidepressant drug treatment in the elderly. Psychogeriatrics. 2014;14:261–8. https://doi.org/10.1111/psyg.12057.
14. Katona C, Hansen T, Olsen CK. A randomized, doubleblind, placebo-controlled, duloxetine-referenced, fixed-dose study comparing the efficacy and safety of Lu AA21004 in elderly patients with major depressive disorder. Int Clin Psychopharmacol. 2012;27:215–23.
15. Bishop MM, Fixen DR, Linnebur SA, Pearson SM. Cognitive effects of vortioxetine in older adults: a systematic review. Ther Adv Psychopharmacol. 2021;11:20451253211026796. https://doi.org/10.1177/20451253211026796. eCollection 2021.
16. Zhang X, Cai Y, Hu X, Lu CY, Nie X, Shi L. Systematic review and meta-analysis of vortioxetine for the treatment of major depressive disorder in adults. Front Psychiatry. 2022;13:922648. https://doi.org/10.3389/fpsyt.2022.922648. eCollection 2022.
17. Benraad CE, Kamerman-Celie F, van Munster BC, Oude Voshaar RC, Spijker J, Olde Rikkert MG. Geriatric characteristics in randomised controlled trials on antidepressant drugs for older adults: a systematic review. Int J Geriatr Psychiatry. 2016;31:990–1003. https://doi.org/10.1002/gps.4443.
18. American Psychiatric Association. Diagnostic and statistical manual of mental disorders. 5th ed. Washington DC: American Psychiatric Association; 2013. https://doi.org/10.1016/j.jagp.2015.05.010.
19. National Institute for health & Care Excellence. Depression in adults: recognition and management. October 2009, updated April 2016. www.nice.org.uk
20. Haute Autorité de Santé. Recommandations pour la pratique clinique. Episode dépressif caractérisé de l'adulte : prise en charge en soins de premier recours (guidelines for the management of depressive episode in primary care). October 2017. 45p. www.has.fr. Accessed 02 Nov 2021.
21. Bonin-Guillaume S, Roche J, Vandel P. Psychotropes. In: Clément JP, Calvet B, editors. Psychiatrie de la personne âgée. 2nd ed. Paris: Lavoisier; 2019. p. 423–42.
22. Pruckner N, Holthoff-Detto V. Antidepressant pharmacotherapy in old-age depression—a review and clinical approach. Eur J Clin Pharmacol. 2017;73:661–7. https://doi.org/10.1007/s00228-017-2219-1.
23. Bonin-Guillaume S, Benoit M. Depression. In: Roller-Wirnsberger R, Singler K, Polidori MC, editors. Learning geriatric medecine. A study guide for medical students. Practical issues in geriatrics. Cham: Springer Nature; 2018. p. 145–50.
24. Kivela SL, Viramo P, Pakhala K. Factors predicting the relapse of depression in old age. Int J Geriatr Psychiatry. 2000;15:112–9. https://doi.org/10.1002/(sici)1099-1166(200002)15:2<112::aid-gps83>3.0.co;2-b.

25. Lu CY, Rougheaud E. New users of antidepressant medications: first episode duration and predictors of discontinuation. Eur J Clin Pharmacol. 2012;68:65–71. https://doi.org/10.1007/s00228-011-1087-3.
26. Braunstein D, Hardy A, Boucherie Q, Frauger E, Blin O, Gentile G, Micallef J. Antidepressant adherence patterns in older patients: use of a clustering method on a prescription database. Fundam Clin Pharmacol. 2017;31:226–36.
27. Bautista LE, Vera-Cala LM, Colombo C, Smith P. Symptoms of depression and anxiety and adherence to antihypertensive medication. Am J Hypertens. 2012;25:505–11. https://doi.org/10.1038//ajh.2011.256.
28. Breining A, Bonnet-Zamponi D, Zerah L, Micheneau C, Riolacci-Dhoyen N, Chan-Chee C, et al. Exposure to psychotropics in the French older population living with dementia: a nationwide population-based study. Int J Geriatr Psychiatry. 2017;32:750–60.
29. Jacquin-Piques A, Sacco G, Tavassoli N, Rouaud O, Bejot Y, Giroud M, et al. Psychotropic drug prescription in patients with dementia: nursing home residents versus patients living at home. J Alzheimers Dis. 2016;49:671–80. https://doi.org/10.3233/JAD-150280.
30. Alexopoulos GS, Abrams RC, Young RC, Shamoian CA. Cornell scale for depression in dementia. Biol Psychiatry. 1988;23:271–81.
31. Banerjee S, Hellier J, Dewey M, Romeo R, Ballard C, Baldwin R, et al. Sertraline or mirtazapine for depression in dementia (HTA-SADD): a randomised, multicentre, double-blind, placebo-controlled trial. Lancet. 2011;378:403–11. https://doi.org/10.1016/S0140-6736(11)60830-1.
32. Dudas R, Malouf R, McCleery J, Dening T. Antidepressants for treating depression in dementia. Cochrane Database Syst Rev. 2018;(8):CD003944. https://doi.org/10.1002/14651858.CD003944.pub2.
33. Lee HB, Lyketsos CG. Depression in Alzheimer disease: heterogeneity and related issues. Biol Psychiatry. 2003;54:353–62. https://doi.org/10.1016/s0006-3223(03)00543-2.
34. Starkstein SE, Jorge R, Mizrahi R, Robinson RG. The construct of minor and major depression in Alzheimer's disease. Am J Psychiatry. 2005;162:2086–93. https://doi.org/10.1176/appi.ajp.162.11.2086.
35. Benoit M, Berrut G, Doussaint J, Bakchine S, Bonin-Guillaume S, Fremont P, et al. Apathy and depression in mild Alzheimer's disease: a cross-sectional study using diagnostic criteria. J Alzheimers Dis. 2012;31:325–34.
36. Haute Autorité de Santé. Recommandation de bonnes pratiques. Maladie D'Alzheimer et Maladies Apparentées : diagnostic et prise en charge de l'apathie. (Guidelines for Alzheimer's disease and related disorders: diagnosis and management of apathy) July 2014; 46p. www.has.fr. Accessed 2 Nov 2021.
37. Sansone RA, Sansone LA. SSRI-induced indifference. Psychiatry. 2010;7:14–8.
38. Fotso Soh J, Klil-Drori S, Rej S. Using lithium in older age bipolar disorder: special considerations. Drugs Aging. 2019;36:147–54. https://doi.org/10.1007/s40266-018-0628-1.
39. Gerhard T, Devanand DP, Huang C, Stephen CS, Olfson M. Lithium treatment and risk for dementia in adults with bipolar disorder: population-based cohort study. Br J Psychiatry. 2015;207:46–51. https://doi.org/10.1192/bjp.bp.114.154047.
40. Wiles N, Thomas L, Abel A, Ridgway N, Turner N, Campbell J, et al. Cognitive behavioural therapy as an adjunct to pharmacotherapy for primary care based patients with treatment resistant depression: results of the CoBalT randomised controlled trial. Lancet. 2013;381:375–84. https://doi.org/10.1016/S0140-6736(12)61552-9.
41. Kerner N, Prudic J. Current electroconvulsive therapy practice and research in the geriatric population. Neuropsychiatry. 2014;4:33–54. https://doi.org/10.2217/npy.14.3.
42. Pinna M, Manchia M, Oppo R, Scano F, Pillai G, Loche AP, et al. Clinical and biological predictors of response to electroconvulsive therapy (ECT): a review. Neurosci Lett. 2018;669:32–42.
43. Stek ML, van der Wurff FB, Uitdehaag BMJ, Beekman ATF, Hoogendijk WJG. ECT in the treatment of depressed elderly: lessons from a terminated clinical trial. Int J Geriatr Psychiatry. 2007;22:1052–4. https://doi.org/10.1002/gps.1800.
44. Jalenques I, Legrand G, Vaille-Perret E, Tourtauchaux R, Galland F. Therapeutic efficacy and safety of repetitive transcranial magnetic stimulation in depression of the elderly: a review. Encéphale. 2010;36(Suppl 2):D105–18. https://doi.org/10.1016/j.encep.2009.10.007.

45. Ren J, Li H, Palaniyappan L, Liu H, Wang J, Li C, et al. Repetitive transcranial magnetic stimulation versus electroconvulsive therapy for major depression: a systematic review and meta-analysis. Prog Neuro-Psychopharmacol Biol Psychiatry. 2014;51:181–9. https://doi.org/10.1016/j.pnpbp.2014.02.004.
46. Chen J-J, Zhao L-B, Liu Y-Y, Fan S-H, Xie P. Comparative efficacy and acceptability of electroconvulsive therapy versus repetitive transcranial magnetic stimulation for major depression: a systematic review and multiple-treatments meta-analysis. Behav Brain Res. 2017;320:30–6. https://doi.org/10.1016/j.bbr.2016.11.028. Epub 2016 Nov 19.
47. Wolitzky-Taylor KB, Castriotta N, Lenze EJ, Stanley MA, Craske MG. Anxiety disorders in older adults: a comprehensive review. Depress Anxiety. 2010;27:190–211. https://doi.org/10.1002/da.20653.
48. Bourgeois J, Elseviers MM, Azermai M, Van Bortel L, Petrovic M, Vander Stichele RR. Barriers to discontinuation of chronic benzodiazepine use in nursing home residents: perceptions of general practitioners and nurses. Eur Ger Med. 2014;5:181–7.
49. Haute Autorité de Santé. Modalités d'arrêt des benzodiazépines et des molécules apparentées chez le sujet âgé. Modalités d'arrêt des benzodiazépines et médicaments apparentés chez le patient âgé (How to discontinue chronically use of Benzodiazepines in older patient). 2007, 143 p (www.has-sante.fr) Accessed 02 Nov 2021.
50. Agence Nationale de Sécurité des Médicaments et des produits de santé. Etat des lieux de la consommation des Benzodiazépines en France, Décembre 2013, 82p. www. ansm.sante.fr. Accessed 02 Nov 2021.
51. Billioti de Gage S, Moride Y, Ducruet T, Kurth T, Verdoux H, Tournier M, et al. Benzodiazepine use and risk of Alzheimer's disease: case-control study. BMJ. 2014 Sep;9:349. https://doi.org/10.1136/bmj.g5205.
52. Wu CS, Ting TT, Wang SC, Chang IS, Lin KM. Effect of benzodiazepine discontinuation on dementia risk. Am J Geriatr Psychiatry. 2011;19:151–9. https://doi.org/10.1097/JGP.0b013e3181e049ca.
53. Beuscart JB, Dupont C, Defebvre MM, Puisieux F. Potentially inappropriate medications (PIMs) and anticholinergic levels in the elderly: a population based study in a French region. Arch Gerontol Geriatr. 2014;59:630–5. https://doi.org/10.1016/j.archger.2014.08.006.
54. Jørgensen VR. Benzodiazepine reduction in general practice. Are the elderly neglected? Affect Disord. 2012;136:1216–21. https://doi.org/10.1016/j.jad.2011.10.016.
55. Hall J, Kellet S, Berrios R, Bains MK, Scott S. Efficacy of cognitive behavioral therapy for generalized anxiety disorder in older adults: systematic review, meta-analysis, and meta-regression. Am J Geriatr Psychiatry. 2016;24:1063–73. https://doi.org/10.1016/j.jagp.2016.06.006.
56. Wurthrich VM, Meuldijk D, Jagielle T, Gonzalez Robles A, Jones MP, Cuijpers P. Efficacy and effectiveness of psychological interventions on co-occurring mood and anxiety disorders in older adults: a systematic review and meta-analysis. Int J Geriatr Psychiatry. 2021;36:858–72. https://doi.org/10.1002/gps.5486.

26 Nutritional Deficiency and Malnutrition

Eva Kiesswetter and Cornel C. Sieber

26.1 Introduction

A balanced nutrition providing sufficient energy and nutrients is considered an important factor contributing to health and well-being throughout life. However, with older age, several physiological, disease-related, functional, mental, and social changes occur making older people more prone to nutritional deficiencies and malnutrition (Box 26.1).

Box 26.1 Definitions of nutritional deficiency and malnutrition

Nutritional deficiencies occur due to an imbalance between energy or nutrient needs and actual intake (needs > intake). This can be due to increased needs, reduced absorption, and/or reduced intake.

Malnutrition is defined as "a state of energy, protein or nutrient deficiency which produces a measurable change in body function, and is associated with a worse outcome from illness as well as being specifically reversible by nutritional support" [1]. This chapter mainly refers to energy-protein malnutrition.

E. Kiesswetter (✉)
Institute for Biomedicine of Aging, Friedrich-Alexander-Universität Erlangen Nürnberg, Nürnberg, Germany
e-mail: eva.kiesswetter@fau.de

C. C. Sieber
Institute for Biomedicine of Aging, Friedrich-Alexander-Universität Erlangen Nürnberg, Nürnberg, Germany

Department of Medicine, Kantonsspital Winterthur, Winterthur, Switzerland
e-mail: cornel.sieber@fau.de

A. Cherubini et al. (eds.), *Optimizing Pharmacotherapy in Older Patients*, Practical Issues in Geriatrics, https://doi.org/10.1007/978-3-031-28061-0_26

In particular, in older people in need of care, with insufficient social support, or with acute medical conditions obtaining an adequate diet is challenging, and insufficient intakes of energy and nutrients are frequently reported [2, 3]. Energy needs are usually reduced in older adults due to changes in body composition and reduced physical activity levels, while nutrient requirements do not decline accordingly making a more nutrient-dense diet necessary [4]. Studies in older adults demonstrate that nutrients such as protein, fiber, vitamin D, B1, B2, B12, folate, calcium, magnesium, and selenium become deficient more readily due to low intakes or suboptimal levels in the body [5–7]. Compared to community-dwelling older adults, older hospitalized patients and nursing home residents experience low intakes of energy and nutrients more frequently [3, 8]. This likely can be attributed to impaired health and function in these populations but also situational or structural aspects related to the settings.

In a recently published meta-analysis of 240 studies which included 113,967 older adults, the prevalence of malnutrition according to the Mini Nutritional Assessment (MNA) was 3% in community-dwelling older adults, 6% in older outpatients, 9% in older adults receiving home care, 18% in nursing home residents, 22% in geriatric inpatients, and 29% in geriatric rehabilitation inpatients [9]. Furthermore, in all settings, high proportions of older persons were identified as being at nutritional risk (27%–55%) [9]. Based on these data, it can be summarized that malnutrition prevalence increases in groups with deteriorated health and functional status. However, based on sampling strategies and diagnostic criteria, differences in prevalence need to be considered.

If nutritional deficiencies and malnutrition are left untreated, numerous negative clinical consequences are more likely, including increased rates of infections and pressure ulcers, longer hospital stays, increased in-hospital complications, increased duration of convalescence after acute illness, and increased all-cause mortality [10–12]. In addition, malnutrition is linked to the common geriatric syndromes of frailty and sarcopenia [13, 14], mainly due to the malnutrition-associated loss of muscle mass and is a risk factor for functional impairment [15, 16] and reduced quality of life [17]. Consequently, malnutrition poses a major burden for the individual and healthcare systems [11].

26.2 Causes of Malnutrition in Older People

At younger ages, the origin of nutritional deficiency and malnutrition is mainly disease-related, while in older people, the causes are commonly multifactorial (Fig. 26.1). Potential causes are:

- Age-related physiological changes (e.g., chemosensory decline, changes in the regulation of hunger and satiety (anorexia of aging))
- Disease-related factors (e.g., dysphagia, multimorbidity, adverse effects of medication, polypharmacy)
- Psychological factors (e.g., depression, impaired cognition, anxiety)

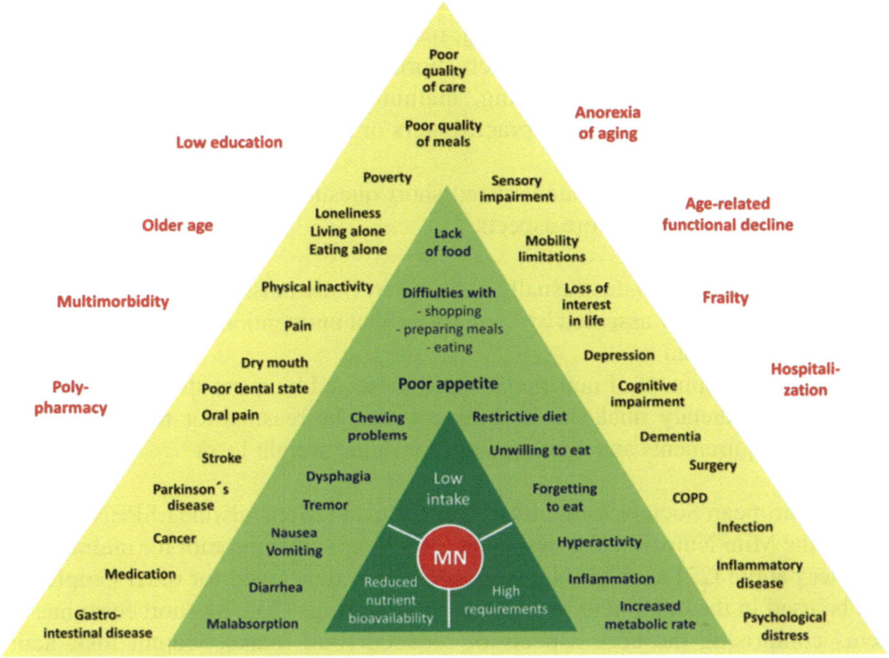

Fig. 26.1 The DoMAP schematic model illustrating the various factors contributing to malnutrition in older people. Level 1 in dark green represents the core etiological mechanisms that lead to malnutrition. Level 2 in light green consists of the factors that lead directly to one or more of the core etiological mechanisms that cause malnutrition. Level 3 in yellow lists the various common conditions that indirectly contribute to malnutrition [18]

- Functional aspects (e.g., oral function, loss of dentition, mobility limitations, eating dependency)
- Socioeconomic factors (e.g., poverty, missing social support)
- Lifestyle factors

Even though there is broad consensus by experts on the multiple causes of malnutrition in older adults, evidence for many of these determinants is low or conflicting [19, 20]. This is mainly due to a different operationalization of determinants and malnutrition among studies, inappropriate confounder control, and lack of longitudinal or randomized trials.

26.3 Screening of Malnutrition

Screening is regarded as a first step in identifying persons at risk of malnutrition or with overt malnutrition. It is recommended to routinely screen older people for their malnutrition risk independent of diagnoses and the presence of overweight and obesity using a validated screening tool [21]. In institutional care settings, screening should be conducted at admission and afterward at regular intervals. In the long-term care setting, intervals of 3 months are recommended, while in the acute care setting, much shorter intervals between screenings are necessary. In the outpatient setting, malnutrition screening in older persons should be conducted by general practitioners or ambulatory nursing staff at least once a year.

For screening purposes, standardized short questionnaires are commonly used focusing on the following core aspects:

- Current nutritional status (usually assessed by body mass index)
- Prehistory (usually assessed by enquiring about unintentional weight loss within the past 3 months)
- Further development of nutritional status (assessed by acute stress/diseases and/or reduced dietary intake as both aspects can be reasons for not meeting the energy requirements and consequently for future weight loss)

The European Society for Clinical Nutrition and Metabolism (ESPEN) recommends the Mini Nutritional Assessment (MNA) as screening tool for malnutrition in older people [22] as the MNA was specifically developed for older people and can be used in the outpatient and institutional settings [23]. Its short form has six items comprising the core aspects of reduced food intake, weight loss, acute stress, and BMI. In addition, there are questions on mobility limitations and neuropsychological problems—two important risk factors for malnutrition in older people. A further feature is the option to exchange the BMI item with calf circumference if BMI assessment is not possible, e.g., due to immobility. According to a sum score ranging from 0 to 14 points, patients are categorized as well-nourished (12–14 points), at risk of malnutrition (8–11 points), or malnourished (<7 points) [24].

A screening alternative in the hospital setting is the Nutritional Risk Screening tool (NRS) [25], specifically developed for the acute care setting and which can be used also in younger patients. The NRS is designed to identify patients who might benefit from nutrition interventions. It is composed of a prescreening with four questions on the core aspects low BMI, recent weight loss, reduced dietary intake, and severe disease. In case of a positive prescreening, the above core elements are quantified during the main screening. The age of patients ($\geq$70 years) is considered as a further risk factor. Three or more points on the NRS indicate nutritional risk.

There are several other screening tools available that are less often used in clinical practice. In a systematic review on the validity of malnutrition screening instruments in older people, 34 different tools that have been used in older people were identified, of which 23 were specifically developed for this age group [26]. The usage of a specific tool often depends on the health policies and guidelines of the respective countries.

26.4 Assessment of Nutritional Status

Following a positive screening result, the nutritional status of an older person needs to be further assessed to form the basis for targeted interventions aiming to improve nutritional status, the overall clinical course of the presenting illness, and the quality of life [21].

26.4.1 Diagnosis of Malnutrition

Both, in research and clinical practice, different criteria and cutoff values are used for the diagnosis of malnutrition. To align the diagnosis of malnutrition, a coalition of several international medical nutrition societies mostly from Europe, the USA, and Asia—the so-called Global Leadership Initiative on Malnutrition (GLIM)—compiled consensus-based criteria for malnutrition [27]. The concept proposes that after a positive screening, the phenotypic criteria "unintentional weight loss," "low BMI," and "low muscle mass" as well as the etiologic criteria "reduced food intake or assimilation" and "inflammation" should be assessed (Table 26.1). If at least one phenotypic and one etiological criterion apply, malnutrition can be assumed. The severity of malnutrition can be further evaluated based on the expression of the phenotypic criteria [27].

In clinical trials, muscle mass or lean body mass and fat-free mass as its proxies are usually assessed by bioelectrical impedance analysis (BIA) or dual-energy

Table 26.1 Phenotypic and etiological criteria to diagnose malnutrition (based on Global Leadership Initiative [27])

Phenotypic criteria	
Weight loss	>5% within past 6 months or >10% beyond 6 months
Low body mass index	<20 kg/m^2, if <70 years or <22 kg/m^2, if ≥70 years
Reduced muscle mass	Depends on the measuring technique, e.g., BIA: FFMI <17 (m), <15 (f) kg/m^2, BIA, DXA: ASMI <7 (m), <6 (f) kg/m^2
Etiologic criteria	
Reduced food intake or assimilation	≤50% of energy needs >1 week or any reduction for >2 weeks or any chronic gastrointestinal condition adversely affecting food assimilation or absorption, e.g., short bowel syndrome or chronic diarrhea
Inflammation	Acute disease/injury, e.g., infections, burns, trauma Chronic diseases, e.g., cancer, chronic obstructive pulmonary disease

BIA Bio-electrical impedance analysis, *DXA* Dual-energy X-ray absorptiometry, *FFMI* Fat free mass index, *ASMI* Appendicular skeletal muscle mass index, *m* male, *f* female

X-ray absorptiometry (DXA). As these methods are often not available in routine clinical practice or are too expensive, calf circumference is often used as an indicator of muscle mass (cutoff <31 cm for both sexes).

26.4.2 Quantification of Energy and Nutrient Deficiency

By quantifying the nutritional deficits, the necessity for and the amount of nutritional interventions can be determined. The fundamental metrics for the determination are the individual's energy and protein intake and the corresponding requirements.

As in routine clinical practice, measurement of energy requirements is usually not possible, formulae to estimate resting energy expenditure, e.g., by Mueller [28] or Harris-and Benedict [29], are used. For this purpose, details of age, sex, and body weight are needed. In combination with the physical activity level (PAL), total energy expenditure can be calculated. A PAL between 1.2 and 1.3 represents a low energy expenditure in frail, immobile, or bedridden older people. For older people, a guiding value for energy intake of 30 kcal/kg body weight (BW)/day is proposed, which needs to be adjusted according to nutritional status, physical activity level, disease status, and tolerance [21].

Protein requirements of older people are currently the subject of the much scientific debate, and reference values differ by country. While the European Food Safety Authority recommends an intake of 0.8 g/kg BW/day for young and older adults [30], expert groups suggest a higher optimal protein intake in older people to prevent decline in muscle mass (1–1.2 g/kg BW/day) [31]. Higher amounts might be needed to compensate for increased metabolic demands due to inflammation, sepsis, or wounds.

Intake can be assessed by dietary records of at least 3 days, where all consumed foods and their quantities are described in detail. An approximate measure of the amount eaten is plate diagrams where the intake is estimated by quarters of the offered amount [nothing, ¼, ½, ¾, all].

26.4.3 Identification of Potential Causes of Malnutrition

The elimination of causes of malnutrition is an important element of nutritional therapy. Therefore, potential causes should be systematically clarified within the assessment, e.g., during interviews with older people and, if necessary, supported by interviewing relatives or care persons of the older person. Summary lists of possible causes can give guidance. An example is the so-called DoMap, a theoretical model on determinants of malnutrition in aged persons, which was developed by experts in the field of geriatric nutrition based on a Delphi validation process [18]. The DoMap displays beside the central etiologic mechanisms of malnutrition, factors directly or indirectly affecting these mechanisms (Fig. 26.1).

26.5 Nutritional Therapy

Based on the nutritional assessment, realistic and individualized goals for nutritional therapy need to be established, considering potential risks, contraindications, benefits as well as resources, needs, and preferences of the older patient. Nutritional interventions generally incorporate the following options:

- Nutritional counseling by a dietitian (provision individualized recommendations to optimize dietary intake)
- Food modification, e.g., by texture modification, energy-dense meals, energy and nutrient (e.g., protein) fortification, additional snacks, or finger food
- Oral nutritional supplements (usually provided if oral intake is insufficient; availability of different products, e.g., low volume or protein-rich)
- Tube feeding (used if oral nutrition is impossible or insufficient for >3 days, having a good overall prognosis for recovery to a degree that allows resumption of sufficient nutritional intake)
- Parenteral feeding (used if oral and enteral nutrition are impossible/insufficient for >3 days, having an overall good prognosis for recovery to a degree that allows resumption of sufficient nutritional intake)

For tube feeding (and parenteral nutrition), end-of-life situations or severe dementia are considered contraindications [21].

Nutritional care goes far beyond simple nutritional interventions, also covering nursing support (e.g., mealtime assistance (verbal prompting or eating support), provision of adequate tools like ergonomic cutlery), the adaption of environmental factors (e.g., avoiding disturbances during mealtimes, pleasant meal ambience), and the treatment of underlying causes [21].

In clinical practice, combinations of different intervention strategies are often needed. Consequently, multidisciplinary contributions of dietitians, nursing and kitchen staff, medical doctors, and therapists (speech, occupational, physio) are vitally important factors for successful nutrition interventions [21]. Detailed evidence-based recommendations for clinical nutrition and hydration in geriatrics can be found in the ESPEN guidelines [21].

26.6 Conclusions

Nutritional deficiency and malnutrition are common in older people in all care settings and are commonly multifactorial. Early detection by a routine screening, a thorough comprehensive nutritional assessment, and an individualized and multidisciplinary therapy regimen can improve nutritional status, related clinical outcomes, and overall prognosis in older people with malnutrition.

References

1. Allison SP. Malnutrition, disease, and outcome. Nutrition. 2000;16(7–8):590–3.
2. Sharkey JR, Branch LG, Zohoori N, Giuliani C, Busby-Whitehead J, Haines PS. Inadequate nutrient intakes among homebound elderly and their correlation with individual characteristics and health-related factors. Am J Clin Nutr. 2002;76(6):1435–45.
3. Rosenberger C, Rechsteiner M, Dietsche R, Breidert M. Energy and protein intake in 330 geriatric orthopaedic patients: are the current nutrition guidelines applicable? Clin Nutr ESPEN. 2019;29:86–91.
4. de Groot CP, van Staveren WA. Nutritional concerns, health and survival in old age. Biogerontology. 2010;11(5):597–602.
5. Hengeveld LM, Boer JMA, Gaudreau P, Heymans MW, Jagger C, Mendonça N, et al. Prevalence of protein intake below recommended in community-dwelling older adults: a meta-analysis across cohorts from the PROMISS consortium. J Cachexia Sarcopenia Muscle. 2020;11(5):1212–22.
6. Kehoe L, Walton J, Flynn A. Nutritional challenges for older adults in Europe: current status and future directions. Proc Nutr Soc. 2019;78(2):221–33.
7. ter Borg S, Verlaan S, Hemsworth J, Mijnarends DM, Schols JM, Luiking YC, et al. Micronutrient intakes and potential inadequacies of community-dwelling older adults: a systematic review. Br J Nutr. 2015;113(8):1195–206.
8. Tieland M, Borgonjen-Van den Berg KJ, Van Loon LJ, de Groot LC. Dietary protein intake in Dutch elderly people: a focus on protein sources. Nutrients. 2015;7(12):9697–706.
9. Cereda E, Pedrolli C, Klersy C, Bonardi C, Quarleri L, Cappello S, et al. Nutritional status in older persons according to healthcare setting: a systematic review and meta-analysis of prevalence data using MNA(R). Clin Nutr. 2016;35(6):1282–90.
10. Marshall S, Bauer J, Isenring E. The consequences of malnutrition following discharge from rehabilitation to the community: a systematic review of current evidence in older adults. J Hum Nutr Diet. 2014;27(2):133–41.
11. Correia MI, Waitzberg DL. The impact of malnutrition on morbidity, mortality, length of hospital stay and costs evaluated through a multivariate model analysis. Clin Nutr. 2003;22(3):235–9.
12. Norman K, Pichard C, Lochs H, Pirlich M. Prognostic impact of disease-related malnutrition. Clin Nutr. 2008;27(1):5–15.
13. Lorenzo-López L, Maseda A, de Labra C, Regueiro-Folgueira L, Rodríguez-Villamil JL, Millán-Calenti JC. Nutritional determinants of frailty in older adults: a systematic review. BMC Geriatr. 2017;17(1):108.
14. Ligthart-Melis GC, Luiking YC, Kakourou A, Cederholm T, Maier AB, de van der Schueren MAE. Frailty, sarcopenia, and malnutrition frequently (co-)occur in hospitalized older adults: a systematic review and meta-analysis. J Am Med Dir Assoc. 2020;21(9):1216–28.
15. Hai S, Gao Q, Gwee X, Chua DQL, Yap KB, Ng TP. Malnutrition risk, physical function decline and disability in middle-aged and older adults followed up in the Singapore longitudinal ageing study. Clin Interv Aging. 2021;16:1527–39.
16. Buurman BM, Hoogerduijn JG, de Haan RJ, Abu-Hanna A, Lagaay AM, Verhaar HJ, et al. Geriatric conditions in acutely hospitalized older patients: prevalence and one-year survival and functional decline. PLoS One. 2011;6(11):e26951.
17. Rasheed S, Woods RT. Malnutrition and quality of life in older people: a systematic review and meta-analysis. Ageing Res Rev. 2013;12(2):561–6.
18. Volkert D, Kiesswetter E, Cederholm T, Donini LM, Eglseer D, Norman K, et al. Development of a model on determinants of malnutrition in aged persons: a MaNuEL project. Gerontol Geriatr Med. 2019;5:2333721419858438.
19. van der Pols-Vijlbrief R, Wijnhoven HA, Schaap LA, Terwee CB, Visser M. Determinants of protein-energy malnutrition in community-dwelling older adults: a systematic review of observational studies. Ageing Res Rev. 2014;18:112–31.

20. O'Keeffe M, Kelly M, O'Herlihy E, O'Toole PW, Kearney PM, Timmons S, et al. Potentially modifiable determinants of malnutrition in older adults: a systematic review. Clin Nutr. 2019;38(6):2477–98.
21. Volkert D, Beck AM, Cederholm T, Cruz-Jentoft A, Goisser S, Hooper L, et al. ESPEN guideline on clinical nutrition and hydration in geriatrics. Clin Nutr. 2019;38(1):10–47.
22. Kondrup J, Allison SP, Elia M, Vellas B, Plauth M. ESPEN guidelines for nutrition screening 2002. Clin Nutr. 2003;22(4):415–21.
23. Guigoz Y, Vellas B, Garry PJ. Mini Nutritional Assessment: A practical assessment tool for grading nutritional state of elderly patients. Facts Res Gerontol. 1994;(Supplement 2):15–59.
24. Kaiser MJ, Bauer JM, Ramsch C, Uter W, Guigoz Y, Cederholm T, et al. Validation of the mini nutritional assessment short-form (MNA-SF): a practical tool for identification of nutritional status. J Nutr Health Aging. 2009;13(9):782–8.
25. Kondrup J, Rasmussen HH, Hamberg O, Stanga Z. Nutritional risk screening (NRS 2002): a new method based on an analysis of controlled clinical trials. Clin Nutr. 2003;22(3):321–36.
26. Power L, Mullally D, Gibney ER, Clarke M, Visser M, Volkert D, et al. A review of the validity of malnutrition screening tools used in older adults in community and healthcare settings—a MaNuEL study. Clin Nutr ESPEN. 2018;24:1–13.
27. Cederholm T, Jensen GL, Correia M, Gonzalez MC, Fukushima R, Higashiguchi T, et al. GLIM criteria for the diagnosis of malnutrition—a consensus report from the global clinical nutrition community. Clin Nutr. 2019;38:1–9.
28. Müller MJ, Bosy-Westphal A, Klaus S, Kreymann G, Lührmann PM, Neuhäuser-Berthold M, et al. World Health Organization equations have shortcomings for predicting resting energy expenditure in persons from a modern, affluent population: generation of a new reference standard from a retrospective analysis of a German database of resting energy expenditure. Am J Clin Nutr. 2004;80(5):1379–90.
29. Harris JA, Benedict FG. A biometric study of human basal metabolism. Proc Natl Acad Sci U S A. 1918;4(12):370–3.
30. European Food Safety Authority EPoDP, Nutrition and Allergies (NDA). Scientific opinion on dietary reference values for protein. EFSA J. 2012;10:1–66.
31. Bauer J, Biolo G, Cederholm T, Cesari M, Cruz-Jentoft AJ, Morley JE, et al. Evidence-based recommendations for optimal dietary protein intake in older people: a position paper from the PROT-AGE Study Group. J Am Med Dir Assoc. 2013;14(8):542–59.

Pharmacotherapy of Insomnia in Older Adults

27

Mirko Petrovic

27.1 Insomnia as the Most Common Sleep Disorder

Separately from age-related changes, sleep problems affect 10–15% of the general population and increase with older age as well [1, 2]. Sleep disturbances include insomnia, as the most common sleep disorder and therefore the most researched one, dyssomnia (restless legs, periodic limb movement, sleep apnoea, narcolepsy) and parasomnia (REM sleep behaviour disorder, night terrors, sleepwalking). Insomnia is often identified as the subjective complaint of problems with initiating or maintaining sleep, or non-restorative sleep, causing significant daytime symptoms such as concentration problems and mood disturbances. The overall prevalence of insomnia symptoms ranges from 30% to 48% among older adults [3–6], while the prevalence of insomnia disorder ranges from 12% to 20% [7]. Insomnia is usually categorised by the predominant symptom of either difficulty in sleep onset or sleep maintenance. Sleep maintenance symptoms are most prevalent among adults complaining of insomnia (50–70%), followed by difficulty in initiating sleep (35–60%) and non-restorative sleep (20–25%). An incidence rate for insomnia symptoms of 5% per year, with a yearly incidence of 8% at 1-year follow-up, has been observed among older adults [8, 9].

27.2 Treatment

Treatment options for insomnia can be categorised into non-pharmacological, foremost cognitive behavioural therapy, and pharmacological options [3, 10–12]. There is large evidence to support the effectiveness and sustainability of non-pharmacologic

M. Petrovic (✉)
Section of Geriatrics, Department of Internal Medicine and Paediatrics, Ghent University, Ghent, Belgium
e-mail: mirko.petrovic@ugent.be

A. Cherubini et al. (eds.), *Optimizing Pharmacotherapy in Older Patients*, Practical Issues in Geriatrics, https://doi.org/10.1007/978-3-031-28061-0_27

interventions for insomnia in adults of all ages. For the purpose of this chapter, however, only the pharmacological options have been discussed here in detail.

27.3 Pharmacological Treatment

Pharmacological treatments are principally categorised as benzodiazepines (BZDs) and non-benzodiazepine receptor agonists (so-called Z-drugs), as the most commonly used drug classes and alternatives including antidepressants, melatonin receptor agonists and orexin receptor antagonists. Recently published clinical practice guidelines of the American Academy of Sleep Medicine for the pharmacological treatment of chronic insomnia represent an evidence-based review of each class of drug commonly used in the treatment of insomnia [13].

27.4 Benzodiazepines and Non-benzodiazepine Receptor Agonists

BZDs and Z-drugs are the most commonly used symptomatic treatment for insomnia. The term benzodiazepine has been related to the portion of the structure composed of a benzene ring fused to a seven-membered diazepine ring. Since almost all BZDs contain a 5-aryl substituent and a 1,4 diazepine ring, the term actually denotes the 5-aryl-1,4-benzodiazepines. Although variations in the structure of the ring systems yield different chemical compounds, pharmacological activity remains similar [29, 30]. Three non-benzodiazepine receptor agonists are now available: zaleplon (a pyrazolopyrimidine), zolpidem (an imidazopyridine) and zopiclone (a cyclopyrrolone). Although termed non-BZD, Z-drugs interact with BZD receptors [14–16].

Almost all the effects of the BZDs result from actions on the central nervous system (CNS).

Molecular targets for BZD actions in the CNS are inhibitory neurotransmitter receptors directly activated by the amino acid gamma-aminobutyric acid (GABA) [14, 15].

Two central BZD receptor subtypes (BZ_1, and BZ_2,) and one peripheral BZD receptor have been categorised. BZ_1, (also called omega 1) receptors are located in the cerebellum. Hypnosedative and anxiolytic actions are mediated mainly through the BZ_1 receptor subtype. BZ_2, (omega 2) receptors, on the other hand, are located predominantly in the spinal cord and striatum. These receptors may be involved in mediating the muscle relaxant actions of BZDs [17]. Most BZDs interact non-selectively with both receptor subtypes, which result in a variety of inhibitory central nervous system effects [18]. The peripheral BZD receptor is located in the kidney. Its role in anxiolytic and hypnosedative actions remains unclear [17].

There are obvious differences in potency between different BZDs. The equivalent dose may differ as much as 20-fold [19, 20]. We should keep this in mind when substituting one BZD by another. These differences in potency relate to differences in affinity for various receptor subtypes.

Almost all of the BZDs are completely absorbed; some of them reach the systemic circulation only in the form of active metabolites. As a result, three categories BZDs are identified based on the elimination half-lives ($t_{1/2}$): short-acting agents ($t_{1/2}$ 2–5 h), intermediate acting agents ($t_{1/2}$ 6–24 h) and long-acting agents ($t_{1/2}$ more than 24 h) [15].

The BZDs and their metabolites have a high affinity for binding to plasma proteins. The degree of binding correlates with lipid solubility and varies from 70 to 99 %. Most BZDs have a large volume of distribution due to their high lipid solubility. The concentration in cerebrospinal fluid is practically the same as the concentration of free drug in plasma [21].

BZDs are metabolised in the liver primarily by oxidation, nitroreduction and glucuronidation [15, 22]. Most of them can be classified as low clearance drugs.

Alterations in BZD *pharmacokinetics* have been observed in older adults. A prolongation of the half-life of the oxidised drugs has been reported in this age group, but the clearance or half-life of the glucuronised drugs is less affected. Consequently, the BZDs metabolised by oxidation (e.g. flurazepam and diazepam) should not be prescribed to older adults, since higher plasma concentrations for a given drug dosage and consequently enhanced clinical effects are expected [21, 23].

Other significant and often seen age-related changes that may alter BZD metabolism include decreased liver blood flow, plasma albumin and lean body mass. Reduced hepatic blood flow can change the plasma concentration-time profile and increase peak concentrations. Decrease in plasma albumin levels may affect protein-binding capacity as well. Distribution volume may increase as a consequence of decreased lean body mass and increased proportion of fat. This results in an increased elimination half-time, prolonged effects after administration and accumulation of active metabolites [24, 25].

Changes in *pharmacodynamics* may also occur, as a result of altered affinity of the receptors, which implies a greater effect for a given plasma concentration. Older adults are more vulnerable to the effects of BZDs on cognitive function, especially at higher dosages. Different researchers report that older adults require both a lower dose and a lower plasma concentration to cause a constant level of sedation [26, 27]. Memory loss, altered balance and high risk of falls and fractures have been reported after short-term administration of BZDs [28, 29].

27.5 Clinical Effects of BZDs

All BZDs are characterised by, in somewhat altering degrees, five major effects: hypnosedative, anxiolytic, anticonvulsant, muscular relaxant and amnesic. In the short term, BZDs may be used safely in certain clinical conditions. With long-term use, tolerance, dependence and withdrawal effects may become major drawbacks [30, 31].

As to hypnotic effects, BZDs accelerate sleep onset, decrease nocturnal arousals and increase total sleep time [23]. However, they change the normal sleep pattern: light sleep is prolonged, while the duration of restorative slow wave sleep and rapid eye movement sleep is reduced. The onset of the first rapid eye movement sleep episode may be delayed [20]. Although some long-term users of BZDs are self-assured that sleep quality and duration are bettered as a result of the treatment, the findings of polysomnographic studies illustrate that the sleep pattern remains clearly different from normal sleep [32]. The aberrant sleep profile possibly results from unselective depression of both arousal and sleep mechanisms in the brainstem [33, 34].

Anxiolytic effects are induced by doses that cause minimal sedation, although the hypnotic, muscular relaxant and amnesic actions may all provide relief of associated tension and insomnia [35]. The effect on anxiety is presumably related to suppressive activity in limbic and other brain areas involved in the development of anxiety. The principal clinical characteristic of BZDs prescribed for anxiety is the rapid onset of action, usually noticeable after a single dose. BZDs provide only symptomatic treatment for anxiety. However, they might be indicated in the initial management of distressing anxiety while awaiting enduring clinical effects from more specific non-pharmacological treatments [17].

As to anticonvulsant effects, BZDs are effective in the treatment of status epilepticus and convulsions due to drug poisoning and, however, can only be used in emergency situations and are not indicated for the long-term treatment of epilepsy because of the development of tolerance in the majority of patients [36, 37].

Muscular relaxant effects of BZDs can sometimes be used in case of different motor disorders (i.e. dystonias and involuntary movements, myoclonus, restless limbs syndrome and muscle spasm associated with pain) [38].

As to amnesic effects, BZDs also cause dose-related anterograde amnesia. These amnesic effects may be clinically significant, particularly in older adults and in those with coexisting medical problems [23, 39].

27.6 Susceptibility of Older Adults to BZDs

Older adults in particular are vulnerable to adverse effects of BZDs. These patients are more sensitive to CNS depression, states of confusion and ataxia that can result in falls and fractures [29, 40]. They are also prone to respiratory depression, decreased ventilatory response, hypercapnia and increased hypopnoeic episodes during sleep [40].

27.7 Side Effects of BZDs

In addition to tolerance to the hypnotic and anxiolytic effects, ageing increases the susceptibility to the side effects of BZDs. The atrophy of neurons and the increased sensitivity of the CNS, together with pharmacokinetic changes, which lead to BZD/Z-drug accumulation, increase the possibility of confusion and CNS side effects, hangover effects and subsequent risk of falling [41–43]. Often falls have no major consequences, but in frail older adults, they can cause injuries and fractures, leading to hospitalisation and serious disability [44]. It has been questioned whether there is an independent association between BZD/Z-drug use and increased fall risk. Not only have falls a multifactorial aetiology but other psychotropic drugs are also associated with a 30–70% increased risk of falls [45–47].

Even though BZDs at first induce and prolong sleep, *tolerance* develops shortly. Sleep latency and duration regress to pre-treatment levels after a few weeks of continued treatment. Sleep quality, on the other hand, does not improve, since deep NREM sleep and REM sleep stages are partially replaced by stage 2 light NREM sleep [23, 48]. *Tolerance* to the anxiolytic properties of BZDs develops more gradually than to the hypnotic effects.

Rebound insomnia refers to an increase in the initial symptom beyond the base level after withdrawal from BZDs. Population surveys and results from large treatment effectiveness studies show rebound insomnia in 14–20% of patients treated with BZDs, a rate indistinguishable from that seen with over-the-counter drugs or placebo [49].

27.8 Rationale for Prescribing BZDs

If cognitive-behavioural therapy alone is not sufficient in alleviating insomnia, beginning of pharmacotherapy might be considered. The decision should be based on the severity of symptoms and on the patient's quality of life [50]. BZDs in low doses for 1 or 2 weeks only may be indicated for short-term insomnia due to temporary stress. Treatment of chronic insomnia secondary to physical, psychological or psychiatric conditions with hypnotics is rarely indicated [23].

Before choosing a hypnotic agent, the types of sleep problems reported by the patient should be taken into consideration and matched to the properties of different available medications. An ideal hypnotic agent should have a rapid onset of action, a duration of action that lasts through the night with no residual and no adverse effects [51]. The most worrying side effects of BZDs in older adults are residual sedation, psychomotor impairment and cognitive impairment, all of which revoke any benefit from obtaining a better night sleep [50]. Another concern with older patients using BZDs is the effect of respiratory depressants on sleep apnoea [52] and the risk of nocturnal falls [29].

BZDs and Z-drugs are effective for short-term treatment of insomnia [53]. Systematic reviews showed that time to fall asleep is decreased and total sleep duration enhanced [54–57]. Polysomnographic research showed also a changed sleep structure, with an increase in NREM, a decrease in deep sleep (SWS) and a prolonged REM latency. A meta-analysis in older adults with insomnia [58] showed an improvement in sleep quality, an increased total sleep time (mean 25 min) and a decreased number of night-time awakenings when using BZDs and/or Z-drugs compared to placebo. Although the effect sizes are statistically significant, their extent is small. Moreover, a meta-analysis indicated that the polysomnographic findings show small improvement in sleep latency and sleep duration, while the patient's reported subjective sleep latency (assessed with sleep diaries or questionnaires) was more optimistic [55]. This indicates that there may be an overestimation of the BZD's effects on sleep outcome parameters. Moreover, the selective reporting and publishing of positive studies and results also indicate that there is an overestimation favouring the BZD/Z-drugs' effects [56, 59]. In addition to the possible overestimation of the BZD/Z-drug's effects, several meta-analyses showed that placebo treatment also improves the sleep significantly [60, 61]. Because BZDs/Z-drugs are not free of side effects, the overall risk/benefit balance must be taken into account. Moreover, all these studies investigated the effect of a short-term treatment. The maximum study duration for BZDs is 8 weeks [62], and for Z-drugs, it is 1 year [63, 64]. Although the majority of BZD/Z-drug users are chronic users, research on long-term BZD or Z-drug use is lacking.

So far, there is a lack of a sound evidence base for the long-term efficacy of BZD/Z-drug use. Because of practical barriers but also because the fact that long-term BZD/Z therapy is not concordant with the guidelines, it is difficult to initiate randomised controlled trials with incident users and follow the sleep longitudinal. The studies that tried to evaluate long-term effectiveness found a worse sleep quality in long-term users [65–67]. After taking into consideration both the short-term and long-term risks of BZD/Z-drug use, and in the light of questionable effect of these drugs on insomnia in the long term, guidelines discourage chronic BZD/Z--drug use.

27.9 Guidance for Withdrawal

This age group, with a higher risk of abovementioned side effects, needs tailored prescribing which also includes deprescribing [68]. Discontinuation of BZDs/Z-drugs is widely advised but has not reached global acceptance among prescribers, caregivers and patients.

There is a general agreement on the notion that most patients who take BZDs regularly should try and discontinue treatment [69, 70]. Many patients who have taken BZDs for years can have these drugs withdrawn successfully. Men under the age of 50 without personality disturbance show particularly good response after withdrawal from BZDs. On the contrary, older women with anxious symptoms and personality disturbance respond less successfully to withdrawing [71].

The factors presumed to affect withdrawal are personality profile, dose and half-life of BZDs, duration of treatment and mode of withdrawal [71, 72]. On the contrary, there are reports suggesting that with the exception of age, withdrawal outcome is not related to any particular variable [72].

Withdrawal symptoms, if any, occur most often after 3 months of habitual use. They may include anxiety, restlessness, sleep disturbance, headache, muscle cramps, nausea, delirium or convulsions.

The treatment of BZD withdrawal symptoms includes appropriate psychological support together with a gradual dosage tapering. The level of psychological support may range from simple encouragement to anxiety management or behavioural therapy. Chronic insomnia can be effectively treated in older subjects with structured and sleep-focused interventions designed to change poor sleep habits [73]. In most of the cases, sleep symptoms progressively improve after withdrawal. It has been demonstrated that older adults tolerate withdrawal as well as if not better than young individuals [74].

There are no unanimous recommendations in the literature with regard to the optimal duration of the withdrawal process. Therefore, a variable withdrawal period ranging from 2 to 12 weeks may be allowed. The size of the stepwise lowering in dosage that should be applied is arguable as well. Some researchers propose a fixed tapering schedule, while others claim that the reduction rate should be titrated against the patient's withdrawal symptoms [75].

In a systematic review of interventions to deprescribe BZDs among older adults, seven studies of benzodiazepines and Z-drug withdrawal were identified. Benzodiazepine discontinuation rates were 64.3% in one study that applied pharmacological substitution with melatonin and 65.0% in a study that applied general practitioner-targeted intervention. Mixed interventions including patient education and tapering ($n = 2$), pharmacological substitution with psychological support ($n = 1$) and tapering with psychological support ($n = 1$) yielded discontinuation rates between 27.0 and 80.0%. Five studies measured clinical outcomes following benzodiazepine discontinuation. Most of the studies ($n = 4$) observed no difference in prevalence of withdrawal symptoms or sleep quality, while one study reported decline in quality of life in those who continued taking benzodiazepine vs. those who discontinued over 8 months [76].

Most older BZD/Z users for the indication insomnia are low-dose users. Although there is not much research done on which BZD/Z-drug is more resistant to withdrawal, generally, short-acting BZD/Z-drugs are more likely to cause withdrawal symptoms upon discontinuation than long-acting BZDs. Therefore, substitution with a long-acting BZD (diazepam) can lessen (and delay) withdrawal symptoms [77]. However, it is not appropriate to use long-acting BZDs/Z-drugs in older adults (in concordance with all explicit criteria). The long half-life can result in accumulation. Therefore, substitution with an intermediate working BZD/Z-drug (lorazepam/lormetazepam) or simply stay with the same product when discontinuing is advised. Psychological interventions which support withdrawal, such as cognitive behavioural therapy (CBT), have shown to be effective, also in older adults [78, 79]. These psychological techniques are intended to facilitate withdrawal and motivate patients to maintain abstinent over time (relapse prevention).

A meta-analysis focusing on older adults showed that the best strategy for discontinuing BZDs/Z-drugs in older adults residing in the nursing home setting was the combination of supervised withdrawal with psychotherapy [80]. Supervising the withdrawal in a setting with supporting care personnel is possible, but delivering psychotherapy seems more difficult to implement. A promising strategy for reducing BZDs/Z-drugs in the nursing home setting was the implementation of a pharmacist medication review [81, 82]. Often, the pharmacists gave recommendations or feedback to the nursing staff and delivered "an educational message". Also, a programme led by a psychologist which educated prescribers and caregivers, offered health education and relaxation training to the residents, reduced the overall prevalence of BZD/Z-drug use (from 70% to 35%) in this setting [83]. The educational tools used in long-term care facilities varied from prescribing algorithms and bulletins to staff meetings and lectures [84]. However, educational interventions alone cannot be expected to change behaviour when healthcare providers do not perceive it to be important, or when the change is complex and dependent on the interaction of too many stakeholders.

Several studies have investigated BZD/Z-drug withdrawal in the nursing home setting and focused on the success rate (focus on residents already willing to discontinue) [83, 85, 86]. However, health policy-makers should have an idea of the extent of the target population and the overall feasibility, including the willingness towards discontinuation in this setting. Therefore, general practitioner, nurse and, more importantly, the patient have to be susceptible towards change. Moreover, a lack of knowledge on non-pharmacological treatments and a lack of their availability and/or time to administer make it difficult for health providers to offer alternatives when withdrawal or rebound symptoms emerge. Some studies show that patients are susceptible towards change. Therefore, it is advised to routinely raise the issue of discontinuation and negotiate dose reduction [87, 88]. Current evidence shows that benzodiazepine withdrawal is feasible in older population, but withdrawal rates vary according to the type of intervention. As the benefits and sustainability of these interventions are unclear, further studies should be conducted to assess this.

27.10 Alternatives to BZDs

There are several pharmacotherapeutic alternatives that are used as alternative for BZDs including antidepressants, melatonin receptor agonists and orexin receptor antagonists. Different antidepressants, including trazodone, tricyclic antidepressants (doxepin) and serotonergic antidepressant (mirtazapine), have sedating properties and are often used for the treatment of insomnia [3].

However, despite the fact that these alternatives have been shown to be more effective than placebo at bettering short-term sleep outcomes, the size of effect is variable; most trials have been industry sponsored, posing questions about publication bias, and the overall estimation of risk-to-benefit ratio is low [13]. The potential benefits of pharmacotherapy on sleep quality and daytime function should always be balanced against the risk of side effects and physical and psychological dependence with long-term use.Trazodone is often prescribed for insomnia in doses of 25–100 mg. A study on trazodone comparing its effect with zolpidem in 21- to 65-year-olds showed a similar efficacy for sleep latency and sleep efficiency; however, both effects decrease after the first week [89]. Adverse effects such as cardiac arrhythmias, orthostatic hypotension, dizziness and potential priapism are well documented and can be important in older population [90]. There is lack of evidence about pharmacotherapy of sleep disorders in older adults with dementia. Several small trials showed certain beneficial effects on sleep outcomes from trazodone, although larger trials are needed to allow more sound conclusions. Systematic assessment of adverse effects in future studies is essential [91]. However, clinical practice guidelines from the American

Academy of Sleep Medicine suggest that trazodone should not be used for treatment of insomnia because its harms prevail over its benefits [13].

Doxepin is the only antidepressant approved by the Food and Drug Administration (FDA) for insomnia at doses of 3–6 mg. Studies of adults aged 65 years and older have shown, based on patient reports, that doxepin in doses of 1 mg and 3 mg, respectively, improved measures of sleep onset, sleep duration, sleep quality and global treatment outcomes over the 12-week study period [92].

Mirtazapine, a serotonergic antidepressant, might also improve insomnia. In a study of adults with mean age of 40.9 years, the mirtazapine group showed improvement in sleep latency, sleep efficiency and awakenings after sleep onset after 2 weeks of treatment. However, because of conflicting evidence and tolerance to its sedative effects, it should not be used to treat insomnia in the absence of depression [93].

Ramelteon is a melatonin receptor agonist. It is approved by the FDA for treatment of insomnia. In a study of older adults, ramelteon reduced patient reports of sleep latency over 5 weeks of treatment with no significant rebound insomnia or withdrawal effects [94, 95].

Melatonin at a dose of 2 mg has been approved by the European Medicines Agency (EMA) for the short-term treatment of primary insomnia in patients aged 55 years and older. However, formal recommendations for the use of melatonin in the treatment of insomnia still require further research [13, 96, 97].

Suvorexant is an orexin receptor antagonist. It is the first FDA-approved dual orexin receptor antagonist and may be prescribed up to a 20-mg dose. It targets wakefulness-promoting neuropeptides that regulate the sleep-wake cycle. It has shown to be effective in decreasing sleep latency and in increasing total sleep time. Suvorexant has been studied in both older (age 65 years or older) and younger (age 18–64 years) patients, showing no significant differences efficacy or safety between these two groups. Long-term data are still lacking [98–100].

27.11 Conclusions

A profound discriminatory history should identify a real cause of insomnia among diverse somatic, psychological and situational factors in order to line up a problem-oriented treatment strategy in older adults.

Despite the fact that pharmacological treatments these alternatives have been shown to be more effective than placebo at bettering short-term sleep outcomes, the size of effect is variable, and the overall benefit-to-risk ratio is low. The potential benefits of pharmacotherapy on sleep quality and daytime function in older adults should always be balanced against the risk of side effects and physical and psychological dependence with long-term use. As to future perspectives, trials should focus on advising and motivating patients already using hypnotic drugs to discontinue these medications, while effective non-pharmacological programs should be given a priority in respect of avoiding the use of hypnotics. Psychological support and follow-up of the patient make herein an important task for caregivers.

References

1. Conn D, Madan R. Use of sleep-promoting medications in nursing home residents: risks versus benefits. Drugs Aging. 2006;23:271–87.
2. Wolkove N, Elkholy O, Baltzan M, Palayew M. Sleep and aging: 1. Sleep disorders commonly found in older people. Can Med Assoc J. 2007;176:1299–304.
3. Patel D, Steinberg J, Patel P. Insomnia in the elderly: a review. J Clin Sleep Med. 2018;14:1017–24.
4. Crowley K. Sleep and sleep disorders in older adults. Neuropsychol Rev. 2011;21:41–53.
5. Ohayon M. Epidemiology of insomnia: what we know and what we still need to learn. Sleep Med Rev. 2002;6(2):97–111.
6. Hillman D, Murphy A, Pezzullo L. The economic cost of sleep disorders. Sleep. 2006;29:299–305.
7. Roth T, Coulouvrat C, Hajak G, Lakoma M, Sampson N, Shahly V, Shillington A, Stephenson J, Walsh J, Kessler R. Prevalence and perceived health associated with insomnia based on DSM-IV-TR; International Statistical Classification of Diseases and Related Health Problems, Tenth Revision; and Research Diagnostic Criteria/International Classification of Sleep Disorders, Second Edition criteria: results from the America Insomnia Survey. Biol Psychiatry. 2011;69:592–600.
8. Foley D, Monjan A, Simonsick E, Wallace R, Blazer D. Incidence and remission of insomnia among elderly adults: an epidemiologic study of 6,800 persons over three years. Sleep. 1999;22(Suppl 2):S366–72.
9. Gureje O, Oladeji B, Abiona T, Lebowitz M. The natural history of insomnia in the Ibadan study of ageing. Sleep. 2011;34:965–73.
10. Naylor E, Penev P, Orbeta L, Janssen I, Ortiz R, Colecchia E, Keng M, Finkel S, Zee P. Daily social and physical activity increases slow wave sleep and daytime neuropsychological performance in the elderly. Sleep. 2000;23:87–95.
11. McCurry S, Logsdon R, Teri L, Vitiello M. Evidence-based psychological treatments for insomnia in older adults. Psychol Aging. 2007;22:18–27.
12. Smith M, Perlis M, Park A, Smith M, Pennington J, Giles D, Buysse D. Comparative meta-analysis of pharmacotherapy and behavior therapy for persistent insomnia. Am J Psychiatry. 2002;159:5–11.
13. Sateia M, Buysse D, Krystal A, Neubauer D, Heald J. Clinical practice guideline for the pharmacologic treatment of chronic insomnia in adults: an American Academy of Sleep Medicine clinical practice guideline. J Clin Sleep Med. 2017;13:307–49.
14. Petrovic M, Mariman A, Warie H, Afschrift M, Pevernagie D. Is there a rationale for prescription of benzodiazepines in the elderly? Review of the literature. Acta Clin Belg. 2003;58:27–36.
15. Hobbs W, Rail T, Verdoom T. Hypnotics and sedatives; ethanol. In: Hardman JG, Gilman AG, Limbird LE, editors. Goodman & Gilman's the pharmacological basis of therapeutics. New York: Me Graw-Hill Health Profession Division; 1996. p. 361–97.
16. Heydom W. Zaleplon—a review of a novel sedative hypnotic used in the treatment of insomnia. Exp Opin Invest Drugs. 2000;9:841–58.
17. Stahl S. Anxiolytic and sedative-hypnotics. In: Stahl SM, editor. Essential psychopharmacology. Cambridge: Cambridge University Press; 2000. p. 297–333.
18. Kirkwood CK. Management of insomnia. J Am Pharm Assoc. 1999;39:688–96.
19. Roth T, Roehrs TA. Issues in the use of benzodiazepine therapy. J Clin Psychiatry 1992; 53 (Suppl 6): 14–18.
20. Ashton H. Guidelines for rational use of benzodiazepines -when and what to use. Drugs. 1994;48:25–40.
21. Hammerlein A, Derendorf H, Lowenthal D. Pharmacokinetic and pharmacodynamic changes in the elderly. Clin Pharmacokinet. 1998;35:49–64.
22. Breiner D. Clinical pharmacokinetics of hypnotics. Clin Pharmacokinet. 1997;2:93–109.

23. Buysse D, Reynolds C. Pharmacologic treatment. In: Lichstein KL, Morin CM, editors. Treatment of late-life insomnia. Thousand Oaks: Sage Publications; 2000. p. 231–67.
24. Greenblatt D, Harmatz J, Shader R. Clinical pharmacokinetics of anxiolytics and hypnotics in the elderly: therapeutic considerations. Clin Pharmacokinet. 1991;21:165–77.
25. Ozdemir V, Fourie J, Busto U, Naranjo A. Pharmacokinetic changes in the elderly. Clin Pharmacokinet. 1996;31:372–85.
26. Feely J, Coakley D. Altered pharmacodynamics in the elderly. Clin Geriatr Med. 1990;6:269–83.
27. Turner N, Scarpace PJ, Lowenthal DT. Geriatric pharmacology: basic and clinical consideration. Annu Rev Pharmacol Toxicol. 1992;32:271–302.
28. Foy A, O'Connell D, Henry D, Kelly J, Cocking S, Halliday J. Benzodiazepine use as a cause of cognitive impairment in elderly hospital inpatients. J Gerontol Med Sci. 1995;50A:M99–M106.
29. Herings R, Strieker B, de Boer A, Bakker A, Sturmans F. Benzodiazepines and the risk of falling leading to femur fractures. Arch Intern Med. 1995;155:1801–7.
30. Swift C, Swift M, Hamley J, Stevenson I, Crooks J. Side-effect 'tolerance' in elderly long-term recipients of benzodiazepine hypnotics. Age Ageing. 1987;13:335–43.
31. Petursson H, Lader M. Benzodiazepine dependence. Br J Addiction. 1984;76:133–45.
32. Schneider-Helmert D. Why low dose benzodiazepine-dependent insomniacs can't escape their sleeping pills. Acta Psychiatr Scand. 1988;78:706–11.
33. Grad R. Benzodiazepines for insomnia in community dwelling elderly: a review of benefit and risk. J Fam Pract. 1995;41:473–81.
34. Wheatley D. Effects of drugs on sleep. In: Wheatley D, editor. Psychopharmacology of sleep. New York: Raven Press; 1981. p. 153–76.
35. Tyrer P. Choices of treatment in anxiety. In: Tyrer P, editor. Psychopharmacology of anxiety. Oxford: Oxford Medical Publications; 1989. p. 255–82.
36. Olivier H, Fitz-Gerald MJ, Babiak B. Benzodiazepines revisited. J La State Med Soc. 1988;150:483–5.
37. Brodie M. Status epilepticus in adults. BMJ. 1990;336:551–2.
38. Herrington R. The use of benzodiazepines in neuropsychiatry. In: Hindmarch I, Bauamont G, Brandon S, Leonard B, editors. Benzodiazepines: current concepts. Chichester: John Wiley & Sons Ltd; 1990. p. 95–110.
39. Buysse D. Drugs affecting sleep, sleepiness and performance. In: Monk TH, editor. Sleep, sleepiness and performance. London: John Wiley & Sons; 1991. p. 249–306.
40. Morgan K. Hypnotics in the elderly: what cause for concern? Drugs. 1990;40:688–96.
41. Mangoni A, Jackson S. Age-related changes in pharmacokinetics and pharmacodynamics: basic principles and practical applications. Br J Clin Pharmacol. 2004;57:6–14.
42. Greenblatt D, Divoll HJ, MacLaughlin D, Shader R. Kinetics and clinical effects of flurazepam in young and elderly noninsomniacs. Clin Pharmacol Ther. 1981;30:475–86.
43. Swift C, Ewen J, Clarke P, Stevenson I. Responsiveness to oral diazepam in the elderly: relationship to total and free plasma concentrations. Br J Clin Pharmacol. 1985;20:111–8.
44. Berry S, Lee Y, Cai S, Dore D. Nonbenzodiazepine sleep medication use and hip fractures in nursing home residents. JAMA Intern Med. 2013;173:754–61.
45. Leipzig R, Cumming R, Tinetti M. Drugs and falls in older people: a systematic review and meta-analysis: I. Psychotropic drugs. J Am Geriatr Soc [Proceedings Paper]. 1999;47:30–9.
46. Woolcott J, Richardson K, Wiens M, Patel B, Marin J, Khan K, Marra C. Meta-analysis of the impact of 9 medication classes on falls in elderly persons. Arch Intern Med. 2009;169:1952–60.
47. Sterke C, Verhagen A, van Beeck E, van der Cammen T. The influence of drug use on fall incidents among nursing home residents: a systematic review. Int Psychogeriatr. 2008;20:890–910.
48. Lucki I, Rickels K, Geller A. Chronic use of benzodiazepines and psychomotor and cognitive test performance. Psychopharmacol. 1986;88:426–33.

49. Hajak G, Clarenbach P, Fischer W, Rodenbeck A, Bandelow B, Broocks A, Ruther E. Rebound insomnia after hypnotic withdrawal in insomniac outpatients. Eur Arch Psychiatry Clin Neurosci. 1998;248:148–56.
50. Ancoli-Israel S. Insomnia in the elderly: a review for the primary care practitioner. Sleep. 2000;23(Suppl 1):S23–9.
51. Mendels J. Criteria for selection of appropriate benzodiazepine hypnotic therapy. J Clin Psychiatry. 1991;52:42–6.
52. Wang S, Chen W, Tang S, Lin H, Peng C, Chu H, Kao C. Benzodiazepines associated with acute respiratory failure in patients with obstructive sleep apnea. Front Pharmacol. 2019;9:1513.
53. Riemann D, Perlis M. The treatments of chronic insomnia: a review of benzodiazepine receptor agonists and psychological and behavioral therapies. Sleep Med Rev. 2009;13:205–14.
54. Buscemi N, Vandermeer B, Friesen C, Bialy L, Tubman M, Ospina M, Klassen T, Witmans M. The efficacy and safety of drug treatments for chronic insomnia in adults: a meta-analysis of RCTs. J Gen Intern Med. 2007;22:1335–50.
55. Holbrook AM, Crowther R, Lotter A, Cheng C, King D. Meta-analysis of benzodiazepine use in the treatment of insomnia. Can Med Assoc J. 2000;162:225–33.
56. Huedo-Medina T, Kirsch I, Middlemass J, Klonizakis M, Siriwardena N. Effectiveness of non-benzodiazepine hypnotics in treatment of adult insomnia: meta-analysis of data submitted to the Food and Drug Administration. Br Med J. 2012;345:e8343.
57. Nowell P, Mazumdar S, Buysse D, Dew M, Reynolds C, Kupfer D. Benzodiazepines and zolpidem for chronic insomnia: a meta-analysis of treatment efficacy. J Am Med Assoc. 1997;278:2170–7.
58. Glass J, Lanctot K, Herrmann N, Sproule B, Busto U. Sedative hypnotics in older people with insomnia: meta-analysis of risks and benefits. Br Med J. 2005;331:1169.
59. Mattila T, Stoyanova V, Elferink A, Gispen-de Wied C, de Boer A, Wohlfarth T. Insomnia medication: do published studies reflect the complete picture of efficacy and safety? Eur Neuropsychopharmacol. 2011;21:500–7.
60. McCall W, D'Agostino R, Dunn A. A meta-analysis of sleep changes associated with placebo in hypnotic clinical trials. Sleep Med. 2003;4:57–62.
61. Belanger L, Vallieres A, Ivers H, Moreau V, Lavigne G, Morin C. Meta-analysis of sleep changes in control groups of insomnia treatment trials. J Sleep Res. 2007;16:77–84.
62. Morin C, Colecchi C, Stone J, Sood R, Brink D. Behavioral and pharmacological therapies for late-life insomnia: a randomized controlled trial. J Am Med Assoc. 1999;281:991–9.
63. Krystal A, Walsh J, Laska E, Caron J, Amato D, Wessel T, Roth T. Sustained efficacy of eszopiclone over 6 months of nightly treatment: results of a randomized, double-blind, placebo-controlled study in adults with chronic insomnia. Sleep. 2003;26:793–9.
64. Ancoli-Israel S, Richardson G, Mangano R, Jenkins L, Hall P, Jones W. Long-term use of sedative hypnotics in older patients with insomnia. Sleep Med. 2005;6:107–13.
65. Ohayon M, Caulet M, Arbus L, Billard M, Coquerel A, Guieu J, Kullmann B, Loffont F, Lemoine P, Paty J, Pechadre J, Vecchierini M, Vespignani H. Are prescribed medications effective in the treatment of insomnia complaints? J Psychosom Res. 1999;47:359–68.
66. Billioti de Gage S, Begaud B, Bazin F, Verdoux H, Dartigues J, Pérès K, Kurth T, Pariente A. Benzodiazepine use and risk of dementia: prospective population based study. Br Med J. 2012;345:e6231.
67. Englert S, Linden M. Differences in self-reported sleep complaints in elderly persons living in the community who do or do not take sleep medication. J Clin Psychiatry. 1998;59:137–44.
68. Ostini R, Jackson C, Hegney D, Tett S. How is medication prescribing ceased? A systematic review. Med Care. 2011;49:24–36.
69. Higgitt A, Lader M, Fonagy P. Clinical management of benzodiazepine dependence. Brit Med J. 1985;291:688–90.
70. Ashton H. Benzodiazepine withdrawal: outcome in 50 patients. Br J Addiction. 1987;82:665–71.

71. Holton A, Riley P, Tyrer P. Factors predicting long-term outcome after chronic benzodiazepine therapy. J Affect Disord. 1992;24:245–52.
72. Roy-Byme P, Hommer D. Benzodiazepine withdrawal: overview and implications for the treatment of anxiety. Am J Med. 1988;84:1041–52.
73. Ancoli-Israel S. Sleep problems in older adults: putting myths to bed. Geriatrics. 1997;52:20–30.
74. Schweizer F, Case W, Rickels K. Benzodiazepine dependence and withdrawal in elderly patients. Am J Psychiatry. 1989;146:529–31.
75. Petrovic M, Pevemagie D, Van Den Noortgate N, Mariman A, Michielsen W, Afschrift M. A programme for short-term withdrawal from benzodiazepines in geriatric hospital inpatients: success rate and effect on sleep quality. Int J Geriatr Psychiatry. 1999;14:754–60.
76. Reeve E, Ong M, Wu A, Jansen J, Petrovic M, Gnjidic D. A systematic review of interventions to deprescribe benzodiazepines and other hypnotics among older people. Eur J Clin Pharmacol. 2017;73:927–35.
77. Lader M, Tylee A, Donoghue J. Withdrawing benzodiazepines in primary care. CNS Drugs. 2009;23:19–34.
78. Morin C, Bastien C, Guay B, Radouco-Thomas M, Leblanc J, Vallières A. Randomized clinical trial of supervised tapering and cognitive behavior therapy to facilitate benzodiazepine discontinuation in older adults with chronic insomnia. Am J Psychiatry. 2004;161:332–42.
79. Lichstein K, Nau S, Wilson N, Aguillard R, Lester K, Bush A, McCrae C. Psychological treatment of hypnotic-dependent insomnia in a primarily older adult sample. Behav Res Ther. 2013;51:787–96.
80. Gould R, Coulson M, Patel N, Highton-Williamson E, Howard R. Interventions for reducing benzodiazepine use in older people: meta-analysis of randomised controlled trials. Br J Psychiatry. 2014;204:98–107.
81. Roberts MS, Stokes JA, King MA, Lynne T, Purdie D, Glasziou P, Wilson D, McCarthy S, Brooks G, de Looze F, Del Mar C. Outcomes of a randomized controlled trial of a clinical pharmacy intervention in 52 nursing homes. Br J Clin Pharmacol. 2001;51:257–65.
82. Forsetlund L, Eike MC, Gjerberg E, Vist G. Effect of interventions to reduce potentially inappropriate use of drugs in nursing homes: a systematic review of randomised controlled trials. BMC Geriatr. 2011;11:16.
83. Gilbert A, Owen N, Innes J, Sansom L. Trial of an intervention to reduce chronic benzodiazepine use among residents of aged-care accommodation. Aust NZ J Med. 1993;23:343–7.
84. Smith A, Tett S. Improving the use of benzodiazepines—is it possible? A non-systematic review of interventions tried in the last 20 years. BMC Health Serv Res. 2010;10:321.
85. Salzman C, Fisher J, Nobel K, Glassman R, Wolfson A, Kelley M. Cognitive improvement following benzodiazepine discontinuation in elderly nursing home residents. Int J Geriatr Psych. 1992;7:89–93.
86. Habraken H, Soenen K, Blondeel L, Van Elsen J, Bourda J, Coppens E, Willeput M. Gradual withdrawal from benzodiazepines in residents of homes for the elderly: experience and suggestions for future research. Eur J Clin Pharmacol. 1997;51:355–8.
87. Parr J, Kavanagh D, Young R, McCafferty K. Views of general practitioners and benzodiazepine users on benzodiazepines: a qualitative analysis. Soc Sci Med. 2006;62:1237–49.
88. Dyas J, Apekey T, Tilling M, Ørner R, Middleton H, Siriwardena N. Patients' and clinicians' experiences of consultations in primary care for sleep problems and insomnia: a focus group study. Br J Gen Pract. 2010;60:e180–200.
89. Walsh J, Erman M, Erwin C, Jamieson A, Mahowald M, Regestein Q, Scharf M, Tigel P, Vogel G, Ware C. Subjective hypnotic efficacy of trazodone and zolpidem in DSMIII-R primary insomnia. Hum Psychopharmacol. 1998;13:191–8.
90. Mendelson W. A review of the evidence for the efficacy and safety of trazodone in insomnia. J Clin Psychiatry. 2005;66:469–76.
91. McCleery J, Sharpley A. Pharmacotherapies for sleep disturbances in dementia. Cochrane Database Syst Rev. 2020;11:CD009178.

92. Krystal A, Durrence H, Scharf M, Jochelson P, Rogowski R, Ludington E, Roth T. Efficacy and safety of doxepin 1 mg and 3 mg in a 12-week sleep laboratory and outpatient trial of elderly subjects with chronic primary insomnia. Sleep. 2010;33:1553–61.
93. Winokur A, DeMartinis N, McNally D, Zary E, Cormier J, Gary K. Comparative effects of mirtazapine and fluoxetine on sleep physiology measures in patients with major depression and insomnia. J Clin Psychiatry. 2003;64:1224–9.
94. Zammit G, Wang-Weigand S, Rosenthal M, Peng X. Effect of ramelteon on middle of the night balance in older adults with chronic insomnia. J Clin Sleep Med. 2009;5:34–40.
95. Mets M, de Vries J, de Senerpont DL, Volkerts E, Olivier B, Verster J. Next-day effects of ramelteon (8 mg), zopiclone (7.5 mg), and placebo on highway driving performance, memory functioning, psychomotor performance, and mood in healthy adult subjects. Sleep. 2011;34:1327–34.
96. Wade A, Crawford G, Ford I, McConnachie A, Nir T, Laudon M, Zisapel N. Prolonged release melatonin in the treatment of primary insomnia: evaluation of the age cut-off for short- and long-term response. Curr Med Res Opin. 2011;7:87–98.
97. Riemersma-van der Lek R, Swaab D, Twisk J, Hol E, Hoogendijk W, Van Someren E. Effect of bright light and melatonin on cognitive and noncognitive function in elderly residents of group care facilities: a randomized controlled trial. JAMA. 2008;299:2642–55.
98. Rhyne D, Anderson S. Suvorexant in insomnia: efficacy, safety and place in therapy. Ther Adv Drug Saf. 2015;6:189–95.
99. Owen R. Suvorexant: efficacy and safety profile of a dual orexin receptor antagonist in treating insomnia. Drugs Today. 2016;52:29–40.
100. Norman JL, Anderson SL. Novel class of medications, orexin receptor antagonists, in the treatment of insomnia—critical appraisal of suvorexant. Nat Sci Sleep. 2016;8:239–47.

Optimizing Pharmacotherapy in Older Patients: An Interdisciplinary Approach: Chronic Kidney Disease

28

Andrea Corsonello, Antonello Rocca, Carmela Lo Russo, and Luca Soraci

28.1 Epidemiology and Staging Issues

Chronic kidney disease (CKD) is defined as the occurrence of abnormalities of kidney structure or function, present for more than 3 months, with implications for health. Such a definition is accompanied by a staging system based on GFR (G1 ≥90, G2 89–60, G3a 59–45, G3b 44–30, G4 29–15, and G5 <15 mL/min/1.73 m^2) and albumin-to-creatinine ratio (ACR) (A1 <30, A2 30–300, A3 >300 mg/g). Different combinations of reduced GFR and increased ACR are able to stratify prognosis and to identify patients carrying high risk of negative outcomes (Fig. 28.1) [1].

Older adults over 65 years encompass the most rapidly growing subset of the end-stage renal disease (ESRD) population. While there has been a significant increase in the prevalence of CKD from 10.3% to 13.1% of the population, the greatest percentage increase was observed in those older than 70 years of age, rising from a prevalence of 37–47% [2, 3]. Additionally, CKD and its complications may significantly impact functional status and health-related quality of life among older people, and geriatric syndromes (including cognitive status, depression, disability, frailty, and sarcopenia) are more and more considered in the assessment of older people with CKD [3, 4].

Accordingly, recognizing CKD is of paramount relevance in order to implement interventions aimed at preventing or delaying disease progression and the development of CKD complications and end-stage renal disease (ESRD), as well as reducing the risk of adverse drug reactions (ADRs) and/or nephrotoxicity. However, several reasons make the diagnosis of CKD in the older population

A. Corsonello · A. Rocca · C. L. Russo · L. Soraci (✉)
Unit of Geriatric Medicine and Laboratory of Geriatric Pharmacoepidemiology, Italian National Research Center on Aging (IRCCS-INRCA), Cosenza, Italy
e-mail: a.corsonello@inrca.it; a.rocca@inrca.it; c.lorusso@inrca.it; l.soraci@inrca.it

A. Cherubini et al. (eds.), *Optimizing Pharmacotherapy in Older Patients*, Practical Issues in Geriatrics, https://doi.org/10.1007/978-3-031-28061-0_28

PATIENT-RELATED FACTORS

Age, CKD, Diabetes, Sepsis, Volume depletion, Sodium depletion, Multiple myeloma, Acid-base disturbances, Hypoalbuminemia, Polypharmacy.

Careful assessment of:

- Age-related diseases (renovascular disease, heart failure)
- CKD, diabetes and sepsis (increased risk of nephrotoxic AKI)
- Volume depletion (NSAID-induced and ACEI/ARB-induced nephrotoxicity)
- Volume and sodium depletion (diuretics-induced nephrotoxicity)
- Hypoalbuminemia (cisplatin- and aminoglycosides-induced nephrotoxicity)
- Polypharmacy (exposure to multiple nephrotoxic drugs)

DRUG-RELATED FACTORS

Intrinsic nephrotoxic potential, Dosage, Frequency of administrations, Duration of treatment, Timing of administration, Route of administration, Pharmaceutical formulation.

Careful assessment of:

- Nephrotoxic potential
- Dose-dependent effect (mainly for drugs causing crystal deposition, tubular toxicity, and hemodynamic toxicity)
- Frequency of administrations (aminoglycosides)
- Route of administration (intra-arterial administration of contrast)
- Pharmaceutical formulation (nephrotoxicity is lower with liposomal amphotericin than for amphotericin lipid complex)

DANGEROUS INTERACTIONS

Avoid specific drug combinations

- NSAIDs and ACEI/ARB (and/or diuretics)
- Cephalosporins and aminoglycosides
- Vancomycin and aminoglycosides
- Cephalosporins and acyclovir

Fig. 28.1 Factors to be considered for preventing nephrotoxic AKI among older patients

cumbersome. Distinguishing age-related decline in kidney function from true CKD may be difficult, and many people with CKD are asymptomatic or have nonspecific symptoms; thus, clinical and laboratory clues are to be searched for to make a diagnosis before symptoms become severe or complications develop. Staging issues should be also taken into consideration. While there is substantial agreement in considering GFR <60 mL/min/1.73 m^2 as a clinically and prognostically relevant reduction of kidney function in the general population, not all older patients with an eGFR <60 mL/min/1.73 m^2 should be labeled as having kidney disease, since this may be part of physiological aging. Indeed, age adaptation of CKD definition is still matter of debate. The lack of an age calibration for CKD diagnosis has been considered as an inherent and potentially serious weakness that might lead to substantial overdiagnosis of CKD in otherwise healthy populations of older subjects [5]. The most common CKD category observed in community-based programs is stage 3A (i.e., GFR of 45–59 mL/min/1.73 m^2), which predominantly affects older persons and is seldom progressive in the absence of significant proteinuria [5]. An age-adjusted definition of CKD based on eGFR less than 45 mL/min/1.73m^2 has been proposed for older patients, but it would only be applicable to those who do not have any other corroborating signs of kidney disease such as proteinuria [6]. However, the KDIGO guidelines do not support the use of age-dependent thresholds for CKD diagnosis [1]. Finally, even older patients with stage 3a CKD need to be always assessed for appropriate use of treatments slowing kidney function decline, correct dosing of kidney cleared drugs, and limited use of nephrotoxic medications.

28.2 Multimorbidity and Polypharmacy

CKD usually coexists with other chronic diseases due to a pathogenetic link, e.g., diabetes and atherosclerosis as the cause of CKD, and to the sharing of risk factors (e.g., age and smoking habits) and pathophysiological pathways described above. Recurrent and highly prevalent clusters of diseases including CKD are the rule according to the multimorbidity approach, which defines the main associations between and among diseases without any hierarchical assumption. According to such approach, Formiga et al. [7] reported that CKD contributes to a multimorbidity cluster including coronary artery disease, hypertension, stroke, and diabetes. Zemedikun et al. [8] showed that the multimorbidity cluster including CKD may be wider than that previously observed, being composed by 26 conditions, among which cardiovascular, liver, neurologic, psychiatric, respiratory, endocrine, and muscle-skeletal diseases. More recently, cluster analysis showed that CKD may cluster with hypertension and sensory impairments, but physical performance as assessed by SPPB may be associated with not negligible changes in multimorbidity clusters. These findings strengthen the need of assessing physical performance and investigating interventions targeting physical function among complex multimorbid patients in an attempt to improve outcomes and reduce costs associated with multimorbidity. Finally, CKD severity may significantly affect patterns of multimorbidity, which should be also taken into account in clinical approach to multimorbid patients [9]. In such a complex scenario, the clinical presentation of CKD may be concealed by coexistent diseases. Thus, fatigue, sarcopenia, dyspnea, and anorexia may be expression of several conditions. As a consequence, CKD may remain unrecognized until blood exams performed for unrelated reasons allow detect it. Furthermore, multimorbidity accounts for polypharmacy which, in turn, is frequently nephrotoxic. The kinetics of many drugs is variously compromised in CKD, and recognizing CKD is mandatory to tailor the doses to actual eGFR values. Thus, renal function should systematically be screened for in the aged and multimorbid patients. Furthermore, sarcopenia and hypoalbuminemia may decrease the distribution volume and the bound fraction of water-soluble drugs and reduce serum creatinine out of proportion to the true eGFR, which defines the condition of concealed renal failure, which may further increase the risk of ADRs [10]. Indeed, diabetes mellitus, musculoskeletal diseases, and COPD are commonly associated with this condition [11]. Not unfrequently, acute kidney injury due to contrast medium unravels CKD [12–14]. Indeed, the inherent risk starts increasing from eGFR <60 mL/min/1.73 m^2 and further increases in patients given metformin or other potentially nephrotoxic drugs as well as in those having anemia, diabetes mellitus, CHF, and hypotension, which are well-known age-related diseases [15].

28.3 Guideline-Based Recommendations and CKD Treatment Among Older Patients

Evidence-based guidelines for managing CKD do not include specific recommendations for older patients. Nevertheless, geriatric issues, such as frailty, quality of life, life expectancy, end of life, and iatrogenic risk, usually challenge physicians and need to be addressed when managing CKD in the older population. In this section, we provide an overview of the impact of these issues on the pharmacological treatment for CKD and its complications.

28.3.1 Hypertension

Hypertension is present in up to 80–85% of CKD patients and can be both a cause and a consequence of CKD. Several mechanisms including sodium retention, fluid overload, and increased activities of sympathetic and renin-angiotensin systems concur to its pathogenesis [16]. Blood pressure control in CKD has shown to be useful to slow progressive renal function loss [17]; however, many of the key studies supporting guideline-based recommendations did not include participants older than 70 [18] which reduces their generalizability [16]. For this reason, individualized antihypertensive approaches are generally advised in older patients with CKD, depending upon concurrent comorbidities and renal function [19]:

- Target BP levels should be 130/70 mmHg (and not below) for older people of 65 years or more; in older patients over 80 years or in all frail older patients, a smaller reduction of SBP is advised according to the benefit/risk ratio of treatment. These target thresholds are higher compared with those suggested from clinical practice guidelines [20] and are derived from independent studies showing how a more intensive BP treatment may worsen prognosis in such populations [21]. Diastolic blood pressure levels <70 mmHg were in fact associated with increased cardiovascular risk [21] and accelerated decline in kidney function in patients aged 85 years or more [22]; similarly, systolic blood pressure <130 mmHg was associated with increased mortality in CKD patients aged 75 years or more [23].
- Angiotensin-converting enzyme inhibitors (ACE-I) and angiotensin II receptor antagonists (ARBs) are still considered first-line agents for patients with diabetic CKD (defined as an eGFR <60 mL/min per 1.73 m^2 or micro- or macroalbuminuria) and nondiabetic proteinuric CKD [24], even in the absence of hypertension [25, 26]. Usage of renin angiotensin system (RAS) blockers is important to slow progression of CKD, thanks to their antiproteinuric effects. However, potential iatrogenic risks related to ACE-I or ARBs should be taken into account. Indeed, prescription of ACE-I and ARBs in older patients with CKD mandates careful monitoring for acute renal failure and hyperkalemia; the occurrence of symptomatic hypotension or eGFR <15 mL/min/1.73 m^2 suggests discontinuation of treatment, whereas reduction of drug doses is indicated for milder renal function

deteriorations; increase in serum potassium levels requires dietary modification and chronic administration of ion-exchange resins and can also limit the use of other medications raising serum potassium (e.g., spironolactone) [24]. Thus, the presence of proteinuria in the context of a clearly progressive CKD, the occurrence of other health concerns or priorities that might make another antihypertensive agent preferable, as well as the patient's acceptance of the additional burden that these agents may impose should always be considered when prescribing an ACE-I or ARB to slow the progression of CKD [24].

- Diuretics should be added to RAS blockers in older CKD patients with fluid overload/edema; additionally, they may be considered the first-line medication in nondiabetic nonproteinuric CKD with fluid retention; loop diuretics are preferred over thiazides when antiproteinuric effects of RAS blockers need to be enhanced; torasemide, which has a longer duration of action than furosemide, may be preferred. Administration of diuretics in older patients needs strict monitoring of serum electrolytes, body weight, and renal function because of increased risk of electrolyte abnormalities and dehydration; additionally, despite thiazides are usually not recommended when eGFR falls below 30 mL/min/1.73 m^2 [24], a recent RCT showed that adding chlortalidone to either ACEi, ARBs, or beta-blockers may improve 24-h systolic blood pressure control in patients with CKD stage 4 and poorly controlled hypertension; indeed, patients receiving chlortalidone underwent a significant reduction of 10.5 mmHg of systolic blood pressure at 3 months, as well as a significant decrease in NT-proBNP, body weight, and albuminuria [27].
- Calcium channel blockers (CCBs) are the second-line medications in BP control in CKD patients. The non-dihydropyridine CCBs, such as diltiazem and verapamil, have significant antiproteinuric effects and are then preferred in older patients with proteinuria; amlodipine is generally preferred in nondiabetic nonproteinuric CKD. However, administration of these drugs in older patients should be carefully monitored as they are associated with several side effects (hypotension, tachycardia, peripheral edema for dihydropyridine CCBs; bradycardia for non-dihydropyridine CCBs) [24].
- Mineralocorticoid receptor antagonists (MRA) can be used in patients with resistant hypertension despite combination therapy; careful monitoring of renal function is suggested; the risk of MRA-related adverse effects, including hyperkalemia and worsening renal function, is amplified in individuals with eGFR <30 mL/min/1.73 m^2 [24].

28.3.2 Diabetes

Glycemic control in diabetic patients also represents an important intervention to reduce the burden of CKD and to slow its progression. Older diabetic patients with stages 3–4 CKD have particular needs that differ from those of younger patients with the same conditions, mainly due to frailty and reduced life expectancy [28]. Therapeutic options for older diabetic patients and CKD are limited because reduced kidney function may result in the accumulation of several drugs and/or their metabolites.

- HbA1c target levels should be individualized: a target from 6.5% to 8.0% in patients with diabetes and CKD not treated with dialysis should be considered; for patients with multiple comorbidities and decreased life expectancy, higher HbA1c targets might be more appropriate [29, 30].
- Metformin is the first-line therapeutic option in older patients with diabetic kidney disease; it should be cautiously used in patients with mild to moderate chronic kidney disease, with appropriate dosage reductions and careful follow-up of kidney function [30, 31].
- Conventional oral hypoglycemic agents, such as sulfonylureas (SUs), are not suitable due to the risk of prolonged hypoglycemia [28, 30]. However, in selected older patients with CKD and adequate hypoglycemia awareness, low-dose glipizide, gliclazide, or glimepiride can be considered [32].
- Glinides are rapid- and short-acting insulinotropic SU receptor ligands, but similar to the Sus, the main concern with repaglinide and nateglinide use in patients with CKD is a potentially increased risk of hypoglycemia [30, 33]. Thus, lower initial doses of these agents are recommended in this population.
- α-glucosidase inhibitors, acarbose and miglitol, are minimally absorbed from the gastrointestinal tract, yet plasma levels can increase in CKD; therefore, caution is advised for the use of these agents in diabetic patients with low eGFR (<30 mL/min/1.73 m^2) [30, 33].
- Thiazolidinediones are known to increase insulin sensitivity and HDL levels in diabetic patients; some of them, namely, rosiglitazone and pioglitazone, are metabolized by the liver and could be preferred in CKD patients; however, these drugs are not generally recommended in CKD because of increased risk of fluid overload, which mandates a close body weight monitoring and checking of fluid retention signs [32]. Additionally, according to a recent metanalysis, the effects on cardiovascular outcomes and hypoglycemia are uncertain [34]. These medications are also contraindicated in all individuals with osteoporosis and NYHA III-IV heart failure, which are frequently associated with CKD in older patients [32].
- Incretin mimetics and dipeptidyl peptidase-4 (DPP-4) inhibitors are changing the paradigm of antidiabetic treatment, especially for older diabetic patients with CKD. Incretin-mimetics are currently the glucose-lowering drugs with the strongest evidence of benefit on cardiovascular and kidney outcomes in patients with preexisting cardiovascular or kidney disease [35]. They are then indicated in patients with type 2 diabetes and CKD who have not achieved glycemic control despite first-line therapy (with metformin and eventually SGLT2 inhibitors) [32]. However, incretin mimetics have important limitations in older patients. Despite recent studies have decreased the eGFR threshold for GLP-1 discontinuation to up to 15 mL/min/1.73 m^2 for liraglutide, semaglutide, and dulaglutide [30], administration of these drugs in older adults needs to take into account the benefit/risk ratio, as several (severe weight loss, vomiting, nausea) may lead to kidney function worsening and AKI development, if not appropriately counteracted

[30]. Conversely, DPP-4 inhibitors are potentially advantageous for older diabetic patients with CKD because they are associated with a lower risk of hypoglycemia compared to other antidiabetic medications [30]. All currently available DPP-4 inhibitors can be used in CKD, but dosage of sitagliptin, saxagliptin, and alogliptin needs to be reduced in patients with GFR <50 mL/min/1.73 m^2 [30, 36]. Linagliptin is not cleared by the kidney and does not require any dosage adjustment in patients with CKD [30, 37].

  - Inhibitors of sodium-glucose cotransporters type 2 (SGLT2) significantly and consistently improve glycemic control with a marginal risk of hypoglycemia, especially when in monotherapy [30]. Furthermore, they have recently emerged as a disease-modifying treatment to counteract the progression of chronic renal disease in patients with or without diabetes [38]. No dose adjustment is required in mild CKD, but current evidence suggests being very cautious in moderate-severe stages of the disease. Indeed, findings from DECLARE-TIMI 58 [39, 40], CREDENCE [41], DAPA-CKD [42], and EMPA-KIDNEY trials have shown that these drugs can be safely prescribed after dose adjustment in patients with eGFR ≥20–30 mL/min/1.73 m^2; conversely, their use in patients with lower eGFR is not recommended. Within this family, canagliflozin has good safety profile in older diabetic patients with macroalbuminuria [43], whereas dapagliflozin can be safely prescribed to decrease the risk of CKD progression irrespective of albuminuria [44]; previous evidence of an increased risk of lower limb amputations in patients taking canagliflozin [35] has not been confirmed by recent RCTs, while concerns of genital mycotic infections and euglycemic diabetic ketoacidosis were confirmed for canagliflozin only [41, 42].

- Insulin remains the mainstay of treatment in diabetic patients with secondary failure and moderate to advanced CKD, especially those undergoing dialysis [30]. About one third of exogenous insulin is cleared by the kidney. Sixty percent of the renal clearance is due to glomerular filtration, while the remaining 40% is secreted after uptake from peritubular vessels. The available long- and short-acting insulin analogues have similar pharmacokinetics in patients with CKD [30]. To reduce the risk of hypoglycemia, insulin dosage reduction of 25% has been recommended in patients with GFR – 10–50 mL/min. However, when the long-acting insulins glargine or detemir are used, it may be wise to start treatment with 50% of the usual initial dosage of 0.1 IU/kg, titrating the dosage until target fasting glucose concentrations are reached [45]. The pharmacokinetics of the ultralong-acting insulin degludec does not change in patients with different degrees of kidney dysfunction [32, 46], thus suggesting that dose adjustments in patients with mild to severe renal impairment should not be required.

28.3.3 Albuminuria

Evidence have clearly shown that renin-angiotensin system blockade by ACE-I or ARBs is associated with a significant decrease in proteinuria and a slower decline in renal function in hypertensive adults. Lowering urinary albumin excretion may slow the progression of diabetic kidney disease and improve clinical outcomes even in the absence of hypertension [47]. Guidelines recommend that normotensive people with diabetes and macroalbuminuria should be treated with ACE-I or ARBs [19]. However, treatment with ACE-I or ARBs was found beneficial even in microalbuminuric normotensive patients, where benefits were more pronounced in diabetic compared to nondiabetic patients and in patients with more severe proteinuria (>3 g/24 h) compared to those with less severe proteinuria (<1 g/24 h) [19, 48]. Evidence from subgroup analysis of older patients from proteinuria-lowering trials suggests a reduced risk of cardiovascular outcomes even in this group of patients compared with that seen in younger subjects [49].

However, concerns related to treatment outcomes in older patients already described above (see paragraph dealing with hypertension) also apply to the use of these medications in normotensive patients. Additionally, combined therapy with ACE-I and ARBs was proposed to treat proteinuria, but the ONTARGET study clearly showed that combining ACE-I and ARBs was associated with faster decline in renal function, more side effects, and worse overall outcome [50, 51]. These findings are of particular concerns for older complex patients who are much more vulnerable to iatrogenic injury.

28.3.4 Hyperlipidemia

Lipid metabolism abnormalities are commonly associated with CKD and contribute to cardiovascular morbidity and mortality in CKD patients.

- Primary prevention: according to current knowledge, statin treatment should not be used for primary prevention in older patients with CKD. A recent metanalysis concerning the efficacy and safety of statin in older people has shown no significant benefit of statins for primary prevention among older individuals of 75 years of age [52].
- Secondary prevention: although secondary prevention trials using LDL-lowering therapies have shown beneficial effects on both cardiac events and all-cause mortality, limited data are available in older subjects. Statin trials in the general population included a variable proportion of older participants [53], but the percentage of older patients in CKD treatment statin trials ranged between 28 and 32% [54–56]. Currently, moderate-intensity statin or statin/ezetimibe treatment is recommended in adults aged 50 years or older, and dose adjustment is necessary with GFR <30 mL/min for statins other than atorvastatin and fluvastatin [57]. Evidence from subgroup analysis of older patients from lipid-lowering trials suggests a similar evidence in terms of reductions in all-cause mortality, major cardiovascular events, and outcomes of revascularization procedures in older compared to younger patients [58]. However, the benefits of treatment need to be weighed carefully against potential risks in older patients. With the exception of non-CYP3A4 substrates pravastatin, rosuvastatin, and fluvastatin, several statins are metabolized by cytochrome P450-CYP3A4 and therefore can interact

with commonly used medications such as amiodarone, macrolides, calcium channel blockers, fibric acid derivatives, and cyclosporine, thus resulting in increased risk of hepatotoxicity and myopathy [59, 60]. Thus, the choice of statin to treat older CKD patients should take into account the additional risk of potentially dangerous drug interactions.

28.3.5 Bone Metabolism

CKD-related mineral bone disorder (CKD-MBD) is characterized by derangements in bone and mineral metabolism leading to abnormal regulation of calcium, phosphorous, vitamin D, and PTH [61]. Whether medications used for osteoporosis in general population should be also used to treat older patients with CKD is not always clear. According to current guidelines, serial assessment of calcium, phosphate, vitamin D, and parathyroid hormone (PTH) levels provides indications for treatment [62].

- Hyperphosphatemia (phosphate serum levels >5.5 mg/dL) develops early in CKD because of decreased filtering of phosphate load, even if overt excess of serum phosphates starts when eGFR falls below 40 mL/min/1.73 m^2 [63]. Low-phosphate diet (<900 mg/day) is the first-line treatment for hyperphosphatemia aiming at maintaining a serum concentration of <4.5 mg/dL [64]; administration of phosphate binders should be reserved to persistent hyperphosphatemia despite lifestyle modifications or severe hyperphosphatemia (>6 mg(dL); non-calcium phosphate binders (sevelamer, lanthanum) are the first-line medications. Calcium-containing binders (calcium carbonate and calcium acetate) may lead several side effects (e.g., hypercalcemia, adynamic bone disease, vascular calcification) [64].
- Vitamin D deficiency: a large proportion of patients with CKD exhibit vitamin D deficiency (plasma 25-OH vitamin D <25–30 nmol/L) [65]. Additionally, older patients with CKD are particularly prone to vitamin D deficiency, as resulting from multiple mechanisms including reduced synthesis, inadequate intake, dietary restrictions, and inactive lifestyle in dialysis patients [66]. 25(OH) vitamin D deficiency may lead to CKD-MBD via increase in iPTH levels, reduced bone mineral density (BMD), and increased rate of hip fractures [65]. For this reason, clinical practice guidelines recommend maintaining 25(OH)vitamin D levels above 30 ng/mL by supplementation with ergocalciferol in moderate-to-severe CKD [61]; caution should be taken in older patients with overt manifestations of CKD-MBD (e.g., hypercalcemia and hyperphosphatemia) [65]. In older patients, vitamin D supplementation should be tailored on the basis of several factors, including food intake, sun exposure, physical activity, and skin pigmentation. Furthermore, vitamin D dose should be increased according to serum 25(OH) vitamin D in patients taking selected medications (e.g., cholestyramine bind vitamin D in the gut, while phenytoin and phenobarbital accelerate the breakdown of vitamin D by inducing the cytochrome P450 pathway) [67]. In

patients with persistently high PTH levels (>2.3–3 times the normal values), despite treatment of hyperphosphatemia and vitamin D deficiency, calcitriol should be administered with a regimen of 0.25 mcg three times a week [64].

- Hypercalcemia: in CKD stages 3 to 5, total elemental calcium intake including dietary and supplements should not exceed 2000 mg/d. The National Osteoporosis Foundation recommends a daily calcium intake of 1200 mg and vitamin D intake of 800–1000 IU/d for adults 50 and older [64, 68]. However, an only modestly increased risk of cardiovascular events in postmenopausal women undergoing calcium supplementation with or without vitamin D was reported in some studies [69, 70], thus suggesting the need to weigh the clinical significance of cardiovascular risks related to calcium supplements against the risks related to osteoporosis and its complications.
- Osteoporosis in CKD patients:
  - Use of bisphosphonates in CKD older patients with osteoporosis is controversial, as it was found associated with progressive renal disease, acute renal failure, and nephrotic syndrome [71]. This finding was not confirmed in other studies showing that even in older, frail, osteoporotic patients with renal impairment, intravenous bisphosphonate therapy did not result in long-term renal function decline [72]. However, it is worth reminding that bisphosphonates are not indicated in adynamic or osteomalacic bone disease. Additionally, calcium-phosphorous alterations, vitamin D deficiency, and hyperparathyroidism should always be addressed before starting bisphosphonates. Finally, there is no evidence that using bisphosphonates for short periods of time (2–3 years) in the CKD population will result in a significantly reduced incidence of fractures [71, 73].
  - The anti-RANKL monoclonal antibody denosumab decreases bone reabsorption, is useful for osteoporosis treatment and prevention of fractures, and is not cleared by the kidney. The efficacy and renal safety of denosumab have been demonstrated in elderly women [74]. However, by inhibiting bone resorption, it may lead to hypocalcemia. For this reason, patients with creatinine clearance <30 mL/min and/or other conditions predisposing to hypocalcemia should be strictly monitored during denosumab treatment [75, 76].
  - The use of selective estrogen receptor modulators (SERM) raloxifene was found associated with increased spine BMD, reduced incidence of vertebral fractures, and no effect on non-vertebral fractures compared with placebo in postmenopausal women with osteoporosis. No safety risk related to raloxifene in patients with mild to moderate CKD over the 2- to 3-year observation period [64, 77]. However, SERMs may increase the risk of deep venous thrombosis (DVT), pulmonary embolism, and fatal stroke in postmenopausal women with coronary heart disease, which raise the need for further investigations about their long-term safety in older patients already carrying increased risk of cardiovascular events [64].
  - Strontium ranelate is able to rebalance bone remodeling without a strong inhibition of bone reabsorption, which could reduce the risk of hypocalcemia during treatment. However, it is cleared by the kidney and is contraindicated in patients with GFR <30 mL/min. Additionally, an increased cardiovascular

risk was observed in a pooled analysis of strontium RCTs [78, 79], which makes this drug less appealing for use in older patients with CKD.

28.3.6 Acidosis

Metabolic acidosis is a common complication associated with progressive loss of kidney function and leading to other complications, including uremic bone disease, muscle catabolism, bone derangement, and increased mortality [80]. Recommendations to treat chronic metabolic acidosis in patients with CKD include the following:

- Start oral alkali therapy with sodium bicarbonate (or citrate) when serum bicarbonate <22 mmol/L [81].
- Therapy should be given to maintain the normal range (23–29 mmol/L) [82], since small clinical trials have reported that treatment within this range may delay CKD progression [83, 84], improve nutrition status [85], increase insulin sensitivity [86], and decrease atherogenic lipid levels [87]. Conversely, the effect on bone health was not fully documented [88]. However, especially in older patients, overcorrection should be avoided because of potentially harmful effects, mainly resulting from the U-shaped relationship between serum bicarbonate levels and mortality [89]. Whether the sodium load that accompanies alkali therapy could cause volume overload and hypertension remains to be determined. Additionally, alkali therapy may lead to hypokalemia, ionized hypocalcemia, and QTc prolongation. The above evidence supports a judicious use of alkali treatment as well as a careful monitoring of serum bicarbonates, electrolytes, and ECG in older patients with acidosis.

28.3.7 Anemia

The association between CKD and anemia is related to several mechanisms such as impaired production of erythropoietin, iron deficiency, and inflammation with increased hepcidin levels [90]. Despite its prevalence increases with decline of eGFR, in some older patients, e.g., those with diabetic kidney disease, impaired production of erythropoietin usually precedes the decline of eGFR, and even mildly depressed eGFR may then be associated with significant anemia of renal origin [91]. Recommendations for treatment of CKD-related anemia are mainly based on clinical practice guidelines, although most studies did not include geriatric populations [92]:

- Consider treating anemia when hemoglobin <10.0 g/dL or symptoms attributable to anemia develop with Hb between 10 and 12–13 g/dL [93].
- Determine individual iron's status and potential responsiveness to iron supplementation by checking the percent hypochromic red cells (%HRC) and reticulocyte hemoglobin content (CHr) to estimate the Hb content in RBCs [92]. Whether

%HRC and CHr are not available or the patient has thalassaemia/thalassaemia trait, check transferrin saturation (TSAT), and ferritin serum levels.
- Start iron supplementation before erythropoiesis stimulating factors (ESAs) in patients with iron responsiveness, defined as having %HRC >6% and CHR >29 pg (or TSAT <20% and ferritin <100 μg/L). Oral iron (ferrous sulfate, fumarate, or gluconate) is the preferred starting treatment, at a daily regimen of 200 mg in up to three divided doses. Target iron status is defined as a %HRC <6% (unless ferritin >800 μg/L) and CHr >29 pg (or TSAT >20% and ferritin >100 μg/L) when above tests are not available or patient has thalassaemia/thalassaemia trait; serum ferritin levels should be checked every 1–3 months to check for potential iron overload.
- Start ESA for patients who are likely to benefit in quality of life and physical function, only after correcting iron status (patients with %HRC >6% and CHr >29 pg). Although patients of 75 years or more were excluded from studies assessing ESA efficacy in the treatment of CKD-related anemia [90], guidelines clearly suggest that age alone should not be a determinant for treating or not treating anemia in CKD [90]. However, long-term treatment with ESA has been associated with increased blood pressure and seizures [94], as well as polyglobulia and increased thrombotic risk. For this reason, older patients should always be closely monitored, and ESAs should be given at the lowest dose capable of (a) maintaining stable Hb between 10.0 and 12.0 g/dL and (b) keeping rate of Hb increase between 1.0 and 2.0 g/dL/month. Caution should be taken in some categories, including patients with previous cancer or previous/current stroke (risk of recurrence) and older patients with increased thrombotic risk, bedridden patients, and individuals with very limited functional capacity (in whom risks clearly outweigh the benefits of treatment).

Among older CKD patients, ESA administration may be not sufficient to counteract anemia due to the coexistence of systemic inflammatory processes blunting response to erythropoietin, and inflammation-induced increased hepcidin production reducing iron absorption and utilization [90], which further strengthen the need for studies in older patients with multimorbidity.

28.4 Nephrotoxicity

Medications can impair any of the kidney functions, including renal arterial blood flow, glomerular filtration, tubular fluid formation, and urine output. While many drugs have a single mechanism of injury, some medications may affect kidney function by multiple pathways. Main mechanisms of nephrotoxicity are summarized in Table 28.1 [95, 96].

Overall, nephrotoxic medications contribute to up to 66% of all acute kidney injuries (AKIs) in older hospitalized patients [97]. Older age is an independent predictor of AKI in several different study populations [98–105]. In particular, the relative risk of developing AKI after myocardial revascularization with or without

Table 28.1 Mechanisms of drug-induced nephrotoxicity [95, 96]

Mechanism	Pathophysiology	Example medication(s)
Hemodynamically mediated damage	Reduced hydrostatic pressure in glomerular capillaries	ACE-I, ARBs
	Imbalance between vasoconstriction/ vasodilation	NSAIDs, cyclosporine, tacrolimus
Tubular epithelial cell damage	Acute tubular necrosis	Aminoglycosides, radiocontrast media, platinum compounds, amphotericin B
	Osmotic nephrosis	Mannitol, LMW-dextran, radiocontrast media, sucrose, propylene glycol
Tubulointerstitial disease	Acute allergic interstitial nephritis	β-Lactams, NSAIDs
	Chronic interstitial nephritis	Lithium, cyclosporine, aristolochic acid
	Nephrocalcinosis	Oral sodium phosphate solutions
	Papillary necrosis	Analgesics
Glomerular disease	Minimal change glomerular injury	NSAIDs
	Focal segmental glomerulosclerosis	Heroine abuse, HIV infection
	Membranous nephropathy	Gold, penicillamine, NSAIDs
Vascular disease	Renal vasculitis and thrombosis	Hydralazine, propylthiouracil, allopurinol, penicillamine, minocycline Mitomycin C, contraceptive agents, cyclosporin, tacrolimus, antineoplastic agents, interferon, ticlopidine, clopidogrel
Obstructive nephropathy	Intratubular obstruction	Rhabdomyolysis from statins,
	Nephrolithiasis	Sulfonamides, antiviral agents, ciprofloxacin, nitrofurantoin

concurrent valvular surgery increases from 1.6 (95% CI, 1.1–2.3) among patients aged 70–79 years to 3.5 (95%CI, 1.9–6.3) among patients aged 80–95 years compared to those aged less than 70 [106]. The risk of developing AKI was 50% higher in patients admitted to intensive care units aged 65 or more compared to younger ones [102]. Nevertheless, only few studies were devoted to address nephrotoxic AKI among older patients. In a single-center Japanese study of hospitalized patients aged 80 or more, the use of nephrotoxic medications (with antibiotics being the most common culprit medications) was among major causes of AKI, together with hypovolemia, cardiac dysfunction, and respiratory failure [107]. In other studies, the relationship between age and risk of nephrotoxic AKI was no longer significant after adjusting for confounders [108, 109]. However, it should be considered that older patients are frequently affected by multiple chronic diseases which need to be treated with complex polypharmacy regimens. In this scenario, both multimorbidity per se and the use of multiple nephrotoxic medications may contribute to increase the risk of AKI [96, 108–110]. Older age is also associated with increased risk of nephrotoxic AKI-related death [96]. More recently, glycopeptide antibiotics, drugs for anti-heart failure, ICU transfer, multi-organ dysfunction, and cardiopulmonary resuscitation were found to be independent risk factors for mortality among people aged 65 or more affected by community-acquired AKI receiving dialysis [111]. Finally, consequences of nephrotoxic AKI among older patients are not limited to negative effects in terms of mortality or risk of developing progressive CKD. Indeed, patients surviving to AKI often experience worsening quality of life and disability, with physical pain, sleep disorders, depression, and loss of mobility and energy reported as the most frequently complaints [96, 112–114]. Additionally, negative effects of AKI in terms of disability are supported by data showing an increased risk of stroke among AKI survivors [115].

28.4.1 Suggestions to Prevent Nephrotoxic AKI

Preventing AKI first involves recognizing the increased vulnerability of the aging kidney to injury due to age-related structural and functional changes. Indeed, age >75 years is a recognized risk factor for nephrotoxicity [110]. However, vulnerability to nephrotoxic injury may be further increased by multiple chronic diseases accumulated over the life span, and especially CKD. Thus, identifying CKD patients may help to individuate patients at greater risk of nephrotoxicity. Other diseases associated with increased risk of developing AKI are diabetes, heart failure, liver disease, peripheral arterial disease, hypotension, hypovolemia, and acid-base disorders [116]. Physicians should be aware of such an increased risk when prescribing a potentially nephrotoxic medication for patients carrying one or more of these conditions.

General rules to reduce the risk of nephrotoxic AKI include assessing baseline renal function and consider patient's renal function when prescribing a new drug, adjusting medication dosages to renal function, avoiding dangerous nephrotoxic combinations (e.g., the triple whammy, cephalosporins plus aminoglycosides, vancomycin plus aminoglycosides, cephalosporins plus acyclovir), and correcting, when possible, risk factors for nephrotoxicity before the initiation of drug therapy. Adequate attention should be also devoted to ensure valid hydration before and during therapy with potential nephrotoxins, use equally effective non-nephrotoxic drugs whenever possible, monitoring drug levels to use the correct dose [117]. Improving overall quality of prescriptions may also contribute to reducing risks. In a study of hospitalized patients with a minimum 0.5 mg/dL change in serum creatinine who were prescribed a nephrotoxic or renal eliminated medication, failure to adjust dosing for kidney function (63%) and the use of nephrotoxic medications during AKI accounted for 63% and 28% of all recorded adverse drug events [118]. Thus, reducing inappropriate prescribing is very likely to represent a good strategy for reducing the risk of nephrotoxicity, and studies using available explicit criteria to target inappropriate medications in older patients [119, 120] are highly desirable. A summary of useful strategies is suggested in Fig. 28.1.

Specific recommendations exist for preventing radiocontrast-induced AKI (CI-AKI), which is among the most common cause of hospital-acquired AKI. Prior to contrast media exposure, serum creatinine must be measured and GFR calculated. Patients with GFR less than 60 mL/min/1.73 m^2 should be considered at risk. Volume expansion with either isotonic sodium chloride or sodium bicarbonate solutions may be useful to prevent CI-AKI in patients with reduced volemia. The use of established nephrotoxic drugs (e.g., cyclosporine, aminoglycoside, NSAIDs, COX-2 inhibitors) should be stopped for at least 2 days. Diabetic patients with pre-existing renal impairment should withhold metformin for 48 h because lactic acidosis may occur once CI-AKI develops [121]. Finally, GFR should always be estimated 48–72 h after receiving contrast media in order to ensure timely CI-AKI detection.

Preventing strategies include isotonic fluid administration, N-acetylcysteine, alkalization of the urine with IV or oral agents, and statins. Volume expansion with either isotonic sodium chloride or sodium bicarbonate solutions may be useful to prevent CI-AKI in patients with reduced volemia. While no specific benefits have been observed when using sodium bicarbonate vs. isotonic saline likely because target urine alkalization was not always reached [122, 123], the combination of oral sodium/potassium citrate and volume expansion with isotonic saline was found to significantly reduce the risk of CI-AKI [124]. Volume expansion often raises the concern related to the risk of fluid overload in patients with impaired renal function or heart failure. Using left ventricular end-diastolic pressure (LVEDP) to guide volume expansion was found to reduce the risk of CI-AKI but not that of stopping fluid administration because of the occurrence of dyspnea [125]. The Prevention of Radiocontrast Induced Nephropathy Clinical Evaluation (PRINCE) trial showed that forcing diuresis with loop diuretics with urinary flow rate >150 mL/h may protect against CI-AKI, even if the risk of volume depletion needs to be taken into account [126]. However, forced diuresis in combination with saline infusion to match the input and maintain iso-volemia was found to lower the risk of CI-AKI [127].

N-acetylcysteine did not show any significant benefit in terms of reduction of CI-AKI risk in both low-risk or high-risk populations [128, 129], while rosuvastatin was found to reduce the likelihood of CI-AKI [130, 131].

28.5 Conclusions

Optimizing pharmacological treatments among older people with chronic kidney disease (CKD) may be very difficult. Main issues faced in clinical practice are related to the observation that CKD is usually observed in the context of complex multimorbidity profiles which may conceal its clinical presentation, delay diagnosis, and make use of kidney-cleared and/or potentially nephrotoxic medications which are a really challenging task. Guidelines not always provide age-specific recommendations for treating CKD and related disorders, and there is substantial evidence suggesting that target of treatments should be carefully adapted to the older population. Taking into account patient- and drug-related factors as well as avoiding potentially dangerous interactions and reducing inappropriate prescribing may be useful to prevent nephrotoxicity.

References

1. KDIGO CKD Work Group. KDIGO 2012 clinical practice guideline for the evaluation and management of chronic kidney disease. Kidney Int Suppl. 2013;3:1–150.
2. Collins AJ, Foley RN, Chavers B, Gilbertson D, Herzog C, Johansen K, et al. United States Renal Data System 2011 Annual Data Report: Atlas of chronic kidney disease & end-stage renal disease in the United States. Am J Kidney Dis. 2012;59(1 Suppl 1):A7, e1–420.
3. Aucella F, Corsonello A, Leosco D, Brunori G, Gesualdo L, Antonelli-Incalzi R. Beyond chronic kidney disease: the diagnosis of Renal Disease in the Elderly as an unmet need. A position paper endorsed by Italian Society of Nephrology (SIN) and Italian Society of Geriatrics and Gerontology (SIGG). J Nephrol. 2019;32(2):165–76.
4. Webster AC, Nagler EV, Morton RL, Masson P. Chronic kidney disease. Lancet. 2017;389(10075):1238–52.
5. Glassock RJ. Con: Thresholds to define chronic kidney disease should not be age dependent. Nephrol Dial Transplant. 2014;29(4):774–9; discussion 9–82.
6. Glassock R, Delanaye P, El Nahas M. An age-calibrated classification of chronic kidney disease. JAMA. 2015;314(6):559–60.
7. Formiga F, Ferrer A, Sanz H, Marengoni A, Alburquerque J, Pujol R, et al. Patterns of comorbidity and multimorbidity in the oldest old: the Octabaix study. Eur J Intern Med. 2013;24(1):40–4.
8. Zemedikun DT, Gray LJ, Khunti K, Davies MJ, Dhalwani NN. Patterns of multimorbidity in middle-aged and older adults: an analysis of the UK Biobank data. Mayo Clin Proc. 2018;93(7):857–66.
9. Corsonello A, Fabbietti P, Formiga F, Moreno-Gonzalez R, Tap L, Mattace-Raso F, et al. Chronic kidney disease in the context of multimorbidity patterns: the role of physical performance : The screening for CKD among older people across Europe (SCOPE) study. BMC Geriatr. 2020;20(Suppl 1):350.
10. Corsonello A, Pedone C, Corica F, Mussi C, Carbonin P, Antonelli Incalzi R, et al. Concealed renal insufficiency and adverse drug reactions in elderly hospitalized patients. Arch Intern Med. 2005;165(7):790–5.
11. Incalzi RA, Corsonello A, Pedone C, Battaglia S, Paglino G, Bellia V, et al. Chronic renal failure: a neglected comorbidity of COPD. Chest. 2010;137(4):831–7.
12. Chawla LS, Amdur RL, Amodeo S, Kimmel PL, Palant CE. The severity of acute kidney injury predicts progression to chronic kidney disease. Kidney Int. 2011;79(12):1361–9.
13. Ishani A, Xue JL, Himmelfarb J, Eggers PW, Kimmel PL, Molitoris BA, et al. Acute kidney injury increases risk of ESRD among elderly. J Am Soc Nephrol. 2009;20(1):223–8.
14. Bucaloiu ID, Kirchner HL, Norfolk ER, Hartle JE 2nd, Perkins RM. Increased risk of death and de novo chronic kidney disease following reversible acute kidney injury. Kidney Int. 2012;81(5):477–85.
15. Mehran R, Aymong ED, Nikolsky E, Lasic Z, Iakovou I, Fahy M, et al. A simple risk score for prediction of contrast-induced nephropathy after percutaneous coronary intervention: development and initial validation. J Am Coll Cardiol. 2004;44(7):1393–9.
16. Ku E, Lee BJ, Wei J, Weir MR. Hypertension in CKD: core curriculum 2019. Am J Kidney Dis. 2019;74(1):120–31.
17. Bakris G, Ali W, Parati G. ACC/AHA versus ESC/ESH on hypertension guidelines: JACC guideline comparison. J Am Coll Cardiol. 2019;73(23):3018–26.
18. Verbeke F, Lindley E, Van Bortel L, Vanholder R, London G, Cochat P, et al. A European Renal Best Practice (ERBP) position statement on the Kidney Disease: Improving Global Outcomes (KDIGO) clinical practice guideline for the management of blood pressure in non-dialysis-dependent chronic kidney disease: an endorsement with some caveats for real-life application. Nephrol Dial Transplant. 2014;29(3):490–6.
19. Cheung A, Chang TI, Cushman W, Furth S, Hou FF, Ix JH, et al. KDIGO (Kidney Disease: Improving Global Outcomes) guideline update on the management of blood pressure in

chronic kidney disease: what's new and what's different from other guidelines. Hypertension. 2021;78(suppl_1):A52. -A.
20. Williams B, Mancia G, Spiering W, Agabiti Rosei E, Azizi M, Burnier M, et al. ESC/ESH Guidelines for the management of arterial hypertension: the task force for the management of arterial hypertension of the European Society of Cardiology (ESC) and the European Society of Hypertension (ESH). Eur Heart J. 2018;39(33):3021–104.
21. Franklin SS, Gokhale SS, Chow VH, Larson MG, Levy D, Vasan RS, et al. Does low diastolic blood pressure contribute to the risk of recurrent hypertensive cardiovascular disease events? Hypertension. 2015;65(2):299–305.
22. van Bemmel T, Woittiez K, Blauw GJ, van der Sman-de BF, Dekker FW, Westendorp RG, et al. Prospective study of the effect of blood pressure on renal function in old age: the Leiden 85-Plus Study. J Am Soc Nephrol. 2006;17(9):2561–6.
23. Weiss JW, Johnson ES, Petrik A, Smith DH, Yang X, Thorp ML. Systolic blood pressure and mortality among older community-dwelling adults with CKD. Am J Kidney Dis. 2010;56(6):1062–71.
24. Cheung AK, Chang TI, Cushman WC, Furth SL, Hou FF, Ix JH, et al. KDIGO 2021 clinical practice guideline for the management of blood pressure in chronic kidney disease. 2021;99(3):S1–S87.
25. Taler SJ, Agarwal R, Bakris GL, Flynn JT, Nilsson PM, Rahman M, et al. KDOQI US commentary on the 2012 KDIGO clinical practice guideline for management of blood pressure in CKD. Am J Kidney Dis. 2013;62(2):201–13.
26. Page MR, The JNC. 8 hypertension guidelines: an in-depth guide. Am J Manag Care. 2014;20(1):E8.
27. Agarwal R, Sinha AD, Cramer AE, Balmes-Fenwick M, Dickinson JH, Ouyang F, et al. Chlorthalidone for hypertension in advanced chronic kidney disease. New Engl J Med. 2021;385(27):2507–19.
28. Douros A, Ebert N, Jakob O, Martus P, Kreutz R, Schaeffner E. Estimating kidney function and use of oral antidiabetic drugs in elderly. Fundam Clin Pharmacol. 2015;29(3):321–8.
29. de Boer IH, Caramori ML, Chan JCN, Heerspink HJL, Hurst C, Khunti K, et al. KDIGO 2020 clinical practice guideline for diabetes management in chronic kidney disease. Kidney Int. 2020;98(4):S1–S115.
30. de Boer IH, Caramori ML, Chan JC, Heerspink HJ, Hurst C, Khunti K, et al. Executive summary of the 2020 KDIGO diabetes management in CKD guideline: evidence-based advances in monitoring and treatment. Kidney Int. 98:2020, 839–848.
31. Inzucchi SE, Lipska KJ, Mayo H, Bailey CJ, McGuire DK. Metformin in patients with type 2 diabetes and kidney disease: a systematic review. JAMA. 2014;312(24):2668–75.
32. Navaneethan SD, Zoungas S, Caramori ML, Chan JC, Heerspink HJ, Hurst C, et al. Diabetes management in chronic kidney disease: synopsis of the 2020 KDIGO clinical practice guideline. 2021;174(3):385–94.
33. KDOQI clinical practice guideline for diabetes and CKD: 2012 Update. Am J Kidney Dis. 2012;60(5):850–86.
34. Wang W, Zhou X, Kwong JSW, Li L, Li Y, Sun X. Efficacy and safety of thiazolidinediones in diabetes patients with renal impairment: a systematic review and meta-analysis. Sci Rep. 2017;7(1):1717.
35. Palmer SC, Tendal B, Mustafa RA, Vandvik PO, Li S, Hao Q, et al. Sodium-glucose cotransporter protein-2 (SGLT-2) inhibitors and glucagon-like peptide-1 (GLP-1) receptor agonists for type 2 diabetes: systematic review and network meta-analysis of randomised controlled trials. BMJ (Clinical research ed). 2021;372:m4573.
36. Aroda VR, Henry RR, Han J, Huang W, DeYoung MB, Darsow T, et al. Efficacy of GLP-1 receptor agonists and DPP-4 inhibitors: meta-analysis and systematic review. Clin Ther. 2012;34(6):1247–58 e22.
37. Giorda CB, Nada E, Tartaglino B. Pharmacokinetics, safety, and efficacy of DPP-4 inhibitors and GLP-1 receptor agonists in patients with type 2 diabetes mellitus and renal or hepatic impairment. A systematic review of the literature. Endocrine. 2014;46(3):406–19.

38. Yau K, Dharia A, Alrowiyti I, Cherney DZI. Prescribing SGLT2 inhibitors in patients with CKD: expanding indications and practical considerations. Kidney Int Rep. 2022;7(7):1463–76.
39. Wiviott SD, Raz I, Bonaca MP, Mosenzon O, Kato ET, Cahn A, et al. Dapagliflozin and cardiovascular outcomes in type 2 diabetes. N Engl J Med. 2019;380(4):347–57.
40. Mosenzon O, Wiviott SD, Cahn A, Rozenberg A, Yanuv I, Goodrich EL, et al. Effects of dapagliflozin on development and progression of kidney disease in patients with type 2 diabetes: an analysis from the DECLARE-TIMI 58 randomised trial. Lancet Diabetes Endocrinol. 2019;7(8):606–17.
41. Perkovic V, Jardine MJ, Neal B, Bompoint S, Heerspink HJL, Charytan DM, et al. Canagliflozin and renal outcomes in type 2 diabetes and nephropathy. N Engl J Med. 2019;380(24):2295–306.
42. Heerspink HJL, Stefánsson BV, Correa-Rotter R, Chertow GM, Greene T, Hou FF, et al. Dapagliflozin in patients with chronic kidney disease. N Engl J Med. 2020;383(15):1436–46.
43. Sehgal V, Bajwa SJ, Sehgal R, Consalvo JA. Management of diabetes in the elderly with canagliflozin: a newer hypoglycemic drug on the horizon. J Pharmacol Pharmacother. 2014;5(4):227–31.
44. Mende CW. Chronic kidney disease and SGLT2 inhibitors: a review of the evolving treatment landscape. Adv Ther. 2022;39(1):148–64.
45. Scheen AJ. Pharmacokinetic considerations for the treatment of diabetes in patients with chronic kidney disease. Expert Opin Drug Metab Toxicol. 2013;9(5):529–50.
46. Kiss I, Arold G, Roepstorff C, Bottcher SG, Klim S, Haahr H. Insulin degludec: pharmacokinetics in patients with renal impairment. Clin Pharmacokinet. 2014;53(2):175–83.
47. Murton M, Goff-Leggett D, Bobrowska A, Garcia Sanchez JJ, James G, Wittbrodt E, et al. Burden of chronic kidney disease by KDIGO categories of glomerular filtration rate and albuminuria: a systematic review. Adv Ther. 2021;38(1):180–200.
48. Verma V, Kant R, Sunnoqrot N, Gambert SR. Proteinuria in the elderly: evaluation and management. Int Urol Nephrol. 2012;44(6):1745–51.
49. Winkelmayer WC, Zhang Z, Shahinfar S, Cooper ME, Avorn J, Brenner BM. Efficacy and safety of angiotensin II receptor blockade in elderly patients with diabetes. Diabetes Care. 2006;29(10):2210–7.
50. Mann JF, Schmieder RE, McQueen M, Dyal L, Schumacher H, Pogue J, et al. Renal outcomes with telmisartan, ramipril, or both, in people at high vascular risk (the ONTARGET study): a multicentre, randomised, double-blind, controlled trial. Lancet. 2008;372(9638):547–53.
51. Ren F, Tang L, Cai Y, Yuan X, Huang W, Luo L, et al. Meta-analysis: the efficacy and safety of combined treatment with ARB and ACEI on diabetic nephropathy. Ren Fail. 2015;37(4):548–61.
52. Armitage J, Baigent C, Barnes E, Betteridge DJ, Blackwell L, Blazing M, et al. Efficacy and safety of statin therapy in older people: a meta-analysis of individual participant data from 28 randomised controlled trials. Lancet. 2019;393(10170):407–15.
53. Shepherd J, Blauw GJ, Murphy MB, Bollen EL, Buckley BM, Cobbe SM, et al. Pravastatin in elderly individuals at risk of vascular disease (PROSPER): a randomised controlled trial. Lancet. 2002;360(9346):1623–30.
54. Wanner C, Krane V, Marz W, Olschewski M, Mann JF, Ruf G, et al. Atorvastatin in patients with type 2 diabetes mellitus undergoing hemodialysis. N Engl J Med. 2005;353(3):238–48.
55. Baigent C, Landray MJ, Reith C, Emberson J, Wheeler DC, Tomson C, et al. The effects of lowering LDL cholesterol with simvastatin plus ezetimibe in patients with chronic kidney disease (Study of Heart and Renal Protection): a randomised placebo-controlled trial. Lancet. 2011;377(9784):2181–92.
56. Fellstrom BC, Jardine AG, Schmieder RE, Holdaas H, Bannister K, Beutler J, et al. Rosuvastatin and cardiovascular events in patients undergoing hemodialysis. N Engl J Med. 2009;360(14):1395–407.
57. Grundy SM, Stone NJ, Bailey AL, Beam C, Birtcher KK, Blumenthal RS, et al. 2018 AHA/ACC/AACVPR/AAPA/ABC/ACPM/ADA/AGS/APhA/ASPC/NLA/PCNA guideline on the management of blood cholesterol: a report of the American College of Cardiology/

American Heart Association Task Force on Clinical Practice Guidelines. Circulation. 2019;139(25):e1082–e143.
58. Afilalo J, Duque G, Steele R, Jukema JW, de Craen AJ, Eisenberg MJ. Statins for secondary prevention in elderly patients: a hierarchical bayesian meta-analysis. J Am Coll Cardiol. 2008;51(1):37–45.
59. Nemerovski CW, Lekura J, Cefaretti M, Mehta PT, Moore CL. Safety and efficacy of statins in patients with end-stage renal disease. Ann Pharmacother. 2013;47(10):1321–9.
60. Horodinschi R-N, Stanescu AMA, Bratu OG, Pantea Stoian A, Radavoi DG, Diaconu CC. Treatment with statins in elderly patients. Medicina (Kaunas). 2019;55(11):721.
61. KDIGO clinical practice guideline for the diagnosis, evaluation, prevention, and treatment of Chronic Kidney Disease-Mineral and Bone Disorder (CKD-MBD). Kidney Int Suppl. 2009;113:S1–130.
62. Kidney Disease: Improving Global Outcomes CKDMBDUWG. KDIGO 2017 clinical practice guideline update for the diagnosis, evaluation, prevention, and treatment of chronic kidney disease-mineral and bone disorder (CKD-MBD). Kidney Int Suppl (2011). 2017;7(1):1–59.
63. Tonelli M. Serum phosphorus in people with chronic kidney disease: you are what you eat. Kidney Int. 2013;84(5):871–3.
64. Ketteler M, Block GA, Evenepoel P, Fukagawa M, Herzog CA, McCann L, et al. Executive summary of the 2017 KDIGO Chronic Kidney Disease-Mineral and Bone Disorder (CKD-MBD) guideline update: what's changed and why it matters. Kidney Int. 2017;92(1):26–36.
65. Christodoulou M, Aspray TJ, Schoenmakers I. Vitamin D supplementation for patients with chronic kidney disease: a systematic review and meta-analyses of trials investigating the response to supplementation and an overview of guidelines. Calcified Tissue Int. 2021;109(2):157–78.
66. Jean G, Souberbielle JC, Chazot C. Vitamin D in chronic kidney disease and dialysis patients. Nutrients. 2017;9(4):328.
67. Recommendations abstracted from the American Geriatrics Society Consensus Statement on vitamin D for Prevention of Falls and Their Consequences. J Am Geriatr Soc. 2014;62(1):147–52.
68. Weaver CM, Alexander DD, Boushey CJ, Dawson-Hughes B, Lappe JM, LeBoff MS, et al. Calcium plus vitamin D supplementation and risk of fractures: an updated meta-analysis from the National Osteoporosis Foundation. Osteoporos Int. 2016;27:367–76.
69. Bolland MJ, Grey A, Avenell A, Gamble GD, Reid IR. Calcium supplements with or without vitamin D and risk of cardiovascular events: reanalysis of the Women's Health Initiative limited access dataset and meta-analysis. BMJ (Clinical Research Ed). 2011;342:d2040.
70. Moe SM. Calcium as a cardiovascular toxin in CKD-MBD. Bone. 2017;100:94–9.
71. Miller PD. Is there a role for bisphosphonates in chronic kidney disease? Semin Dial. 2007;20(3):186–90.
72. Black DM, Delmas PD, Eastell R, Reid IR, Boonen S, Cauley JA, et al. Once-yearly zoledronic acid for treatment of postmenopausal osteoporosis. N Engl J Med. 2007;356(18):1809–22.
73. Nitta K, Yajima A, Tsuchiya K. Management of osteoporosis in chronic kidney disease. Intern Med. 2017;56(24):3271–6.
74. Jamal SA, Ljunggren O, Stehman-Breen C, Cummings SR, McClung MR, Goemaere S, et al. Effects of denosumab on fracture and bone mineral density by level of kidney function. J Bone Miner Res. 2011;26(8):1829–35.
75. Gopaul A, Kanagalingam T, Thain J, Khan T, Cowan A, Sultan N, et al. Denosumab in chronic kidney disease: a narrative review of treatment efficacy and safety. 2021;16(1):1–9.
76. Bhanot RD, Kaur J, Bhat Z. Severe hypocalcemia and dramatic increase in parathyroid hormone after denosumab in a dialysis patient: a case report and review of the literature. Case Rep Nephrol. 2019;2019:3027419.
77. Ishani A, Blackwell T, Jamal SA, Cummings SR, Ensrud KE. The effect of raloxifene treatment in postmenopausal women with CKD. J Am Soc Nephrol. 2008;19(7):1430–8.
78. European Medicines Agency recommends that Protelos/Osseor remain available but with further restrictions. EMA/84749/2014. Published on line 21 February 2014.

79. Ott SMJNRN. Therapy for patients with CKD and low bone mineral density. Nat Rev Nephrol. 2013;9(11):681–92.
80. Sy J, Chen JLT, Kalantar-Zadeh K. New solutions to old problems-metabolic acidosis in chronic kidney disease. Ann Transl Med. 2020;8(19):1256.
81. Andrassy KM. Comments on 'KDIGO 2012 clinical practice guideline for the evaluation and management of chronic kidney disease'. Kidney Int. 2013;84(3):622–3.
82. Melamed ML, Raphael KL. Metabolic acidosis in CKD: a review of recent findings. Kidney Med. 2021;3(2):267–77.
83. Mannon EC, O'Connor PM. Alkali supplementation as a therapeutic in chronic kidney disease: what mediates protection? Am J Physiol-Renal Physiol. 2020;319(6):F1090–F104.
84. Di Iorio BR, Bellasi A, Raphael KL, Santoro D, Aucella F, Garofano L, et al. Treatment of metabolic acidosis with sodium bicarbonate delays progression of chronic kidney disease: the UBI Study. J Nephrol. 2019;32(6):989–1001.
85. Mathur RP, Dash SC, Gupta N, Prakash S, Saxena S, Bhowmik D. Effects of correction of metabolic acidosis on blood urea and bone metabolism in patients with mild to moderate chronic kidney disease: a prospective randomized single blind controlled trial. Renal Fail. 2006;28(1):1–5.
86. Bellasi A, Di Micco L, Santoro D, Marzocco S, De Simone E, Cozzolino M, et al. Correction of metabolic acidosis improves insulin resistance in chronic kidney disease. BMC Nephrol. 2016;17(1):158.
87. Rizzetto F, Mafra D, Barra AB, Pires de Melo G, Abdalla DSP, Leite M Jr. One-year conservative care using sodium bicarbonate supplementation is associated with a decrease in electronegative LDL in chronic kidney disease patients: a pilot study. Cardiorenal Med. 2017;7(4):334–41.
88. Melamed ML, Horwitz EJ, Dobre MA, Abramowitz MK, Zhang L, Lo Y, et al. Effects of sodium bicarbonate in CKD stages 3 and 4: a randomized, placebo-controlled, multicenter clinical trial. Am J Kidney Dis. 2020;75(2):225–34.
89. Kovesdy CP, Anderson JE, Kalantar-Zadeh K. Association of serum bicarbonate levels with mortality in patients with non-dialysis-dependent CKD. Nephrol Dial Transplant. 2009;24(4):1232–7.
90. Portolés J, Martín L, Broseta JJ, Cases A. Anemia in chronic kidney disease: from pathophysiology and current treatments, to future agents. Front Med (Lausanne). 2021;8(328). [Review].
91. Bosman DR, Winkler AS, Marsden JT, Macdougall IC, Watkins PJ. Anemia with erythropoietin deficiency occurs early in diabetic nephropathy. Diabetes Care. 2001;24(3):495–9.
92. Ratcliffe LE, Thomas W, Glen J, Padhi S, Pordes BA, Wonderling D, et al. Diagnosis and management of iron deficiency in CKD: a summary of the NICE guideline recommendations and their rationale. Am J Kidney Dis. 2016;67(4):548–58.
93. National Clinical Guideline Centre (UK). National Institute for Health and Care Excellence: clinical guidelines. anaemia management in chronic kidney disease: partial Update 2015. London: Royal College of Physicians (UK); 2015.
94. Solomon SD, Uno H, Lewis EF, Eckardt KU, Lin J, Burdmann EA, et al. Erythropoietic response and outcomes in kidney disease and type 2 diabetes. N Engl J Med. 2010;363(12):1146–55.
95. Nolin TD, Himmelfarb J. Mechanisms of drug-induced nephrotoxicity. Handb Exp Pharmacol. 2010;196:111–30.
96. Fusco S, Garasto S, Corsonello A, Vena S, Mari V, Gareri P, et al. Medication-induced nephrotoxicity in older patients. Curr Drug Metab. 2016;17(6):608–25.
97. Kohli HS, Bhaskaran MC, Muthukumar T, Thennarasu K, Sud K, Jha V, et al. Treatment-related acute renal failure in the elderly: a hospital-based prospective study. Nephrol Dial Transplant. 2000;15(2):212–7.
98. Groeneveld AB, Tran DD, van der Meulen J, Nauta JJ, Thijs LG. Acute renal failure in the medical intensive care unit: predisposing, complicating factors and outcome. Nephron. 1991;59(4):602–10.

99. Zanardo G, Michielon P, Paccagnella A, Rosi P, Calo M, Salandin V, et al. Acute renal failure in the patient undergoing cardiac operation. Prevalence, mortality rate, and main risk factors. J Thorac Cardiovasc Surg. 1994;107(6):1489–95.
100. Vivino G, Antonelli M, Moro ML, Cottini F, Conti G, Bufi M, et al. Risk factors for acute renal failure in trauma patients. Intensive Care Med. 1998;24(8):808–14.
101. Conlon PJ, Stafford-Smith M, White WD, Newman MF, King S, Winn MP, et al. Acute renal failure following cardiac surgery. Nephrol Dial Transplant. 1999;14(5):1158–62.
102. de Mendonca A, Vincent JL, Suter PM, Moreno R, Dearden NM, Antonelli M, et al. Acute renal failure in the ICU: risk factors and outcome evaluated by the SOFA score. Intensive Care Med. 2000;26(7):915–21.
103. Bove T, Calabro MG, Landoni G, Aletti G, Marino G, Crescenzi G, et al. The incidence and risk of acute renal failure after cardiac surgery. J Cardiothorac Vasc Anesth. 2004;18(4):442–5.
104. Bahar I, Akgul A, Ozatik MA, Vural KM, Demirbag AE, Boran M, et al. Acute renal failure following open heart surgery: risk factors and prognosis. Perfusion. 2005;20(6):317–22.
105. Landoni G, Bove T, Crivellari M, Poli D, Fochi O, Marchetti C, et al. Acute renal failure after isolated CABG surgery: six years of experience. Minerva Anestesiol. 2007;73(11):559–65.
106. Mangano CM, Diamondstone LS, Ramsay JG, Aggarwal A, Herskowitz A, Mangano DT. Renal dysfunction after myocardial revascularization: risk factors, adverse outcomes, and hospital resource utilization. The Multicenter Study of Perioperative Ischemia Research Group. Ann Intern Med. 1998;128(3):194–203.
107. Wen J, Cheng Q, Zhao J, Ma Q, Song T, Liu S, et al. Hospital-acquired acute kidney injury in Chinese very elderly persons. J Nephrol. 2013;26(3):572–9.
108. Oliveira JF, Silva CA, Barbieri CD, Oliveira GM, Zanetta DM, Burdmann EA. Prevalence and risk factors for aminoglycoside nephrotoxicity in intensive care units. Antimicrob Agents Chemother. 2009;53(7):2887–91.
109. Mendes CA, Cordeiro JA, Burdmann EA. Prevalence and risk factors for acute kidney injury associated with parenteral polymyxin B use. Ann Pharmacother. 2009;43(12):1948–55.
110. Wang X, Bonventre JV, Parrish AR. The aging kidney: increased susceptibility to nephrotoxicity. Int J Mol Sci. 2014;15(9):15358–76.
111. Li G, Lian X, Hao W, Hu W. Clinical characteristics and risk factors for mortality in older patients with dialysis-receiving community-acquired acute kidney injury. Int J Gen Med. 2021;14:5693–701.
112. Bagshaw SM. The long-term outcome after acute renal failure. Curr Opin Crit Care. 2006;12(6):561–6.
113. Morgera S, Schneider M, Neumayer HH. Long-term outcomes after acute kidney injury. Crit Care Med. 2008;36(4 Suppl):S193–7.
114. Coca SG. Acute kidney injury in elderly persons. Am J Kidney Dis. 2010;56(1):122–31.
115. Wu VC, Wu PC, Wu CH, Huang TM, Chang CH, Tsai PR, et al. The impact of acute kidney injury on the long-term risk of stroke. J Am Heart Assoc. 2014;3(4)
116. Eftekhari P. Evaluation of acute kidney injury in the hospital setting. Prim Care. 2014;41(4):779–802.
117. Philips BJ, Lane K, Dixon J, Macphee I. The effects of acute renal failure on drug metabolism. Expert Opin Drug Metab Toxicol. 2014;10(1):11–23.
118. Cox ZL, McCoy AB, Matheny ME, Bhave G, Peterson NB, Siew ED, et al. Adverse drug events during AKI and its recovery. Clin J Am Soc Nephrol. 2013;8(7):1070–8.
119. American Geriatrics Society updated Beers Criteria for potentially inappropriate medication use in older adults. J Am Geriatr Soc. 2012;60(4):616–31.
120. Gallagher P, O'Mahony D. STOPP (Screening Tool of Older Persons' potentially inappropriate Prescriptions): application to acutely ill elderly patients and comparison with Beers' criteria. Age Ageing. 2008;37(6):673–9.
121. Nawaz S, Cleveland T, Gaines PA, Chan P. Clinical risk associated with contrast angiography in metformin treated patients: a clinical review. Clin Radiol. 1998;53(5):342–4.

122. Subramaniam RM, Wilson RF, Turban S, et al. AHRQ comparative effectiveness reviews. In: Contrast-induced nephropathy: comparative effectiveness of preventive measures. Rockville, MD: Agency for Healthcare Research and Quality (US); 2016.
123. Jang JS, Jin HY, Seo JS, Yang TH, Kim DK, Kim TH, et al. Sodium bicarbonate therapy for the prevention of contrast-induced acute kidney injury—a systematic review and meta-analysis. Circ J. 2012;76(9):2255–65.
124. Markota D, Markota I, Starcevic B, Tomic M, Prskalo Z, Brizic I. Prevention of contrast-induced nephropathy with Na/K citrate. Eur Heart J. 2013;34(30):2362–7.
125. Brar SS, Aharonian V, Mansukhani P, Moore N, Shen AY, Jorgensen M, et al. Haemodynamic-guided fluid administration for the prevention of contrast-induced acute kidney injury: the POSEIDON randomised controlled trial. Lancet. 2014;383(9931):1814–23.
126. Stevens MA, McCullough PA, Tobin KJ, Speck JP, Westveer DC, Guido-Allen DA, et al. A prospective randomized trial of prevention measures in patients at high risk for contrast nephropathy: results of the P.R.I.N.C.E. Study. Prevention of radiocontrast induced nephropathy clinical evaluation. J Am Coll Cardiol. 1999;33(2):403–11.
127. Briguori C, Visconti G, Focaccio A, Airoldi F, Valgimigli M, Sangiorgi GM, et al. Renal Insufficiency After Contrast Media Administration Trial II (REMEDIAL II): RenalGuard System in high-risk patients for contrast-induced acute kidney injury. Circulation. 2011;124(11):1260–9.
128. Investigators ACT. Acetylcysteine for prevention of renal outcomes in patients undergoing coronary and peripheral vascular angiography: main results from the randomized Acetylcysteine for Contrast-induced nephropathy Trial (ACT). Circulation. 2011;124(11):1250–9.
129. Weisbord SD, Gallagher M, Jneid H, Garcia S, Cass A, Thwin SS, et al. Outcomes after angiography with sodium bicarbonate and acetylcysteine. N Engl J Med. 2018;378(7):603–14.
130. Leoncini M, Toso A, Maioli M, Tropeano F, Villani S, Bellandi F. Early high-dose rosuvastatin for contrast-induced nephropathy prevention in acute coronary syndrome: Results from the PRATO-ACS Study (Protective Effect of Rosuvastatin and Antiplatelet Therapy On contrast-induced acute kidney injury and myocardial damage in patients with Acute Coronary Syndrome). J Am Coll Cardiol. 2014;63(1):71–9.
131. Zhou X, Dai J, Xu X, Wang Z, Xu H, Chen J, et al. Comparative efficacy of statins for prevention of contrast-induced acute kidney injury in patients with chronic kidney disease: a network meta-analysis. Angiology. 2019;70(4):305–16.

Palliation at End of Life

29

Joanne Droney, Phoebe Wright, and Dola Awoyemi

29.1 Introduction: Palliative Care for Older Patients

Palliative care is a multidisciplinary approach that improves the quality of life of patients and their families when faced with complex chronic or acute, life-threatening illness or life-limiting health conditions. It involves early identification, assessment and management of pain and other symptoms and provision of emotional, spiritual, psychological and social support [1, 2]. All healthcare and social care providers, with some basic training, should be able to provide palliative care. Specialist multi-professional palliative care teams focus mainly on complex cases. The role of geriatricians in the provision of palliative and end of life care is well described, and there is an increased recognition of the benefits of collaboration with specialist palliative care teams [3, 4]. Specialist palliative care complements geriatric medicine in several ways, principally:

- It can be provided in any healthcare setting and also in extended care facilities and patients' own homes [1, 2] with integration between services and settings leading to improved quality of life [5].
- Palliative care can be beneficial for patients with a wide range of serious illnesses, including cancer, chronic organ failure [6], dementia and progressive neurological disorders. Palliative care has traditionally focused on patients who

J. Droney (✉) · P. Wright · D. Awoyemi
Symptom Control and Palliative Care Team, Royal Marsden NHS Foundation Trust, London, UK
e-mail: joanne.droney@rmh.nhs.uk; phoebewright@nhs.net; dola.awoyemi@rmh.nhs.uk

A. Cherubini et al. (eds.), *Optimizing Pharmacotherapy in Older Patients*, Practical Issues in Geriatrics, https://doi.org/10.1007/978-3-031-28061-0_29

are imminently dying. However, palliative care is also increasingly recognised as adding value at any stage of illness and is applicable early in the course of illness, alongside other life prolonging therapies [1].

- Early involvement of palliative care for patients improves patient experience and quality of life, supports communication and promotes patient choice and decision-making [7, 8]. Early palliative care has also been shown to reduce the use of unplanned acute hospital admissions and emergency department attendances [9].

There have been several recent initiatives specifically designed to enhance palliative care provision for older patients. These include the following:

- Palliative care as a core component of care for older patients with cancer [10]
- Integrated community-based palliative care for older patients with chronic non-cancer diagnoses [11]
- Palliative care in long-term care facilities and nursing homes [12–16]

In many countries, there is an aging population, and older people are living longer with a high burden of serious health-related suffering [1, 17, 18]. Palliative care is particularly relevant for patients with multi-morbidities, chronic illnesses with fluctuant and unpredictable disease trajectories [19] and patients with complex clinical conditions manifested in severe physical and psychosocial needs [20].

Over the next two to three decades, with major demographic changes expected in most countries, there is likely to be a significant increase in the need for palliative and end-of-life care for older patients, especially for those being cared for and dying at home and in care homes [17, 21].

29.2 Approach to Prescribing Medications to Palliate Symptoms at End of Life in Older Patients

Palliative care is considered "an essential component of comprehensive care" [1]. Core principles of palliative care include communication, advance care planning and setting goals of treatment, provision of care that is centred around the needs and priorities of the individual patient and careful and judicious use of medications to alleviate symptoms [7]. Unmanaged symptoms are common in older people as they approach the end of life. Patients with advanced dementia have a similar symptom burden to those with advanced cancer [22]. Pain and breathlessness are most prevalent in this population, and other common symptoms include nausea, respiratory secretions and agitated delirium. Impeccable assessment of symptoms and response to medication is the mainstay of palliative care. To support this, validated pain assessment tools can be used to quantify the severity of pain [23] and are available for assessing pain in patients with dementia [24]. Ongoing assessment is required to ensure pain remains controlled, and adverse effects are managed.

In addition to its being a physical symptom, pain is an outcome of a person's psychological, social, spiritual and cultural circumstances, a concept sometimes known as "Total Pain" [25]. Holistic assessment and management of all potential areas of suffering is required.

Studies of pharmacological agents have mostly excluded older patients with multi-morbidity [4]. There are little specific data about the pharmacological management of symptoms at end of life in older people, and much of the information available is extrapolated from studies of and experience with younger patients. When using medications to manage symptoms in older patients, especially those who are dying, there is a need for regular review of drugs and doses against symptoms, adverse effects and individualised goals of treatment.

There are a number of specialist pharmacotherapy resources available for reference when prescribing in palliative care; the reader is referred to these for greater detail [26, 27].

29.3 Route and Mode of Administration of Medications at End of Life

The paradigm for treating pain—by mouth, by the clock (on a regular basis), individualised and with attention to detail [28]—holds true for most medications used for symptom control. Patients suffering from pain, nausea, agitation, constipation or respiratory secretions should have medications administered regularly to *prevent* rather than to merely alleviate symptoms, with "when required" doses available. This is particularly relevant in the frail elderly population: it has been demonstrated that medications prescribed "when required" in residential homes are not given as often as clinicians anticipate [29].

The preferred route for medication administration in palliative care is by mouth [30]. However, if absorption is compromised, for example, by vomiting or intestinal obstruction, or when swallowing is difficult in the last days of life, an alternative route may be more appropriate, e.g. the subcutaneous route. The daily dose of medication can be given as a continuous subcutaneous infusion over 24 hours, and "when required" medication as subcutaneous injections. A number of the medications used frequently at the end of life can be combined within one infusion to ensure symptoms are managed effectively. For most medications, this route of administration is off licence. Syringe driver compatibility charts are available to guide drug choice [26].

29.4 Managing Symptoms in Last Days of Life

This section presents a concise guide to the use of some key medications in the management of specific symptoms in the last days of life, including pain, dyspnoea, nausea, anxiety and agitation.

29.4.1 The Use of Opioids for Pain Management at End of Life

Pain is common in the elderly, with around half of care home residents experiencing pain which often remains under detected and undertreated especially in those with dementia [29]. There is an association between pain and behavioural and psychological symptoms of dementia including agitation and anxiety [31].

29.4.2 Starting Opioids in a Patient Who Is Approaching End of Life

For patients who are in moderate-severe pain and who have not been prescribed a regular opioid previously, a low-dose strong opioid such as morphine should be initiated and up-titrated, based on response, until a balance is achieved between acceptable pain control and medication side effects. It is generally accepted that there is little or no pharmacological indication for weak opioids in cancer pain, as low-dose morphine (or other strong opioids) often provides better pain relief with a lower adverse effect burden [26].

Opioids should generally be administered at regular intervals, with "as required" doses also available for breakthrough pain. If appropriate, the oral route is preferable for initial up-titration of opioids, for example, 2.5–5 mg immediate release morphine 4 hourly by mouth. For frail older patients, it is recommended that the starting dose is reduced by 30–50% [32] and that a more cautious approach is taken in up-titration. For morphine, an appropriate "as required" dose is usually 1/6th of the total 24-h morphine dose. Once the opioid has been up-titrated to a point where good pain relief is achieved, this may be converted to either a modified release formulation (which is administered less frequently) or, if a non-oral route is preferred, to a transdermal patch, such as a buprenorphine or fentanyl patch [33]. If the patient is imminently dying, a subcutaneous syringe driver may be more appropriate.

29.4.3 Morphine and Alternative Opioids for Dying Patients

On a population level, there is no difference between any of the strong opioids in terms of effectiveness or tolerability [34]. For moderate to severe cancer pain, morphine is often the initial opioid of choice [23, 33], a decision commonly based on cost, availability and familiarity.

However, there is marked inter-individual variation in response to opioids for pain. This inter-individual variability means that there is no predetermined dose to manage a particular patient's pain and individualised titration according to medication effect is required [35]. Most patients respond well to whichever opioid they are started on, that is, they achieve adequate analgesia without significant side effects. However, some patients experience either inadequate analgesia despite upward dose titration and/or intolerable side effects. In these cases, switching to an alternative opioid can be beneficial to improve analgesia and minimise adverse effects [36].

Alternative strong opioids include oxycodone, fentanyl, buprenorphine and methadone, to mention more commonly prescribed drugs in this category. These drugs have different potencies and bioavailability compared to morphine, which must be taken into consideration when switching between opioids. For example, oral oxycodone is considered 1.5–2 times more potent, milligram for milligram, than oral morphine [26]. Therefore 60 mg of oral morphine is the equivalent of 30–40 mg of oral oxycodone. Transdermal fentanyl (as in fentanyl patches) is 100–150 times more potent than oral morphine. A fentanyl patch 25 mcg/h is roughly equivalent to 60–90 mg oral morphine in 24 h [27]. A buprenorphine patch 5 mcg/h is roughly equivalent to 12 mg oral morphine in 24 h (based on dose conversion ratio of oral morphine to transdermal buprenorphine of 100:1) [26].

Opioids also differ in their side effects and how they are metabolised. Methadone is associated with QT prolongation and has a long plasma half-life, making it more likely to accumulate in frailer older people [44]. Oxycodone, unlike morphine, is metabolised via the Cytochrome P450 system with potential for multiple drug interactions, especially in patients with multi-morbidity and polypharmacy [37]. Differences in the pharmacodynamic and pharmacokinetic properties of opioids and the phenomenon of incomplete cross tolerance make switching between opioids sometimes challenging and unpredictable, requiring careful supervision, regular review and cautious dose titration.

Published opioid "equianalgesic" conversion ratios are merely guidelines to the relative potencies of different opioids and are often taken from single-dose studies that cannot be fully extrapolated into clinical practice. Importantly, these guides do not take into account individual patient factors which may contribute to effect, such as genetic variation, pharmacokinetics, previous opioid therapy, opioid tolerance, concomitant medication and disease status [38].

When switching between opioids, it is recommended that the equivalent opioid dose is reduced by 33–50% before the second opioid is initiated, especially in patients who are older and frailer, and titrated according to desired effect [35, 39]. Opioid switching should be carried out with caution and in challenging cases, with advice and supervision from a specialist palliative care team.

29.4.4 Subcutaneous Opioids for Dying Patients Who Are No Longer Able to Take Oral Medications

Patients who are no longer able to take oral medications can be given morphine (and certain other strong opioids) administered as a continuous 24-h subcutaneous syringe driver infusion. The bioavailability of subcutaneous opioids is often much higher than oral opioids, and therefore the total 24-h subcutaneous dose will differ from the oral equivalent. For example, 60 mg of oral morphine in a 24-h period is approximately equivalent to 30 mg of subcutaneous morphine administered by continuous infusion over 24 h [26]. Opioids can often be combined with other necessary medications, e.g. anti-emetics, anti-secretory agents in a single syringe driver delivery system.

29.4.5 The Use of Transdermal Opioid Patches in a Patient Who Is Imminently Dying

Transdermal opioids (e.g. transdermal fentanyl or buprenorphine) are not suitable for rapid titration in a patient with acute or severe pain or for whom prognosis is very short. Effective systemic analgesic concentrations of fentanyl are generally not reached until approximately 12 h after dose change and steady-state plasma concentrations of fentanyl are not achieved for at least 36–48 h. Substantial plasma concentrations of fentanyl can persist for at least 24 h after removal of the transdermal patch.

Due to the high potency and risk of overdose, transdermal fentanyl is usually not recommended pharmacotherapy in opioid naïve patients. Drug absorption from transdermal opioid patches can be increased by heat (e.g. electric blanket, hot water bottles), resulting in an increased risk of opioid adverse effects, toxicity and overdose.

In dying patients who are already on a stable fentanyl or buprenorphine patch, if pain is controlled, it is sensible to continue the transdermal patch and provide additional subcutaneous (SC) morphine on an "as required" basis. The appropriate SC morphine dose can be calculated based on one-sixth of the total oral morphine equivalent dose of the fentanyl patch. In this circumstance, careful and regular review of the patient is required, and specialist palliative care advice is recommended.

29.4.6 Opioid Adverse Effects

The majority of patients taking morphine for cancer pain achieve good analgesia with minimal adverse effects. Common and predictable adverse effects include constipation and dry mouth, the former being largely avoidable with co-prescription of laxatives. Other adverse effects such as nausea and vomiting are usually temporary, following initiation of the opioid, and can be managed with a suitable antiemetic. This may need to be added to the syringe driver if the patient is no longer able to take oral medications. Central adverse effects, such as severe drowsiness, confusion, myoclonus or hallucinations, are more concerning and suggestive of opioid toxicity. Prompt assessment of the patient is necessary to determine the dose reduction that is required and assessment of potential precipitants, e.g. renal impairment, infection or interacting medicines. Respiratory depression is rare if strong opioids are titrated carefully according to individual patient response. If this occurs, the opioid should be stopped, and the use of naloxone considered; however, this must be judged carefully in the palliative patient population due to the risk of opioid withdrawal syndrome and severe pain.

Renal and hepatic impairment is more prevalent in the older patient population and can increase the risk of opioid toxicity. This risk varies between opioids; thus, caution is required, and an alternate formulation or dose adjustment will often be required [26]. Some alternate strong opioids may be indicated in specific circumstances, for example, fentanyl and alfentanil are safer than morphine in patients with renal failure.

Non-opioids and adjuvants can be used to better target pain with an opioid sparing intent; this is discussed in more detail elsewhere in this book.

29.4.7 Medications for Nausea and Vomiting at End of Life

Reversible causes of nausea and vomiting, such as hypercalcaemia, should be corrected with specific treatments. The most appropriate antiemetic can be selected based on the likely cause of the nausea and the mechanism of action of the drug [40, 41]; see Table 29.1. If the initial antiemetic is not successful then a second, more broadly active choice (e.g. levomepromazine) may be used. A combination of antiemetics with different mechanisms of action may be useful for persistent nausea.

Table 29.1 Commonly used antiemetics at end of life: mechanisms of action, indications and cautions

Antiemetic	Principle mechanism of action	Main indication	Cautions and contraindications	Starting "as required" dose for frail elderly
Haloperidol [42]	D_2 antagonist. Acts in the chemoreceptor trigger zone	Chemical causes of nausea, e.g. renal failure, hypercalcaemia, medication-induced	Parkinson's disease; dementia; epilepsy; renal and liver impairment; cardiac disease	0.5 mg
Cyclizine [43]	H_1 and muscarinic receptor antagonist	Raised intracranial pressure or vestibular symptoms	Severe heart failure; liver disease	50 mg
Metoclopramide [44, 45]	D_2 antagonist. Acts as prokinetic, also 5HT3 receptor antagonist and 5HT4 agonist	Gastritis, gastric stasis, functional bowel obstruction	Heart disease; bowel obstruction; Parkinson's disease. Avoid long-term treatment in older people Can cause acute dystonia in older patients	10 mg
Levomepromazine [46]	D_2, H_1, $5HT_2$ and muscarinic antagonist	Second-line or for nausea of unclear aetiology	Parkinson's disease; dementia. Can be sedating	3.125 mg

D_2 Dopamine type 2, *H_1* Histamine type 1, *5HT* 5′hydroxytryptamine (serotonin)

The listed antiemetics can be given orally, subcutaneously or via syringe driver in equivalent dose (although in some specialist centres, it is advised to dose reduce levomepromazine by 50% when converting from oral to subcutaneous).

The choice and dose of antiemetic might be influenced by several factors in older patients. Firstly, physiological changes in the frail elderly can lead to a potential need for dose reduction [47]. In addition, comorbidities and concurrent use of medications that might influence antiemetic choice are more common in older people. For example, medications with dopamine antagonist activity such as metoclopramide and haloperidol should be avoided in Parkinson's disease patients and used with caution in frail older people due to increased risk of extra-pyramidal adverse effects [48]. In heart failure, cyclizine should be avoided. Those with pre-existing risk factors for ventricular arrhythmia should be prescribed with caution antiemetics that prolong the QT interval (e.g. domperidone, ondansetron or haloperidol). Furthermore, co-prescription of some antiemetics should be avoided, for example, cyclizine with metoclopramide, where cyclizine can be expected to block the prokinetic action of metoclopramide.

29.4.8 Management of Respiratory Secretions at End of Life

Respiratory secretions at end of life, sometimes called the "death rattle", are thought to be due to an accumulation of secretions in the airways and are common in the last hours of life, usually when the patient has become unconscious. Prior to commencing medications, non-pharmacological interventions such as repositioning can be useful. While it is unclear if clinically assisted hydration worsens respiratory secretions [49], the need for this should be regularly reviewed. In addition, it is important to address any concerns and to provide reassurance to family members and others present that the noisy breathing is generally not thought to be distressing to the patient [50].

Anticholinergic medications are commonly used to reduce secretions [50]. As older people are at increased risk, monitoring for adverse effects such as severe xerostomia (dry mouth) and urinary retention is necessary.

Commonly used non-sedating medications include glycopyrronium and hyoscine butylbromide. Neither is known to be more efficacious than the other [50]. Both have poor bioavailability and therefore are given subcutaneously, either "as required" or in a syringe driver over 24 h. The usual "as required" dose for glycopyrronium is 200–400 micrograms, with a maximum recommended dose of 1.2 mg over 24 h; for hyoscine butylbromide, this is 20 mg with a maximum recommended dose of 60–120 mg over 24 h [51] (some specialist centres use higher maximum doses).

Hyoscine hydrobromide crosses the blood brain barrier and can cause central adverse effects including sedation and delirium, especially in patients with renal and liver failure. This drug can be administered subcutaneously. It is also available as a transdermal patch, which is changed every 3 days. This may be useful in settings such as nursing homes, where access to syringe drivers may be more of a challenge [52]. For patients with fluid overload secondary to heart failure, this can contribute to respiratory symptoms so can be managed with furosemide, which can be given subcutaneously in the community setting [53].

29.4.9 Management of Dyspnoea at End of Life

Breathlessness is a common symptom in the last week of life. As with other symptoms, careful assessment is required to understand the most likely aetiology and to ensure that any reversible causes are treated, including using supplemental oxygen in hypoxia. Simple, instant non-pharmacological interventions can be trialled, such as handheld or electric fans. If these are not effective, then pharmacological measures include low-dose morphine should be applied. For patients who are not imminently dying, the published evidence demonstrates improvement with regular low-dose morphine, e.g. modified release morphine, starting at 5 mg twice a day, which can be up-titrated weekly to a maximum of 15 mg twice a day. Within these doses, there is no evidence of excess hospital admissions or mortality [54]. The oral route is preferred, but if a patient is thought to be in the final days of life, low-dose morphine can be given subcutaneously for breathlessness, e.g. 5–10 mg over 24 h via syringe driver.

Benzodiazepines are used to relieve the sensation of breathlessness especially where there is associated anxiety [55], most commonly sublingual lorazepam or subcutaneous midazolam. However there is no evidence in the literature to support this approach [56].

29.4.10 The Use of Medications to Relieve Agitation at End of Life

Sometimes patients can become agitated and restless when they are imminently dying. This is called "terminal agitation" and may be a feature of delirium at end of life. It can also be due to uncontrolled physical symptoms or psychological or spiritual distress. Reversible causes of agitation should be investigated and treated where appropriate and when possible, e.g. hypercalcaemia and urinary retention.

The main types of medications that are used to relieve terminal agitation are benzodiazepines and antipsychotics. It is generally not appropriate to use opioids for this purpose [57].

Benzodiazepines, such as midazolam, can be used if anxiety is a predominant symptom. If refractory symptoms of delirium including confusion and hallucinations are predominant, then antipsychotics such as haloperidol or levomepromazine are preferable treatment options [58]. There has been a recent move away from the use of neuroleptics in older patients and in palliative care patients with delirium due to a lack of high-quality evidence [59]. However, if a patient is thought to be imminently dying and is exhibiting severe distress and agitation, then drug treatment can be considered with the aim of relieving symptoms [60]. Ideally, this should be carried out with specialist palliative care support.

Patients who are sufficiently distressed and agitated to require medications to manage their symptoms are often not able to take oral medications. In such cases, medications may be administered by intermittent subcutaneous bolus or by continuous subcutaneous infusion.

Refractory agitation in a dying patient should be treated with a low dose of medication, which should be reviewed regularly and titrated as necessary. In frail older patients, the starting dose should be reduced, with cautious up-titration, aiming to relieve symptoms. For example, a starting single dose of haloperidol would be 0.5 mg subcutaneously and levomepromazine 6.25 mg subcutaneously [61, 62]. Usually, low doses of medications are sufficient to relieve symptoms. A national audit of the care of dying patients in UK hospitals found that the final median dose of midazolam prescribed prior to death was 10 mg subcutaneously over 24 h, (interquartile range of 5–15 mg) [63].

Many of the medications used to treat terminal agitation can be sedating. Palliative sedation is the monitored use of medications intended to induce a state of decreased or absent awareness (unconsciousness) in order to relieve intractable and intolerable symptoms or distress in a patient close to death [58, 64], usually in the last hours and days of life. Palliative sedation should be carried out with support from the specialist palliative care team.

The aim of palliative sedation is patient comfort at end of life, not to hasten death. When used appropriately, palliative sedation does not appear to have any detrimental effect on survival of patients with terminal cancer. Palliative sedation differs from euthanasia in its intentions, procedures and results [57]. The level of sedation should be proportional, i.e. the lowest necessary to provide adequate relief of suffering [65–67]. Good symptom relief may be attainable with light sedation, where the patient is still able to communicate. Continuous sedation should only be considered if the patient is in the very terminal stages of their illness with an expected prognosis of hours, or a short number of days at most.

The decision to use medications to sedate a patient at end of life should be made in conjunction with the multidisciplinary team involved in the care of that patient including senior clinicians, ward staff and, if possible, the patient and his/her close family members [64]. Where possible and appropriate, clinicians should have a pre-emptive discussion of the potential role of sedation with the patient and his/her family particularly for patients at risk of catastrophic end-of-life events such as major bleeding [67]. Patients requiring sedation need ongoing regular review and assessment to ensure that the level of sedation is adequately controlling their symptoms. The need for continued palliative sedation should be re-evaluated regularly. Management of pain and other symptoms should be continued. The need for and appropriateness of artificial hydration should be considered in each individual case [67].

Delirium is a neurocognitive syndrome that commonly occurs in older populations and people with cancer, particularly in those with advanced disease and in the last hours or days of life [68]. Up to 88% of patients suffer from delirium in their final weeks of life [69]. As cognitive impairment, comorbidity and increased age are independent risk factors for delirium, an understanding of this condition is particularly important for the older patient population. Management of agitated delirium in palliative care involves optimising patient environment; treating causes such as infection, constipation and urinary retention and pain [70]; and careful explanatory communication with patients and their families [60]. Sedation should only be used for patients with delirium who are imminently dying and whose distress and suffering cannot be alleviated by any other means.

29.5 Using Medications for Palliation at End of Life: Summary

Medications may be used to relieve symptoms for patients who are approaching the end of life. Careful assessment of cause, regular review of effect and a clear understanding of pharmacokinetics and pharmacodynamics of individual drugs can guide rational and effective prescribing.

References

1. Knaul FM, Farmer PE, Krakauer EL, De Lima L, Bhadelia A, Jiang Kwete X, et al. Alleviating the access abyss in palliative care and pain relief—an imperative of universal health coverage: the Lancet Commission report. Lancet. 2018;391(10128):1391–454.
2. Radbruch L, De Lima L, Knaul F, Wenk R, Ali Z, Bhatnaghar S, et al. Redefining palliative care—a new consensus-based definition. J Pain Symptom Manage. 2020;60(4):754–64.
3. Runacres F, Poon P, King S, Lustig J, Ugalde A. Examining the role of specialist palliative care in geriatric care to inform collaborations: a survey on the knowledge, practice and attitudes of geriatricians in providing palliative care. Age Ageing. 2021;50(5):1792–801.
4. Voumard R, Rubli Truchard E, Benaroyo L, Borasio GD, Büla C, Jox RJ. Geriatric palliative care: a view of its concept, challenges and strategies. BMC Geriatr. 2018;18(1):1–6.
5. Bayly J, Bone AE, Ellis- C, Yaqub S, Yi D, Nkhoma KB, et al. Common elements of service delivery models that optimise quality of life and health service use among older people with advanced progressive conditions: a tertiary systematic review. BMJ Open. 2021;11:e048417.
6. Brännström M, Boman K. Effects of person-centred and integrated chronic heart failure and palliative home care. PREFER: A randomized controlled study. Eur J Heart Failure. 2014;16:1142–51.
7. Van Der Steen JT, Radbruch L, Hertogh CM, De Boer ME, Hughes JC, Larkin P, et al. White paper defining optimal palliative care in older people with dementia: a Delphi study and recommendations from the European Association for Palliative Care. Palliat Med. 2014;28(3):197–209.
8. Temel J, Greer J, Muzikansky A, Gallagher E, Admane S, Jackson V. Early palliative care for patients with metastatic non-small-cell lung cancer. N Engl J Med. 2010;363(8):733–42.
9. Sahlollbey N, Lee CKS, Shirin A, Joseph P. The impact of palliative care on clinical and patient-centred outcomes in patients with advanced heart failure: a systematic review of randomized controlled trials. Eur J Heart Fail. 2020;22(12):2340–6.
10. VanderWalde N, Jagsi R, Dotan E, Baumgartner J, Browner IS, Burhenn P, et al. NCCN guidelines insights: older adult oncology, version 2.2016. J Natl Compr Cancer Network. 2016;14(11):1357–70.
11. Evans CJ, Bone AE, Yi D, Gao W, Morgan M, Taherzadeh S, et al. Community-based short-term integrated palliative and supportive care reduces symptom distress for older people with chronic noncancer conditions compared with usual care: a randomised controlled single-blind mixed method trial. Int J Nurs Stud. 2021;120:103978.

12. Oosterveld-Vlug M, Onwuteaka-Philipsen B, Ten Koppel M, Van Hout H, Smets T, Pivodic L, et al. Evaluating the implementation of the PACE Steps to Success Programme in long-term care facilities in seven countries according to the RE-AIM framework. Implementation Sci. 2019;14(1):1–19.
13. Van Den Block L, Honinx E, Pivodic L, Miranda R, Onwuteaka-Philipsen BD, Van Hout H, et al. Evaluation of a palliative care program for nursing homes in 7 countries: the PACE cluster-randomized clinical trial. JAMA Intern Med. 2020;180(2):233–42.
14. Froggatt KA, Moore DC, Van den Block L, Ling J, Payne SA, Arrue B, et al. Palliative care implementation in long-term care facilities: European Association for Palliative Care White Paper. J Am Med Dir Assoc. 2020;21(8):1051–7.
15. Mota-Romero E, Esteban-Burgos AA, Puente-Fernández D, García-Caro MP, Hueso-Montoro C, Herrero-Hahn RM, et al. NUrsing Homes End of Life care Program (NUHELP): developing a complex intervention. BMC Palliat Care. 2021;20(1):98.
16. Froggatt K, Best A, Bunn F, Burnside G, Coast J, Dunleavy L, et al. A group intervention to improve quality of life for people with advanced dementia living in care homes: The namaste feasibility cluster RCT. Health Technol Assess (Rockv). 2020;24(6):vii–139.
17. Bone AE, Gomes B, Etkind SN, Verne J, Murtagh FEM, Evans CJ, et al. What is the impact of population ageing on the future provision of end-of-life care? Population-based projections of place of death. Palliat Med. 2018;32(2):329–36.
18. Nguyen H, Wu YT, Dregan A, Vitoratou S, Chua KC, Prina AM. Multimorbidity patterns, all-cause mortality and healthy aging in older English adults: results from the English longitudinal study of aging. Geriatr Gerontol Int. 2020;20(12):1126–32.
19. Nicholson C, Davies JM, George R, Smith B, Pace V, Harris L, et al. What are the main palliative care symptoms and concerns of older people with multimorbidity?—A comparative cross-sectional study using routinely collected phase of illness, Australia-modified karnofsky performance status and integrated palliative care out. Ann Cardiothorac Surg. 2018;7(Suppl 3):S164–75.
20. Etkind SN, Bone AE, Gomes B, Lovell N, Evans CJ, Higginson IJ, et al. How many people will need palliative care in 2040? Past trends, future projections and implications for services. BMC Med. 2017;15(1):102.
21. Williams N, Hermans K, Stevens T, Hirdes JP, Declercq A, Cohen J, et al. Prognosis does not change the landscape: palliative home care clients experience high rates of pain and nausea, regardless of prognosis. BMC Palliat Care. 2021;20(1):1–10.
22. Sampson EL. Palliative care for people with dementia. Br Med Bull. 2010;96(1):159–74.
23. Fallon M, Giusti R, Aielli F, Hoskin P, Rolke R, Sharma M, et al. Management of cancer pain in adult patients: ESMO Clinical Practice Guidelines. Ann Oncol. 2018;29:iv166–91.
24. Zwakhalen SMG, Hamers JPH, Abu-Saad HH, Berger MPF. Pain in elderly people with severe dementia: a systematic review of behavioural pain assessment tools. BMC Geriatr. 2006:6, 3.
25. Saunders C, Dbe Frcp OM. The evolution of palliative care. J R Soc Med. 2001;94:430–2.
26. Wilcock A, Howard P, Charlesworth S. Palliative care formulary. 8th ed. Pharmaceutical Press. 2022.
27. Watson M, Armstrong P, Back I, Gannon C, Sykes N. Palliative adult network guidelines. 4th ed. Lisburn, NI: Tricord; 2016.
28. World Health Organization. WHO guidelines for the pharmacological and radiotherapeutic management of cancer pain in adults and adolescents. Geneva: World Health Organization; 2018.
29. La Frenais F, Vickerstaff V, Cooper C, Livingston G, Stone P, Sampson EL. Factors influencing prescription and administration of analgesic medication: a longitudinal study of people with dementia living in care homes. Int J Geriatr Psychiatry. 2021;36:1354–61.
30. Doyle D, Hanks G, Cherny N, Calman K. Oxford textbook of palliative medicine. 3rd ed. Oxford University Press; 2006. p. 288–438.
31. Sampson EL, White N, Lord K, Leurent B, Vickerstaff V, Scott S, et al. Pain, agitation, and behavioural problems in people with dementia admitted to general hospital wards: a longitudinal cohort study. Pain. 2015;156(4):675–83.

32. Jones MR, Ehrhardt KP, Ripoll JG, Sharma B, Padnos IW, Kaye RJ, et al. Pain in the elderly. Vol. 20, Current pain and headache reports. Current Medicine Group LLC 1; 2016. p. 1–9.
33. Caraceni A, Hanks G, Kaasa S, Bennett MI, Brunelli C, Cherny N, et al. Use of opioid analgesics in the treatment of cancer pain: evidence-based recommendations from the EAPC. Lancet Oncol. 2012;13:e58–68.
34. Bekkering GE, Soares-Weiser K, Reid K, Kessels AG, Dahan A, Treede RD, et al. Can morphine still be considered to be the standard for treating chronic pain? A systematic review including pair-wise and network meta-analyses. Curr Med Res Opin. 2011;27(7):1477–91.
35. Drewes AM, Jensen RD, Nielsen LM, Droney J, Christrup LL, Arendt-Nielsen L, et al. Differences between opioids: pharmacological, experimental, clinical and economical perspectives. Br J Clin Pharmacol. 2013;75(1):60–78.
36. Riley J, Branford R, Droney J, Gretton S, Sato H, Kennett A, et al. Morphine or oxycodone for cancer-related pain? A randomized, open-label, controlled trial. J Pain Symptom Manage. 2015;49(2):161–72.
37. Gudin J. Opioid therapies and cytochrome P450 interactions. J Pain Symptom Manage. 2012;44(6 Suppl):S4–14.
38. Gammaitoni A, Fine P, Alvarez N, McPherson LM, Bergmark S. Clinical application of opioid equianalgesic data. Clin J Pain. 2003;19(5):286–97.
39. Fine PG, Portenoy RK. Establishing "Best Practices" for opioid rotation: conclusions of an expert panel. J Pain Symptom Manage. 2009;38(3):418–25.
40. Stephenson J, Davies A. An assessment of aetiology-based guidelines for the management of nausea and vomiting in patients with advanced cancer. Supportive Care Cancer. 2006;14(4):348–53.
41. Mannix K. Palliation of nausea and vomiting. In: Doyle D, Hanks G, Cherny N, Calman K, editors. Oxford textbook of palliative medicine. 3rd ed. Oxford: Oxford University Press; 2015. p. 459–68.
42. Hardy JR, O'Shea A, White C, Gilshenan K, Welch L, Douglas C. The efficacy of haloperidol in the management of nausea and vomiting in patients with cancer. J Pain Symptom Manage. 2010;40(1):111–6.
43. Bentley A, Boyd K. Use of clinical pictures in the management of nausea and vomiting: a prospective audit. Palliat Med. 2001;15(3):247–53.
44. Davis MP, Hallerberg G. A systematic review of the treatment of nausea and/or vomiting in cancer unrelated to chemotherapy or radiation. J Pain Symptom Manage. 2010;39(4):756–67.
45. Bruera E, Belzile M, Neumann C, Harsanyi Z, Babul N, Darke A. A double-blind, crossover study of controlled-release metoclopramide and placebo for the chronic nausea and dyspepsia of advanced cancer. J Pain Symptom Manage. 2000;19(6):427–35.
46. Dietz I, Schmitz A, Lampey I, Schulz C. Evidence for the use of Levomepromazine for symptom control in the palliative care setting: a systematic review. BMC Palliat Care. 2013;12(1)
47. Gridelli C. Antiemetic therapy in older cancer patients. Aging Health. 2006;2(3):449–59.
48. Glare P, Miller J, Nikolova T, Tickoo R. Treating nausea and vomiting in palliative care: a review. Clin Interv Aging. 2011;6(1):243–59.
49. Kingdon A, Spathis A, Brodrick R, Clarke G, Kuhn I, Barclay S. What is the impact of clinically assisted hydration in the last days of life? A systematic literature review and narrative synthesis. BMJ Support Palliat Care. 2021;11(1):68–74.
50. Wee B, Hillier R. Interventions for noisy breathing in patients near to death. Cochrane Database Syst Rev. 2008;1
51. Wildiers H, Menten J. Death rattle: prevalence, prevention and treatment. J Pain Symptom Manage. 2002;23(4):310–7.
52. Spiller JA, Fallon M. The use of Scopoderm in palliative care. Hospital Med. 2000;61(11):782–4.
53. Birch F, Boam E, Parsons S, Ghosh J, Johnson MJ. Subcutaneous furosemide in advanced heart failure: service improvement project. BMJ Support Palliat Care. 2021:1–5.
54. Johnson MJ, Currow DC. Opioids for breathlessness: A narrative review. BMJ Support Palliat Care. 2020;10(3):287–95.

55. Hui D, Maddocks M, Johnson MJ, Ekström M, Simon ST, Ogliari AC, et al. Management of breathlessness in patients with cancer: ESMO Clinical Practice Guidelines. ESMO Open. 2020;5(6):1–13.
56. Simon S, Higginson I, Booth S, Harding R, Weingärtner V, Bausewein C. Benzodiazepines for the relief of breathlessness in advanced malignant and non-malignant diseases in adults (Review). Cochrane Database Syst Rev. 2016;10(10)
57. Garetto F, Cancelli F, Rossi R, Maltoni M. Palliative sedation for the terminally ill patient. CNS Drugs. 2018;32:951–61.
58. Cherny NI, Radbruch L, Chasen M, Coyle N, Charles D, Dean M, et al. European Association for Palliative Care (EAPC) recommended framework for the use of sedation in palliative care. Palliat Med. 2009;23(7):581–93.
59. Finucane AM, Jones L, Leurent B, Sampson EL, Stone P, Tookman A, et al. Drug therapy for delirium in terminally ill adults. Cochrane Database Syst Rev. 2020;2020(1)
60. Hosker CMG, Bennett MI. Delirium and agitation at the end of life. BMJ (Online). 2016;353:1–6.
61. NHS Scotland. Levomepromazine [Internet]. Scottish Palliative Care Guidelines. 2021 [cited 2021 Nov 24]. https://www.palliativecareguidelines.scot.nhs.uk/guidelines/medicine-information-sheets/levomepromazine.aspx
62. Zaporowska-Stachowiak I, Stachowiak-Szymczak K, Oduah MT, Sopata M. Haloperidol in palliative care: Indications and risks. Biomed Pharmacother. 2020;132(October):110772.
63. "Royal College of Physicians." National care of the dying audit for hospitals, England Executive summary; 2014.
64. Kirk TW, Mahon MM. National Hospice and Palliative Care Organization (NHPCO) position statement and commentary on the use of palliative sedation in imminently dying terminally ill patients. J Pain Symptom Manage. 2010;39(5):914–23.
65. Maltoni M, Scarpi E, Rosati M, Derni S, Fabbri L, Amadori FM, et al. Palliative sedation in end-of-life care and survival: a systematic review. J Clin Oncol. 2012;30(27)
66. Beller EM, van Driel ML, Mcgregor L, Truong S, Mitchell G. Palliative pharmacological sedation for terminally ill adults. Cochrane Database Syst Rev. 2015;2017(6)
67. Cherny N. ESMO clinical practice guidelines for the management of refractory symptoms at the end of life and the use of palliative sedation. Ann Oncol. 2014;25(July):iii143–52.
68. Bush SH, Lawlor PG, Ryan K, Centeno C, Lucchesi M, Kanji S, et al. Delirium in adult cancer patients: ESMO Clinical Practice Guidelines. Ann Oncol. 2018 Oct;1(29):iv143–65.
69. Hosie A, Davidson PM, Agar M, Sanderson CR, Phillips J. Delirium prevalence, incidence, and implications for screening in specialist palliative care inpatient settings: a systematic review. Palliat Med. 2013;27(6):486–98.
70. Sampson EL, West E, Fischer T. Pain and delirium: mechanisms, assessment, and management. Eur Geriatr Med. 2020;11(1):45–52.

Index

A. Cherubini et al. (eds.), *Optimizing Pharmacotherapy in Older Patients*, Practical Issues in Geriatrics, https://doi.org/10.1007/978-3-031-28061-0

GPSR Compliance

The European Union's (EU) General Product Safety Regulation (GPSR) is a set of rules that requires consumer products to be safe and our obligations to ensure this.

If you have any concerns about our products, you can contact us on ProductSafety@springernature.com

In case Publisher is established outside the EU, the EU authorized representative is:

Springer Nature Customer Service Center GmbH
Europaplatz 3
69115 Heidelberg, Germany

Batch number: 10732031

Printed by Printforce, the Netherlands